3, 5, 10
14

THE STIMULATED BRAIN

Cognitive Enhancement Using Non-invasive Brain Stimulation

THE STIMULATED BRAIN

Cognitive Enhancement Using Non-Invasive Brain Stimulation

Edited by

ROI COHEN KADOSH

Department of Experimental Psychology,
University of Oxford, Oxford, UK

AMSTERDAM • BOSTON • HEIDELBERG • LONDON
NEW YORK • OXFORD • PARIS • SAN DIEGO
SAN FRANCISCO • SINGAPORE • SYDNEY • TOKYO

Academic Press is an imprint of Elsevier

Academic Press is an imprint of Elsevier
32 Jamestown Road, London NW1 7BY, UK
225 Wyman Street, Waltham, MA 02451, USA
525 B Street, Suite 1800, San Diego, CA 92101-4495, USA

British Library Cataloguing-in-Publication Data
A catalogue record for this book is available from the British Library

Library of Congress Cataloging-in-Publication Data
A catalog record for this book is available from the Library of Congress

ISBN: 978-0-12-404704-4

For information on all Academic Press publications
visit our website at elsevierdirect.com

Typeset by SPi Global, India

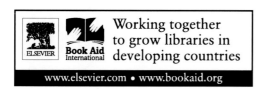

Dedication

To my father Mordechai, a man with a spark

Contents

II

IMPROVING FUNCTIONS IN THE TYPICAL BRAIN

7. Effects of Transcranial Electrical Stimulation on Sensory Functions   181

LEILA CHAIEB, CATARINA SAIOTE, WALTER PAULUS, AND ANDREA ANTAL

8. Motor System   207

JANINE REIS, GEORGE PRICHARD, AND BRITA FRITSCH

9. Effects of Brain Stimulation on Declarative and Procedural Memories   237

MARCO SANDRINI AND LEONARDO G. COHEN

III

IMPROVING FUNCTIONS IN THE ATYPICAL BRAIN

13. Transcranial Direct Current Stimulation and Cognition in the Elderly   371

FRANCESCA MAMELI, MANUELA FUMAGALLI, ROBERTA FERRUCCI, AND ALBERTO PRIORI

14. Clinical use of Transcranial Direct Current Stimulation in Psychiatry   397

ANDRE BRUNONI AND PAULO BOGGIO

15. The Use of Non-Invasive Brain Stimulation in Drug Addictions   425

ANTOINE HONE-BLANCHET AND SHIRLEY FECTEAU

IV

FUTURE PERSPECTIVES

16. Transcranial Electrical Stimulation to Enhance Cognitive Abilities in the Atypically Developing Brain   455

BEATRIX KRAUSE, CHUNG YEN LOOI, AND ROI COHEN KADOSH

17. A Brief Guide to the Scientific Entrepreneur 485
SOUHILE ASSAF AND JOSEPH KERR

18. The Neuroethics of Transcranial Electrical Stimulation 499
NEIL LEVY AND JULIAN SAVULESCU

19. The Future Usage and Challenges of Brain Stimulation 523
ROI COHEN KADOSH

Contributors

Andrea Antal   Georg-August-University, Department of Clinical Neurophysiology, Göttingen, Germany

Souhile Assaf   Medtrode Inc., London, Ontario, Canada and XLR Imaging Unit 116, Stiller Centre, London, Ontario, Canada

Marom Bikson   Department of Biomedical Engineering, The City College of New York of CUNY, New York, NY, USA

Paulo Boggio   Social and Cognitive Neuroscience Laboratory, Center for Health and Biological Sciences, Mackenzie Presbyterian University, São Paulo, Brazil

Andre Brunoni   Center for Clinical and Epidemiological Research & Interdisciplinary Center for Applied Neuromodulation, University Hospital, and University of São Paulo Medical School, University of São Paulo, São Paulo, Brazil

Leila Chaieb   Clinic for Epileptology, University Clinic of Bonn, Bonn, Germany

Leonardo G. Cohen   Human Cortical Physiology and Stroke Neurorehabilitation Section, National Institute of Neurological Disorders and Stroke, National Institutes of Health, Bethesda, MD, USA

Roi Cohen Kadosh   Department of Experimental Psychology, University of Oxford, Oxford, UK

José María Delgado-García   Division of Neurosciences, University of Pablo de Olavide, Seville, Spain

Paul Elliott   School of Humanities, University of Derby, Derby, UK

Shirley Fecteau   Centre Interdisciplinaire de Recherche en Réadaptation et Intégration Sociale, Centre de Recherche de l'Institut Universitaire en Santé Mentale de Québec, Medical School, Laval University, Québec, Canada and Berenson-Allen Center for Noninvasive Brain Stimulation, Beth Israel Deaconess Medical Center, Harvard Medical School, Harvard University, Boston, MA

Roberta Ferrucci   Centro Clinico per la Neurostimolazione, le Neurotecnologie ed i Disordini del Movimento, Fondazione IRCCS Ca' Granda, Ospedale Maggiore Policlinico, Milan, Italy and Dipartimento di Fisiopatologia Medico-Chirurgica e dei Trapianti, Università degli Studi di Milano, Milan, Italy

Gereon R. Fink   Cognitive Neuroscience, Institute of Neuroscience and Medicine (INM3), Research Center Juelich, Juelich, Germany; and Department of Neurology, University of Cologne, Germany

Nicholas S. Fitz   National Core for Neuroethics, The University of British Columbia, Vancouver, BC, Canada

Felipe Fregni Laboratory of Neuromodulation, Department of Physical Medicine and Rehabilitation, Spaulding Rehabilitation Hospital and Massachusetts General Hospital, Harvard Medical School, Boston, MA, USA

Brita Fritsch Albert-Ludwigs-University Freiburg, Department of Neurology, Freiburg, Germany

Manuela Fumagalli Centro Clinico per la Neurostimolazione, le Neurotecnologie ed i Disordini del Movimento, Fondazione IRCCS Ca' Granda, Ospedale Maggiore Policlinico, Milan, Italy

Nigel Gebodh Laboratory of Neuromodulation, Department of Physical Medicine and Rehabilitation, Spaulding Rehabilitation Hospital and Massachusetts General Hospital, Harvard Medical School, Boston, MA, USA and Department of Biomedical Engineering, The City College of the City University of New York, New York, NY, USA

Agnès Gruart Division of Neurosciences, University of Pablo de Olavide, Seville, Spain

Berkan Guleyupoglu Department of Biomedical Engineering, The City College of the City University of New York, New York, NY, USA

Maike D. Hesse Cognitive Neuroscience, Institute of Neuroscience and Medicine (INM3), Research Center Juelich, Juelich, Germany; and Department of Neurology, University of Cologne, Germany

Antoine Hone-Blanchet Centre Interdisciplinaire de Recherche en Réadaptation et Intégration Sociale, Centre de Recherche de l'Institut Universitaire en Santé Mentale de Québec, Medical School, Laval University, Québec, Canada

Friedhelm C. Hummel Brain Imaging and Neuro-Stimulation (BINS) Laboratory, Department of Neurology, University Medical Center Hamburg-Eppendorf, Hamburg, Germany and Favoloro University, Medical School, Buenos Aires, Argentina

Joseph Kerr XLR Imaging Unit 116, Stiller Centre, London, Ontario, Canada

Beatrix Krause Department of Experimental Psychology, University of Oxford, Oxford, UK

Michal Lavidor Department of Psychology, and The Gonda Multidisciplinary Brain Research Center, Bar Ilan University, Ramat Gan, Israel

Rocío Leal-Campanario Division of Neurosciences, University of Pablo de Olavide, Seville, Spain

Neil Levy Florey Institute of Neuroscience and Mental Health, Melbourne, Victoria, Australia and Oxford Centre for Neuroethics, University of Oxford, Oxford, UK

Chung Yen Looi Department of Experimental Psychology, University of Oxford, Oxford, UK

Francesca Mameli Centro Clinico per la Neurostimolazione, le Neurotecnologie ed i Disordini del Movimento, Fondazione IRCCS Ca' Granda, Ospedale Maggiore Policlinico, Milan, Italy

Javier Márquez-Ruiz   Division of Neurosciences, University of Pablo de Olavide, Seville, Spain

Preet Minhas   Department of Biomedical Engineering, The City College of New York of CUNY, New York, NY, USA

Ingrid Moreno-Duarte   Laboratory of Neuromodulation, Department of Physical Medicine and Rehabilitation, Spaulding Rehabilitation Hospital and Massachusetts General Hospital, Harvard Medical School, Boston, MA, USA

Abhilash Nair   Department of Biomedical Engineering, The City College of New York of CUNY, New York, NY, USA

Walter Paulus   Georg-August-University, Department of Clinical Neurophysiology, Göttingen, Germany

George Prichard   Albert-Ludwigs-University Freiburg, Department of Neurology, Freiburg, Germany and Institute of Cognitive Neuroscience, UCL, London, UK

Alberto Priori   Centro Clinico per la Neurostimolazione, le Neurotecnologie ed i Disordini del Movimento, Fondazione IRCCS Ca' Granda, Ospedale Maggiore Policlinico, Milan, Italy and Dipartimento di Fisiopatologia Medico-Chirurgica e dei Trapianti, Università degli Studi di Milano, Milan, Italy

Davide Reato   Department of Biomedical Engineering, The City College of the City University of New York, New York, NY, USA

Peter B. Reiner   National Core for Neuroethics, The University of British Columbia, Vancouver, BC, Canada

Janine Reis   Albert-Ludwigs-University Freiburg, Department of Neurology, Freiburg, Germany

Giulio Ruffini   Starlab Barcelona SL, Barcelona, Spain

Catarina Saiote   Georg-August-University, Department of Clinical Neurophysiology, Göttingen, Germany

Marco Sandrini   Human Cortical Physiology and Stroke Neurorehabilitation Section, National Institute of Neurological Disorders and Stroke, National Institutes of Health, Bethesda, MD, USA and Center for Neuroscience and Regenerative Medicine at Uniformed Services University of Health Sciences, Bethesda, MD, USA

Julian Savulescu   Oxford Centre for Neuroethics, University of Oxford, Oxford, UK

Pedro Schestatsky   Laboratory of Neuromodulation, Department of Physical Medicine and Rehabilitation, Spaulding Rehabilitation Hospital and Massachusetts General Hospital, Harvard Medical School, Boston, MA, USA and Programa de Pós-Graduação em Ciências Médicas da Universidade Federal do Rio Grande do Sul, Brasil; Coordenação de Aperfeiçoamento de Pessoal de Nível Superior (CAPES), Brazil

Tal Sela   Department of Psychology, and The Gonda Multidisciplinary Brain Research Center, Bar Ilan University, Ramat Gan, Israel

Charlotte J. Stagg   Oxford Centre for Functional MRI of the Brain (FMRIB), Department of Clinical Neuroscience, University of Oxford, Oxford, UK

Dennis Truong Department of Biomedical Engineering, The City College of New York of CUNY, New York, NY, USA

Fabrice Wendling INSERM, Rennes, France and Université de Rennes, Rennes, France

Maximo Zimerman Brain Imaging and Neuro-Stimulation (BINS) Laboratory, Department of Neurology, University Medical Center, Hamburg, Germany and Institute of Cognitive Neurology (INECO), Buenos Aires, Argentina

Preface

In 2007, I sat in my office thinking about how to conduct a research project which would combine brain stimulation with daily cognitive training. I was compelled to put it aside, as transcranial magnetic stimulation (TMS), the most known method for non-invasive brain stimulation, is not recommended to be applied on a daily basis, and causes mild discomfort, which is not optimal for cognitive training. When a colleague returned from a research visit to Göttingen and told me about his collaboration on a project that involved transcranial direct current stimulation (tDCS) and transcranial alternating current stimulation (tACS), I immediately knew that these methods could be the perfect tools to get my research finally on the way. Indeed, not many people had heard back then about transcranial electrical stimulation (tES) methods such as tDCS or tACS, and when scientists in the field used to tell their colleagues about their work with tES, the Pavlovian response usually was "so, you are working with TMS . . ."

Therefore, it is with great enthusiasm that I present *The Stimulated Brain*, the first book that focuses on the key aspects of tES in experimental and clinical research. It details the most important mechanistic advances and discusses the impact of these findings for clinical and basic researchers, while also providing a prospective for the future research, translation, and application of these methods.

Although parts of these topics have been presented in a few books, it is important to bring them together in a volume that focuses on tES in its own right. In fact, tES research is no longer esoteric. People in diverse fields are working with this tool, and interest in tES is growing into excellent and exciting lines of research all around the world. It attracts attention from the research community and the public, as it encompasses the realms of both basic science and clinical viewpoints, and its implications can go beyond these to the healthy population.

The first part of the book is devoted to the basic knowledge of tES, from a fascinating first chapter on its history, to a comprehensive introduction of the different methods in use, to a fresh insight on safety at the physical and psychological level, as well as modeling work, animal studies, and the physiological bases. My expectation is that these chapters will not only be of interest to scientists who are already working with tES, but will also offer a good kick-start to those who are less familiar with it but want to increase their knowledge and possibly to use this tool in their future research. In this respect I, with the help of the authors of the various chapters, have made all efforts to ensure that the chapters in this section and in the other parts in the book are accessible to all those from the various fields of medicine, psychology, neuroscience, physiology, pharmacology, and biochemistry.

Following this introduction, the second part of the book focuses on research on the typical brain and how its modulation using tES has been shown to improve various functions, including sensory, motor, memory, and high-level cognitive functions such as executive function, attention, mathematics, and language. The third section is dedicated to studies that have aimed to improve functions in the atypical brain. These chapters include work on neurological disorders such as stroke, dysfunctions in the elderly, and psychiatric illnesses. The final section concludes with chapters that discuss future perspectives, including commercialization, neuroethics, the application of tES in the field of education, and a concluding chapter on the future usage of tES and its challenges.

This book could have not been produced by myself alone, and I am honored and privileged to have engaged scientists whose valuable contributions have advanced and elucidated these areas of research. These researchers have paved the way to several of the most relevant discoveries in the field, and have provided excellent chapters that provide state-of-the-art knowledge.

Undoubtedly, as much as I wanted to, I could not cover all topics or involve all researchers in the field in this volume, and some of those who did not contribute to this book as authors were courteous enough to serve as reviewers and provide excellent feedback that improved the chapters in this book.

I wish to thank all the authors for their contributions, which also increased my knowledge of the field. I would also like to thank the reviewers who gave their time to provide excellent feedback for the various chapters. I am grateful to Mica Haley, the acquisitions editor at Elsevier, for her brilliant idea and offer to edit this book, and to April Farr, the Editorial Project Manager, for all the support during the various stages of this project. Thanks are due to the Wellcome Trust for its support, which allowed me to complete this book. Finally, I would like to thank the members of my laboratory, my wife Kathrin, and my children Jonathan and Itamar for their patience and support.

I trust that this book provides a valuable contribution in promoting future discoveries, providing material for critical discussions, and educating readers about this fascinating and promising field. I am sure that this book will be stimulating.

Roi Cohen Kadosh

PART I

THE BASIS

CHAPTER

1

Electricity and the Brain: An Historical Evaluation

Paul Elliott

School of Humanities, University of Derby, Derby, UK

OUTLINE

INTRODUCTION

Since the mid-18th century there has been a persistent though much contested belief in the efficacy of electrotherapy as a treatment for various conditions and, to a lesser extent, a belief that electrical stimulation of the mind and body also conferred various benefits. Consistent evidence for

3

the latter emerges from accounts of electrotherapy, which will be the focus of this chapter, although it is important to note that the widespread private domestic usage can only briefly be covered here. These convictions were supported by changing theories of the nature of electricity and developments in electrical technology, which were invariably intertwined. Usually regarded as a form of fire in the early 18th century, following Isaac Newton's work electricity was perceived as a subtle ethereal fluid akin to magnetism or gravity, and the Queries in the fourth edition of Newton's *Optics* (1730) helped to inspire many experimenters to investigate its properties. Only after the development of modern mathematical physics was it treated as a force susceptible to understanding according to mathematical laws which defined its behavior in different mediums. Between 1750 and 1900, galvanism, electrotherapy, and transcranial electrical stimulation fostered theoretical conceptions of a vital fluid intended to bridge the division between mentalism and physicality, which excited philosophical and political attacks in the febrile and fractured political climate of the revolutionary era. As we shall see, electrotherapy was promoted and marketed as a popular and less expensive alternative to standard treatments used by medical professionals, such as bleeding, blistering, and opium, but also encountered considerable opposition from some of the faculty and some patients. Electrotherapeutic machines came to be widely available, and for thousands suffering from all manner of painful and debilitating health conditions electrotherapy offered the hope of relief. Electrical stimulation was used across the social spectrum, from wealthy European aristocrats to the laboring poor, for general mental and bodily stimulation and for a wide variety of conditions ranging from epilepsy to impotence and tapeworms to toothache. Some patients claimed that electrotherapy induced a general sense of mental improvement and enhanced their powers of judgment. Whilst these historical instances of usage do not generally, of course, conform to modern clinical investigative standards, nevertheless they merit more systematic scrutiny, and we can only hope to scratch the surface here of what is a vast body of evidence in the medical literature, institutional records, and private accounts of transcranial electrical stimulation.

After briefly exploring how medical electricity was employed by medical practitioners, healers, and patients themselves through self medication, and the evidence for related transcranial electrical stimulation, we will then examine how and why electricity was used for the treatment of psychiatric disorders, and how a belief in the more general efficacy of transcranial electrical stimulation arose. The history of transcranial electrical stimulation illustrates very clearly the permeability of boundaries and reciprocal stimulation between professional and private medicine, and between professional and popular science. Numerous types of electrical machine and electrical apparatus were produced for professional and popular medical markets between 1800 and the 1930s, and there was a close relationship between technological development and clinical electricity. In the 20th century, electrotherapy was used as a form of shock therapy during World War I and, from the 1930s, as electroconvulsive therapy (ECT).

For the purposes of this historical evaluation, transcranial electrical stimulation denotes all applications of electricity to the head, whilst electrotherapy refers to applications of electricity to the body for the purpose of curing or relieving mental or physical conditions. ECT is the use of sufficient electricity to induce seizures to relieve or cure psychological problems in controlled conditions. As we shall see, between 1750 and 1950 three different kinds of electricity were employed in transcranial electrical stimulation. Static or frictional electricity was generated by belt-driven frictional electrical machines and stored in the Leyden jar. After 1800, current electricity generated by the voltaic pile or battery was also utilized (see Fig. 1.1), whilst alternating current (faradic electricity) generated by electromagnetic induction generally became the most favored electrotherapeutic agent from the 1840 s onwards (see Figs 1.1–1.3). In practice,

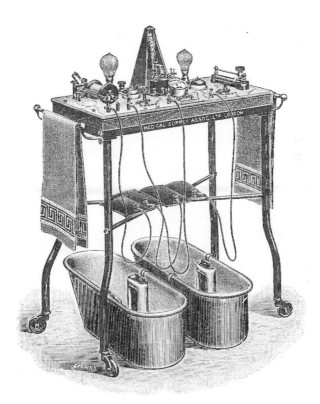

FIGURE 1.1 Combined table apparatus with galvanic battery, metronome, and faradic-coil. *Figure from Browne, 1931: 106.*

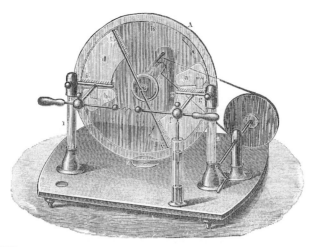

FIGURE 1.2   Holtz electrical generating machine. *Figure from Jones, 1904: 155.*

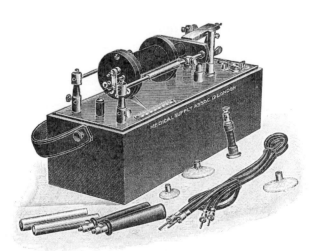

FIGURE 1.3   Physio faradic wave coil showing different sized button electrodes, electrode handles, and wires. *Figure from Browne, 1931: 94.*

historically there was often no clear distinction (if there ever has been) between mental and physical causes of psychiatric problems, or agreement on whether particular conditions were primarily psychological or physical in nature. Likewise, alterations in scientific, medical, and psychological terms and concepts mean that whenever possible original terminology from the historical sources has been employed, helping to avoid whiggishness.

ENLIGHTENMENT ELECTROTHERAPY AND TRANSCRANIAL ELECTRICAL STIMULATION

Electricity became one of the most popular and fashionable scientific pursuits of the Enlightenment in the colonies, including North America, and in Europe, with experiments and demonstrations being performed in a variety of spaces from theaters and assembly rooms to taverns and private homes. Domestic experiments were encouraged by the adaptation of household objects as electrical instruments, whilst electric experiments were promoted as a form of natural philosophy appropriate for female education and entertainment, and in many philosophical associations such as the Lunar Society in England. Electrical experiments and demonstrations were relatively easy to perform and could be undertaken at home with everyday objects such as glass jars, wool, and metal rods. Once Benjamin Franklin had demonstrated that electricity in the natural world was the same kind of substance as that encountered in the laboratory or domestic experiments, the operation of electricity in phenomena as diverse as earthquakes, fireballs, precipitation, and plant growth suggested that it was one of the primary powers in the divine economy. The bodily and sensory experiences were always central to Enlightenment electrical demonstrations and experiments, and some of the more popular demonstrations involved electrifying individuals or groups of people. It is therefore likely that these first suggested that the application of electricity might have medical benefits. Electric shocks from torpedo fish had been applied for medical purposes at least since antiquity, and may also have been suggestive, although the power or force induced by the fish was not demonstrated to be the same phenomenon as the force from rubbed amber or lightning until much later (Elliott, 2008, pp. 196, 207–212; Finger, 2006, pp. 89–91; Finger & Piccolini, 2011; Mottelay, 1922, p. 20).

Encouraged by the German physician and naturalist Johann Gottlob Krüger (1715–1759), his student Christian Gottlieb Kratzenstein (1723–1795) discovered that the electric fluid appeared to relieve paralyses of the finger caused by arthritis, which encouraged others to experiment with medical electricity in Europe and North America, including the French philosopher Abbé Nollet (1700–1770). Subsequently, Enlightenment natural philosophers and medical practitioners, including Benjamin Franklin (1706–1790), John Birch (1745–1815), and Erasmus Darwin (1731–1802), were measured advocates of electrotherapy which was used in some hospitals, although not usually as a treatment of first resort. There was disagreement amongst Enlightenment medical practitioners about which conditions electrotherapy treated best and exactly why it appeared to be effective. The Italian philosopher Tiberius Cavallo (1749–1809), for instance, believed that electrotherapy was most useful for conditions "arising from obstructions and nervous affections" when used in moderation, whilst Darwin believed that, like alcohol and opium, it increased the "exertions of all irritative motions" and could therefore be useful for paralysis, torpor, and sometimes pain relief. He also took full advantage of the invention of the pile by Alessandro Volta (1745–1827) to recommend it for electrotherapy. Other individuals were even more enthusiastic. John Wesley (1703–1791), for instance, believed that electrotherapy was the key to a new form of popular medicine, whilst natural philosophers, quacks, and healers such as the celebrated Scottish physician James Graham (1745–1794) and the Prussian lecturer and showman Gustavus Katterfelto (c. 1743–1799) recommended it for all kinds of stimulation and innumerable medical problems. Static electric machines and other apparatus such as Leyden jars became widely available, and efforts were made to modify these to improve the design, portability, and effectiveness of such instruments so that the amount and strength of the fluid could be regulated (Adams, 1799, pp. 483–558; Bertucci, 2001, 2006; Elliott, 2008; Finger, 2006, pp. 80–114; Schiffer, 2003, pp.133–160).

Many Enlightenment medical practitioners and philosophers believed the body to be a closely integrated system that was interdependent with the mind. This meant that, as Scull has contended, "medical theory and its associated remedies were ... readily adapted to the understanding and treatment of insanity," and that remedies used apparently efficaciously for other illnesses could be applied for the relief of madness (Scull, 1993, p. 184). Medical men such as Thomas Arnold (1742–1816) in Leicester, England, claimed they were best placed to treat madness, and specialized as "mad doctors" using the stock interventions of Georgian medical practice, including the administration of Peruvian bark, opium, bleedings, blistering, purging, vomiting, and, quite often, electricity – all of which were reassuringly interventionist and dramatic. Whilst there was some initial reluctance to apply electricity to the head because of the perceived dangers, some of these also began to use electrotherapy to treat psychiatric conditions (Beaudreau & Finger, 2006; Porter, 1990, pp. 12, 184–185; Scull, 1993, pp. 183–184). Birch, for instance, surgeon at St Thomas's Hospital in London, experimented with applications of electricity from the Leyden jar for melancholy during the 1780s. He was surprised to find that very "strong shocks" from a Leyden jar with 112 square inches of coated surface and larger could be applied to the head without apparent injury (Adams, 1799, pp. 549–552). Encouraged by electrical applications to the head by Birch and others, by successful recoveries from accidental shocks and the mental stimulation these sometimes induced, it was found that the electric fluid could be safely and beneficially administered. Philosophers such as Franklin and the Dutch physician Jan Ingenhousz (1730–1799) advised that such treatments were worth giving to the mad, or for specific conditions such as melancholia and hysteria. The power of electric shocks to the head was demonstrated by accounts of memory loss and sometimes of mental stimulation or improvement that they had apparently induced. Ingenhousz described in a letter to Franklin one such accidental electric shock received at Vienna in 1783. According to Ingenhousz, the electrical explosion caused by touching a charged Leyden jar and which passed through his hat, forehead, and left hand, caused him to be struck down and lose all his senses, "memory, understanding and even sound judgement," such that he could not answer questions put to him by others in the room, or read or write. Having retired to bed, he awoke several hours later to find that his "mental faculties were at that time not only returned, but I felt the most lively joye in finding, as I thought at the time, my judgement infinitely more acute." He now "saw much clearer the difficulties of every thing, and what did formerly seem to me difficult to comprehend, was now become of an easy solution," whilst feeling "a liveliness in my whole frame, which I never had observed before" (Finger, 2006, pp. 111–112). Similarly, the German physician Friedrich Ludwig Augustin (1776–1854) reported in 1803 that a boy experienced improved mental performance after being galvanized. The boy suffered from cataleptic attacks resulting from ague (malarial fever) which caused paralysis in the arms and legs and periodic insanity. However, after 3 weeks of galvanization, Augustin claimed that the boy had not only been cured of paralysis but also become "quicker of mind" as a result (Arndt, 1892, p. 427).

The apparent kinship between electricity, magnetism, and other ethereal substances such as fire suggested that electricity might be inherent in all bodies and be synonymous with the vital spirit or spark of divinity mediating between matter and God. Supporters of such theories during the 18th century believed that the ethereal qualities of electricity bridged the divide between the physical and spiritual without interposing mechanistic limitations on the divine. Stimulated by electrotherapy and observations of the effects of electricity upon animate bodies, Deists believed that electricity provided an explanation for animation in a mechanistic universe. Such claims excited considerable argument, with some natural philosophers, theologians, and writers invoking electricity in natural theology as evidence for divine power, whilst others accused electricians of infidel materialism (Elliott, 2008, pp. 196, 207–212; Finger, 2006, pp. 89–91; Finger & Piccolini, 2011; Mottelay, 1922, p. 20).

The physician Erasmus Darwin, for instance, regarded the vital principle which interfaced between senses, nerves, and the brain as closely analogous to electricity. Inspired by his use of medical electricity, work on natural and artificial electricity and knowledge of the physiology of Albrecht von Haller (1708–1777) and psychology of David Hartley (1705–1757), Darwin defined an ethereal "spirit of animation" in his medical treatise the *Zoonomia* which acted through the "sensorium," interfaced between mentalism and physicality, and had qualities remarkably similar to those of the electrical fluid. He defined the sensorium within the body as "not only the medullary part of the brain, spinal marrow, nerves, organs of sense, and of the muscles" but simultaneously as the "living principle, or spirit of animation, which resides throughout the body, without being cognizable to our senses, except by its effects." In support of this Darwin adduced the external similarity of the brain to the pancreas, the way in which "the electric fluid itself is actually accumulated and given out voluntarily by the torpedo and the *gymnotus electricus,*" the electrical stimulation of paralytic limbs and the "singular figure of the brain and nervous system," which appeared to be "well adapted to distribute it over every part of the body" (Darwin, 1801, Vol. 1, pp. 9–10; Elliott, 2008, pp. 202, 207–219; Porter, 1989).

The Italian natural philosopher Luigi Galvani (1737–1798) believed that his dramatic experiments on frogs' legs demonstrated the existence of a special animal electricity. Making full use of the voltaic pile, Galvani's nephew Giovanni Aldini (1762–1834) mounted a strong defense of animal electricity internationally, utilizing dramatic experiments on animal heads and the corpses of recently deceased criminals to demonstrate the potential that the wonderful fluid offered for the revival of victims of drowning. In 1818 at Glasgow, the Scottish philosopher Andrew Ure (1778–1857) performed similar and more extensive galvanic experiments upon the body of a murderer Matthew Clydesdale, inducing wild contortions and facial expressions, some of which drove audience members from the room. Whilst exploiting the dramatic and macabre quality of galvanic effects to demonstrate the potential medical efficacy of galvanism, Aldini and Ure also excited revulsion and fear, associating them with materialism and helping to increase suspicion and political opposition towards medical galvanism and vitalism. Aldini claimed to have "perfectly cured" two patients at Bologna of "melancholic insanity" using galvanism, whilst the English chemist William Nicholson (1753–1815) believed that these widely reported experiments and demonstrations provided "very encouraging prospects for the benefit of mankind in disorders prominent of the head and in apoplexies." Whilst "many precautions are necessary to be used in the administration of this powerful remedy in lunacy or apoplexy," Nicholson argued that "the application of galvanism in melancholic insanity is absolutely new, and of great interest," recommending further trials of galvanism for "melancholic insanity," it being "an affliction so distressing, against which the present system of physic has so little to offer" (Morus, 1998, pp. 126–130; Nicholson, 1802; Ure, 1819).

NINETEENTH-CENTURY PSYCHIATRY AND THE PSYCHIATRIC PROFESSIONS

During the 19th century traditional medical structures in Britain, Europe, and North America underwent radical transformation induced by the medical sciences, industrialization, urbanization, and pressures for social and political reforms, and these changes helped to explain the growing popularity (and subsequent decline) of electrotherapy. Professionalization reinforced the male domination of the medical professions, which sought to regulate and control medical education, to exclude women from the higher echelons, and to differentiate themselves and their methods from other healers and quacks. Institutionalization gathered apace and hospitals and asylums assumed ever greater importance in medical careers whilst, especially in the second half of the century, nursing was reformed and new medical occupations appeared. Government regulation of medical institutions was undertaken in Britain, the USA, and Europe, although there was greater state intervention in medicine in the latter. Hospitals came to occupy an even more significant place in medical careers, growing in size and range as specialist and teaching institutions appeared. Most hospitals in Britain, the British colonies, and the USA remained charitable institutions, but treated a growing proportion of private patients. Aspiring doctors forged lucrative practices, whilst competition for wealthier middle-class patients grew as hospital treatment became more accepted (Porter, 1997, pp. 348–427; Waddington, 1984). Psychiatry as a discipline devoted to the diagnosis, analysis, treatment, and prevention of mental disorders took shape, although it was only at the end of the century that psychiatrists were labeled as such, and practitioners continued to be called "alienists" until the early 20th century. Organizations such as the British Psychological Association (1841) and American Psychiatric Association (1844) and specialist publications such as the *Asylum Journal* (1853) helped to forge the discipline and profession. These agencies also facilitated the exchange of psychiatric ideas, including the use of electrotherapy and its equipment. Efforts were made to place psychiatry upon a more systematic footing, with clearly defined conditions modeled on general medical nosology and based upon clinical case studies. The use of electrotherapy in psychiatry emerged as part of these processes, as the possibility of physical treatment seemed to offer considerable potential for professional medical practice and institutional control (Beveridge & Renvoize, 1988, p. 158; Colwell, 1922; Porter, 1997, pp. 493–524; Rowbottom & Susskind, 1984; Shorter, 1997, pp. 16–17, 100–109).

ELECTRICITY IN CULTURE AND SOCIETY

At the same time, the period after 1850 saw large-scale development of the electrical industry, which fostered the belief that electricity might be the key to social as well as technological progress. In 1892, William Crookes (1832–1919), physicist and President of the British Institution of Electrical Engineers, believed that there were almost boundless opportunities for exploring the interaction of electricity in nature. A decade later, John Arthur Thomson (1861–1933), Regius Professor of Natural History at the University of Aberdeen, argued that the development of electromagnetism had "initiated the movement which has made the word electricity almost as characteristic of the 19th century as the word evolution." According to Thomson, both "as regards theory and as regards practical applications" for electricity there had been "astounding progress," and the next century was "pregnant with possibilities of development" (Crookes, 1892; Thomson, 1906, pp. 158, 165).

The major expansion of the electrical, chemical, and automotive industries has been defined as a second industrial revolution, and initially provided major encouragement for the adoption of electrotherapy. The production of electrical generating machines and apparatus passed from the province of mechanics and instrument makers to that of instrument manufacturers. The invention of the voltaic pile or battery and Michael Faraday's development of the induction coil made possible the production of portable supplies of electrical current (see Figs 1.1 and 1.3). Important theoretical and mathematical changes regarding the way that electricity was understood occurred, but these did not impact beyond the scientific community until the end of the century, and most continued to regard electricity as an extremely subtle ethereal fluid. Most fundamentally, the physicist James Clerk Maxwell (1831–1879) argued that electricity should be regarded as a field of force rather than an extremely refined fluid, although he accepted that the analogy with fluids could be useful. Faraday and Hermann Von Helmholtz (1821–1894) demonstrated experimentally, and Clerk Maxwell theoretically, that "light and electromagnetic radiation are alike due to rhythmical disturbances in the ether, differing only in their wave lengths," which Thomson believed was "one of the most unifying ideas in modern science" and "raised" electricity from the "observation and classificatory level" into an "integral part of a unified" science. Whilst the 19th century had remained "ignorant" of "what is meant by an electric charge," yet "many laws of electrical phenomena" had been discovered, and the fact that "electrical radiations are best interpreted in terms of ethereal waves" had been "generally conceded" by the early 1900s (Thomson, 1906, pp. 156, 158, 165). Powered by the first permanent urban electricity-generating networks from the 1880s, electric power took over urban and domestic living as towns were bathed in electric light, and communication over distance was transformed through the telegraph, telephone and, subsequently, radio transmitters. Electric trams supplanted horse-drawn vehicles and the steam trains of the London underground began to be replaced with electric versions, whilst in the early years of motoring electric cars bid fair to supplant the internal combustion engine as the preferred source of power. Giant hydro-electric power stations such as that on Niagara Falls in North America were the wonders of the age as the wonderful possibilities of electricity were celebrated in a series of international exhibitions, including those in the Crystal Palace, London (1892), and the Columbian Exposition in Chicago, USA (1893). Modern late Victorian and Edwardian middle-class households could have their rooms illuminated by electric light and warmed by electric heaters, their clothes ironed by an electric iron and repaired by electric sewing machine, their water boiled in electric kettles, their food cooked on an electric kitchen range, their cigar lit by an electric lighter, and their bed warmed by an electric blanket (see Fig. 1.4).

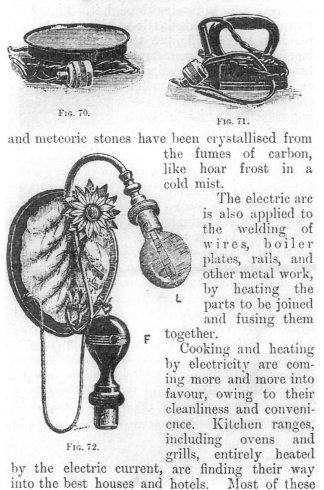

metals are now smelted by its means, and rough brilliants such as those found in diamond mines

FIG. 70.

FIG. 71.

and meteoric stones have been crystallised from the fumes of carbon, like hoar frost in a cold mist.

The electric arc is also applied to the welding of wires, boiler plates, rails, and other metal work, by heating the parts to be joined and fusing them together.

Cooking and heating by electricity are coming more and more into favour, owing to their cleanliness and convenience. Kitchen ranges, including ovens and grills, entirely heated by the electric current, are finding their way into the best houses and hotels. Most of these

FIG. 72.

FIGURE 1.4 Electric saucepan, flat iron, and cigar lighter. *Figure from Munro, 1898: 127.*

I. THE BASIS

The association of electricity with modernity, progress, and comfort, reinforced by its increasing industrial significance, helped to allay safety fears and initially encouraged therapeutic applications (Beauchamp, 1997; Bowers, 1982; Gooday, 2004, 2007; Hughes, 1983; Marvin, 1988; Morus, 1998, p. 231; Munro, 1898, pp. 85–185; Nye, 1990).

NINETEENTH-CENTURY ELECTROTHERAPY

Nineteenth-century medical practitioners who advocated electrotherapy for different conditions used various means to try and distinguish themselves and their truth claims from those made by numerous healers, instrument makers, and other electrotherapists operating in the medical marketplace. These included publishing detailed accounts of their work in the medical journals, in which the exact condition, number of patients and their characteristics were recorded, such as age, occupation, symptoms, and physical appearance. However, there was some disagreement within the medical fraternity and beyond about which conditions were best treated with electricity. Morus has shown how Henry Marshall Hughes (1805–1858), physician at Guy's Hospital in London, published summaries of his electrotherapeutic applications in the "electrifying room" in medical periodicals, claiming that these demonstrated the efficacy of galvanism for the treatment of chorea (involuntary writhing movements) and, especially, hysteria in young women (Morus, 1998, pp. 237, 238). Between the 1830s and 1850s, other London electrotherapists from the faculty, such as the physician Golding Bird (1814–1854), made more effort to engage with popular electricians such as those involved with the London Electrical Society. In the electrifying room at Guy's, Bird tried to systematize and integrate electrotherapy "into the hospital's everyday routine" and sought to overcome resistance from his medical colleagues. Outpatients and residential patients had to attend the room regularly whilst careful notes were taken recording progress. Electricity was administered from a range of static frictional machines, galvanic batteries and, increasingly, electromagnetic apparatus, often by medical assistants, details of which are evident from instrument maker's advertisements and textbooks of electrotherapy such as Alfred Smee's *Elements of Electro-Biology* (London, 1849). Although smaller and cheaper than plate electrical machines and Leyden jars, the first voltaic or galvanic piles were large, cumbrous, and only available to relatively wealthy individuals or institutions, requiring much continuous effort and attention to function, which initially limited their medical application. Similarly, it was initially difficult to regulate and replicate the strength or amount of electricity administered to suit particular patients or conditions, which increased the dangers of galvanism and discouraged applications to the head. As the *Medical and Physical Journal* emphasized in 1803, "one of the principal difficulties in instituting comparative experiments on the operation of galvanism is the perpetually varying energy of the pile or battery." This was "a difficulty which it is the less easy to remove, as the test and measure of this influence in exciting muscular contraction is equally variable, according to the original force of vital action, or remaining susceptibility to stimuli which the animal organ possesses and retains" (*Medical and Physical Journal*, 1803, p. 385). The development of more portable, adjustable, cheaper, and specialist machines encouraged psychiatric applications of galvanism and electromagnetism to the head.

One way of applying electrotherapy was by seating patients on an insulating stool connected to the prime conductor of the electrical machine and then electrifying their skin surfaces. Alternatively, galvanic or electromagnetic apparatus provided larger doses of electricity using a range of different types of electrodes for different parts of the body. As Morus has shown, the application of these treatments was largely limited to nervous disorders, especially chorea or hysterical paralysis. The range of conditions for which electricity was utilized was clearly defined, which helped to present it as careful and rational rather than random, and distinguished the process from more popular usage (Morus, 1998, pp. 231–240). The development of the electromagnetic induction coil provided more portable and manageable supplies of electric fluid, and medical men and instrument makers devised improvements for automating the making and breaking of the current using an electromagnet and spring (Fig. 1.3). Other improvements included Henry Letheby's unidirectional induction coil, which allowed only a succession of shocks in a single direction to be felt; this, he suggested, was crucial so that the current be passed "in the route of the *vis nervosa*" from center to periphery in "motor paralysis" but from "extremities to centres when the sensitive nerves are affected." It was also noted that the break-current shock was more severe than that from the make-current, so the former was believed to be better for over-sensitive nerves and the latter for motor nerve disorders (Morus, 1998, pp. 249–254).

After 1850, electrotherapy was used more extensively in European, British, and North American asylums. The period saw some of the largest mental hospitals constructed on the periphery of urban centers, whilst psychiatry itself crystallized as a discipline and the profession and term "psychiatrist" was coined. With large-scale incarceration of the insane away from the "sane," doctors faced the problem of managing numerous residential patients. They believed that structure, discipline, and routine provided much of the solution, and major asylums were constructed and based upon the pavilion plan and often on the periphery of urban centers with extensive lands and gardens around, shielded by dense planting or high walls and fences. Asylums were secure institutions with hundreds and sometimes thousands of patients and staff, locked rooms, and almost endless corridors, imposing clock towers, and regulated routines and environments. Patients could often reside in these institutions for decades and sometimes lifetimes (Scull, 1993, pp. 267–333; Shorter, 1997, pp. 33–68). Whilst architecture, discipline, routines, and carefully regulated activities were thought to be beneficial for the insane, there was frustration that long-established treatments were proving inefficacious, including drugs and other techniques which were limited to controlling and sedating patients rather than curing them. Psychiatrists were keen to emulate some of the success that had occurred in medicine through the use of antiseptics and anesthetics. There were international differences; in Britain madness tended to be regarded as a disease of the brain rather than one of the mind, and it was therefore believed that physical interventions such as electrotherapy would be efficacious, as accounts of its successful use in continental Europe seemed to confirm. In some European countries, such as France, there was a greater tendency to regard psychiatric problems as disorders of the mind, and therefore there was greater receptivity to Freudian psychoanalysis by the late 19th and early 20th centuries (Beveridge & Renvoize, 1988, p. 158; Scull, 1993, pp. 267–333).

New research regarding the physiological impact of electricity on the head and brain from the middle of the 19th century helped to encourage psychological applications of electrotherapy and its use as a diagnostic tool. Ernst Heinrich Weber (1795–1878), the German physician and professor of anatomy at Leipzig University, examined the impact of electricity upon the brain of living animals as part of his investigations into neural structures and sensation, whilst from the 1830s, inspired by the work of Galvani and his followers, the Italian natural philosopher Carlo Matteucci (1811–1868) examined electricity produced by wounds in the body and also the responses of living animal brains to electrical stimulation, whilst the French neurologist Guillaume-Benjamin-Amand Duchenne (1806–1875) studied many areas of electrophysiology and muscle stimulation. Citing their work, in 1870 the German/English physician Julius Althaus (1833–1900) asserted that continuous galvanic (direct) current caused a distinct "physiological action" on the brain of a living man. However, static electricity and electromagnetic current had to be applied too powerfully to be useful, which caused a danger to health. He believed that a "gentle, continuous current, directed to the face, scalp or neck" caused negligible pain yet was "readily transmitted" through the skull and muscle tissue to the "cerebral substance," which was demonstrated by the sensations that it induced in the subject, including a distinctive light, sound, smell, and taste (Althaus, 1870, pp. 130–131). Althaus found that more powerful shocks impacted strongly on the cerebral matter, as experiments using frogs legs on the brains of corpses, and feelings of dizziness, giddiness, sickness, fainting, vomiting, and "even convulsions" induced in living patients, demonstrated (Althaus, 1870, pp. 129–131, 132–136).

Whilst trial and error were an important part of the electrotherapy process in 19th-century asylums, there was a growing body of experience and knowledge which was communicated through textbooks, professional journals, and interaction between medical practitioners, manufacturers of electrotherapeutic equipment, and other interested parties. The range of equipment and methods of application in the period varied, but broad trends can be discerned. Treatment tended to be sustained for days, weeks, or months rather than being limited to a single application, whilst sessions might typically occupy 10 or 20 minutes at a time. Victorian doctors observed that electrotherapy could cause epileptic convulsions if the current was strong enough, but it was believed that weaker currents applied over sustained periods were more clinically effective. Whilst various parts of the body would be electrified for psychiatric disorders, including the spine and hands, subsequently electrodes were typically applied to the head (Fig. 1.3). This has been described as the "cephalic shift," and seems to have paralleled some of the developments in neurophysiology discussed above (Beveridge & Renvoize, 1988, p. 159; Stainbrook, 1948).

From 1857, US electrotherapists George Miller Beard (1839–1883) and Alphonso David Rockwell (1840–1933) began to experiment with using electrical current for the treatment of indigestion, nervousness, and general debility using methods "substantially modelled" on the "localized electrization" of Duchenne. From 1866 they tried "general electrization" for cases of indigestion and "general debility," and found this to be much more effective (Beard & Rockwell, 1867, pp. iii–iv). Beard and Rockwell regarded applications of electrotherapy to the head as "perhaps the best tests both of the efficiency of general electrisation and of the skill of the operator." They recommended that galvanism was best applied to the head through the temples, forehead, or over the ears, using a moistened hand or "large soft sponge" which was usually "the first step in the process of general electrification," and that negative electricity was usually best from an electrode placed near the neck and positive from another on the forehead, which was "far more sensitive to the electric current than any other portion of the surface of the body" (Beard & Rockwell, 1871, pp. 198–199, 174–178). In many asylums, hospitals, clinics, and spas electricity was applied in special electrical rooms whilst "electric baths" were also employed, which provided stimulation for limbs by propelling current through water. One example was the four-cell Schnee bath for treating general rheumatic conditions, painful joints, and poor blood circulation, invented by German physician Emil Schnee in the important Bohemian (Czech Republic) spa town of Karlovy Vary (Carlsbad) and used widely across Europe and North America (see Fig. 1.5). This

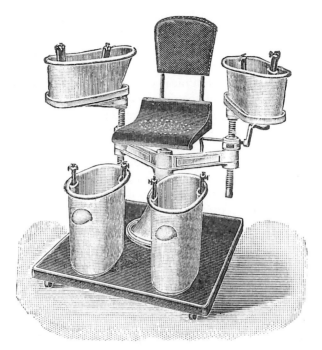

FIGURE 1.5   Schnee four-cell bath. *Figure from Browne, 1931: 186.*

provided four small containers for separate limb immersion, allowed strong currents to be employed (variable for each cell), did not require connection to the water supply, allowed patient use while fully clothed, and had other practical advantages. The perception that electricity functioned as a stimulus was inherited from the 18th century, and it was suggested that it therefore heightened blood flow, especially to the brain, but there was no consensus as to whether galvanic, induction, or static current was the best stimulant. It was also suggested that electricity could be a sedative (Beveridge & Renvoize, 1988, pp. 160–161; Browne, 1931, pp. 182–186; Jones, 1904, pp. 206–221).

Electrotherapy was believed to be particularly effective in cases of severe mental depression or melancholia. During the 1870s, the German physician Rudolph Gottfried Arndt (1835–1900) examined the impact on the brain of electrotherapy in patients suffering from severe psychoses with serious depression and delusions. He concluded that faradic electricity was best applied for severe inactivity, stupor, weakness, and manic depression, whilst galvanic current could relieve affective disorders and psychoses (Arndt, 1892, pp. 428–431; Steinberg, 2013). At the Rainhill Asylum in England in 1887, 11 women were treated with galvanism by Dr Joseph Wigglesworth, who found that 3 had been cured, 3 improved, and 5 received no apparent benefit from the treatment. Most of kinds of disorders of behavior, paralysis, headaches, neuralgia, and sometimes also chorea and epilepsy, were also treated by electrotherapy, as even were bedwetting and "sexual neurasthenia." There are also many Victorian accounts of electrotherapy being used to treat hysteria in Britain, Europe, and North America, and generally female patients were more likely to receive electrotherapy in asylums than men (Beveridge & Renvoize, 1988, pp. 159–160; Stainbrook, 1948, pp. 172, 173–174). As Morus shows, electrotherapy was favored as a treatment for mental and physical conditions associated with women, notably hysterical nervous conditions often resulting in irregular menstruation. A number of these had clear psychological origins, such as the case of Sarah Wheeler, whose involuntary motion of the right arm and shoulder was attributed to "fear, produced by the threats of her schoolmistress" (Morus, 1998, pp. 237, 239). Finally, electricity was increasingly utilized as a diagnostic tool for identifying nerve and muscle damage or degeneration for treatment through electrotherapy or other means. It was also employed in this way to measure the rate of improvement or nerve regeneration after treatment. Motor points of the body where the motor nerve entered the muscle were identified and mapped so that electrodes could be positioned to observe responses to the application of galvanic or faradic current (see Fig. 1.6). By the 1920s, such diagnostic applications of medical electricity had become far more significant than electrotherapy (Browne, 1931, pp. 158–181; Jones, 1904, pp. 257–280).

ELECTRICAL STIMULATION AND MENTAL ENERGY

Between 1750 and 1914, doctors, electrotherapists, and patients often found that electricity caused feelings of euphoria and sometimes appeared to improve mental performance, although it was known that this could occur merely through suggestion. This was underpinned by a somatic approach to functional disorders and Victorian physiological psychology. According to the writer and novelist Grant Allen (1848–1899), "modern scientific psychology based upon an accurate physiology, has roughly demonstrated that all mental phenomena are the subjective sides of what are objectively cognised as nervous functions." These were therefore "as rigorously limited by natural laws as the physical processes whose correlatives they are," as had been "abundantly illustrated" in respect to "those psychical functions (such as sensations and voluntary motions) which are ordinarily regarded as of purely bodily origin" (Allen, 1877, p. 2). The concept of mental energy underpinned much contemporary psychology which emphasized that the mind could be fatigued or exhausted by excessive mental exertion. In 1852, the philosopher

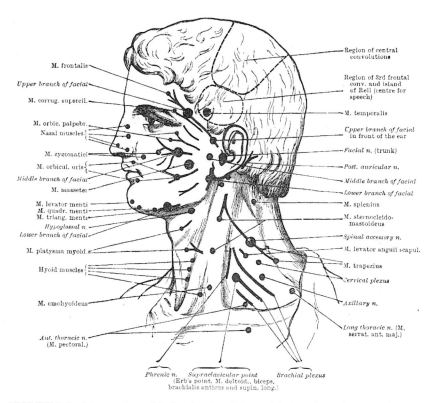

FIGURE 1.6   Motor points of the head and neck for positioning electrodes to test for nerve or muscle damage. *Figure from Browne, 1931: 164.*

Herbert Spencer (1820–1903) argued that verbal and literary style could be understood in terms of the "economy of … mental energy" which was "the cause of force" because "every faculty," including "reflective faculties, the imagination, the perceptions of the beautiful," are "exhausted by exercise." Like muscles in the body, exercised faculties always strive "to resume their original states" and require "continued rest" in order to "regain their full powers" (Spencer, 1852, pp. 356, 362). It was believed that the need to preserve psychological equilibrium encouraged actions and thoughts that expended the least mental energy, which seemed to provide a useful explanation for much of human culture and behavior and for the dangers of mental fatigue. It was also highly consonant with Victorian middle-class values of thrift, hard work, economy, and careful management of resources expounded by authors such as Samuel Smiles. Encouraged by Spencer and others, the concept of mental energy became an important part of Victorian evolutionary associational psychophysiology.

Although sometimes interpreted as an analogy, the concept of mental energy posited the existence of an extremely rarified or ethereal substance and appeared to equate thoughts or ideas with material substance. It therefore provided a justification for somatic treatments for mental illness, such as the use of electrotherapy, and electrotherapists often claimed to be replenishing or restimulating lost mental energies.

The physician Althaus claimed that galvanism applied along the spine was able to restore the "power of memory" and alleviate other symptoms in one 42-year-old musician who returned to work after a few weeks of the process. Likewise, a merchant whose symptoms included impairment of memory and "power of application" was able to go back to business after 10 weeks of galvanization through the spine, cerebral hemispheres and ganglia or sympathetic (autonomic) nervous system (Althaus, 1870, pp. 438–440). Beard and Rockwell's standard textbook on electrotherapy asserted that "many patients, perhaps the majority" experienced feelings of "enlivenment and exhilaration that often last for several hours" from galvanization, which "very" frequently provided "relief of pain and local or general weariness." Unpleasant effects were more likely with the galvanic than the faradic current. The "permanent or tonic effects" of electricity included an "increased disposition and capacity for labour ... of the brain," including improvements in the strength of "will and the capacity for exertion ... that is sometimes surprising" (Beard & Rockwell, 1871, pp. 222–223, 227, 231). For these doctors, the evidence for transcranial electrical stimulation induced by electrotherapy therefore provided additional evidence for the power of "neurasthenia," the debilitating psychopathological condition defined by Beard in 1869, symptoms of which included depression, fatigue, neuralgia, and tiredness, and which came to be particularly associated with modern American urban existence. They claimed that patients suffering from neurasthenia "find that they can read with closer attention and with greater zest; that they can pursue connected thought without fatigue, and endure mental, toil and anxiety that was once intolerable" (Beard & Rockwell, 1871, p. 231). The language employed by Beard to describe neurasthenia as an exhaustion of energy reserves in the nervous system paralleled that used to describe the physiological impact of electrotherapy, but both the condition of neurasthenia and the claim that it could be relieved by electricity attracted much contemporary criticism.

Similar observations were recorded by British and European doctors and psychiatrists. In 1899, Stéphane Leduc (1853–1939) of the École de Médecine de Nantes in France described how an elderly judge under his care for facial paralysis had continued to receive treatment even after this was cured because of the "comfortable feeling of increased mental rigour" afforded by the galvanization of his head and neck. The judge claimed that he felt lighter, and my ideas are more clear. I can concentrate my attention more closely upon my work, I struggle more successfully against the sleep-producing effect of long pleadings; I grasp more clearly the arguments which are advanced before me, and I can weigh them more exactly; in fact, I find my intelligence is brighter and my work is more easy to do, and for that reason I come to you for an electrical application whenever I am confronted by a fatiguing or difficult piece of work.

The British electrotherapist Henry Lewis Jones (1857–1915), for instance, Chief Medical Officer at the Electrical Department of St Bartholomew's Hospital in London and President of the British Electrotherapeutic Society, found that one of his patients receiving electricity for "nerve deafness" became "so conscious of the good effect produced upon her general condition as to be most anxious that her husband" receive similar treatment even though it had little improved her condition (Jones, 1904, pp. 301–302). Jones believed that after over 150 year's development, electrotherapy had made "steady progress" in Britain, Europe, and North America. Furthermore, despite the "passive resistance" of some medical practitioners, it would "continue to advance with the advance of general electrical knowledge." At St Bartholomew's, he oversaw the transformation of what was an "neglected, ill-equipped and unimportant branch of the hospital" into a "vigorous, progressive" department "rated as high as any similar department in the country" (Jones, 1904, p. 3; Medvei & Thornton, 1974, p. 187).

Although Leduc found that transverse current from side to side or in an oblique direction could produce unpleasant sensations, if the current was applied from front to back with one electrode bandaged into the forehead and the other applied to the nape of the neck no discomfort would occur. He concluded that application of battery current to the brain was free from danger if carefully applied, whilst negative current appeared to "excite the functions" and positive appeared to have "a calming and depressing action." He believed that negative applications provided probably the best means of "relieving the effects of mental overwork, and of raising the intellectual powers to their highest level" (Browne, 1931, p. 145; Jones, 1904, p. 102). Based upon observations from doctors, the accounts of patients or introspection, such accounts of the mental efficacy of transcranial electrical stimulation were widely reported but do not appear to have been subjected to systematic experimental investigation.

Studies of galvanism and electrotherapy by Giovanni Aldini and his followers did eventually help to foster the development of neurology, and in turn encouraged the application of neurology to psychiatry. With antiseptics, anesthetics, and the development of new surgical techniques from the mid-19th century, limited brain surgery became possible, which allowed living human brains to be observed for the first time. Attempts were made to apply electricity directly to animal and human brains, to determine the "situation of motor centres in the exposed cerebral cortex," by neurologists, medical men, and scientists such as Eduard Hitzig (1838–1907), Gustav Fritsch (1838–1927), and David Ferrier (1842–1928) (Jones, 1904, p. 246). Current and faradic electricity was used to induce convulsions, unconsciousness and revival in animals. In 1902, for instance, Stéphane Leduc described how he had achieved some "remarkable effects" by employing "rapidly interrupted currents passed longitudinally through the nerve centres." Having shaved a dog, he placed one anode onto the hind part of its back and the cathode on the skull, increasing the current gradually until general convulsions began producing unconsciousness, relaxation of the sphincter, and a halt to respiration. At this point, he discovered that "the current could be reduced in part, and respiration then commenced, and a state of tranquil sleep" and esthesia was induced until the current ceased. In this state it was found that no injuries appeared to have occurred and "the animal jumps up and seems quite well," and it was generally concluded that an epileptic state had been induced by the application of electrical current (Jones, 1904, pp. 246–247).

POPULAR ELECTROTHERAPY

During the Victorian and Edwardian eras, machines for transcranial electrical stimulation and electrotherapy that dispensed static or frictional, faradic or battery current electricity were available everywhere from London department stores to seaside resorts, and used in the home. The number of newspaper advertisements for electrotherapeutic apparatus, instrument-makers' catalogs and devices featured in shop catalogs demonstrate the extent of the market across Britain, Europe, and North America. One good example of a popular and longstanding piece of electrical equipment is Pulvermacher's Patent Galvanic Chain, which was invented by a Viennese engineer and healer, Isaac Lewis Pulvermacher, around 1850 and promoted by him in Britain, Europe, and North America from the early 1850s. Pulvermacher managed to obtain endorsement from numerous medical practitioners who supplied testimonials which featured in his pamphlets and newspaper advertisements. Available in various sizes, including pocket versions, the Pulvermacher chain consisted of a belt with multiple links and two insulated handles. It came in a box with an instruction booklet and series of testimonials from individuals who had claimed to benefit from its use. Effectively a voltaic pile or battery, the chain was originally constructed of copper (the anode) and zinc (the cathode) over wooden dowels which, after the application of vinegar or salt solution using sponges, absorbed the acid to become the electrolyte. The Pulvermacher chain was placed upon part of the body, to which it supplied a continuous flow of the electric fluid. The numerous interlinked cells in the chain made it strong, flexible, and comfortable, so it could easily be worn for long periods, whilst it was probably less intimidating in appearance than other electrical apparatus, which helps to explain its popularity. The strength of the battery could be altered easily by removing or adding the chains, and various different types of machine were produced by the company over the ensuing decades. Some designs claimed to obviate the need for vinegar by using bodily sweat as an electrolyte, whilst the interposition of interrupters – some of which were worked by patient movements and, later, clockwork – allowed alternating instead of continuous current to be supplied. The market for popular electrotherapeutic and transcranial electrical stimulation apparatus remained strong until the 1920s (Coley, 1969, pp. 369–370; de la Peña, 2005, pp. 110–111, 138–140, 150–153, 264–266; Morus, 2011, pp. 107–108, 145–182).

After examining and testing what he described as an "ingenious modification" of Volta's pile in 1851, the physician Golding Bird of Guy's Hospital, London, found that Pulvermacher's chain was "capable of producing all the physiological effects of the well-known galvanic battery," which was "cumbrous" and "inconvenient" for medical purposes. It was an "ingenious invention" which provided "an apparatus of the smallest possible bulk capable of evolving a constant or uninterrupted current of electricity of moderate tension and always in one direction," which he strongly recommended to his "medical brethren." Electric current from the chain was believed to be efficacious in applications to the head, and to stimulate mental performance. Samuel Patterson Evans, MD, Physician to the Newmarket-on-Fergus Dispensary, County Clare, Ireland, for instance, reported to Pulvermacher that it had successfully been used to restore mental energy. According to Evans, he advised one man who was not very strong intellectually, and whose mind became "tired and incapable of continued thought" after fatigue, to try the chain "applied round the head and forehead" on the basis that "the energy of the brain becomes exhausted, either from bodily labor or mental fatigue." After undertaking the treatment, Evans believed that he had become "capable of more continued application in either thinking or writing since," which he attributed to the fact that "the brain becomes stimulated by the outward dose of galvanic or electric energy supplied by the [Pulvermacher] Chain in action" which it had previously lost "either by its own loss of power directly, or indirectly by bodily fatigue." Whilst warning that "its application in such cases should not be continued too long" in case the "constant and forced stimulation" caused serious injury to the brain, Evans believed that the application of the chain deserved to be "closely studied in relation to its action on the brains of intellectual individuals" and for all types of nervous condition (Pulvermacher, 1853, pp. 15, 16–17).

SKEPTICISM TOWARDS ELECTROTHERAPY

Partly because it became associated with popular quackery, there remained considerable opposition to transcranial electrical stimulation and electrotherapy; even amongst supportive medical practitioners there was much disagreement about the reasons for its apparent efficacy in psychiatry and the best mode of application for each condition. After a systematic review of the clinical literature and extensive and enthusiastic electrotherapeutic practice, the German neurophysiologist Paul Julius Möbius (1853–1907) attributed the undoubted curative effects of transcranial electrical stimulation to the power of suggestion rather than exogenous physiological change induced by current. His ideas were strongly opposed by a congress of 35 electrotherapists and neuropsychiatrists led by Ludwig Edinger (1855–1918), Leopold Laquer, and Ernst Asche at Frankfurt in 1891, who argued that the efficacy of electrotherapy against a range of nervous or neuropathological conditions was a hard empirical fact supported by overwhelming evidence from numerous researchers, practitioners, and patients (Killen, 2006, pp. 48–80; Steinberg, 2011). The decline of physiological models of thought and the concept of mental energy, and somatic approaches to psychological problems and the rise of psychiatry and psychoanalysis, also contributed towards the decline of electrotherapy, as Sigmund Freud's rejection of electrotherapy as a treatment for neuroses during the 1890 s demonstrates (Gilman, 2008, pp. 344–345).

There were also continuing professional medical concerns that electrotherapy was being left to individuals with insufficient training, knowledge, and experience rather than being supervised by qualified practitioners. Golding Bird complained in the *Lancet* about the number of self-styled galvanists across the capital who, he claimed, could make thousands of pounds a year, whilst many parts of London had at least two or three of these "irregulars." He also blamed fellow medical practitioners for not educating themselves enough about electricity and galvanism, and for failing to stake out the territory professionally (Morus, 1998, p. 249). At Frankfurt in 1891, Laquer noted it was commonplace knowledge that electrotherapy was usually left in the hands of nurses, assistants, and students, which he advanced as an argument against suggestibility. In the early 1900s Lewis Jones worried that electrotherapy had passed through "many vicissitudes," being embraced by hospitals and then rejected and then "left in the hands of ignorant persons, who continue to perpetrate the grossest impositions in the name of electricity." In his article on electricity and psychiatry in Daniel Hack Tuke's influential *Dictionary of Psychological Medicine* (1892), the physician Rudolf Arndt observed that electrotherapy was a "two edged sword" which, he accepted, might "aggravate some forms of mental derangement and even make them incurable" when "great care, patience and confidence" were required, "qualities only found in those convinced of the final effect of the treatment." He urged that electrotherapy should never be left in the hand of "mere attendants, nurses or assistants, who simply do what they are told ... because it is their duty" (Arndt, 1892, pp. 428, 429; Beveridge & Renvoize, 1988, p. 161; Stainbrook, 1948, p. 174; Steinberg, 2011, p. 1235).

WORLD WAR I

The unprecedented demands of fighting in World War I, of course, stretched the limits of medicine and psychiatry in all combatant nations, resulting in experimentation with a range of shock and electrotherapeutic therapies. The industrial scale of death, conscription, and the relaxation in the criteria governing entry into the forces forced all combatant countries to make judgments about the effectiveness of individuals crippled by fear, suspected of cowardice, or who appeared to be suffering from mental illness. In practice, in Austria-Hungary, Britain, France, and Germany, distinctions between medicine and punishment, and between debilitating terror, cowardice, and mental illness, were frequently blurred, and the latter was sometimes regarded as a cover for fear, weakness, or a reversion to childhood. In these cases, doctors and psychiatrists were required by states – and considered it their responsibility – to make judgments about the reasons why men were unfit or unable to fight. Electrotherapy and various forms of shock therapy came to be seen as useful for distinguishing between these claims and different conditions. The most important consideration was, of course, to get men back to the front, but curing or relieving mental illnesses to equip them for future civilian life and helping the government control post-war expenditure by limiting claims for war pensions were also significant objectives (Adrian & Yealland, 1917; Killen, 2006, pp. 127–161; Leese, 2001; Linden, Jones, & Lees 2013, pp. 1976–1977; Scull, 2007, p. 279; Steinberg, 2011, pp. 1239–1240; Van Bergen, 2009, pp. 376–381, 399).

On the German side, the psychiatrist Fritz Kaufmann believed that applications of electric current strong enough to be effective but not quite enough to cause loss of consciousness to the head and body parts most apparently effected, combined with suggestion, was useful for treating neurosis and returning men to the front (Lerner, 2003, pp. 102–113; Killen, 2006, pp. 127–161; Steinberg, 2011, pp. 1239–1240; Van Bergen, 2009, pp. 378–383, 385). On the French and British side, there remained a conflict between neurological and psychological explanations for neuroses. French doctors and psychiatrists were more inclined to seek psychological explanations than their British counterparts, and this was reflected in their respective clinical language. The French formed a Centre for Psychoneuroses to treat soldiers disturbed by their fighting experiences, and psychiatrists such as Clovis Vincent (1879–1947) and Gustave Roussy (1874–1948) employed faradization to treat hysterical, paralyzed, and neurotic patients (Bogousslavsky & Tatu, 2013). One account of the application of electricity by French doctors was provided by the novelist and physician Louis-Ferdinand Céline in his semi-autobiographical novel *Voyage au Bout de la Nuit* (1932), which described how an army doctor "had installed a complicated assortment of gleaming electrical contraptions which periodically pumped us full of shocks" that he claimed "had a tonic effect" (Van Bergen, 2009, pp. 386–388). On the British side, once specialist psychiatric hospitals began to be provided close to the Western Front, electricity was used to treat a variety of patients, including those suffering from "shell shock" as well as other psychological problems, those with epilepsy, and some prisoners. Doctors such as the Canadian neurosurgeon Lewis Ralph Yealland (1884–1954) employed electric shocks for soldiers both on the Continent and at home. Working at the National Hospital for the Paralysed and Epileptic in London, Yealland treated 196 soldiers with functional motor and sensory symptoms, functional seizures, and somatoform disorders, integrating peripheral and central electrical stimulation with various other psychological and physical interventions. His methods appeared to work, at least in the short term, and, in contrast to most French and German doctors, Yealland claimed that they were equally applicable for civilian medicine. Whilst he has been regarded as one of the most zealous advocates of electricity as a form of discipline therapy, in fact (as Linden and colleagues demonstrate) Yealland mainly favored weaker faradic currents as part of a broader suggestive therapy, only resorting to stronger currents if this failed. His methods were fairly similar to those of other neurologists, and he only sent a small proportion of patients back to the front (Linden et al., 2013, pp. 1977–1987; Van Bergen, 2009, pp. 389–391).

Whilst the use of electric "cures" for war neurosis was generally accepted, some patients died as a result of the shock treatment and others committed suicide, and opposition came from some doctors such as the German Jewish psychiatrist Kurt Goldstein (1878–1965), who believed that the power of suggestion provided a much more efficient, less painful, and more effective form of treatment (Lerner, 2003, pp. 113–114; Van Bergen, 2009, pp. 383–384). It is significant that electrotherapy was not usually applied to officers. William Bailey, a British doctor treating soldiers in the British army for "neurological" problems, for instance, argued that electrotherapy was most effective for ordinary soldiers, as the superior intelligence and education of officers and other qualities associated with their social class meant that their conditions were invariably more complex, requiring greater time and patience for successful treatment

(Van Bergen, 2009, p. 391). Van Bergen and others have argued that for a variety of reasons, including the brutality and barbarism of trench fighting (which caused far more neuroses than normal in civilian life), the demands of "total war," the vulnerability and docility of mentally ill soldiers, and the requirement to return troops to the front and minimize pension costs, electrotherapy was used more aggressively than before World War I. However, as the case of Yealland and his low-current faradic treatments and suggestive therapy demonstrates, there was also much continuity with pre-war electrotherapeutic practices, and a general acceptance that electrotherapy and transcranial electrical stimulation could be useful.

CONCLUSIONS

Electrotherapy in medicine and psychiatry has faced opposition partly because it appears to reinforce the asymmetrical power relationship between medical practitioners and their patients, but also because the more general electrostimulative applications have been comparatively neglected. Although numerous individuals have claimed to benefit from transcranial electrical stimulation, there has been a tendency to downplay these accounts or attribute them to the power of suggestion, because of the professional knowledge and status of doctors, the investment in pain and discomfort made by patients, and also the multisensory drama and power of electrotherapeutic processes. Some historians of electrotherapy have emphasized the extent to which electrotherapy was conducted on relatively powerless subjects, whether (frequently young) women with hysteria between 1750 and 1914, Victorian and Edwardian asylum patients, or soldiers during the Great War suffering from war neuroses or "shell shock." It has been argued that Victorian patients were experimental objects "invariably drawn from the poorer sections of the working classes," and therefore objects of charity and thus "docile bodies" unlikely to resist (Morus, 1998, pp. 237, 239). In Britain, prior to the formation of the National Health Service in 1948, most hospitals and asylums were wholly or partly charitable institutions, and until the late 19th century were largely the preserve of the "deserving" poor. With their system of rules, regulations, and recommendations, many people were typically excluded, including those convicted of crimes, prostitutes, pregnant women, children, and any thought to be wealthy enough to pay for private medicine. Those admitted were supposed to gain moral and spiritual guidance as well as treatment, and charitable hospitals and asylums provided opportunities for medical experimentation on subservient subjects whilst providing a market incentive for the sale and improvement of electrotherapeutic instruments and equipment. However, for various reasons, including professionalism, natural human sympathy, and the demands of competition in the medical marketplace, many medical practitioners paid considerable attention to applying electricity carefully and sensitively, with full consent from patients. The Georgian surgeon John Birch (1745–1815), for instance, when treating a man for "severe melancholy" with electricity from a Leyden jar applied through the "frontal to the occipital bone and from one temporal bone to the other," increased the power of the shock very carefully in stages in close consultation with the patient, only recommending the "electrical experiment" after more conventional treatments had failed (Adams, 1799, pp. 551–552).

Certainly, the development of electrotherapy was partly driven by professionalization of the medical and psychiatric occupations. Doctors and psychiatrists who promoted it strove to differentiate themselves from the numerous quacks, healers, and instrument makers active in the medical marketplace by various means, including claiming superior knowledge, education, qualifications, and expertise. However, there is overwhelming evidence from patients, medical professionals, and other users that many – perhaps even a majority – believed that electrotherapy provided effective relief for some illnesses, including severe depression, whilst inducing a feeling of well being and sometimes improving mental performance. There should be a presumption of sincerity unless evidence suggests otherwise (manufacturers of electrical apparatus, for instance, had a clear incentive to extol and exaggerate the benefits of their machines). It is also evident that even the strongest proponents of electrotherapy were not blind to its faults, and many had a healthy skepticism towards more inflated claims made on its behalf. Even where it did not cure immediately, electricity usually induced highly visible immediate effects, including hot flushes and a quickening of the pulse, which were often taken as evidence of its clinical potency. Some Georgian and Victorian doctors were also well aware of the power of suggestion and the fact that electrotherapeutic apparatus could arouse fear in patients. Lewis Jones, for instance, noted that after electrodes had been placed upon the body some patients claimed to be cured before the electricity had even been turned on (Jones, 1904, p. 306).

As we have seen, electrotherapy was employed for a variety of medical and psychiatric purposes across Europe and in North America between 1750 and 1950, through the activities of scientific lecturers, natural philosophers, electricians, medical practitioners, and the incentives of the medical marketplace. This was encouraged by an emphasis upon the role of ethereal powers in the natural world and the divine economy, the generally accepted kinship or consonance between electricity and the nervous fluid, and the assumption that all physiological processes within the body were fundamentally electrical in nature. The apparent efficacy of electricity for a range of psychiatric conditions, activities of humane societies, and galvanic experiments on corpses all seemed to suggest that electricity was a potent force that offered power over life and death. The adoption and pervasiveness of electrotherapy in private and institutional medical practice and the medical marketplace helped to foster a belief that electricity could induce more general mental improvement – a fact asserted by many patients, medical practitioners, and electrotherapeutic textbooks. When the popularity of electrotherapy declined during the first decades of the 20th century, so likewise did belief in the efficacy of electricity for mental stimulation. Whilst electricity remained fundamental to modern living, as just one wave force on the electromagnetic spectrum rather than the wonderful ethereal fluid of the 18th or 19th centuries, and neurology was supplanted by psychiatric and behavioral cures, so it appeared less physiologically and even ontologically and metaphysically significant. Although ECT emerged from the 1930s to become a standard psychiatric intervention, the trauma and side effects of the convulsive process did not initially make it an attractive option for those merely seeking mental improvement rather than relief from severe neuroses. However, it is clear that for about 150 years many practitioners, patients, and users found the induction of low- and high-level electrical current a useful means of relieving symptoms, and sometimes a source of mental improvement and rejuvenation. This in itself provides a significant incentive for more systematic scientific investigations into transcranial electrical stimulation.

References and Further Reading

References

Adams, G. (1799). *An essay on electricity* (5th ed.). London, UK: J. Dillon & Co, with corrections and additions by W. Jones.

Adrian, A. D., & Yealland, L. R. (1917). Treatment of some common war neuroses. *The Lancet*, 1, 867–872.

Allen, G. (1877). *Physiological aesthetics.* London, UK: Henry King & Co.

Althaus, J. (1870). *A treatise on medical electricity theoretical and practical* (2nd ed.). London, UK: Longmans, Green & Co.

Arndt, R. (1892). Electricity, use of in the treatment of the insane. In D. H. Tuke (Ed.), *Dictionary of psychological medicine: 2 Vols.; Vol. 1.* (pp. 427–433). London, UK: Churchill.

Beard, G. M., & Rockwell, A. M. (1867). *The medical use of electricity with special reference to general electrisation as a tonic.* New York, NY: W. Wood.

Beard, G. M., & Rockwell, A. M. (1871). *A practical treatise on the medical and surgical uses of electricity.* New York, NY: William Wood & Company.

Beauchamp, K. (1997). *Exhibiting electricity.* London: Institution of Electrical Engineers.

Beaudreau, S. A., & Finger, S. (2006). Medical electricity and madness the eighteenth century: The legacies of Benjamin Franklin and Jan Ingenhousz. *Perspectives in Biology and Medicine*, 49, 330–345.

Bertucci, P. (2001). *Sparks of life: Medical electricity and natural philosophy in England, c. 1746–1792.* unpublished DPhil thesis, University of Oxford.

Bertucci, P. (2006). Revealing sparks: John Wesley and the religious utility of electrical healing. *British Journal for the History of Science, 39*, 341–362.

Beveridge, A. W., & Renvoize, E. B. (1988). Electricity: A history of its use in the treatment of mental illness in Britain during the second half of the 19th century. *British Journal of Psychiatry, 153*, 157–162.

Bogousslavsky, J., & Tatu, L. (2013). French neuropsychiatry in the Great War: Between moral support and electricity. *Journal of the History of the Neurosciences, 22*, 144–154.

Bowers, B. (1982). *A history of electric light and power*. London, UK: Institution of Engineering and Technology.

Bradley, T., Batty, R., & Noehden, A. A. (1803). Review of An account of the galvanic experiments performed by John Aldini, Professor of Experimental Philosophy in the University of Bologna, on the body of a malefactor. *Medical and Physical Journal, 9*, 382–385.

Browne, A. R. I. (1931). *Medical electricity for students* (3rd ed.). London, UK: Humphrey Milford, Oxford University Press.

Coley, N. G. (1969). The collateral sciences in the work of Golding Bird (1814–1854). *Medical History, 13*, 363–376.

Colwell, H. A. (1922). *An essay on the history of electrotherapy and diagnosis*. London, UK: William Heinemann.

Crookes, W. (1892). Some possibilities of electricity. *Fortnightly Review, 51*, 173–181.

Darwin, E. (1801). In *Zoonomia; or the laws of organic life: Four vols* (3rd ed.). London, UK: J. Johnson.

de la Peña, C. T. (2005). *The body electric: How strange machines built the modern American*. New York, NY: New York University Press.

Elliott, P. (2008). "More subtle than the electric aura": Georgian medical electricity, the spirit of animation and the development of Erasmus Darwin's psychophysiology. *Medical History, 52*, 195–220.

Finger, S. (2006). *Doctor Franklin's medicine*. Philadelphia, PA: University of Pennsylvania Press.

Finger, S., & Piccolino, M. (2011). *The shocking history of electric fishes: From ancient epochs to the birth of modern neurophysiology*. New York, NY: Oxford University Press.

Gilman, S. L. (2008). Electrotherapy and mental illness: Then and now. *History of Psychiatry, 19*, 339–357.

Gooday, G. (2004). *The morals of measurement: Accuracy, irony, and trust in late Victorian electrical practice*. Cambridge, UK: Cambridge University Press.

Gooday, G. (2007). Illuminating the expert–consumer relationship in domestic electricity. In A. Fyfe & B. Lightman (Eds.), *Science in the market place: Nineteenth-century sites and experiences* (pp. 231–268). Chicago, IL: Chicago University Press.

Hughes, T. (1983). *Networks of power: Electrification in western society*. Baltimore, MD: Johns Hopkins University Press.

Jones, H. L. (1904). *Medical electricity: A practical handbook for students and Practitioners* (4th ed.). London, UK: H. K. Lewis.

Killen, A. (2006). *Berlin electropolis: Shock, nerves and German modernity*. Berkeley and Los Angeles, CA: University of California Press.

Leese, P. (2001). "Why are they not cured?": British shell-shock treatment during the Great War. In M. S. Micale & P. Lerner (Eds.), *Traumatic pasts: History, psychiatry and trauma in the modern age, 1870–1930* (pp. 205–221). Cambridge, UK: Cambridge University Press.

Lerner, P. (2003). *Hysterical men: War, psychiatry and the politics of trauma in Germany, 1890–1930*. Ithaca, NY: Cornell University Press.

Linden, S. C., Jones, E., & Lees, A. J. (2013). Shell shock at Queen Square: Lewis Yealland 100 years on. *Brain, 136*, 1976–1988.

Marvin, C. (1988). *When old technologies were new*. Oxford, UK: Oxford University Press.

Medvei, V. C., & Thornton, J. L. (Eds.). (1974). *The royal hospital of Saint Bartholomew, 1123–1973*. London, UK: The Royal Hospital of Saint Bartholomew.

Morus, I. R. (1998). *Frankenstein's children: Electricity, exhibition, and experiment in early nineteenth-century London*. Princeton, NJ: Princeton University Press.

Morus, I. R. (2011). *Shocking bodies: Life, death and electricity in Victorian England*. Stroud, UK: History Press.

Mottelay, P. F. (1922). *Bibliographical history of electricity and magnetism*. London, UK: Charles Griffon.

Munro, J. (1898). *The story of electricity*. London, UK: George Newnes.

Nicholson, W. (1802). Abstract of the late experiments of Professor Aldini on galvanism. *Journal of Natural Philosophy, 3*, 298–300.

Nye, D. (1990). *Electrifying America: Social meanings of a new technology*. Cambridge, MA: MIT Press.

Porter, R. (1989). Erasmus Darwin: doctor of evolution? In J. R. Moore (Ed.), *History, humanity and evolution: Essays for John C. Greene* (pp. 39–69). Cambridge, UK: Cambridge University.

Porter, R. (1990). *Mind-forged manacles: A history of madness in England from the Restoration to the Regency*. Harmondsworth, UK: Penguin Books.

Porter, R. (1997). *The greatest benefit to mankind: A medical history of humanity from Antiquity to the present*. London, UK: Harper Collins Publishers.

Pulvermacher, I. L. (1853). *I. L. Pulvermacher's patent portable hydro-electric voltaic chain batteries*. New York, NY: C. Dinsmore & Company.

Rowbottom, M., & Susskind, C. (1984). *Electricity and medicine: History of their interaction*. San Francisco, CA: San Francisco Press.

Schiffer, M. B. (2003). *Draw the lightning down: Benjamin Franklin and electrical technology in the age of enlightenment*. Berkeley, CA: University of California Press.

Scull, A. (1993). *The most solitary of afflictions: Madness and society in Britain, 1700–1900*. New Haven, CT: Yale University Press.

Scull, A. (2007). *Madhouse: A tragic tale of megalomania and modern medicine*. New Haven, CT: Yale University Press.

Shorter, E. (1997). *A history of psychiatry: From the age of the asylum to the age of Prozac*. New York, NY: John Wiley & Sons.

Spencer, H. ([1891]1852). *The philosophy of style. Essays: Scientific, political and speculative* London, UK: Williams & Norgate, pp. 333–369.

Stainbrook, E. (1948). The use of electricity in psychiatric treatment during the nineteenth century. *Bulletin of the History of Medicine, 22*, 156–177.

Steinberg, H. (2011). Electrotherapeutic disputes: The "Frankfurt Council" of 1891. *Brain, 134*, 1229–1243.

Steinberg, H. A. (2013). A pioneer work on electric brain stimulation in psychotic patients: Rudolph Gottfried Arndt and his 1870 s studies. *Brain Stimulation, 6*, 477–481.

Thomson, J. A. (1906). *Progress of science in the century*. Edinburgh, UK: W. & R. Chambers Ltd.

Ure, A. (1819). An account of some experiments made on the body of a criminal immediately after execution with physiological and practical observations. *Quarterly Journal of Science, 6*, 283–294.

Van Bergen, L. (2009). *Before my helpless sight suffering, dying and military medicine on the Western Front, 1914–1918*. Aldershot, UK: Ashgate.

Waddington, I. (1984). *The medical profession in the Industrial Revolution*. Dublin: Gill & Macmillan.

Further Reading

Aldini, J. (1803). *An account of the galvanic experiments performed by John Aldini, Professor of Experimental Philosophy in the University of Bologna, on the Body of a Malefactor executed at Newgate, January 17, 1803*. London, UK: Cuthel Martin.

Berkwitz, N. J. (1939). Faradic shock treatment of the "functional psychoses". *The Lancet, 59*, 351–355.

Berrios, G. E. (1997). The scientific origins of electroconvulsive therapy. *History of Psychiatry*, *8*, 105–119.

Buckmaster, J. C., & Buckmaster, C. A. (1881). *The elements of magnetism and electricity* (10th ed.). London, UK: Simpkin, Marshall and Company.

Cerletti, U. (1956). Electroshock therapy. In F. Marti-Ibanez, A. M. Sackler, M. D. Sackler, & R. R. Sackler (Eds.), *The great physiodynamic therapies in psychiatry: An historical appraisal* (pp. 91–120). New York, NY: Hoeber-Harper.

Clare, A. (1980). *Psychiatry in dissent: Controversial issues in thought and practice* (2nd ed.). London, UK: Tavistock Publications, 229–277.

Currier, D. P. (2004). *Guide to electrotherapy instruments and history of their American makers.* West Conshohocken, PA: Infinity Publishing.

Eysenck, H. J. (1952). The effectiveness of psychotherapy: An evaluation. *Journal of Consulting Psychology*, *16*, 319–324.

Fink, M. (1984). The origins of convulsive therapy. *American Journal of Psychiatry, 141*, 1034–1041.

Haüy, R. J. (1807). *An elementary treatise upon natural philosophy.* (Olinthus Gregory, Trans.) London, UK: George Kearlsey..

Heilbron, J. (1999). *Electricity in the seventeenth and eighteenth centuries.* New York, NY: Dover Publications, Inc.

Milner, D. (2009). *From the rainforests of South America to the operating room: A history of curare.* Available at: http://www.med.uottawa.ca/historyofmedicine/hetenyi/milner.html.

Oliver, W. (1785). Account of the effects of *camphor* in a case of insanity. *London Medical Journal*, *6*, 120–130.

Pancaldi, G. (2003). *Volta: Science and culture in the age of enlightenment.* Princeton, NJ: Princeton University Press.

Pera, M. (1992). *The ambiguous frog: The Galvani-Volta controversy on animal electricity.* (J. Mandelbaum, Trans.) Princeton, NJ: Princeton University Press.

Rifkin, A. (2008). Review of E. Shorter and D. Healey, *Shock therapy.* (2007). *New England Journal of Medicine*, *358*, 205–206.

Rudorfer, M. V., Henry, M. E., & Sackeim, H. A. (2003). Electroconvulsive therapy. In A. Tasman, J. Kay, & J. A. Lieberman (Eds.), *Psychiatry* (pp. 1865–1901) (2nd ed.). Chichester, UK: John Wiley & Sons Ltd.

Schaffer, S. (1983). Natural philosophy and public spectacle in the eighteenth century. *History of Science*, *21*, 1–43.

Schlesinger, H. (2010). *The battery: How portable power sparked a technological revolution.* Washington, DC: Smithsonian Books.

Shorter, E., & Healy, D. (2007). *Shock therapy: A history of electroconvulsive treatment in mental illness.* New Brunswick, Canada: Rutgers University Press.

Stainbrook, E. (1946). Shock therapy: Psychologic theory and research. *Psychological Bulletin*, *43*, 21–60.

Whittaker, H., Smith, C. U. M., & Finger, S. (Eds.). (2007). *Brain, mind and medicine: Neuroscience in the 18th century.* New York, NY: Springer Science and Business Media.

Transcranial Electrical Stimulation: Transcranial Direct Current Stimulation (tDCS), Transcranial Alternating Current Stimulation (tACS), Transcranial Pulsed Current Stimulation (tPCS), and Transcranial Random Noise Stimulation (tRNS)

Ingrid Moreno-Duarte[1], Nigel Gebodh[1,2], Pedro Schestatsky[1,3], Berkan Guleyupoglu[2], Davide Reato[2], Marom Bikson[2], and Felipe Fregni[1]

[1]Laboratory of Neuromodulation, Department of Physical Medicine and Rehabilitation, Spaulding Rehabilitation Hospital and Massachusetts General Hospital, Harvard Medical School, Boston, MA, USA
[2]Department of Biomedical Engineering, The City College of the City University of New York, New York, NY, USA
[3]Programa de Pós-Graduação em Ciências Médicas da Universidade Federal do Rio Grande do Sul, Brasil; Coordenação de Aperfeiçoamento de Pessoal de Nível Superior (CAPES), Brazil

HISTORY OF TRANSCRANIAL ELECTRICAL STIMULATION (tES)

The historical origins of using transcranial electrical stimulation (tES) for therapy follow the history of the discovery of electricity itself. Though with (uncontrolled) dose bearing little resemblance to modern techniques, early attempts utilized electrosensitive animals such as the torpedo fish (*T. torpedo*), and examined the effects of electrical discharge over the scalp on headache pain reduction (Priori, 2003). With the development of man-made electric sources, studies in the 19th and early 20th centuries implemented the use of galvanic currents in the treatment of psychiatric disorders (see also Chapter 1). Electroconvulsive therapy (ECT) emerged in the 1930s (Abrams, 2002; Baghai, Lieb, & Rupprecht, 2012; Gilula & Kirsch, 2005), with the first treatment of a patient occurring in 1939 (Bini, 1995), and was shown to induce epileptogenic activity via the use of strong electrical currents. Variations of the technique continue to be used today with significant effects on psychiatric conditions but with some side effects, in particular memory loss (Gitlin, 2006; Lauber, Nordt, & Rossler, 2005; Lisanby, Kinnunen, & Crupain, 2002; Stagg & Nitsche, 2011; Uk ECT Review Group, 2003; Vitalucci, Coppola, Mirra, Maina, & Bogetto, 2013). In parallel, research using low-intensity currents continued throughout the 20th century with a recent resurgence in the investigation of weak direct and alternating currents (Nitsche & Paulus, 2000). Four main methods of low-intensity tES have been intensively investigated over the past decade: transcranial direct current stimulation (tDCS), transcranial pulsed current stimulation (tPCS), transcranial alternating current stimulation (tACS), and transcranial random noise stimulation (tRNS) (Fig. 2.1). All four techniques are considered well tolerated (where precise established protocols are followed), and operate by influencing spontaneous and sometimes non-spontaneous (if coupled with a cognitive task) neuronal activity, generating gradual changes in neural networks. Here we consider the basis, dose (Peterchev et al., 2012), methods, and applications of each of the approaches.

TRANSCRANIAL DIRECT CURRENT STIMULATION (tDCS)

tDCS uses a low-intensity (0.5–2 mA; Zaghi, Acar, Hultgren, Boggio, & Fregni, 2010) constant current (see anodal and cathodal tDCS diagrams in Fig 2.1), which is applied directly to the head, partially penetrates the skull, and enters the brain. This non-invasive method of stimulation has been shown to be a reliable method of modulating cortical excitability (Nitsche & Paulus, 2000), producing changes of up to 40% that can last for between 30 and 120 minutes (Kuo et al., 2013) after the end of stimulation (depending on the parameters used for stimulation). Computer modeling studies have shown that this type of stimulation can induce significant currents in superficial cortical areas (Datta et al., 2009; Miranda, Lomarev, & Hallett, 2006; Wagner, Valero-Cabre, & Pascual-Leone, 2007; see also Chapter 4) and influence neuronal excitability without eliciting action potentials (Bikson et al., 2004). As with other tES approaches, tDCS does pose some limitations, including limits on focality when conventional large electrodes (e.g., 5 × 7 cm) are used. Various methods to shape the outcomes of stimulation using large electrodes have been proposed (Nitsche et al., 2007), as well as approaches to focalize stimulation using smaller (e.g., 1 cm) arrays of high-definition electrodes (HD-tDCS; Bikson et al., 2004; Edwards et al., 2013). Despite the limited focality of conventional montages used in tDCS, global current flow patterns and resulting behavioral and clinical outcomes are montage specific.

Basic Principles

The parameters for dosage in tDCS take into account the amount of current delivered (in mA), the duration of the stimulation (in minutes), and the size and placement of the electrodes (see Fig. 2.1). From the electrode size and applied current, the average current density at the electrode can be

	tDCS	tACS	tPCS	tRNS
Typical electrode size (if present)	Two electrodes, 20–35 cm² each*	16 cm²*	16 cm²*	16 cm²
Typical type of current delivered	Small direct constant current at 0.5–2 mA	Bidirectional, biphasic current in sinusoidal waves. Average intensity, 0.25–1 mA; frequency, 1, 10, 15, 30, and 45 Hz; voltage, 5–15 mV	Unidirectional, monophasic current pulses in typically rectangular waves; can be bidirectional/biphasic. Average intensity, 0.6–1 mA; frequency, 1 Hz – 167 kHz	Alternate current along with random amplitude and frequency (between 0.1 and 640 Hz); intensity between −500 and +500 μA with a sampling rate of 1280 samples/s providing a current of 1 mA
Typical time for stimulation	20 min	2 and 5 min	20 min	10 min
NEUROMODEC Classification	tES technique where DC is sustained for greater than 1 minute with amplitude greater than 0.1 mA where current level does not change significantly (>5%)	tES technique where biphasic sinusoidal AC current is sustained for greater than 1 minute with amplitude greater than 0.1 mA peak-to-peak	tES technique in which current with rectangular pulses or trains of pulses, either monophasic or biphasic, is sustained for greater than 1 minute with amplitude greater than 0.1 mA peak-to-peak	tES technique in which AC is sustained for greater than 1 minute with a random and constantly changing amplitude greater than 0.1 mA RMS
Side effects	Tingling, itching, redness	Tingling, itching, redness	Tingling, itching, redness	Tingling, itching
EEG	Increased slow oscillatory activity (3 Hz)	Increased low alpha (8–12 Hz) and high theta (3–8 Hz) activity (Antal, Boros et al., 2008)	Increased slow oscillatory activity (<1 Hz) with 0.75-Hz stimulation (Marshall, Helgadottir, Molle, & Born, 2006)	No change
Cortical excitability	Increased excitability with anodal stimulation (Boros, Poreisz, Munchau, Paulus, & Nitsche, 2008; Nitsche et al., 2003) and decreased excitability with cathodal stimulation (Ardolino, Bossi, Barbieri, & Priori et al., 2005).	No change (Antal, Boros et al., 2008)	No known changes	Apparently enhances corticospinal excitability (Terney, Chaieb, Moliadze, Antal, & Paulus, 2008); although other studies do not support this finding (Fertonani, Pirulli, & Miniussi, 2011), Snowball et al. (2013) suggest modulation of cortical excitability with reduction of regional cerebral blood flow without affecting regional cerebral metabolic rate of oxygen consumption

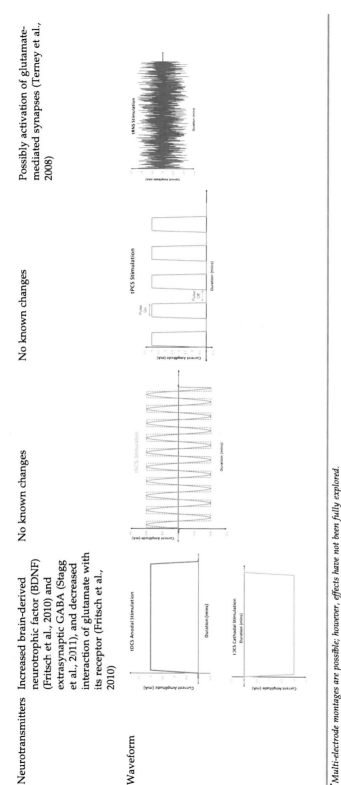

Neurotransmitters	Increased brain-derived neurotrophic factor (BDNF) (Fritsch et al., 2010) and extrasynaptic GABA (Stagg et al., 2011), and decreased interaction of glutamate with its receptor (Fritsch et al., 2010)	No known changes	No known changes	Possibly activation of glutamate-mediated synapses (Terney et al., 2008)

Waveform

Multi-electrode montages are possible; however, effects have not been fully explored.

FIGURE 2.1   Summary of non-invasive brain stimulation techniques: tDCS, tACS, tPCS, and tRNS.

calculated (the current delivered divided by the size of the electrode). The most commonly used equipment for tDCS involves two saline-soaked sponges, electrodes (typically conductive rubber), non-conductive elastic straps, cables, and a battery powered tDCS current stimulating device (DaSilva, Volz, Bikson, & Fregni, 2011). The two saline-soaked sponges are usually 20–35 cm^2 in area and contain slits into which electrodes (an anode and cathode) are placed, creating an electrode–sponge unit (Fig. 2.2).

The shape and size of the sponges is designed so that they promote a uniform distribution of current over the stimulation area, reducing the risk of skin burns caused by electricity concentrations (or "hot spots") in areas of the sponge/skin interface (Furubayashi et al., 2008; Kronberg & Bikson, 2012). These electrodes are concurrently attached to a battery-operated tDCS current stimulating device, which delivers a constant flow of weak current (up to 2 mA depending on the device) to the electrode–sponge units for a desired amount of time (Fig. 2.3).

The electrode placement on the scalp is usually derived from the International EEG 10–20 System. At least one of the electrode–sponge units is placed on the scalp, whereas the second can be placed at another cephalic location (known as a bipolar or bicepahlic montage) or extracephalic location (known as a unipolar or monocephalic montage), usually the shoulder or upper arm (Datta, Baker, Bikson, & Fridriksson, 2011). The electrode–sponge units, which are secured by non-conducting rubber elastic straps, can also be placed in configurations where the reference electrode is placed over the forehead (above the supraorbital ridge) and the active electrode is placed over the contralateral hemisphere, commonly over the motor cortex (M1) or the dorsolateral prefrontal cortex (DLPFC), depending on the design (Fig. 2.4; Nitsche & Paulus, 2000).

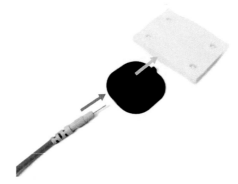

FIGURE 2.2   Electrode–sponge unit setup in tDCS. The metallic end of the cable is plugged into the carbon rubber electrode, which is then placed between the slits of the saline soaked sponge.

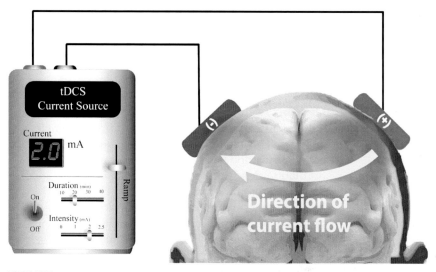

FIGURE 2.3 Parameters of current intensity (mA), duration (min) and direction of current flow in tDCS. The current delivered by the tDCS current stimulating device, enters the brain through the anode (+), passes through cortical and subcortical regions then leaves through the cathode (−).

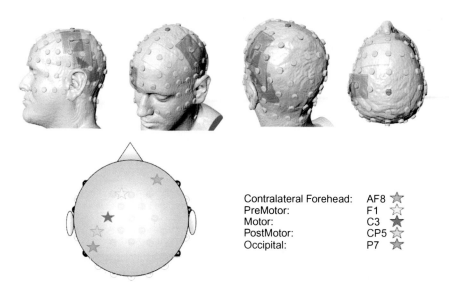

Contralateral Forehead: AF8
PreMotor: F1
Motor: C3
PostMotor: CP5
Occipital: P7

FIGURE 2.4 Common electrode placement for tDCS based on the International EEG10–20 system. The reference electrode is placed over the contralateral forehead (AF8), whereas the active electrode can be placed over the premotor (F1), motor (C3), postmotor (CP5), or occipital (P7) area.

The duration of the stimulation most often ranges between 20 and 40 minutes (Brunoni et al., 2012; Paulus, 2011).

Although some parameters of stimulation may vary, the outcomes have been strongly associated with the current density, duration of stimulation, polarity, and location of stimulation (Zaghi, Acar, Hultgren, Boggio, & Fregni, 2010). In particular, electrode polarity will influence the effects on cortical excitability. For example, for currents up to 1 mA and duration less than 20 minutes, anodal stimulation over the motor cortex increases the motor evoked potential (MEP) and results in an opposite effect when the polarity is changed to cathodal stimulation (Paulus, 2011). Importantly, changing stimulation dose, including increasing duration and/or intensity, or alterations in ongoing brain activity, can change and even invert the direction of excitability modulation (Batsikadze, Moliadze, Paulus, Kuo, & Nitsche, 2013). The amount of current that reaches neuronal tissue, though, is dependent on several uncontrollable factors, including the resistance of several cephalic structures such as skin, skull, blood vessels, and brain tissue (Brunoni et al., 2012).

Neurophysiological Mechanisms of tDCS

While the use of surface electrodes results in some shunting of current at the scalp as well as cerebrospinal fluid (CSF), a portion of current will penetrate to the brain, producing a peak electric field of approximately 0.3 V/m per 1 mA applied. While the resulting electric fields are low intensity (for comparison, TMS produces an almost 100-V/m electric field), the sustained electric field produced during tDCS will modify the transmembrane neuronal potential and can influence the level of excitability and the responsiveness to synaptic input (Rahman et al., 2013), and modulate the firing rate of individual neurons (Miranda et al., 2006; Wagner et al., 2007). tDCS-induced neuroplastic changes may be associated with modulation of neuronal ionic channels, specifically the L-type voltage gated calcium channel (L-VGCC), and N-methyl-D-aspartate (NMDA) receptors (Paulus, 2011). Mechanisms analogous to long-term potentiation (LTP) or long-term depression (LTD) have been attributed to tDCS effects on plasticity (see Chapter 5).

Importantly, since the current used in tDCS is subthreshold, it does not induce action potentials (Bikson et al., 2004); instead it modulates spontaneous neuronal activity (evoked, ongoing/endogenous activity) in a polarity-dependent fashion (Fig. 2.5). Surface anodal stimulation will typically produce inward current flow at the cortex, which is expected due to somatic depolarization of pyramidal cortical neurons and apical dendrite hyperpolarization, while surface cathodal stimulation will typically produce outward current flow at the cortex and is expected to result in somatic hyperpolarization of pyramidal cortical neurons and apical

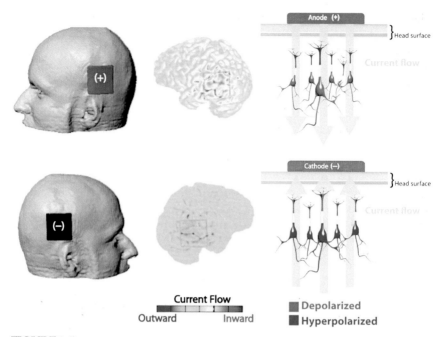

FIGURE 2.5   With tDCS, electrode polarity determines current direction of flow in the brain. The polarity also influences the cortical and sub cortical regions that are activated by the stimulation. *Upper right*: Direction of current flow through the anode (+) in tDCS. The current passes through structures, including the scalp and bone, before reaching cortical and subcortical regions. In the pyramidal cortical neurons under the anode, apical dendritic regions of the neuron become hyperpolarized (blue) whereas the somatic regions become depolarized (red). *Lower right*: Direction of current flow through the cathode (−) in tDCS. The current passes through cortical and subcortical structures, then through the bone and scalp, before reaching the cathode. In the pyramidal cortical neurons under the cathode, apical dendritic regions of the neuron become depolarized (red) whereas the somatic regions become hyperpolarized (blue).

dendrite depolarization (Radman, Ramos, Brumberg, & Bikson, 2009; Zaghi, Acar, Hultgren, Boggio, & Fregni, 2010).

Changes in brain excitability are assumed to track somatic polarization, at least at moderate stimulation intensities and durations. For example, 1-mA, 20-minute anodal tDCS applied over the motor cortex increases, whereas cathodal tDCS at the same intensities decreases, the excitability of the said region (Nitsche & Paulus, 2000; Wassermann & Grafman, 2005).

While the nominal targets of tDCS are often under the electrodes, the current flow produced using conventional tDCS spans all cortical regions between and around the electrodes and is thus not restricted to the area under the electrodes (Nitsche et al., 2004). It is therefore important to take care to distinguish between stimulating with an electrode "over" a region and specifically targeting that region. Moreover, current flow with conventional montages is expected to reach deep structures and, with extracephalic electrodes, the midbrain and spinal cord (Bikson, Datta, Rahman, & Scaturro, 2010; Brunoni et al., 2012; DaSilva et al., 2012; Keeser et al., 2011; Miranda et al., 2006; Salvador, Mekonnen, Ruffini, & Miranda, 2010; Zaghi, Acar, Hultgren, Boggio, & Fregni, 2010). This far-reaching activation is thought to be due to the stimulation of regions on alternate neural networks (Nitsche et al., 2005). In fact, tDCS has been found to modulate resting-state functional connectivity after prefrontal stimulation (Keeser et al., 2011). However, as noted above, the diffuse nature of current flow does not mean that (even small) changes in montage can change the *pattern* of current flow leading to significant changes in specific outcome measures (Nitsche & Paulus, 2000; Mendonca et al., 2011).In addition, tDCS may be "functionally" focalized by timing stimu-lation with specific tasks (Cano, Morales-Quezada, Bikson, & Fregni, 2013, Cohen Kadosh, Soskic, Iuculano, Kanai, & Walsh, 2010).

Clinical Applications of tDCS

Due to the pronounced neuromodulatory effects of tDCS, specifically its effects on modulating rate of learning, tDCS has been tested with sev-eral neuropsychiatric disorders (see Table 2.1). For instance, tDCS has been used for motor learning enhancement in stroke rehabilitation (Schlaug, Renga, & Nair, 2008), for behavioral performance enhancement with Alzheimer's patients (Boggio, Khoury et al., 2009; Ferrucci et al., 2008; see also Chapter 13), for modulation of emotional affective neural circuits in depression patients (Boggio, Zaghi, & Fregni, 2009; Bueno et al., 2011; Kalu, Sexton, Loo, & Ebmeier, 2012; Loo et al., 2012; see also Chapter 14), and for patients with chronic pain (Boggio, Zaghi, Lopes, & Fregni, 2008; Fenton, Palmieri, Boggio, Fanning, & Fregni, 2009; Fregni, Marcondes, Boggio, Marcolin, Rigonatti et al., 2006; Gabis et al., 2009; Zaghi, Thiele, Pimentel, Pimentel, & Fregni, 2011). In stroke neurorehabilitation, tDCS has shown benefits when used together with other interventions such as rehabilitatory training, in primates (Plautz et al., 2003; see Chapter 12) or occupational therapy in humans (Nair, Renga, Lindenberg, Zhu, & Schlaug, 2011). In terms of pain, tDCS has been applied to cases of chronic pain refractory to pharmacologic interventions (Lefaucheur et al., 2008; Nizard, Lefaucheur, Helbert, de Chauvigny, & Nguyen, 2012) and for a number of different pain conditions such as fibro-myalgia, pelvic pain, and neuropathic pain (DaSilva et al., 2012; Fenton et al., 2009; Fregni, Boggio, Santos, Lima, Vieira et al., 2006). Some studies have also examined the effects of anodal tDCS on learning in healthy sub-jects, showing improvement in implicit learning (Kincses, Antal, Nitsche, Bartfai, & Paulus, 2004), motor memory (Galea & Celnik, 2009), working memory (Mulquiney, Hoy, Daskalakis, & Fitzgerald, 2011; Ohn et al.,

TABLE 2.1   Examples of tDCS Electrode Montages in Different Clinical Conditions

Disease	Authors	Anode	Cathode
Depression	Boggio, Bermpohl et al., 2007; Boggio, Rigonatti et al., 2008; Loo et al., 2012	DLPFC	Supraorbital
Stroke	Lindenberg, Renga, Zhu, Nair, & Schlaug, 2010	M1	Contralateral M1
	Boggio, Nunes et al., 2007	M1 (affected side)	Supraorbital
		Supraorbital	M1 (non-affected side)
Tinnitus	Fregni, Gimenes, Valle, Ferreira, Rocha et al., 2006	LTA	Supraorbital
Parkinson	Benninger et al., 2010	M1/DLPFC	Mastoid
	Fregni, Boggio, Nitsche, Marcolin, Rigonatti et al., 2006; Fregni, Boggio, Nitsche, Rigonatti, & Pascual-Leone, 2006; Fregni, Boggio, Santos, Lima, Vieira et al., 2006; Boggio et al., 2006	M1	Supraorbital
Migraine	Antal, Kincses, Nitsche, & Paulus, 2003; Antal, Lang et al., 2008; Antal, Kriener, Lang, Boros, & Paulus, 2011; Chadaide et al., 2007; Antal et al., 2011	V1	Oz
Alcohol abuse	Boggio, Sultani et al., 2008	R/L – DLPFC	L/R – DLPFC

LTA, left temporoparietal area; V1, visual cortex; DLPFC, dorsolateral prefrontal cortex; M1, motor cortex; R, right; L, left; Oz, occipital lobe at midline (EEG 10/20 system).

2008), and memory retrieval (Boggio, Nunes et al., 2007; Boggio, Fregni et al., 2009; Chi, Fregni, & Snyder, 2010; see also Chapter 9).

Although the majority of the preliminary clinical results show positive outcomes, it should be noted that in most cases stimulation parameters were varied across clinical studies. It should also be noted that these studies contained small sample sizes with relatively homogeneous populations, and used mostly surrogate outcomes.

The field of tDCS is, however, ever advancing, with a new method of tDCS having been recently developed. This method, known as "high definition" tDCS (HD-tDCS), utilizes an array of smaller electrodes (Fig. 2.6). The position and current at each electrode can be optimized for intensity or targeting (Dmochowski, Datta, Bikson, Su, & Parra, 2011). One HD-tDCS, the "4 × 1 ring" electrode montage, has been shown to be a more focused method of stimulation compared to conventional tDCS (Fig. 2.7; Datta et al., 2009; Edwards et al., 2013). Though relatively few

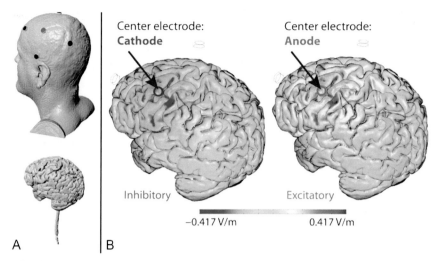

FIGURE 2.6   HD-tDCS setup and current penetration. (A) One center electrode (red) is placed over the area of stimulation and four return electrodes (black) are placed around it. The radius of the ring around the center electrode determines the modulation of the area of interest. (B) An inhibitory effect is achieved with the center electrode as a cathode, whereas an excitatory effect is achieved with the center electrode as an anode.

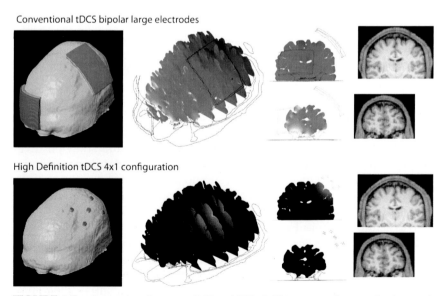

FIGURE 2.7   Comparison between tDCS and HD-tDCS in terms of set-up, focality, and depth of current penetration. tDCS is shown to activate the region of interest as well as other cortical and subcortical areas, whereas HD-tDCS focuses the stimulation to the cortical region of the area of stimulation.

HD-tDCS studies have been published as of yet, 4 × 1 HD-tDCS has been shown to be a reliable method of targeting specific cortical areas, can produce plasticity changes that may outlast conventional tDCS (Kuo et al., 2013), and has even been shown to reduce the perception on pain in fibromyalgia patients (Villamar, Volz et al., 2013; Villamar, Wivatvongvana et al., 2013) and in experimental pain (Borckardt et al., 2012). In the coming decades we can expect the field of tDCS to see advancements in areas like methods of deeper current penetration, more specific cortical targeting, more specific patient dosage parameters, and a larger shift of the use of tDCS in clinical environments.

TRANSCRANIAL ALTERNATING CURRENT STIMULATION (tACS)

Basic Principles

Broadly, alternating current (AC) stimulation is a method of delivering a non-constant current to the brain. This method of stimulation is accomplished by using pulses of current in either rectangular waves (the intensity reaches a certain amplitude, is held at that amplitude for a short duration of time, is then interrupted by zero current, the polarity of the current changes, and the process repeats) or sinusoidal waves (Zaghi, Acar, Hultgren, Boggio, & Fregni, 2010). For a recent review of the cellular mechanisms of tACS, see Reato, Rahman, Bikson, and Parra (2013). Briefly, as for DC (Bikson et al., 2004), AC stimulation alters the transmembrane potential of single neurons, with maximal effects when currents are directed along the somatodendritic axis. The polarization profile tracks the applied current – so, for example, sinusoidal stimulation leads to a sinusoidal fluctuation of the membrane potential. The polarization is linearly proportional to the current applied but is also frequency-dependent (Deans et al., 2007; Reato, Rahman, Bikson, & Parra, 2010). Therefore, AC stimulation at low frequencies induces bigger polarizations than stimulation at high frequencies.

Stimulation with alternating current is used in deep brain stimulation, motor cortex stimulation, spinal cord stimulation, transcutaneous nerve stimulation, vagal nerve stimulation, transcranial magnetic stimulation, and electroconvulsive therapy. Among the variety of methods of low-intensity non-invasive AC stimulation in this chapter we will focus on tACS, which typically consists of biphasic sine waves (Fig. 2.1), albeit other methods with established clinical effects, including cranial electrotherapy stimulation (CES), transcutaneous electrical stimulation (TCES) with Limoge's current, and transcranial electrical stimulation (tES) with Lebedev's current, exist.

Transcranial Alternating Current Stimulation (tACS)

Low-intensity AC methods use different electrode montages and current characteristics. The use of alternating currents with a similar montage as that used in tDCS is known as transcranial alternating current stimulation (tACS; Antal, Boros et al., 2008) (see tACS diagram in Fig. 2.1). Antal, Boros et al. (2008) applied tACS for 2 and 5 minutes, with a current intensity of 0.25–0.40 mA using a 16-cm^2 electrode (current density = 25 μA/cm^2) at several frequencies (1, 10, 15, 30, and 45 Hz). The study claimed not to have an effect on cortical excitability, as assessed by MEPs and electroencephalogram power; however, it did show that 5 minutes of tACS at 10 Hz applied at the motor cortex was related to improvement in implicit motor learning while other studies have claimed effects on cortical excitability, as mentioned in the next section, using higher frequencies. Moreover, Kanai, Chaieb, Antal, Walsh, and Paulus (2008) applied tACS to the visual cortex at 5–30 Hz and 250 μA to 1000 μA to assess the visual phosphene threshold. The study showed the influence of tACS on inducing phosphenes at 20 Hz (beta frequency range) when applied in an illuminated room, and 10 Hz (alpha frequency range) in darkness. These studies suggest that the effects seen as a result of this type of stimulation are dependent on the intensity of the current, and the frequencies and duration of the stimulation. However, the direction of the effect (either increasing or decreasing cortical excitability) is not clear yet. Note, however, that a later study has attributed Kanai et al.'s results to retinal rather than cortical effects (Schutter & Hortensius, 2010). Recent studies also extended the usage of tACS to the high-level cognitive domain (e.g., Santarnecchi et al., 2013; see also Chapter 11).

Proposed Mechanisms of Action in AC Stimulation with Weak Electric Current

Changes in Cortical Excitability

Several studies performed with tACS have used a variety of current intensities and frequencies, showing contradictory results on cortical excitability. Using a current density of 25 μA/cm^2 at 1, 10, 15, 30, and 45 Hz for 5 minutes, Antal, Boros et al. (2008) showed that AC stimulation did not result in significant changes to cortical excitability as measured by TMS evoked motor potentials. Another study, by Zaghi, de Freitas Rezende et al. (2010), showed differing results. The latter authors tested tACS with a lower current density (0.08 μA/cm^2) at a frequency of 15 Hz and for a longer duration (20 minutes) than previously used (i.e., around 0.16–0.25 mA/m^2 for current and 2–5 minutes for timing) (Antal, Boros et al., 2008). With the aforementioned parameters of stimulation, Zaghi et al.

found a decrease in MEPs and intracortical facilitation, reflecting a change in the cortical excitability. Alternatively, Chaieb, Antal, and Paulus (2011) used high frequencies (1, 2, and 5 kHz) for 10 minutes at 1 mA (current density 20.8 μA/cm^2) and found increased amplitude in the MEPs at all frequencies compared to baseline, suggesting that high frequencies might be associated with increased excitability of the motor cortex. Regarding the intensity of the current, Moliadze, Atalay, Antal, and Paulus (2012) showed that 1 mA is associated with increased cortical excitability, while lower intensities close to 0.4 mA promote a switch to inhibition. All these studies found different results, suggesting that changes in the cortical excitability due to AC stimulation are frequency and intensity specific.

Changes in Brain Electrical Activity

Electroencephalography (EEG) changes during cranial stimulation with low-intensity AC have been seen. An early EEG study found that one 30-minute session of cranial AC stimulation daily for 5 days increased the amplitude of slower EEG frequencies with increased alpha wave (8–12 Hz) activity (McKenzie, Rosenthal, & Driessner, 1971). In contrast, Schroeder and Barr (2001) compared EEG activity in sham and active CES (at frequencies of 0.5 and 100 Hz), showing a decrease of the alpha band median frequency and beta band power fraction in the active group. As for tACS, Zaehle, Rach, and Herrmann (2010) performed a study investigating tACS over the occipital cortex while measuring alpha activity on EEG. They found that tACS increased alpha activity, which could be potentially useful for treating patients with cognitive dysfunction due to the modulatory effects of tACS seen in this and previous studies. The effects observed in the EEG recordings provide initial mechanistic data to explain tACS results, in particular presenting additional evidence of the frequency and intensity-specific effect of this technique; however, further studies are needed to clarify the cellular mechanisms of this intervention.

Biochemical Changes

There is evidence that AC stimulation is associated with changes in neurotransmitters such as urinary free catecholamines, 17-ketosteroids (Briones & Rosenthal, 1973), and endorphin release. A study by Kirsch and Smith (2004), analyzed presynaptic membranes before, during, and after cranial AC stimulation in monkeys. They showed a reduction in the number of vesicles at the beginning of stimulation, then an increase after 5 minutes, and finally a regression to normal shortly after the end of stimulation. These changes were believed be related to serotonin-releasing raphe nuclei, norepinephrine-releasing locus ceruleus, or the cholinergic laterodorsal tegmental and pediculo-pontine nuclei of the brainstem (Giordano, 2006; Kirsch, 2002). Plasmatic and CSF levels of endorphins have been found to increase during cranial AC stimulation

(Limoge, Robert, & Stanley, 1999). In fact, there are reports on naloxone antagonizing the analgesic effects of stimulation, which might account for its effects on endorphins (Limoge et al., 1999). Although some controversy exists regarding the findings of such studies, they do suggest that there might be an association between cranial AC stimulation and neurotransmitter release (Zaghi, Acar, Hultgren, Boggio, & Fregni, 2010).

Basic Principles

Pulsed current stimulation is a non-invasive brain stimulation technique that uses repeated bursts or pulses of current to induce changes over cortical and subcortical brain structures (see tPCS diagram in Fig. 2.1; Datta, Dmochowski, Guleyupoglu, Bikson, & Fregni, 2012). Much like tDCS, it is possible to use many different electrode placements on the head as well as high-definition electrodes to make it more focal. The introduction of pulses, rather than sine waves as traditionally used in tACS, in stimulation allows for different waveforms to be used for optimized dosage considerations. CES is the most common form of modern pulsed current stimulation, and involves the application of current to infra- or supra-auricular structures such as the ear lobes, mastoid processes, zygomatic arches, or maxillo-occipital junction (Ferdjallah, Bostick, & Barr, 1996). Current is usually applied through saline-soaked clips or pads.

Modeling studies predict that, for common CES montages, intensities between 0.2–0.6 V/m are produced in cortical and subcortical structures (Datta et al., 2012; Guleyupoglu, Schestatsky, Edwards, Fregni, & Bikson, 2013). These intensities are near the limit of those established to modulate the waveform of active neuronal networks (Deans, Powell, & Jefferys, 2007; Francis, Gluckman, & Schiff, 2003; Reato, Gasca et al., 2013). As such, the term CES (with "transcranial") may suggest the possibility of actions through stimulation of peripheral nerves (Zaghi, Acar, Hultgren, Boggio, & Fregni, 2010). Thus, CES can also be considered a form of peripheral nerve stimulation due to the electrode locations. Studies with CES have used variable parameters of stimulation, including duration, current density, intensity, and electrode size for the treatment of anxiety, depression, stress, and insomnia (Kirsch & Smith, 2004; Smith, 2007). These studies have shown differing results that could be due to variation in the parameters of stimulation, which include frequency ranges of 0.5–167 kHz, intensities of 0.1–4 mA, and durations ranging from 5 minutes to 6 consecutive days.

Other Methods of Pulsed Current Stimulation

Limoge's current (or "transcutaneous electrical stimulation," TCES; Guleyupoglu et al., 2013) applies a current transmitted over three cutaneous electrodes: one negative (cathode), which is placed between the eyebrows, and two positive (anodes), which are placed in the mastoid regions. Stimulation carries a voltage ranging from 30 to 35 V, an average intensity of 2 mA, and a frequency of 166 kHz with 4 ms ON and 8 ms OFF (Guleyupoglu et al., 2013; Zaghi, Acar, Hultgren, Boggio, & Fregni, 2010). The waveform of this type of stimulation includes trains of successive impulse waves of a particular shape: one positive impulse (S1) of high intensity and short duration, followed by a negative impulse (S2) of weak intensity and long duration (Zaghi, Acar, Hultgren, Boggio, & Fregni, 2010). This form of transcranial stimulation has been suggested to decrease the amount of narcotics required to maintain anesthesia during surgical procedures (Limoge, 1999).

Lebedev used Limoge's electrode positions, but combined AC and DC current at a 2:1 ratio. First, a pulse train of AC is delivered at a frequency of 77.5 Hz for 3.5–4.0 ms and then is separated from the next train by 8 ms. Two trains of AC stimulation are then followed by 4 ms of constant DC (Zaghi, Acar, Hultgren, Boggio, & Fregni, 2010). Lebedev's current has been suggested to be effective for the treatment of stress and affective disturbances (Lebedev et al., 2002).

TRANSCRANIAL RANDOM NOISE STIMULATION (tRNS)

Transcranial random noise stimulation (tRNS) has not been extensively investigated, but preliminary results are encouraging. Terney et al. (2008) were among the first to recently revisit the use of this technique. They showed that by using an alternate current along with random amplitude and frequency (between 0.1 and 640 Hz; see tRNS diagram in Fig. 2.1) on healthy subjects, the motor cortex excitability increased significantly, but this effect was limited to high frequencies. The effects lasted for approximately 60 minutes after 10 minutes of stimulation. The physiological mechanisms underlying the effects of tRNS are not well known, but it is suspected that they may be due to the repeated opening of sodium channels (Paulus, 2011) or to the increased sensitivity of neuronal networks to modulation (Francis et al., 2003). The technique includes all the frequencies up to half of the sampling rate (1280 samples/s) – i.e., 640 Hz (Moliadze, Antal, & Paulus, 2010). Compared to tDCS it has the advantage of being more comfortable (Moliadze et al., 2010), which makes it potentially advantageous for setting and blinding studies (Ambrus, Paulus, & Antal, 2010). Studies with fMRI have shown a reduction of the blood oxygen level dependence (BOLD) after the use of tRNS, relating the change in blood flow to the energy used by brain cells (Chaieb et al., 2009). The same authors also studied the effect of tRNS at frequencies of 100–640 Hz and with decreasing duration of the stimulation (4, 5, and 6 minutes) on motor cortical excitability (Chaieb, Paulus, & Antal, 2011). They found significant increased facilitation at 5 and 6 minutes and none at 4 minutes, suggesting that a minimal duration of 5 minutes is necessary to observe an effect. Mulquiney et al. (2011) used tRNS in the dorsolateral prefrontal cortex to assess its effects on working memory. They used a randomly alternating level of current of between -500 and $+500\,\mu A$ with a sampling rate of 1280 samples/s and high range frequencies (101–640 Hz), providing a current of 1 mA. This study did not find any significant changes in working memory with the use of tRNS. Fertonani et al. (2011) tested the role of high- and low-frequency tRNS on perceptual learning compared to anodal and cathodal tDCS. The parameters used for tRNS were a duration of approximately 4 minutes in five experimental blocks (22 minutes total), with a current of 1.5 mA and frequencies in the low (0.1–100 Hz) and high range (100–640 Hz). The study concluded that high-frequency tRNS subjects showed better accuracy on the perceptual task compared with the other groups. Low-frequency tRNS subjects did not show any difference compared to sham or high-frequency tRNS, which supports the consideration that this stimulation might be useful in the high-frequency range. However, the optimal parameters of stimulation for tRNS as well as the potential clinical effects of this technique remain unclear. tRNS has been coupled with near-infrared spectroscopy to evaluate the hemodynamic changes in the prefrontal cortex. Snowball et al. (2013) reported an improvement on calculation- and memory-recall based arithmetic learning with tRNS that was associated with hemodynamic responses suggesting an efficient neurovascular coupling on the dorsolateral prefrontal cortex. These changes were maintained up to 6 months after the stimulation, implying that the neuromodulatory effects are seen over the long-term.

CONCLUSION

Interest in neuromodulatory interventions has increased in recent decades, as it is considered a promising tool for the management of numerous conditions that range from psychiatric diseases to chronic pain. Studies on non-invasive brain stimulation with weak electrical currents have shown potential benefits by the induction of changes in cortical excitability and, consequently, in neuroplasticity. The effects catalyzed by these techniques seem to depend on the parameters of the stimulation, including intensity, duration, and frequency, which explains the variability of the results. While there is an increased understanding of the mechanisms of tDCS, the mechanisms that underline other methods described here are poorly understood. Therefore, more research is needed, which will lead to a better understanding of the neurophysiological effects and mechanisms of transcranial stimulation (see also Chapters 4–6), and the suitability of each method to enhance the human brain, as indicated by the various chapters in this book.

References

Abrams, R. (2002). *Electroconvulsive therapy* (4th ed.). New York, NY: Oxford University Press.

Ambrus, G. G., Paulus, W., & Antal, A. (2010). Cutaneous perception thresholds of electrical stimulation methods: Comparison of tDCS and tRNS. *Clinical Neurophysiology, 121*(11), 1908–1914.

Antal, A., Boros, K., Poreisz, C., Chaieb, L., Terney, D., & Paulus, W. (2008). Comparatively weak after-effects of transcranial alternating current stimulation (tACS) on cortical excitability in humans. *Brain Stimulation, 1*(2), 97–105.

Antal, A., Kincses, T. Z., Nitsche, M. A., & Paulus, W. (2003). Manipulation of phosphene thresholds by transcranial direct current stimulation in man. *Experimental Brain Research, 150*(3), 375–378.

Antal, A., Kriener, N., Lang, N., Boros, K., & Paulus, W. (2011). Cathodal transcranial direct current stimulation of the visual cortex in the prophylactic treatment of migraine. *Cephalalgia, 31*(7), 820–828.

Antal, A., Lang, N., Boros, K., Nitsche, M., Siebner, H. R., & Paulus, W. (2008). Homeostatic metaplasticity of the motor cortex is altered during headache-free intervals in migraine with aura. *Cerebral Cortex, 18*(11), 2701–2705.

Ardolino, G., Bossi, B., Barbieri, S., & Priori, A. (2005). Non-synaptic mechanisms underlie the after-effects of cathodal transcutaneous direct current stimulation of the human brain. *The Journal of Physiology, 568*(Pt 2), 653–663.

Baghai, T. C., Lieb, M., & Rupprecht, R. (2012). Electroconvulsive therapy - Indications and practical use for pharmacotherapy resistant depressive disorders [Elektrokonvulsionstherapie – Indikationsstellung und Durchfuhrung bei pharmakotherapieresistenten psychiatrischen Erkrankungen]. *Fortschritte Der Neurologie-Psychiatrie, 80*(12), 720–731.

Batsikadze, G., Moliadze, V., Paulus, W., Kuo, M. F., & Nitsche, M. A. (2013). Partially non-linear stimulation intensity-dependent effects of direct current stimulation on motor cortex excitability in humans. *The Journal of Physiology, 591*(Pt 7), 1987–2000.

Benninger, D. H., Lomarev, M., Lopez, G., Wassermann, E. M., Li, X., Considine, E., et al. (2010). Transcranial direct current stimulation for the treatment of Parkinson's disease. *Journal of Neurology, Neurosurgery, and Psychiatry, 81*(10), 1105–1111.

Bikson, M., Datta, A., Rahman, A., & Scaturro, J. (2010). Electrode montages for tDCS and weak transcranial electrical stimulation: Role of "return" electrodes' position and size. *Clinical Neurophysiology, 121*(12), 1976–1978.

Bikson, M., Inoue, M., Akiyama, H., Deans, J. K., Fox, J. E., Miyakawa, H., et al. (2004). Effects of uniform extracellular DC electric fields on excitability in rat hippocampal slices *in vitro*. *The Journal of Physiology, 557*(Pt 1), 175–190.

Bini, L. (1995). Professor bini's notes on the first electro-shock experiment. *Convulsive Therapy, 11*(4), 260–261.

Boggio, P. S., Bermpohl, F., Vergara, A. O., Muniz, A. L., Nahas, F. H., Leme, P. B., et al. (2007). Go-no-go task performance improvement after anodal transcranial DC stimulation of the left dorsolateral prefrontal cortex in major depression. *Journal of Affective Disorders, 101* (1–3), 91–98.

Boggio, P. S., Ferrucci, R., Rigonatti, S. P., Covre, P., Nitsche, M., Pascual-Leone, A., et al. (2006). Effects of transcranial direct current stimulation on working memory in patients with Parkinson's disease. *Journal of the Neurological Sciences, 249*(1), 31–38.

Boggio, P. S., Fregni, F., Valasek, C., Ellwood, S., Chi, R., Gallate, J., et al. (2009). Temporal lobe cortical electrical stimulation during the encoding and retrieval phase reduces false memories. *PloS One, 4*(3), e4959.

Boggio, P. S., Khoury, L. P., Martins, D. C., Martins, O. E., de Macedo, E. C., & Fregni, F. (2009). Temporal cortex direct current stimulation enhances performance on a visual recognition memory task in Alzheimer disease. *Journal of Neurology, Neurosurgery, and Psychiatry, 80*(4), 444–447.

Boggio, P. S., Nunes, A., Rigonatti, S. P., Nitsche, M. A., Pascual-Leone, A., & Fregni, F. (2007). Repeated sessions of noninvasive brain DC stimulation is associated with motor function improvement in stroke patients. *Restorative Neurology and Neuroscience*, 25(2), 123–129.

Boggio, P. S., Rigonatti, S. P., Ribeiro, R. B., Myczkowski, M. L., Nitsche, M. A., Pascual-Leone, A., et al. (2008). A randomized, double-blind clinical trial on the efficacy of cortical direct current stimulation for the treatment of major depression. *The International Journal of Neuropsychopharmacology*, 11(2), 249–254.

Boggio, P. S., Sultani, N., Fecteau, S., Merabet, L., Mecca, T., Pascual-Leone, A., et al. (2008). Prefrontal cortex modulation using transcranial DC stimulation reduces alcohol craving: A double-blind, sham-controlled study. *Drug and Alcohol Dependence*, 92(1–3), 55–60.

Boggio, P. S., Zaghi, S., & Fregni, F. (2009). Modulation of emotions associated with images of human pain using anodal transcranial direct current stimulation (tDCS). *Neuropsychologia*, 47(1), 212–217.

Boggio, P. S., Zaghi, S., Lopes, M., & Fregni, F. (2008). Modulatory effects of anodal transcranial direct current stimulation on perception and pain thresholds in healthy volunteers. *European Journal of Neurology*, 15(10), 1124–1130.

Borckardt, J. J., Bikson, M., Frohman, H., Reeves, S. T., Datta, A., Bansal, V., et al. (2012). A pilot study of the tolerability and effects of high-definition transcranial direct current stimulation (HD-tDCS) on pain perception. *The Journal of Pain*, 13(2), 112–120.

Boros, K., Poreisz, C., Munchau, A., Paulus, W., & Nitsche, M. A. (2008). Premotor transcranial direct current stimulation (tDCS) affects primary motor excitability in humans. *The European Journal of Neuroscience*, 27(5), 1292–1300.

Briones, D. F., & Rosenthal, S. H. (1973). Changes in urinary free catecholamines and 17-ketosteroids with cerebral electrotherapy (electrosleep). *Diseases of the Nervous System*, 34(1), 57–58.

Brunoni, A. R., Nitsche, M. A., Bolognini, N., Bikson, M., Wagner, T., Merabet, L., et al. (2012). Clinical research with transcranial direct current stimulation (tDCS): Challenges and future directions. *Brain Stimulation*, 5(3), 175–195.

Bueno, V. F., Brunoni, A. R., Boggio, P. S., Bensenor, I. M., & Fregni, F. (2011). Mood and cognitive effects of transcranial direct current stimulation in post-stroke depression. *Neurocase*, 17(4), 318–322.

Cano, T., Morales-Quezada, J. L., Bikson, M., & Fregni, F. (2013). Methods to focalize non-invasive electrical brain stimulation: Principles and future clinical development for the treatment of pain. *Expert Review of Neurotherapeutics*, 13(5), 465–467.

Chadaide, Z., Arlt, S., Antal, A., Nitsche, M. A., Lang, N., & Paulus, W. (2007). Transcranial direct current stimulation reveals inhibitory deficiency in migraine. *Cephalalgia*, 27(7), 833–839.

Chaieb, L., Antal, A., & Paulus, W. (2011). Transcranial alternating current stimulation in the low kHz range increases motor cortex excitability. *Restorative Neurology and Neuroscience*, 29(3), 167–175.

Chaieb, L., Kovacs, G., Cziraki, C., Greenlee, M., Paulus, W., & Antal, A. (2009). Short-duration transcranial random noise stimulation induces blood oxygenation level dependent response attenuation in the human motor cortex. *Experimental Brain Research Experimentelle Hirnforschung Experimentation Cerebrale*, 198(4), 439–444.

Chaieb, L., Paulus, W., & Antal, A. (2011). Evaluating after effects of short-duration transcranial random noise stimulation on cortical excitability. *Neural Plasticity*, 2011, 105927.

Chi, R. P., Fregni, F., & Snyder, A. W. (2010). Visual memory improved by non-invasive brain stimulation. *Brain Research*, 1353, 168–175.

Cohen Kadosh, R., Soskic, S., Iuculano, T., Kanai, R., & Walsh, V. (2010). Modulating neuronal activity produces specific and long-lasting changes in numerical competence. *Current Biology: CB*, 20(22), 2016–2020.

DaSilva, A. F., Mendonca, M. E., Zaghi, S., Lopes, M., Dossantos, M. F., Spierings, E. L., et al. (2012). tDCS-induced analgesia and electrical fields in pain-related neural networks in chronic migraine. *Headache*, 52(8), 1283–1295.

DaSilva, A. F., Volz, M. S., Bikson, M., & Fregni, F. (2011). Electrode positioning and montage in transcranial direct current stimulation. *Journal of Visualized Experiments: JoVE*, (51), pii, 2744. doi:10.3791/2744.

Datta, A., Baker, J. M., Bikson, M., & Fridriksson, J. (2011). Individualized model predicts brain current flow during transcranial direct-current stimulation treatment in responsive stroke patient. *Brain Stimulation*, 4(3), 169–174.

Datta, A., Bansal, V., Diaz, J., Patel, J., Reato, D., & Bikson, M. (2009). Gyri-precise head model of transcranial direct current stimulation: Improved spatial focality using a ring electrode versus conventional rectangular pad. *Brain Stimulation*, 2(4), 201–207, 207.e1.

Datta, A., Dmochowski, J. P., Guleyupoglu, B., Bikson, M., & Fregni, F. (2012). Cranial electrotherapy stimulation and transcranial pulsed current stimulation: A computer based high-resolution modeling study. *NeuroImage*, 65C, 280–287.

Deans, J. K., Powell, A. D., & Jefferys, J. G. (2007). Sensitivity of coherent oscillations in rat hippocampus to AC electric fields. *The Journal of Physiology*, 583(Pt 2), 555–565.

Dmochowski, J. P., Datta, A., Bikson, M., Su, Y., & Parra, L. C. (2011). Optimized multi-electrode stimulation increases focality and intensity at target. *Journal of Neural Engineering*, 8(4), 046011.

Edwards, D., Cortes, M., Datta, A., Minhas, P., Wassermann, E. M., & Bikson, M. (2013). Physiological and modeling evidence for focal transcranial electrical brain stimulation in humans: A basis for high-definition tDCS. *NeuroImage*, 74, 266–275.

Fenton, B. W., Palmieri, P. A., Boggio, P., Fanning, J., & Fregni, F. (2009). A preliminary study of transcranial direct current stimulation for the treatment of refractory chronic pelvic pain. *Brain Stimulation*, 2(2), 103–107.

Ferdjallah, M., Bostick, F. X., Jr., & Barr, R. E. (1996). Potential and current density distributions of cranial electrotherapy stimulation (CES) in a four-concentric-spheres model. *IEEE Transactions on Bio-Medical Engineering*, 43(9), 939–943.

Ferrucci, R., Mameli, F., Guidi, I., Mrakic-Sposta, S., Vergari, M., Marceglia, S., et al. (2008). Transcranial direct current stimulation improves recognition memory in alzheimer disease. *Neurology*, 71(7), 493–498.

Fertonani, A., Pirulli, C., & Miniussi, C. (2011). Random noise stimulation improves neuroplasticity in perceptual learning. *The Journal of Neuroscience*, 31(43), 15416–15423.

Francis, J. T., Gluckman, B. J., & Schiff, S. J. (2003). Sensitivity of neurons to weak electric fields. *The Journal of Neuroscience*, 23(19), 7255–7261.

Fregni, F., Boggio, P. S., Nitsche, M. A., Marcolin, M. A., Rigonatti, S. P., & Pascual-Leone, A. (2006). Treatment of major depression with transcranial direct current stimulation. *Bipolar Disorders*, 8(2), 203–204.

Fregni, F., Boggio, P. S., Nitsche, M. A., Rigonatti, S. P., & Pascual-Leone, A. (2006). Cognitive effects of repeated sessions of transcranial direct current stimulation in patients with depression. *Depression and Anxiety*, 23(8), 482–484.

Fregni, F., Boggio, P. S., Santos, M. C., Lima, M., Vieira, A. L., Rigonatti, S. P., et al. (2006). Noninvasive cortical stimulation with transcranial direct current stimulation in parkinson.s disease. *Movement Disorders*, 21(10), 1693–1702.

Fregni, F., Gimenes, R., Valle, A. C., Ferreira, M. J., Rocha, R. R., Natalle, L., et al. (2006). A randomized, sham-controlled, proof of principle study of transcranial direct current stimulation for the treatment of pain in fibromyalgia. *Arthritis and Rheumatism*, 54(12), 3988–3998.

Fregni, F., Marcondes, R., Boggio, P. S., Marcolin, M. A., Rigonatti, S. P., Sanchez, T. G., et al. (2006). Transient tinnitus suppression induced by repetitive transcranial magnetic stimulation and transcranial direct current stimulation. *European Journal of Neurology*, 13(9), 996–1001.

Fritsch, B., Reis, J., Martinowich, K., Schambra, H. M., Ji, Y., Cohen, L. G., et al. (2010). Direct current stimulation promotes BDNF-dependent synaptic plasticity: Potential implications for motor learning. *Neuron, 66*(2), 198–204.

Furubayashi, T., Terao, Y., Arai, N., Okabe, S., Mochizuki, H., Hanajima, R., et al. (2008). Short and long duration transcranial direct current stimulation (tDCS) over the human hand motor area. *Experimental Brain Research Experimentelle Hirnforschung Experimentation Cerebrale, 185*(2), 279–286.

Gabis, L., Shklar, B., Baruch, Y. K., Raz, R., Gabis, E., & Geva, D. (2009). Pain reduction using transcranial electrostimulation: A double blind "active placebo" controlled trial. *Journal of Rehabilitation Medicine, 41*(4), 256–261.

Galea, J. M., & Celnik, P. (2009). Brain polarization enhances the formation and retention of motor memories. *Journal of Neurophysiology, 102*(1), 294–301.

Gilula, M. F., & Kirsch, D. L. (2005). Cranial electrotherapy stimulation review: A safer alternative to psychopharmaceuticals in the treatment of depression. *Journal of Neurotherapy, 9*(2), 7–26.

Giordano, J. (2006). *How Alpha-Stim. Cranial electrotherapy stimulation (CES) works* (Internet). Mineral Wells, TX: Electromedical Products International, Inc. [cited 2009 May 5]. Available at, http://www.alpha-stim.com/repository/assets/pdf/howasworks.pdf.

Gitlin, M. (2006). Treatment-resistant bipolar disorder. *Molecular Psychiatry, 11*(3), 227–240.

Guleyupoglu, B., Schestatsky, P., Edwards, D., Fregni, F., & Bikson, M. (2013). Classification of methods in transcranial electrical stimulation (tES) and evolving strategy from historical approaches to contemporary innovations. *Journal of Neuroscience Methods, 219*(2), 297–311.

Kalu, U. G., Sexton, C. E., Loo, C. K., & Ebmeier, K. P. (2012). Transcranial direct current stimulation in the treatment of major depression: A meta-analysis. *Psychological Medicine, 42* (9), 1791–1800.

Kanai, R., Chaieb, L., Antal, A., Walsh, V., & Paulus, W. (2008). Frequency-dependent electrical stimulation of the visual cortex. *Current Biology: CB, 18*(23), 1839–1843.

Keeser, D., Meindl, T., Bor, J., Palm, U., Pogarell, O., Mulert, C., et al. (2011). Prefrontal transcranial direct current stimulation changes connectivity of resting-state networks during fMRI. *The Journal of Neuroscience, 31*(43), 15284–15293.

Kincses, T. Z., Antal, A., Nitsche, M. A., Bartfai, O., & Paulus, W. (2004). Facilitation of probabilistic classification learning by transcranial direct current stimulation of the prefrontal cortex in the human. *Neuropsychologia, 42*(1), 113–117.

Kirsch, D. L. (2002). *The science behind cranial electrotherapy stimulation.* Edmonton, Alberta: Medical Scope Publishing.

Kirsch, D. L., & Smith, R. B. (2004). Cranial electrotherapy stimulation for anxiety depression, insomnia, cognitive dysfunction, and pain. In P. Rosch (Ed.), *Bioelectromagnetic medicine* (pp. 727–740). New York: Marcel Dekker, Inc.

Kronberg, G., & Bikson, M. (2012). Electrode assembly design for transcranial direct current stimulation: A FEM modeling study. *Conference Proceedings: Annual International Conference of the IEEE Engineering in Medicine and Biology Society. IEEE Engineering in Medicine and Biology Society. Conference, 2012,* 891–895.

Kuo, H. I., Bikson, M., Datta, A., Minhas, P., Paulus, W., Kuo, M. F., et al. (2013). Comparing cortical plasticity induced by conventional and high-definition 4 × 1 ring tDCS: A neurophysiological study. *Brain Stimulation, 6*(4), 644–648.

Lauber, C., Nordt, C., & Rossler, W. (2005). Recommendations of mental health professionals and the general population on how to treat mental disorders. *Social Psychiatry and Psychiatric Epidemiology, 40*(10), 835–843.

Lebedev, V. P., Malygin, A. V., Kovalevski, A. V., Rychkova, S. V., Sisoev, V. N., Kropotov, S. P., et al. (2002). Devices for noninvasive transcranial electrostimulation of the brain endorphinergic system: Application for improvement of human psychophysiological status. *Artificial Organs, 26*(3), 248–251.

Lefaucheur, J. P., Antal, A., Ahdab, R., Ciampi de Andrade, D., Fregni, F., Khedr, E. M., et al. (2008). The use of repetitive transcranial magnetic stimulation (rTMS) and transcranial direct current stimulation (tDCS) to relieve pain. *Brain Stimulation, 1*(4), 337–344.

Limoge, A. (1999). Electricity in pain management [L'electricite pour le traitement de la douleur]. *Presse Medicale (Paris, France: 1983), 28*(39), 2197–2203.

Limoge, A., Robert, C., & Stanley, T. H. (1999). Transcutaneous cranial electrical stimulation (TCES): A review 1998. *Neuroscience and Biobehavioral Reviews, 23*(4), 529–538.

Lindenberg, R., Renga, V., Zhu, L. L., Nair, D., & Schlaug, G. (2010). Bihemispheric brain stimulation facilitates motor recovery in chronic stroke patients. *Neurology, 75*(24), 2176–2184.

Lisanby, S. H., Kinnunen, L. H., & Crupain, M. J. (2002). Applications of TMS to therapy in psychiatry. *Journal of Clinical Neurophysiology: Official Publication of the American Electroencephalographic Society, 19*(4), 344–360.

Loo, C. K., Alonzo, A., Martin, D., Mitchell, P. B., Galvez, V., & Sachdev, P. (2012). Transcranial direct current stimulation for depression: 3-week, randomised, sham-controlled trial. *The British Journal of Psychiatry, 200*(1), 52–59.

Marshall, L., Helgadottir, H., Molle, M., & Born, J. (2006). Boosting slow oscillations during sleep potentiates memory. *Nature, 444*(7119), 610–613.

McKenzie, R. E., Rosenthal, S. H., & Driessner, J. S. (1971). Some psychophysiologic effects of electrical transcranial stimulation (electrosleep). In N. L. Wulfsohn & A. Sances (Eds.), *The nervous system and electric currents* (pp. 163–167). New York: Plenum.

Mendonca, M. E., Santana, M. B., Baptista, A. F., Datta, A., Bikson, M., Fregni, F., et al. (2011). Transcranial DC stimulation in fibromyalgia: Optimized cortical target supported by high-resolution computational models. *The Journal of Pain, 12*(5), 610–617.

Miranda, P. C., Lomarev, M., & Hallett, M. (2006). Modeling the current distribution during transcranial direct current stimulation. *Clinical Neurophysiology, 117*(7), 1623–1629.

Moliadze, V., Antal, A., & Paulus, W. (2010). Electrode-distance dependent after-effects of transcranial direct and random noise stimulation with extracephalic reference electrodes. *Clinical Neurophysiology, 121*(12), 2165–2171.

Moliadze, V., Atalay, D., Antal, A., & Paulus, W. (2012). Close to threshold transcranial electrical stimulation preferentially activates inhibitory networks before switching to excitation with higher intensities. *Brain Stimulation, 5*(4), 505–511.

Mulquiney, P. G., Hoy, K. E., Daskalakis, Z. J., & Fitzgerald, P. B. (2011). Improving working memory: Exploring the effect of transcranial random noise stimulation and transcranial direct current stimulation on the dorsolateral prefrontal cortex. *Clinical Neurophysiology, 122*(12), 2384–2389.

Nair, D. G., Renga, V., Lindenberg, R., Zhu, L., & Schlaug, G. (2011). Optimizing recovery potential through simultaneous occupational therapy and non-invasive brain-stimulation using tDCS. *Restorative Neurology and Neuroscience, 29*(6), 411–420.

Nitsche, M. A., Doemkes, S., Karakose, T., Antal, A., Liebetanz, D., Lang, N., et al. (2007). Shaping the effects of transcranial direct current stimulation of the human motor cortex. *Journal of Neurophysiology, 97*(4), 3109–3117.

Nitsche, M. A., Fricke, K., Henschke, U., Schlitterlau, A., Liebetanz, D., Lang, N., et al. (2003). Pharmacological modulation of cortical excitability shifts induced by transcranial direct current stimulation in humans. *The Journal of Physiology, 553*(Pt 1), 293–301.

Nitsche, M. A., Grundey, J., Liebetanz, D., Lang, N., Tergau, F., & Paulus, W. (2004). Catecholaminergic consolidation of motor cortical neuroplasticity in humans. *Cerebral Cortex (New York, NY: 1991), 14*(11), 1240–1245.

Nitsche, M. A., & Paulus, W. (2000). Excitability changes induced in the human motor cortex by weak transcranial direct current stimulation. *The Journal of Physiology, 527*(Pt 3), 633–639.

Nitsche, M. A., Seeber, A., Frommann, K., Klein, C. C., Rochford, C., Nitsche, M. S., et al. (2005). Modulating parameters of excitability during and after transcranial direct current stimulation of the human motor cortex. *The Journal of Physiology, 568*(Pt 1), 291–303.

Nizard, J., Lefaucheur, J. P., Helbert, M., de Chauvigny, E., & Nguyen, J. P. (2012). Non-invasive stimulation therapies for the treatment of refractory pain. *Discovery Medicine, 14*(74), 21–31.

Ohn, S. H., Park, C. I., Yoo, W. K., Ko, M. H., Choi, K. P., Kim, G. M., et al. (2008). Time-dependent effect of transcranial direct current stimulation on the enhancement of working memory. *Neuroreport, 19*(1), 43–47.

Paulus, W. (2011). Transcranial electrical stimulation (tES – tDCS; tRNS, tACS) methods. *Neuropsychological Rehabilitation, 21*(5), 602–617.

Peterchev, A. V., Wagner, T. A., Miranda, P. C., Nitsche, M. A., Paulus, W., Lisanby, S. H., et al. (2012). Fundamentals of transcranial electric and magnetic stimulation dose: Definition, selection, and reporting practices. *Brain Stimulation, 5*(4), 435–453.

Plautz, E. J., Barbay, S., Frost, S. B., Friel, K. M., Dancause, N., Zoubina, E. V., et al. (2003). Post-infarct cortical plasticity and behavioral recovery using concurrent cortical stimulation and rehabilitative training: A feasibility study in primates. *Neurological Research, 25*(8), 801–810.

Priori, A. (2003). Brain polarization in humans: A reappraisal of an old tool for prolonged non-invasive modulation of brain excitability. *Clinical Neurophysiology, 114*, 589–595.

Radman, T., Ramos, R. L., Brumberg, J. C., & Bikson, M. (2009). Role of cortical cell type and morphology in subthreshold and suprathreshold uniform electric field stimulation in vitro. *Brain Stimulation, 2*(4), 215–228. e1-3.

Rahman, A., Reato, D., Arlotti, M., Gasca, F., Datta, A., Parra, L. C., et al. (2013). Cellular effects of acute direct current stimulation: Somatic and synaptic terminal effects. *The Journal of Physiology, 591*(Pt 10), 2563–2578.

Reato, D., Gasca, F., Datta, A., Bikson, M., Marshall, L., & Parra, L. C. (2013). Transcranial electrical stimulation accelerates human sleep homeostasis. *PLoS Computational Biology, 9*(2), e1002898.

Reato, D., Rahman, A., Bikson, M., & Parra, L. C. (2010). Low-intensity electrical stimulation affects network dynamics by modulating population rate and spike timing. *The Journal of Neuroscience, 30*(45), 15067–15079.

Reato, D., Rahman, A., Bikson, M., & Parra, L. C. (2013). Effects of weak transcranial alternating current stimulation on brain activity – A review of known mechanisms from animal studies. *Frontiers in Human Neuroscience, 7*, 687.

Salvador, R., Mekonnen, A., Ruffini, G., & Miranda, P. C. (2010). Modeling the electric field induced in a high resolution realistic head model during transcranial current stimulation. *Conference Proceedings: Annual International Conference of the IEEE Engineering in Medicine and Biology Society. IEEE Engineering in Medicine and Biology Society. Conference, 2010*, 2073–2076.

Santarnecchi, E., Polizzotto, N. R., Godone, M., Giovannelli, F., Feurra, M., Matzen, L., et al. (2013). Frequency-dependent enhancement of fluid intelligence induced by transcranial oscillatory potentials. *Current Biology, 23*, 1449–1453.

Schlaug, G., Renga, V., & Nair, D. (2008). Transcranial direct current stimulation in stroke recovery. *Archives of Neurology, 65*(12), 1571–1576.

Schroeder, M. J., & Barr, R. E. (2001). Quantitative analysis of the electroencephalogram during cranial electrotherapy stimulation. *Clinical Neurophysiology, 112*(11), 2075–2083.

Schutter, D. J., & Hortensius, R. (2010). Retinal origin of phosphenes to transcranial alternating current stimulation. *Clinical Neurophysiology, 121*(7), 1080–1084.

Smith, R. B. (2007). *Cranial electrotherapy stimulation: Its first fifty years, plus three: A monograph (paperback).* Mustang (OK): Tate Publishing & Enterprises.

Snowball, A., Tachtsidis, I., Popescu, T., Thompson, J., Delazer, M., Zamarian, L., et al. (2013). Long-term enhancement of brain function and cognition using cognitive training and brain stimulation. *Current Biology: CB, 23*(11), 987–992.

Stagg, C. J., Bestmann, S., Constantinescu, A. O., Moreno, L. M., Allman, C., Mekle, R., et al. (2011). Relationship between physiological measures of excitability and levels of glutamate and GABA in the human motor cortex. *The Journal of Physiology, 589*(Pt 23), 5845–5855.

Stagg, C. J., & Nitsche, M. A. (2011). Physiological basis of transcranial direct current stimulation. *The Neuroscientist, 17*(1), 37–53.

Terney, D., Chaieb, L., Moliadze, V., Antal, A., & Paulus, W. (2008). Increasing human brain excitability by transcranial high-frequency random noise stimulation. *The Journal of Neuroscience, 28*(52), 14147–14155.

Uk ECT Review Group. (2003). Efficacy and safety of electroconvulsive therapy in depressive disorders: A systematic review and meta-analysis. *Lancet, 361*(9360), 799–808.

Villamar, M. F., Volz, M. S., Bikson, M., Datta, A., Dasilva, A. F., & Fregni, F. (2013). Technique and considerations in the use of 4 × ring high-definition transcranial direct current stimulation (HD-tDCS). *Journal of Visualized Experiments: JoVE,* (77), e50309, doi(77), e50309.

Villamar, M. F., Wivatvongvana, P., Patumanond, J., Bikson, M., Truong, D. Q., Datta, A., et al. (2013). Focal modulation of the primary motor cortex in fibromyalgia using 4 × 1-ring high-definition transcranial direct current stimulation (HD-tDCS): Immediate and delayed analgesic effects of cathodal and anodal stimulation. *The Journal of Pain: Official Journal of the American Pain Society, 14*(4), 371–383.

Vitalucci, A., Coppola, I., Mirra, M., Maina, G., & Bogetto, F. (2013). Brain stimulation therapies for treatment-resistant depression [Tecniche di stimolazione cerebrale nel trattamento della depressione resistente]. *Rivista Di Psichiatria, 48*(3), 175–181.

Wagner, T., Valero-Cabre, A., & Pascual-Leone, A. (2007). Noninvasive human brain stimulation. *Annual Review of Biomedical Engineering, 9*, 527–565.

Wassermann, E. M., & Grafman, J. (2005). Recharging cognition with DC brain polarization. *Trends in Cognitive Sciences, 9*(11), 503–505.

Zaehle, T., Rach, S., & Herrmann, C. S. (2010). Transcranial alternating current stimulation enhances individual alpha activity in human EEG. *PloS One, 5*(11), e13766.

Zaghi, S., Acar, M., Hultgren, B., Boggio, P. S., & Fregni, F. (2010). Noninvasive brain stimulation with low-intensity electrical currents: Putative mechanisms of action for direct and alternating current stimulation. *The Neuroscientist, 16*(3), 285–307.

Zaghi, S., de Freitas Rezende, L., de Oliveira, L. M., El-Nazer, R., Menning, S., Tadini, L., et al. (2010). Inhibition of motor cortex excitability with 15Hz transcranial alternating current stimulation (tACS). *Neuroscience Letters, 479*(3), 211–214.

Zaghi, S., Thiele, B., Pimentel, D., Pimentel, T., & Fregni, F. (2011). *Restorative Neurology and Neuroscience, 29*(6), 439–451.

The Perils of Using Electrical Stimulation to Change Human Brains

Nicholas S. Fitz and Peter B. Reiner

National Core for Neuroethics, The University of British Columbia, Vancouver, BC, Canada

OUTLINE

THE UNIQUE TOOL

The modern visage of transcranial direct current stimulation (tDCS), born anew in the scientific community, has electrified the cognitive enhancement scene. At this nascent stage, this simple yet elegant technique has been shown to be relatively safe in the laboratory, rather effective in certain domains, and reasonably inexpensive to obtain and operate. Though the exact mechanisms are formally unknown, tDCS is thought to modify the excitability of neuronal membranes (depending on the polarity and montage of the electrodes), thereby facilitating or reducing plasticity in response to endogenous neural activity. The technique is often described as non-invasive, as the devices work by sending modest currents ($\sim$1–2 mA) from the outside of the head to the brain through saline-soaked pads. Today, tDCS generates excitement as: (1) a unique investigative tool in clinical and cognitive neuroscience, (2) a budding treatment for various neurologic and psychiatric conditions, and (3) a would-be cognitive enhancer for "normal," healthy adults and children.

It is natural to be excited about the possible applications for tDCS, in particular as the technique holds great promise for advancing our understanding of the normal function of the human brain as well as opening the door to novel treatments for disease (Nitsche et al., 2008; Stagg & Nitsche, 2011). If tDCS does indeed prove to be as effective as those treatments available via pharmacology, it may well change the modern practices of neurology and psychiatry, especially if it is safer and less expensive than the current standard of care. tDCS might even bridge new ethical terrain: a potential cognitive enhancer that by virtue of its simplicity and modest cost *promotes* fair distribution in society (Cohen Kadosh, Levy, O'Shea, Shea, & Savulescu, 2012). This is quite novel considering that distributive justice, the fair allocation of benefits (and burdens), is often among the most salient concerns in the debate over the propriety of cognitive enhancement, particularly in the face of growing achievement, economic, and social disparity (Murray, 2012; Stiglitz, 2012). Not only are tDCS devices inexpensive, but they are also relatively simple to operate[1], which marks them as a useful tool in areas that lack the requisite financial and technical resources for more advanced treatment (Pascal-Leone, Fregni, Steven-Wheeler, & Forrow, 2011).

Given its potential, investigators have explored tDCS for: motor learning (Boros, Poreisz, Münchau, Paulus, & Nitsche, 2008; Nitsche, Fricke, et al., 2003; Nitsche et al., 2007; Reis et al., 2008), numerical ability (Cohen Kadosh, Soskic, Iuculano, Kanai, & Walsh, 2010), episodic memory (Penolazzi et al., 2010), working memory (Fregni et al., 2005; Ohn et al., 2008), motor memory (Galea & Celnik, 2009), sleep-dependent consolidation of declarative memory (Marshall, 2004), learning and memory writ large (Brasil-Neto, 2012), attention (Coffman, Trumbo, & Clark, 2012), decision-making and risk (Coricelli & Rusconi, 2011; Fecteau et al., 2007), planning ability (Dockery, Hueckel-Weng, Birbaumer, & Plewnia, 2009), complex and creative problem-solving (Cerruti & Schlaug, 2009; Chi & Snyder 2012; Snyder, 2009), grammar (de Vries et al., 2010; Floel, Rösser, Michka, Knecht, & Breitenstein, 2008), object naming (Fertonani, Rosini, Cotelli, Rossini, & Miniussi, 2010; Sparing, Dafotakis, & Meister 2008), word retrieval (Fiori et al., 2011), verbal fluency (Iyer et al., 2005), reading efficiency (Turkeltaub et al., 2011), lying (Mameli et al., 2010; Priori et al., 2007), and the likelihood of utilitarian judgments (Fumagalli et al., 2010), to name but the most prominent applications of this exciting technique.

DIY ENHANCEMENT WITH tDCS

The very same qualities that constitute the egalitarian promise of tDCS – its efficacy and access – simultaneously give rise to its peril: the potential for long-lasting, and potentially irreversible, changes in the DIY home experimenter community. We encourage the thoughtful use of tDCS by professionals in the laboratory and clinic, and regulatory preparation for the potentially significant usage by *the public* at large. The scientific and popular interest in tDCS has kindled a fire: the rapidly increasing presence of tDCS in both the peer-reviewed literature and the popular press is contributing to the increase of DIY tDCS.

The emerging epistemic setting of tDCS might best be understood by considering the inception of functional magnetic resonance imaging (fMRI) in the latter half of the 20th century. While the introduction of magnetic resonance imaging itself had already substantially changed the medical diagnostic landscape, it was not until the 1990s that fMRI emerged as a powerful tool for brain mapping in living humans (Illes & Sahakian, 2011). Today, fMRI wields much explanatory power for public(s) of all stripes (Racine, Bar-Ilan, & Illes, 2005), and the scientific community has left very few experimental stones unturned in classical fMRI investigations. In much the same way as fMRI is a technique for observing the neural activity in behaving humans, tDCS is a technique for manipulating the neural activity of living people. Given the versatility of tDCS, it is reasonable to predict that it will similarly be used as an "uncover everything" investigational tool. The deep fascination with fMRI stems not only from its versatility but also from the putative ability to directly *see* the human mind, further bolstered by the visually arresting pseudocolor images (Dumit, 2004). While tDCS lacks the seductive allure of imaging, the seemingly endless potential to manipulate the human mind represents the opposite side of the fMRI coin.

The excitement bespeaks responsibility: without proper regulatory review, it will prove difficult to balance both the enthusiasms and safety of the public.

As a part of the broader conversation on human enhancement, tDCS raises many of the same concerns – for example, safety, peer pressure, distributive justice, authenticity, medicalization, and more (Bostrom & Sandberg, 2009; Chatterjee, 2004; Conrad, 2007; Degrazia, 2005; Farah et al., 2004; Forlini & Racine, 2009; Greely et al., 2008; Hyman, 2011; Reiner, 2010; Turner & Sahakian, 2006) – seen in the debate over pharmacological cognitive enhancement (PCE). However, the ethical implications of tDCS differ from those of PCE in important ways (Cohen Kadosh et al., 2012; Hamilton, Messing, & Chatterjee, 2011), and, in our view, among the most important of these is DIY enhancement with tDCS. Notably, interest in cognitive enhancement has not engendered any substantial DIY ethos toward PCEs. While there has been concern surrounding the sale of PCEs from those with prescriptions to those without prescriptions (DeSantis, Webb, & Noar, 2008; McCabe, Knight, Teter, & Wechsler, 2005; Vidourek, King, & Knopf, 2010), there has never been a real worry about "home brewing" PCEs. Moreover, and contrary to popular thought, existing PCEs are only modestly successful at enhancing cognitive skills (Greely, 2010; Ilieva, Boland, & Farah, 2012; Smith & Farah, 2011). Already, brain stimulation technologies might be more effective (Cohen Kadosh et al., 2010; Floel et al., 2008; Marshall, 2004; Ukueberuwa & Wassermann, 2010) – and less value-laden or stigmatized (Forlini & Racine, 2011; Franke, Lieb, & Hildt, 2012; Heinrichs, 2012; Outram, 2012; Pillow, Naylor, & Malone, 2012) – than PCEs we might develop in the near future. To be sure, self-medication of individuals using drugs such as methylphenidate intended for the treatment of ADHD without the requisite prescription is, in some ways, akin to DIY tDCS: both scenarios feature an untutored individual making a decision about changing his or her brain using technology without the supervision of a medical professional. The key difference lies in the scope of individual power to manipulate the technology itself. In the case of PCE, prospective users have only the most basic morphological freedom: to take, or not take, the pill. While tDCS might be safer *prima facie*, the mounting concern stems from the unchecked morphological freedom of an uninformed public to modulate polarity, current intensity, stimulation duration and frequency, and electrode size and placement, as well as alterations in endogenous neural activity or employing the technique upon a background of neuroactive pharmaceuticals. In this analysis, we assess the unique, unprecedented, and potentially widespread rise of the DIY world.

FROM BENCH TO HOME: THE GOOD, THE BAD, AND THE UGLY

The first waves of results with respect to therapy and enhancement using tDCS are quite encouraging. The potential of a minimally invasive, non-pharmacological approach is rather exciting, and more research is in the pipeline. In terms of explicit physical side effects in the short term, tDCS appears to be remarkably safe: adverse effects, if reported at all (Brunoni et al., 2011), tend to include mild headache and irritation of the skin under the electrodes (Arul-Anandam, Loo, & Sachdev, 2009; Tadini et al., 2011). Nitsche et al. originally developed what has become the standard of safety criteria for the field, eruditely summarizing safety thresholds for relevant parameters (Nitsche, Liebetanz, et al., 2003). Given their careful awareness of inducing long-term effects, admittedly necessary for possible clinical application, they conclude with a call for more research on safety (Nitsche, Liebetanz, et al., 2003).

Bikson et al. update the safety limits for tDCS, opining that "it is neither accurate nor prudent to determine quantitative safety standards for tDCS from these [existing] reports," and conclude with a call for further research (Bikson, Datta, & Elwassif, 2009). In the same edition of *Clinical Neurophysiology*, an oft-cited experiment appeared that explored the level of current density necessary for inducing overt damage to brain tissue: $142.9 \, A/m^2$ for durations greater than 10 minutes (Liebetanz et al., 2009). Given that researchers employ significantly less current density – usually between 0.029 and 0.08 mA/m^2 (Nitsche et al., 2008) – this study is suitable for ameliorating tissue damage concerns in the laboratory, and sets a useful parameter for future research. However, there may yet be concern in the DIY world about the likelihood of inducing brain damage as users will undoubtedly modify much of the protocol, in particular by manipulating current density, total charge, stimulation duration, electrode location, drug–device interaction, handedness (including some lateralized function), and more. In ensuring the safety of *the public*, we focus on *plausible* scenarios detailing the neurobiological sequelae of using tDCS. Though it is still early days in the development of guidelines for tDCS, we do not currently possess strong data that might inform situations such as these that are likely to arise if and when the public embraces this technology. Today, almost a decade after Nitsche et al.'s safety criteria, most of the literature continues to include a quick caveat on the lack of longitudinal work and/or the possibility of unsuspected side effects (Cohen Kadosh et al., 2012; Hamilton et al., 2011; Utz, Dimova, Oppenländer, & Kerkhoff, 2010). As we detail below, there is an urgent need to investigate these questions now.

To be quite clear, the current discourse on safety is openly intended for the experimental or clinical setting, and is not meant to assess potential safety concerns for the growing demographic of individuals in the DIY sphere. While tDCS seems safe *prima facie* (Nitsche, Liebetanz, et al., 2003), certain aspects of the technology raise legitimate concerns that would be relevant for the DIY demographic: the current data (and prevailing ethos) regarding the safety of tDCS are gleaned from a nascent body of literature that (1) was conducted in the laboratory, not in the field, (2) offers no longitudinal perspective as of yet, (3) contains issues in properly blinding experiments (O'Connell et al., 2012), and (4) appears to show rather malleable effects (from polarity, electrode montage, or stimulation duration). The vast majority of researchers in the field are aware of these concerns as they move forward in their exciting tDCS investigations, but the lay public remains in the dark.

THE POTENTIAL ROOTS OF UNINTENDED CHANGE

Of primary concern is the potential abuse of the technology beyond the purview of the experimental world – a possibility all the more likely without proper supervision and education in best practices. Many have quickly embraced tDCS technology as perfectly safe, quite effective, operationally flexible, and capable of instantiating long-lasting changes in the brain (Cohen Kadosh et al., 2010). For most, the enthusiasm is purely evidence-based, while the eagerness of others arises from biopolitical or financial interest. Indeed, its potential is certainly exciting; we simply advocate thoughtful reflection in light of some important concerns. Taken individually, the claims about tDCS – that it is safe, effective, and long lasting – are certainly data driven. Yet ethical analysis is often tasked with parsing the aggregate effect(s) whilst navigating the slippery slope of incrementalist findings. Although proponents tout tDCS as extremely safe, even the most ardent advocates would not claim that it is unequivocally safe. Adopting an approach that includes humility – recognizing that we understand a great deal about the structure and function of the brain, but we still have even more to learn – will prove indispensable in averting unexpected, unwanted, and perhaps even enduring changes in brains.

Reversing Polarity Can Impair Function

By simply reversing the polarity (from anodal to cathodal or *vice versa*) of tDCS stimulation, one may sometimes impair the targeted function, as the direction of neuronal excitability depends upon – among other factors – polarity (Nitsche, Liebetanz, et al., 2003). In one widely discussed paper on tDCS in enhancing cognitive ability, it was found that left cathodal stimulation caused better performance in numerical tasks while the opposite configuration "led to underperformance, comparable to that observed in young children" (Cohen Kadosh et al., 2010). In verbal testing, anodal tDCS led to better accuracy and speed while cathodal tDCS led to significantly worse performance on those measures (Javadi, Cheng, & Walsh, 2012), and authors have found that stimulation leads to "enhancement or impairment of verbal memorization depending on the polarity of the stimulation" (Javadi & Cheng, 2012; Javadi & Walsh, 2012). In some cases, reversing the polarity appears to affect only certain groups of individuals, e.g., women (Fumagalli et al., 2010), and in other cases, cathodal stimulation unexpectedly leads to better performance (Antal et al., 2004; Dockery et al., 2009).

Building on earlier literature suggesting that TMS over the DLPFC affects decision-making (Knoch, Gianotti, et al., 2006; Knoch, Schneider, Schunk, Hohmann, & Fehr, 2009; Knoch, Pascual-Leone, Meyer, Treyer, & Fehr, 2006; van 't Wout, Kahn, Sanfey, & Aleman, 2005), Fecteau et al. investigated the effects of tDCS over the DLFPC on decision-making in healthy participants (Fecteau et al., 2007). The results quite cleanly reveal the possibility of impairment due simply to the specific polarity configuration: in comparison to the sham group, those receiving anodal stimulation over the right DLPFC chose safe prospects more often, were faster to make that choice, and were not nearly as influenced by the magnitude of the reward. Participants receiving the opposite polarity configuration (anodal stimulation over left DLPFC; cathodal stimulation over right DLPFC) did not differ in their choice of risk, but were significantly slower to come to their decision. Research of this ilk elucidates the capability of tDCS to impair higher-order judgment. In a recent meta-analysis, this trend appears most commonly in motor functions and less commonly in cognitive functions (Jacobson, Koslowsky, & Lavidor, 2012). In an exhaustive review, by the authors, of the effects of tDCS stimulation parameters upon enhancement and impairment, we found numerous studies that either did not follow up with the impaired (or just non-enhanced) group or did not run an opposite-polarity configuration. To be clear, reversing polarity does not necessarily modify the effect (Antal, Terney, Poreisz, & Paulus, 2007; Boggio et al., 2007). In some instances it has shown to have no effect, or, at least, no effect on the *specific domain that was measured* – (see "The Underappreciated Peril," below).

Electrode Placement is Important

The specific placement of electrodes affects different brain regions in different ways – positioning is "of crucial significance for the spatial distribution and direction of the flow of current which together determine the effectiveness of the stimulation" (Utz et al., 2010; see also Chapter 4). This simple notion is essential in considering the use of tDCS by an uninformed lay public. The two early flag-carrying investigations of tDCS in modern investigations reveal the malleable nature of its effects. Priori et al. used a weak direct current (less than 0.5 mA for 7 s) to explore changes in motor evoked potentials (MEP) from TMS, and found that anodal stimulation significantly *depressed* the excitability of the motor cortex (Priori, Berardelli, Rona, Accornero, & Manfredi, 1998). Nitsche and Paulus found that anodal stimulation *enhanced* excitability of the motor cortex whereas cathodal stimulation diminished excitability (again, measured by MEP during TMS) (Nitsche & Paulus, 2000). Traditionally considered irrelevant, the only salient difference between the two experiments, aside from the current level, was the placement of the *reference* electrode (under the chin in the former, and over the contralateral supraorbital in the latter). At the very least, this exemplar illuminates the unknown function of underlying neurophysiological mechanisms active in tDCS.

Most tDCS studies so far show positive effects of anodal stimulation on the left DLPFC for working memory (Brasil-Neto, 2012). This effect may not occur, or may even be reversed, with different electrode montages, such as bilateral anodal prefrontal stimulation (Marshall, Mölle, Siebner, & Born, 2005) or use of a non-cephalic cathode (Ferrucci et al., 2008). We do know that the location of electrodes affects how – and through which neural networks – current travels in the brain, but "little is known about the practical consequences of this for therapy" (Rothwell, 2012).

For an example of import of electrode placement in practice, consider handedness. Most study participant pools select for right-handedness, given that left-handed participants may have lateralized brain function. Of course, not everyone in the world is right handed, and tDCS may differentially activate neural networks in those that have partially lateralized function. Underscoring this point, experimenters have demonstrated that the modulating effects of tDCS on excitability differ moderately in the left- and mixed-handed population compared to right-handed subjects, and that this needs to be taken into account in future work (Schade, Moliadze, Paulus, & Antal, 2012). How this will affect those left-handed experimenters in the DIY world who are stimulating using protocols created for right-handed laboratory participants and not mapping their brains to account for any lateralization is unknown.

Brain Stimulation Interacts with Pharmacology

When changing the brain with tDCS, there is a very real potential for interaction effects with neuroactive pharmaceuticals. It is already established that certain medications modulate the effects of tDCS, "such as neuroleptic and antiepileptic drugs, antidepressants, benzodiazepines and L-Dopa" (Utz et al., 2010), and other studies have shown that in the presence of several different psychoactive drugs the specific polarity montage results in unexpected (and often opposite) function than that observed in healthy subjects (Kuo, Paulus, & Nitsche, 2008; Kuo, Datta, Bikson, Paulus, & Kuo 2013; Liebetanz, Nitsche, Tergau, & Paulus, 2002; Nardone et al., 2012; Nitsche, Schauenburg, et al., 2003; Nitsche et al., 2006). These observations are instructive, but the extent of such interactions with the wide array of prescription medications that modify brain function is unknown. At a minimum, the existing data suggest that the underlying pharmacological status of the brain may have an impact on the specific effects of tDCS.

Not only are there concerns with respect to prescription medications; there is also the possibility that the effects of tDCS interact with non-prescription drugs that are in wide use in the population. For example, nicotine usage can modulate excitability caused by tDCS (Grundey et al., 2012). In a study of the effects of tDCS in chronic users of marijuana (the most widely used illicit substance in the world, with 125–203 million users [Degenhardt & Hall, 2012]) investigators found that: (1) chronic marijuana users demonstrated more conservative decision-making than the normal population (comparing the sham stimulation groups), (2) while right anodal stimulation of the DLPFC enhanced conservative decision-making in healthy volunteers, both right anodal and left anodal DLPFC stimulation *increased* the propensity for risk-taking in marijuana users, and (3) right anodal/left cathodal tDCS of DLPFC is significantly associated with a diminished craving for marijuana (Boggio et al., 2010). While many research laboratories exclude individuals who have used recreational drugs in the past 24 hours (Roi Cohen Kadosh, personal communication), much more research on these interactions is needed. In particular, given the likelihood that the DIY crowd includes individuals who use psychoactive agents, it seems important to communicate these findings to the public.

Long-Lasting Changes

One of the key unknowns in the use of tDCS is the duration of the evoked changes. In their safety guidelines for the field, Nitsche, Liebetanz, et al., (2003) warn against stimulation durations that would result in excitability changes of more than an hour as excitability changes lasting for that long "could be dysfunctional." Indeed, studies have shown that the timing and duration of a tDCS session can lead to effects lasting up to several months (Cohen Kadosh et al., 2010; Dockery et al., 2009; John, 2012; Monte-Silva, Kuo, Liebetanz, Paulus, & Nitsche, 2010; Nitsche, Liebetanz, et al., 2003; Reis et al., 2009). For many, more is better[2]. People experimenting with tDCS might intuitively posit that more current will result in larger effects (John, 2012), but we have no data on more powerful currents[3]. The brain is quite plastic, and though tDCS is quite safe under certain conditions, we are in need of more data overall. As Reis et al., (2009) eloquently opine: *"if there is an evolutionary reason why maximal potential levels of learning are not reached in the absence of stimulation, then there could be a hidden cost to learning enhancement that we do not currently appreciate"* (p. 1593).

In principle, the kinds of effects that have been seen – improvements in cognitive function – are based upon facilitating plasticity in the brain. Since it is well established that short-term changes in plasticity can morph into long-term changes (McGaugh, 2000), there is no neurobiological reason why tDCS will not result in long-lasting changes in the brain. Such changes may be too subtle to measure with extant cognitive tests, but the possibility of the sequelae of unwise use of tDCS – as might occur in the DIY community – makes this issue much more than an academic concern. In order to mitigate the potential for damage in the growing DIY population, we will need sound regulatory policy that creates an environment of safe use.

THE UNDERAPPRECIATED PERIL: IF tDCS CAN CHANGE ONE FUNCTION, IT CAN CHANGE ANOTHER

The nature of tDCS is that it causes modest changes in membrane potential of many neurons (probably millions) (Creutzfeldt, Fromm, & Kapp, 1962; Purpura & McMurtry, 1965) that lie within the effective penumbra of the electrodes. Some but not all of those neuronal membranes may be involved in the functions being targeted, while an unknown number of them may be involved in other functions. From these observations derives an underappreciated peril in the use of tDCS: it may alter neuronal function in unintended ways. While experimenters have generally been meticulous in documenting the effects of tDCS upon specific cognitive functions, it is impossible for them to comment upon effects that the stimulation protocol had upon cognitive functions that were not measured. Even more insidious, tDCS may produce occult effects that do not manifest in overt changes in cognitive function, yet may still be of significance to individuals[4].

The movie *The Fly* depicts a scientist who has perfected a teleportation machine, but when he uses the machine himself, a fly is inadvertently included in the final product. The film is hyperbolic, but it illustrates a quandary that bedevils both the community of professionals employing tDCS, and even more so for DIY tDCS: the prospect of enhancing (or reinforcing) unwanted neural activity.

To test the hypothesis that this might already be at play, we carried out a meta-analysis of the extant literature on tDCS and observed several instances in which it seemed likely that such unintended changes were occurring. We parsed 112 well-cited papers in the literature experimenting with tDCS into brain region, stimulation polarity, and observed effects[5]. From this, we are able to compare, across the literature, the range of effects found from the stimulation of a specific cortical structure for many different domains of cognition. In the hypothetical: if an experimental group studies the effect of anodal stimulation of the DLPFC for craving, and then someone else studies the effect of anodal stimulation of the DLPFC for deception, we might observe (through this aggregate analysis) that a multitude of effects were occurring for each participant – and could occur for anyone employing stimulation of the DLPFC – and yet the unintended effects might not be measured.

A couple of examples illustrate the issue. Numerous experiments have investigated applying anodal stimulation to the left DLPFC and have found similar stimulation paradigms to result in reduction of risk-taking behavior (Fecteau et al., 2007), reduction in smoking craving (Fregni et al., 2008), facilitated recall of unpleasant images (Penolazzi et al., 2010), enhanced verbal fluency (Iyer et al., 2005), and decrease in sleep efficiency (Roizenblatt et al., 2007; see also Fig. 3.1). A similar situation holds when we examined cathodal stimulation to the left DLPFC; investigators have reported decreased verbal fluency, increase in safe choices (Fecteau et al., 2007), impaired declarative memory (Javadi & Walsh 2012), selectively facilitated pleasant image recall (Penolazzi et al., 2010), and impaired verbal memory (Javadi et al., 2012). Finally, Iuculano and Cohen Kadosh have recently demonstrated that a tDCS protocol, which enhanced numerical learning, impaired automaticity for the learned material, while a different protocol that enhanced automaticity impaired numerical learning (Iuculano & Cohen Kadosh, 2013). Such observations provide strong empirical evidence in support of our suggestion that unintended changes in cognitive function may ensue from tDCS.

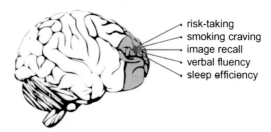

FIGURE 3.1   The shaded section marks the prefrontal cortex and the arrows point to the dorsolateral prefrontal cortex.

The current consensus is that tDCS proves most effective when coupled with some form of behavioral training (Cohen Kadosh et al., 2012). Indeed, mental activity has been shown to alter the efficacy of tDCS (Antal et al., 2007), and part of the elegance of the technique is that it is thought to affect mostly those circuits that are active while the stimulation is being applied. If tDCS is most effective when one is actively engaged in thought, the concern of intention arises: people may be enhancing unwanted extant neural activity. For example, one may be stimulating neural structures associated with memory or self-control, and an unanticipated environmental event might cause anxiety during the session. It is plausible that the presence of tDCS under such conditions may transform a transient event such as this into a long-lasting memory. In a similar fashion, tDCS might also modify the brain's response to uncontrolled internal thoughts. This is a modest problem in the case of the well-controlled laboratory experiment; it is a disaster waiting to happen in the case of DIY tDCS.

tDCS appears to be safe under certain conditions, but this is *provisional*. If, as an experimental community, we are inducing changes – whether transient or long lasting – that we are not aware of in our experimental paradigm, what might be the unintended effects? Fortunately, the institution of scientific inquiry is built in a way that will slowly shine the light over the entire walkway of effects. Unfortunately, there may be widespread use in the public – with effects both unanticipated and unwanted – well before experimenters develop this wider knowledge base. To say that it would be helpful to know what these effects might be would be an understatement.

DIY tDCS IS ONLINE RIGHT NOW

The world of DIY tDCS is quite alive: conversations online and experiments offline are taking place at this very moment. Many in this community are realistically informed, but, as is surely the case for any DIY community in its early stages, some are not (Schmidt 2008; Wohlsen, 2011). To contextualize the growing DIY tDCS within the larger do-it-yourself zeitgeist, consider the following[6]:

- The Maker Community, an extensive "directory of hackerspaces, chaptered geek orgs like Dorkbot, our 'own' independent Make: City groups, and other, similar DIY organizations," created "to support and foster the maker community world-wide" (http://makezine.com/groups/index.csp).
- DIY Bio, a thoughtful[7] organization "dedicated to making biology an accessible pursuit for citizen scientists, amateur biologists and biological engineers who value openness and safety" (http://diybio.org).

- DIY Genomics, a "non-profit research organization founded in March 2010 to realize personalized medicine through crowd sourced health studies and apps" (http://www.diygenomics.org/about.php).
- Genspace, the self-proclaimed "first-ever community biotechnology laboratory, a Biosafety Level One facility" which offers "hands-on courses to the public, provide extracurricular experiences for students, and encourage scientific entrepreneurship, particularly in the fields of molecular and synthetic biology" (http://genspace.org/page/About)[8], created in December 2010.
- DIY Drones (http://diydrones.com), a social networking community (based on the Ning platform) "focused on non-commercial ('recreational') projects by amateurs" (http://diydrones.com/profiles/blog/show?id=705844:BlogPost:17789), with the aim of creating new amateur Unmanned Aerial Vehicle platforms.
- The Hackerspace Prague brmlab, which, since 2010, has been "a place to meet and hack for all people interested in computers, electronics, science, digital art and inventing stuff in general" (https://brmlab.cz/start). Hackerspace Prague brmlab has a lengthy, open, and active wiki on tDCS (https://brmlab.cz/project/brain_hacking/tdcs).
- DIY tDCS, a blog with the purpose of "keeping tabs" on tDCS for the DIY audience (http://www.diytdcs.com).

If DIY tDCS does indeed go viral[9], how should we approach the deluge of people using tDCS devices at home? The answers range from the conservative and reactive (i.e., *laissez-faire* or watchful waiting attitudes) to the pre-emptively active (i.e., running around with our hair on fire because of concerns). We do not want the latter, but we certainly cannot sit back and allow the former. Unfortunately, the time for discussion has already passed – tDCS devices are already being sold to the public in the United States and Canada (www.foc.us). Given some real concerns, our ethos is one akin to managed technological optimism: a perspective which acknowledges both (1) the promise of great benefit from technology, and (2) the role of an active government in making that promise a reality (Sarewitz & Karas 2007)[10].

While the concern of safety in human enhancement is by no means unique to tDCS, its unique access and application (stemming from its low cost and its ease of use) might easily translate into widespread usage. Indeed, the plausibility of widespread availability and usage of tDCS in the short term raises pressing safety issues. In the egalitarian world of tDCS, we are not concerned with the safety of a small demographic (namely, those with sufficient socioeconomic resources to obtain current – and expensive – cognitive enhancement technologies), but rather with the entire populous. As mentioned, those same ingredients that ameliorated concerns about distributive justice ([relatively] safe, effective, inexpensive, and easy/portable) have already resulted in an easily accessible world of DIY tDCS enhancement. Essentially, one needs only a 9-V battery, simple electronic parts, and basic instruction (found online) to build and operate an individual tDCS device, as hobbyists are doing now (Fox, 2011). The rise of the DIY sphere presents a very real concern in the near term.

Already, there are a number of online sources providing information (or even materials) for the purposes of obtaining a tDCS device for home use[11]. The amateur community is quite varied in ideology[12], but the prevailing ethos is one of fast-paced trial-by-fire activity, and the community is growing rapidly. We have no interest in restricting individual autonomy. However, the time is ripe to create policy that safely governs tDCS for all involved in the field.

REGULATION OR LACK THEREOF

At this juncture – the intersection of public health, market forces, and knowledge dissemination – the time is right for the regulatory authorities to enter the picture. The key questions are: (1) how *is* tDCS regulated? (2) what is the likelihood that tDCS devices will be brought before the regulatory authorities? and (3) how *should* tDCS be regulated?

The answer to the first question is clear, at least in the US: at present there is no regulatory framework in place for tDCS devices for either therapeutic or enhancement uses (Marjenin, 2012). The FDA does regulate Cranial Electrotherapy Stimulator (CES) devices, but does not consider tDCS to be CES, given that tDCS utilizes direct current (CES uses an alternating signal), and the electrode placement of a tDCS device may be different from that of cleared CES devices (Marjenin, 2012). Here, two important questions arise: (1) will tDCS rise to the level of concern that the FDA has about devices that affect humans? and (2) would the FDA regulate an enhancement? The answer to (1) is certainly yes, but we do not yet know the answer to (2), given the FDA's mandated reactive focus on therapeutic devices. Indeed, given its wide jurisdiction over medical devices, it appears likely that the FDA will regulate tDCS devices when faced with device applications. Given that, as of February 2012, the FDA does not consider tDCS to be a CES device (Marjenin, 2012), those with an interest in bringing tDCS devices to market might need to apply for the more costly Premarket Approval process, costing $5–300 million depending on the complexity of the device and FDA regulatory approval path, in order to gain access to commercial markets.

While some have opined that, due to the device's low cost and simplicity, tDCS is not of interest to the medical industry (Heinrichs, 2012), we believe just the opposite: there is likely to be significant interest from private industry, given how quickly and easily tDCS might spread in the public domain.

It is always speculative to predict the future, but consider the ways in which the introduction of the iPhone has revolutionized markets ranging from desktop computers to advertising on a global basis. Given the value people put on cognitive ability (Brooks, 2008), the potential size of the market for cognitive enhancement (Stix, 2009), and the resources that the private sector has available to pursue tDCS as a new market, the potential for the emergence of a lucrative market for home tDCS is substantial.

The regulatory authorities face at least two new challenges with tDCS. The first of these is that the technology engages extant neural function by way of a device that places control in the hands of the user. On the one hand, this offers more individual autonomy – users have an unprecedented amount of discretion over their treatment. On the other, this opens a Pandora's Box of safety concerns. Consider the case of existing PCEs: the user either takes the pill or does not take the pill. The pill is "safe and effective" – that is, it does what the company claims that it does. This is a simple and workable model: one might break the pill down or modify it in some way, but there is really not much room for tampering – the pill is what it is, so to speak. This is quite different with tDCS: in the hands of a user, tDCS might be utilized for any number of purposes – some of which (but not all) are safe, and some of which (but not all) are effective. This is what is so hard about creating a prudent regulatory environment for tDCS: so much is left up to the nuanced details – and user control – of polarity, electrode placement, duration, and extant neural function.

The second challenge is even more daunting: tDCS may be the technology that forces the regulatory authorities to directly confront the full range of issues that have been swirling in the enhancement debate. While it seems unlikely that tDCS devices will be submitted specifically for the purposes of enhancement, the freedom to use the devices for such purposes cannot escape the notice of anyone who has been following the subject. As the regulatory authorities begin to grapple with this issue, they will be well advised to engage the neuroethics community to integrate ethical analysis in their regulatory deliberations.

RECOMMENDATIONS

We offer three recommendations for thoughtful reflection to help individuals communicating the excitement of tDCS better able to be deliberate about the messages they offer.

1. *Balance Enthusiasm with Restraint.* The promise of tDCS has caught the eye of many in the popular press (Adee, 2012; Belluck, 2013; Fields, 2011; Lewis, 2012). Certainly, some unique implications of tDCS merit attention in the lab, the home, the clinic, and the medical industry.

Rarely, however, is there more than passing mention of concerns that might arise with use. For those using tDCS without professional supervision, these include the placement of electrodes, impairment from reversing polarity, interaction effects with other brain-changing agents, and potentially lasting effects. Those who speak about the promise of this new technology might take pains to balance their enthusiasm with discussion of the perils of tDCS, and authors, both in the scientific literature and in the popular press, might consider the impact of their diction. A particularly important example is the repeated use of the phrase "non-invasive." Deriving as it does from the surgical literature, the term distinguishes tDCS from technologies such as DBS that penetrate the brain. However, the innocuous nature of the term carries rhetorical power that affects everyone: journalists, home enthusiasts, policy-makers, practicing physicians, and more. To be clear, scholars were well intentioned in using the phrase (Chi & Snyder, 2011; Cohen Kadosh et al., 2012; Heinrichs, 2012; Priori, 2003; Sparing et al., 2008; Utz et al., 2010), but, given the surge in lay interest, it is time to switch to a more nuanced and appropriate term to encourage thoughtful use. As an insightful commentator on such matters has put it: "if thought corrupts language, language can also corrupt thought. A bad usage can spread by tradition and imitation even among people who should and do know better" (Orwell, 1946).

2. *Develop Robust Safety Standards.* The absence of overt physical side effects when using tDCS is quite promising for improving the current state of medical care. However, tDCS can enhance one function *at the expense of another unintended function* (Iuculano & Cohen Kadosh, 2013). From the standpoint of basic neurobiology, the worry is that non-targeted functions that happen to share neural elements which extend into the penumbra of the stimulated area are unintentionally affected in some way during stimulation. If the technique enjoys widespread use in the home, this worry becomes a real concern. We call on the scientific community to put a premium on carefully designed long-term studies.

3. *Engage and Regulate.* We advocate bringing tDCS under regulatory review to create an ethical climate of safe use (Fitz & Reiner, 2013; for a similar view see Maslen, Savulescu, Douglas, Levy, & Cohen Kadosh, 2013; Maslen, Douglas, Cohen Kadosh, Levy, & Savulescu, 2013). We eschew paternalistic control over individual freedom, but thoughtful and balanced regulation can generate best practices, which, at the very least, create guidelines that biohackers might incorporate into the DIY field. At its best, regulation should not constrain the promise of tDCS but rather propagate norms of safe use, offering tools to those interested in experimenting carefully. The approach that we advocate is one of safety, humility, and realism, bolstered by the excitement of scientific exploration – the key drivers of ingenuity and innovation.

ENDNOTES

1. The ease with which one can set up a tDCS device differentiates the technique from even transcranial magnetic stimulation (TMS). The ethical issues surrounding TMS are quite relevant (Horvath, Perez, Forrow, Fregni, & Pascual-Leone, 2011; Illes, Gallo, & Kirschen, 2006), but do not capture all that deserves reflection for tDCS.
2. Specifically, the humans living within the modern capitalistic market society.
3. However, adverse effects were reported more often in studies using higher current densities (Brunoni et al., 2011).
4. To illustrate this, Hamilton et al. have offered the example of adjusting the weights on a complicated mobile: "pushing on one piece may have inadvertent effects on the others" (Hamilton et al., 2011).
5. Inclusive of other relevant data: domain of cognition, duration, current density, side effects, and notes on patients and montage.
6. This list is meant to paint the picture of the growing DIY world writ large, and is not representative of *all* of the relevant DIY movements in existence today.
7. Indeed, they feature the statement that: "this project will require mechanisms for amateurs to increase their knowledge and skills, access to a community of experts, the development of a code of ethics, responsible oversight, and leadership on issues that are unique to doing biology outside of traditional professional settings" (http://diybio.org).
8. And "for a $100-per-month membership, anyone can use the space for whatever experiments they dream up" (http://www.wired.com/wiredscience/2010/12/genspace-diy-science-laboratory/).
9. Recall that it is inexpensive, online, and considered safe and effective under certain conditions.
10. And ideally, distributing the benefit(s) equally for the public.
11. (DaSilva, Volz, Bikson, & Fregni, 2011; "GoFlow: World's First tDCS Kit", 2012 [tdcsdevicekit.com]) (http://www.youtube.com/watch?v=hgFWEBwT6BE). Moreover, a video in the open-access *Journal of Visualized Experiments* is a comprehensive and insightful piece on tDCS operation (DaSilva et al., 2011), and functions as the most complete (albeit advanced) guide to constructing and using a tDCS device at home.
12. As well as in terminology, from libertarian "biohacker" to citizen scientist "home experimenter."

Acknowledgment

This work was supported by a grant from the Medical Research Council of Canada.

References

Adee, S. (2012). How electrical brain stimulation can change the way we think. *The Week*, Available at, http://theweek.com/article/index/226196/how-electrical-brain-stimulation-can-change-the-way-we-think.

Antal, A., Nitsche, M. D., Kruse, W., Kincses, T. Z., Hoffman, K. -P., & Paulus, W. (2004). Direct current stimulation over V5 enhances visuomotor coordination by improving motion perception in humans. *Journal of Cognitive Neuroscience, 16*(4), 521–527.

Antal, A., Terney, D., Poreisz, C., & Paulus, W. (2007). Towards unravelling task-related modulations of neuroplastic changes induced in the human motor cortex. *European Journal of Neuroscience, 26*(9), 2687–2691.

Arul-Anandam, A. P., Loo, C., & Sachdev, P. (2009). Transcranial direct current stimulation – What is the evidence for its efficacy and safety? *F 1000 Medicine Reports, 1*, .

Belluck, P. (2013). New therapy for depression. *New York Times: Well Blog*, 20 March, http://well.blogs.nytimes.com/2013/02/11/promising-depression-therapy/.

Bikson, M., Datta, A., & Elwassif, M. (2009). Establishing safety limits for transcranial direct current stimulation. *Clinical Neurophysiology, 120*(6), 1033–1034.

Boggio, P. S., Rigonatti, S. P., Ribeiro, R. B., Myczkowski, M. L., Nitsche, M. A., Pascual-Leone, A., et al. (2007). A randomized, double-blind clinical trial on the efficacy of cortical direct current stimulation for the treatment of major depression. *The International Journal of Neuropsychopharmacology, 11*(02).

Boggio, P. S., Zaghi, S., Villani, A. B., Fecteau, S., Pascual-Leone, A., & Fregni, F. (2010). Modulation of risk-taking in marijuana users by transcranial direct current stimulation (tDCS) of the dorsolateral prefrontal cortex (DLPFC). *Drug and Alcohol Dependence, 112*(3), 220–225.

Boros, K., Poreisz, C., Münchau, A., Paulus, W., & Nitsche, M. A. (2008). Premotor transcranial direct current stimulation (tDCS) affects primary motor excitability in humans. *European Journal of Neuroscience, 27*(5), 1292–1300.

Bostrom, N., & Sandberg, A. (2009). Cognitive enhancement: Methods, ethics, regulatory challenges. *Science and Engineering Ethics, 15*(3), 311–341.

Brasil-Neto, J. P. (2012). Learning, memory, and transcranial direct current stimulation. *Frontiers in Psychiatry / Frontiers Research Foundation, 3*, 80.

Brooks, D. (2008). The cognitive age. *The New York Times*, 2 May.

Brunoni, A. R., Amadera, J., Berbel, B., Volz, M. S., Rizzerio, B. G., & Fregni, F. (2011). A systematic review on reporting and assessment of adverse effects associated with transcranial direct current stimulation. *The International Journal of Neuropsychopharmacology, 14*(8), 1133–1145.

Cerruti, C., & Schlaug, G. (2009). Anodal transcranial direct current stimulation of the prefrontal cortex enhances complex verbal associative thought. *Journal of Cognitive Neuroscience, 21*(10), 1980–1987.

Chatterjee, A. (2004). Cosmetic neurology. *Neurology, 63*(6), 968–974.

Chi, R. P., & Snyder, A. W. (2011). Facilitate insight by non-invasive brain stimulation. *PLoS One, 6*(2), e16655.

Chi, R. P., & Snyder, A. W. (2012). Brain stimulation enables the solution of an inherently difficult problem. *Neuroscience Letters, 515*(2), 121–124.

Coffman, B. A., Trumbo, M. C., & Clark, V. P. (2012). Enhancement of object detection with transcranial direct current stimulation is associated with increased attention. *BMC Neuroscience, 13*(1), 108.

Cohen Kadosh, R., Levy, N., O'Shea, J., Shea, N., & Savulescu, J. (2012). The neuroethics of non-invasive brain stimulation. *Current Biology: CB, 22*(4), R108–R111.

Cohen Kadosh, R., Soskic, S., Iuculano, T., Kanai, R., & Walsh, V. (2010). Modulating neuronal activity produces specific and long-lasting changes in numerical competence. *Current Biology, 20*(22), 2016–2020.

Conrad, P. (2007). *The medicalization of society*. Baltimore, MD: Johns Hopkins University Press.

Coricelli, G., & Rusconi, E. (2011). Probing the decisional brain with rTMS and tDCS. In *A handbook of process tracing methods for decision research: A critical review and user's guide*. Boca Raton, FL: Taylor & Francis.

Creutzfeldt, O. D., Fromm, G. H., & Kapp, H. (1962). Influence of transcortical d-c currents on cortical neuronal activity. *Experimental Neurology, 5*, 436–452.

DaSilva, A. F., Volz, M. S., Bikson, M., & Fregni, F. (2011). Electrode positioning and montage in transcranial direct current stimulation. *Journal of Visualized Experiments, 51*, e2744.

de Vries, M. H., Barth, A. C. R., Maiworm, S., Knecht, S., Zwitserlood, P., & Floel, A. (2010). Electrical stimulation of broca's area enhances implicit learning of an artificial grammar. *Journal of Cognitive Neuroscience, 22*(11), 2427–2436.

Degenhardt, L., & Hall, W. (2012). Extent of illicit drug use and dependence, and their contribution to the global burden of disease. *The Lancet, 379*(9810), 55–70.

Degrazia, D. (2005). Enhancement technologies and human identity. *Journal of Medicine and Philosophy, 30*(3), 261–283.

DeSantis, A. D., Webb, E. M., & Noar, S. M. (2008). Illicit use of prescription ADHD medications on a college campus: A multimethodological approach. *Journal of American College Health, 57*(3), 315–324.

Dockery, C. A., Hueckel-Weng, R., Birbaumer, N., & Plewnia, C. (2009). Enhancement of planning ability by transcranial direct current stimulation. *Journal of Neuroscience, 29*(22), 7271–7277.

Dumit, J. (2004). *Picturing personhood*. Princeton, NJ: Princeton University Press.

Farah, M. J., Illes, J., Cook-Deegan, R., Gardner, H., Kandel, E., King, P., et al. (2004). Neurocognitive enhancement: What can we do and what should we do? *Nature Reviews Neuroscience, 5*(5), 421–425.

Fecteau, S., Knoch, D., Fregni, F., Sultani, N., Boggio, P., & Pascual-Leone, A. (2007). Diminishing risk-taking behavior by modulating activity in the prefrontal cortex: A direct current stimulation study. *Journal of Neuroscience, 27*(46), 12500–12505.

Ferrucci, R., Mameli, F., Guidi, I., Mrakic-Sposta, S., Vergari, M., Marceglia, S., et al. (2008). Transcranial direct current stimulation improves recognition memory in Alzheimer disease. *Neurology, 71*(7), 493–498.

Fertonani, A., Rosini, S., Cotelli, M., Rossini, P. M., & Miniussi, C. (2010). Naming facilitation induced by transcranial direct current stimulation. *Behavioural Brain Research, 208*(2), 311–318.

Fields, D. R. (2011). Amping up brain function: Transcranial stimulation shows promise in speeding up learning. *Scientific American*, 25 November.

Fiori, V., Coccia, M., Marinelli, C. V., Vecchi, V., Bonifazi, S., Ceravolo, M. G., et al. (2011). Transcranial direct current stimulation improves word retrieval in healthy and nonfluent aphasic subjects. *Journal of Cognitive Neuroscience, 23*(9), 2309–2323.

Fitz, N. S., & Reiner, P. B. (2013). The challenge of crafting policy for do-it-yourself brain stimulation. *Journal of Medical Ethics*, 3 June (epub) 2013.

Floel, A., Rösser, N., Michka, O., Knecht, S., & Breitenstein, C. (2008). Noninvasive brain stimulation improves language learning. *Journal of Cognitive Neuroscience, 20*(8), 1415–1422.

Forlini, C., & Racine, E. (2009). Autonomy and coercion in academic "Cognitive Enhancement" using methylphenidate: Perspectives of key stakeholders. *Neuroethics, 2*(3), 163–177.

Forlini, C., & Racine, E. (2011). Considering the causes and implications of ambivalence in using medicine for enhancement. *American Journal of Bioethics, 11*(1), 15–17.

Fox, D. (2011). Brain buzz. *Nature, 472*(7342), 156–158.

Franke, A. G., Lieb, K., & Hildt, E. (2012). What users think about the differences between caffeine and illicit/prescription stimulants for cognitive enhancement. *PLoS ONE, 7*(6), e40047.

Fregni, F., Boggio, P. S., Nitsche, M., Bermpohl, F., Antal, A., Feredoes, E., et al. (2005). Anodal transcranial direct current stimulation of prefrontal cortex enhances working memory. *Experimental Brain Research, 166*(1), 23–30.

Fregni, F., Liguori, P., Fecteau, S., Nitsche, M. A., Pascual-Leone, A., & Boggio, P. S. (2008). Cortical stimulation of the prefrontal cortex with transcranial direct current stimulation reduces cue-provoked smoking craving: A randomized, sham-controlled study. *Journal of Clinical Psychiatry, 69*(1), 32–40.

Fumagalli, M., Vergari, M., Pasqualetti, P., Marceglia, S., Mameli, F., Ferrucci, R., et al. (2010). Brain switches utilitarian behavior: Does gender make the difference? *PLoS One, 5*(1), e8865.

Galea, J. M., & Celnik, P. (2009). Brain polarization enhances the formation and retention of motor memories. *Journal of Neurophysiology, 102*(1), 294–301.

GoFlow: World's First tDCS Kit. (2012, June 4). GoFlow: World's first tDCS kit. *GoFlow*, Retrieved June 4, 2012, from, http://flowstateengaged.com.

Greely, H. (2010, July). Enhancing brains: What are we afraid of? *Cerebrum*, Retrieved April 3, 2012, from, http://dana.org/news/cerebrum/detail.aspx?id=28786.

Greely, H., Sahakian, B., Harris, J., Kessler, R. C., Gazzaniga, M., Campbell, P., et al. (2008). Commentary: Towards responsible use of cognitive-enhancing drugs by the healthy. *Nature, 456*(7223), 702–705.

Grundey, J., Thirugnanasambandam, N., Kaminsky, K., Drees, A., Skwirba, A. C., Lang, N., et al. (2012). Neuroplasticity in cigarette smokers is altered under withdrawal and partially restituted by nicotine exposition. *Journal of Neuroscience, 32*(12), 4156–4162.

Hamilton, R., Messing, S., & Chatterjee, A. (2011). Rethinking the thinking cap: Ethics of neural enhancement using noninvasive brain stimulation. *Neurology, 76*(2), 187–193.

Heinrichs, J. -H. (2012). The promises and perils of non-invasive brain stimulation. *International Journal of Law and Psychiatry, 35*(2), 121–129.

Horvath, J. C., Perez, J. M., Forrow, L., Fregni, F., & Pascual-Leone, A. (2011). Transcranial magnetic stimulation: A historical evaluation and future prognosis of therapeutically relevant ethical concerns. *Journal of Medical Ethics, 37*(3), 137–143.

Hyman, S. E. (2011). Cognitive enhancement: Promises and perils. *Neuron, 69*(4), 595–598.

Ilieva, I., Boland, J., & Farah, M. J. (2012). Objective and subjective cognitive enhancing effects of mixed amphetamine salts in healthy people. *Neuropharmacology, 64*, 496–505.

Illes, J., Gallo, M., & Kirschen, M. P. (2006). An ethics perspective on transcranial magnetic stimulation (TMS) and human neuromodulation. *Behavioural Neurology, 17*(3–4), 149–157.

Illes, J., & Sahakian, B. J. (2011). *Oxford handbook of neuroethics*. Oxford, UK: Oxford University Press.

Iuculano, T., & Cohen Kadosh, R. (2013). The mental cost of cognitive enhancement. *Journal of Neuroscience, 1–25,* .

Iyer, M. B., Mattu, U., Grafman, J., Lomarev, M., Sato, S., & Wassermann, E. M. (2005). Safety and cognitive effect of frontal DC brain polarization in healthy individuals. *Neurology, 64* (5), 872–875.

Jacobson, L., Koslowsky, M., & Lavidor, M. (2012). tDCS polarity effects in motor and cognitive domains: A meta-analytical review. *Experimental Brain Research, 216*(1), 1–10.

Javadi, A. H., & Cheng, P. (2012). Transcranial direct current stimulation (tDCS) enhances reconsolidation of long-term memory. *Brain Stimulation, 1–7,* .

Javadi, A. H., Cheng, P., & Walsh, V. (2012). Short duration transcranial direct current stimulation (tDCS) modulates verbal memory. *Brain Stimulation, 5*(4), 468–474.

Javadi, A. H., & Walsh, V. (2012). Transcranial direct current stimulation (tDCS) of the left dorsolateral prefrontal cortex modulates declarative memory. *Brain Stimulation, 5*(3), 231–241.

John. (2012, October 25). Transcranial direct current stimulation intensity and duration effects on tinnitus suppression. *DIY tDCS*, Retrieved October 25, 2012, from, http://www.

diytdcs.com/2012/10/transcranial-direct-current-stimulation-intensity-and-duration-effects-on-tinnitus-suppression/.

Knoch, D., Gianotti, L. R. R., Pascual-Leone, A., Treyer, V., Regard, M., Hohmann, M., et al. (2006). Disruption of right prefrontal cortex by low-frequency repetitive transcranial magnetic stimulation induces risk-taking behavior. *Journal of Neuroscience, 2006*(26), 6469–6472.

Knoch, D., Pascual-Leone, A., Meyer, K., Treyer, V., & Fehr, E. (2006). Diminishing reciprocal fairness by disrupting the right prefrontal cortex. *Science, 314*(5800), 829–832.

Knoch, D., Schneider, F., Schunk, D., Hohmann, M., & Fehr, E. (2009). Disrupting the prefrontal cortex diminishes the human ability to build a good reputation. *Proceedings of the National Academy of Sciences, 106*(49), 20895–20899.

Kuo, H. I., Datta, A., Bikson, M., Paulus, W., & Kuo, M. F. (2013). Comparing cortical plasticity induced by conventional and high-definition 4 × 1 ring tDCS: A neurophysiological study. *Brain Stimulation, 6*(4), 644–648.

Kuo, M. -F., Paulus, W., & Nitsche, M. A. (2008). Boosting focally-induced brain plasticity by dopamine. *Cerebral Cortex, 18*(3), 648–651.

Lewis, T. (2012, July 26). Unlock your inner rain man by electrically zapping your brain. *Wired Science*, Retrieved July 26, 2012, from, http://www.wired.com/wiredscience/2012/07/unlock-inner-savant/.

Liebetanz, D., Koch, R., Mayenfels, S., König, F., Paulus, W., & Nitsche, M. A. (2009). Safety limits of cathodal transcranial direct current stimulation in rats. *Clinical Neurophysiology: Official Journal of the International Federation of Clinical Neurophysiology, 120*(6), 1161–1167.

Liebetanz, D., Nitsche, M. A., Tergau, F., & Paulus, W. (2002). Pharmacological approach to the mechanisms of transcranial DC-stimulation-induced after-effects of human motor cortex excitability. *Brain, 125*(10), 2238–2247.

Mameli, F., Mrakic-Sposta, S., Vergari, M., Fumagalli, M., Macis, M., Ferrucci, R., et al. (2010). Dorsolateral prefrontal cortex specifically processes general – But not personal – Knowledge deception: Multiple brain networks for lying. *Behavioural Brain Research, 211*(2), 164–168.

Marjenin, T. (2012). *FDA executive summary: Prepared for the February 10, 2012 meeting of the neurologic devices panel*. Washington, DC: FDA, pp. 1–83.

Marshall, L. (2004). Transcranial direct current stimulation during sleep improves declarative memory. *Journal of Neuroscience, 24*(44), 9985–9992.

Marshall, L., Mölle, M., Siebner, H. R., & Born, J. (2005). *BMC Neuroscience, 6*(1), 23.

Maslen, H., Douglas, T., Cohen Kadosh, R., Levy, N., & Savulescu, J. (2013). Do-it-yourself brain stimulation: A regulatory model. *Journal of Medical Ethics*, (in press).

Maslen, H., Savulescu, J., Douglas, T., Levy, N., & Cohen Kadosh, R. (2013). Regulation of devices for cognitive enhancement. *The Lancet, 382*, 938–939.

McCabe, S. E., Knight, J. R., Teter, C. J., & Wechsler, H. (2005). Non-medical use of prescription stimulants among US college students: Prevalence and correlates from a national survey. *Addiction, 100*(1), 96–106.

McGaugh, J. L. (2000). Memory – A century of consolidation. *Science, 287*(5451), 248–251.

Monte-Silva, K., Kuo, M. -F., Liebetanz, D., Paulus, W., & Nitsche, M. A. (2010). Shaping the optimal repetition interval for cathodal transcranial direct current stimulation (tDCS). *Journal of Neurophysiology, 103*(4), 1735–1740.

Murray, C. (2012). *Coming apart*. New York, NY: Crown Forum.

Nardone, R., Bergmann, J., Christova, M., Caleri, F., Tezzon, F., Ladurner, G., et al. (2012). Effect of transcranial brain stimulation for the treatment of Alzheimer disease: A review. *International Journal of Alzheimer's Disease*, ID 687909.

Nitsche, M. A., Cohen, L. G., Wassermann, E. M., Priori, A., Lang, N., Antal, A., et al. (2008). Transcranial direct current stimulation: State of the art 2008. *Brain Stimulation, 1*(3), 206–223.

Nitsche, M. A., Doemkes, S., Karaköse, T., Antal, A., Liebetanz, D., Lang, N., et al. (2007). Shaping the effects of transcranial direct current stimulation of the human motor cortex. *Journal of Neurophysiology, 97*(4), 3109–3117.

Nitsche, M. A., Fricke, K., Henschke, U., Schlitterlau, A., Liebetanz, D., Lang, N., et al. (2003). Pharmacological modulation of cortical excitability shifts induced by transcranial direct current stimulation in humans. *The Journal of Physiology, 553*(Pt 1), 293–301.

Nitsche, M. A., Lampe, C., Antal, A., Liebetanz, D., Lang, N., Tergau, F., et al. (2006). Dopaminergic modulation of long-lasting direct current-induced cortical excitability changes in the human motor cortex. *European Journal of Neuroscience, 23*(6), 1651–1657.

Nitsche, M. A., Liebetanz, D., Lang, N., Antal, A., Tergau, F., & Paulus, W. (2003). Safety criteria for transcranial direct current stimulation (tDCS) in humans. *Clinical Neurophysiology, 114*(11), 2220–2222.

Nitsche, M. A., & Paulus, W. (2000). Excitability changes induced in the human motor cortex by weak transcranial direct current stimulation. *Journal of Physiology, 527*(Pt 3), 633–639.

Nitsche, M. A., Schauenburg, A., Lang, N., Liebetanz, D., Exner, C., Paulus, W., et al. (2003). Facilitation of implicit motor learning by weak transcranial direct current stimulation of the primary motor cortex in the human. *Journal of Cognitive Neuroscience, 15*(4), 619–626.

O'Connell, N. E., Cossar, J., Marston, L., Wand, B. M., Bunce, D., Moseley, G. L., et al. (2012). Rethinking clinical trials of transcranial direct current stimulation: Participant and assessor blinding Is inadequate at intensities of 2 mA. *PLoS One, 7*(10), e47514.

Ohn, S. H., Park, C. -I., Yoo, W. -K., Ko, M. -H., Choi, K. P., Kim, G. -M., et al. (2008). Time-dependent effect of transcranial direct current stimulation on the enhancement of working memory. *Neuroreport, 19*(1), 43–47.

Orwell, G. (1946). Politics and the English language. *Horizon,* (1946).

Outram, S. M. (2012). Ethical considerations in the framing of the cognitive enhancement debate. *Neuroethics, 5*(2), 173–184.

Pascal-Leone, A., Fregni, F., Steven-Wheeler, M., & Forrow, L. (2011). Non-invasive brain stimulation as a therapeutic and investigative tool: An ethical appraisal. In J. Illes & B. Sahakian (Eds.), *Oxford handbook of neuroethics* (pp. 417–439). Oxford, UK: Oxford University Press.

Penolazzi, B., Di Domenico, A., Marzoli, D., Mammarella, N., Fairfield, B., Franciotti, R., et al. (2010). Effects of transcranial direct current stimulation on episodic memory related to emotional visual stimuli. *PLoS One, 5*(5), e10623.

Pillow, D. R., Naylor, L. J., & Malone, G. P. (2012). Beliefs regarding stimulant medication effects among college students with a history of past or current usage. *Journal of Attention Disorders,* October 9, 1087054712459755.

Priori, A. (2003). Brain polarization in humans: A reappraisal of an old tool for prolonged non-invasive modulation of brain excitability. *Clinical Neurophysiology, 114*(4), 589–595.

Priori, A., Berardelli, A., Rona, S., Accornero, N., & Manfredi, M. (1998). Polarization of the human motor cortex through the scalp. *Neuroreport, 9*(10), 2257–2260.

Priori, A., Mameli, F., Cogiamanian, F., Marceglia, S., Tiriticco, M., Mrakic-Sposta, S., et al. (2007). Lie-specific involvement of dorsolateral prefrontal cortex in deception. *Cerebral Cortex, 18*(2), 451–455.

Purpura, D. P., & McMurtry, J. G. (1965). Intracellular activities and evoked potential changes during polarization of motor cortex. *Journal of Neurophysiology, 28,* 166–185.

Racine, E., Bar-Ilan, O., & Illes, J. (2005). Science and society: fMRI in the public eye. *Nature Reviews Neuroscience, 6*(2), 159–164.

Reiner, P. B. (2010). Distinguishing between restoration and enhancement in neuropharmacology. *Virtual Mentor, 12*(11), 885.

Reis, J., Robertson, E. M., Krakauer, J. W., Rothwell, J., Marshall, L., Gerloff, C., et al. (2008). Consensus: Can transcranial direct current stimulation and transcranial magnetic stimulation enhance motor learning and memory formation? *Brain Stimulation, 1*(4), 363–369.

Reis, J., Schambra, H. M., Cohen, L. G., Buch, E. R., Fritsch, B., Zarahn, E., et al. (2009). Noninvasive cortical stimulation enhances motor skill acquisition over multiple days through an effect on consolidation. *Proceedings of the National Academy of Sciences, 106*(5), 1590–1595.

Roizenblatt, S., Fregni, F., Gimenez, R., Wetzel, T., Rigonatti, S. P., Tufik, S., et al. (2007). Site-specific effects of transcranial direct current stimulation on sleep and pain in fibromyalgia: A randomized, sham-controlled study. *Pain Practice: The Official Journal of World Institute of Pain, 7*(4), 297–306.

Rothwell, J. C. (2012). Clinical applications of noninvasive electrical stimulation: Problems and potential. *Clinical EEG and Neuroscience, 43*, 209–214.

Sarewitz, D., & Karas, T. H. (2007). *Policy implications of technologies for cognitive enhancement.* (No. SAND2006-7609). Albuquerque, NM: Sandia National Laboratories.

Schade, S., Moliadze, V., Paulus, W., & Antal, A. (2012). Modulating neuronal excitability in the motor cortex with tDCS shows moderate hemispheric asymmetry due to subjects' handedness: A pilot study. *Restorative Neurology and Neuroscience, 30*(3), 191–198.

Schmidt, M. (2008). Diffusion of synthetic biology: A challenge to biosafety. *Systems and Synthetic Biology, 2*(1–2), 1–6.

Smith, M. E., & Farah, M. J. (2011). Are prescription stimulants "smart pills"? The epidemiology and cognitive neuroscience of prescription stimulant use by normal healthy individuals. *Psychological Bulletin, 137*(5), 717–741.

Snyder, A. (2009). Explaining and inducing savant skills: Privileged access to lower level, less-processed information. *Philosophical Transactions of the Royal Society, B: Biological Sciences, 364*(1522), 1399–1405.

Sparing, R., Dafotakis, M., & Meister, I. (2008). Enhancing language performance with noninvasive brain stimulation – A transcranial direct current stimulation study in healthy humans. *Neuropsychologia, 46*(1), 261–268.

Stagg, C. J., & Nitsche, M. A. (2011). Physiological basis of transcranial direct current stimulation. *The Neuroscientist, 17*(1), 37–53.

Stiglitz, J. E. (2012). *The price of inequality.* London, UK: W. W. Norton.

Stix, G. (2009). Turbocharging the brain. *Scientific American, 301*(4), 46–55.

Tadini, L., El-Nazer, R., Brunoni, A. R., Williams, J., Carvas, M., Boggio, P., et al. (2011). Cognitive, mood, and electroencephalographic effects of noninvasive cortical stimulation with weak electrical currents. *The Journal of ECT, 27*(2), 134–140.

Turkeltaub, P. E., Benson, J., Hamilton, R. H., Datta, A., Bikson, M., & Coslett, H. B. (2011). Left lateralizing transcranial direct current stimulation improves reading efficiency. *Brain Stimulation, 5*(3), 201–207.

Turner, D. C., & Sahakian, B. J. (2006). Neuroethics of cognitive enhancement. *BioSocieties, 1*(1), 113–123.

Ukueberuwa, D., & Wassermann, E. M. (2010). Direct current brain polarization: A simple, noninvasive technique for human neuromodulation. *Neuromodulation: Technology at the Neural Interface, 13*(3), 168–173.

Utz, K. S., Dimova, V., Oppenländer, K., & Kerkhoff, G. (2010). Electrified minds: Transcranial direct current stimulation (tDCS) and Galvanic Vestibular Stimulation (GVS) as methods of non-invasive brain stimulation in neuropsychology—A review of current data and future implications. *Neuropsychologia, 48*(10), 2789–2810.

van 't Wout, M., Kahn, R. S., Sanfey, A. G., & Aleman, A. (2005). Repetitive transcranial magnetic stimulation over the right dorsolateral prefrontal cortex affects strategic decision-making. *Neuroreport, 16*(16), 1849.

Vidourek, R. A., King, K. A., & Knopf, E. E. (2010). Non-medical prescription drug use among university students. *American Journal of Health Education, 41*(6), 345–352.

Wohlsen, M. (2011). *Biopunk: Kitchen-counter scientists hack the software of life.* Harmondsworth, UK: Penguin Books.

4

Computational Modeling Assisted Design of Optimized and Individualized Transcranial Direct Current Stimulation Protocols

Dennis Truong, Preet Minhas, Abhilash Nair, and Marom Bikson

Department of Biomedical Engineering, The City College of New York of CUNY, New York, NY, USA

OUTLINE

INTRODUCTION TO COMPUTATIONAL MODELS OF NON-INVASIVE NEUROMODULATION

This chapter is intended to provide a broad introduction to both clinical researchers and engineers interested in translational work to develop and apply computational models to inform and optimize tDCS. This first section introduces the rationale for modeling, the next two sections address technical features of modeling relevant to engineers (and to clinicians interested in the limitations of modeling), the next three sections address the use of modeling in clinical practice, and the final section illustrates the application of models in dose design through case studies.

Transcranial electrical stimulation is a promising tool in rehabilitation, based on the growing evidence that delivery of current to specific brain regions can promote desirable plastic changes (Ardolino, Bossi, Barbieri, & Priori, 2005; Zentner, 1989). Of particular interest are neurostimulation modalities that are low cost, portable, and simple to implement. Furthermore, stimulation should be applied using low-intensity current in a manner that is safe, well tolerated, and can be delivered concurrently with physical or cognitive rehabilitation and other therapies. In complement to other brain stimulation approaches (Fig. 4.1), transcranial direct current stimulation (tDCS) has been gaining considerable interest because it possesses all these desired qualities (Brunoni et al., 2012).

In contrast to pharmacotherapy, non-invasive electrotherapy offers the potential for both anatomically specific brain activation and complete temporal control anatomical targeting, which can be achieved through the rational selection of electrode number, shape, and position. In training applications such as rehabilitation, neuromodulatory techniques such as tDCS can combine focal stimulation with "focused" training to reinforce a particular region of activation (Edwards et al., 2009). Temporal control is possible due to the practically instantaneous delivery of electrical dose. There is no electrical "residue," no lingering half-life, as the generated brain current dissipates without stimulation. tDCS dose can be modeled for specific subjects and targets in ways not possible with other

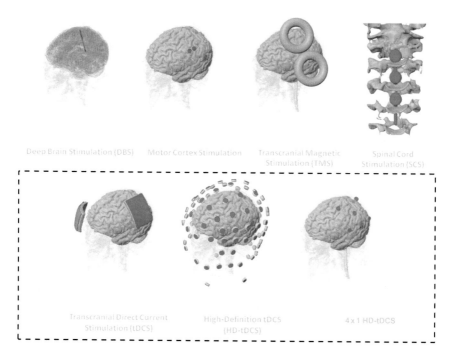

FIGURE 4.1   **Comparable stimulation techniques.** Deep brain stimulation, motor cortex stimulation, transcranial magnetic stimulation, and spinal cord stimulation (top row); classic transcranial direct current stimulation (tDCS) via sponge pads, optimized high definition-tDCS (HD-tDCS), and 4 × 1 HD-tDCS (bottom row). Transcranial direct current stimulation is an increasingly popular investigational form of brain stimulation, in part due to its low cost, portability, usability, and safety. However, there are still many unanswered questions. The number of potential stimulation doses is practically limitless. Stimulation can be varied by simply changing the electric current waveform, and electrode shape, size, and position. These variations can thus be analyzed through computational modeling studies that have resulted in montages such as HD-tDCS and 4 × 1 HD-tDCS.

interventions. Specifically, the "dose" of electrotherapy (see Peterchev et al., 2011, for definition) is readily adjustable by determining the location of electrodes (which determines spatial targeting) and selecting the stimulation waveform (which determines the nature and timing of neuromodulation). Indeed, a single programmable electrotherapy device can be simply configured to provide a diversity of dosages. Though this flexibility underpins the utility of neuromodulation, the myriad of potential dosages (stimulator settings and combinations of electrode placements) makes it difficult to readily ascertain the optimal choice. The essential issue in dose design is to relate each externally controlled dose with the associated brain regions targeted (and spared) by the resulting current flow – and hence the desired clinical outcome. Computational forward models aim to provide precisely these answers to the first part of this

Rational Neuromodulation

Application/outcome specific
neuropsychiatric, rehabilitation, cognitive
performance
Individualized therapy
customized & tune-able
Targeted brain modulation
space + time
Safe
reversible, no residue, minimal complications +
counter-indications
Cost/access
multi-use, production, treatment infrastructure

Pharmacological activity
(efficacy & safety) is determined ◀▶
by drug concentration at tissue

Clinical dose is set by
systemic application
(pills)

Electrical activity
(efficacy & safety) is determined ◀▶
by electric fields at tissue

Clinical dose is set by
systemic application
(stimulators & pads/coils)

Computational models are critical tools for clinicians to understand and improve the neuromodulation outcomes	Computational models predict the electric field generated across the brain for a *specific* stimulation configuration or setting

FIGURE 4.2   **Role of computational models in rational electrotherapy.** (Left) Neuromodulation is a promising therapeutic modality, as it affects the brain in a way not possible with other techniques with a high degree of individualized optimization. The goal of computational models is to assist clinicians in leveraging the power and flexibility of neuromodulation (right). Computational forward models are used to predict brain current flow during transcranial stimulation to guide clinical practice. As with pharmacotherapy, electrotherapy dose is controlled by the operator and leads to a complex pattern of internal current flow that is described by the model. In this way, clinicians can apply computational models to determine which dose will activate (or avoid) brain regions of interest.

question (Fig. 4.2), and thus need to be leveraged in the rational design, interpretation, and optimization of neuromodulation.

The precise pattern of current flow through the brain is determined not only by the stimulation dose (e.g., the positions of the electrodes) but also by the underlying anatomy and tissue properties. In predicting brain current flow using computational models, it is thus important to model precisely both the stimulation itself and the relevant anatomy upon which it is delivered on an individual basis. The latter issue remains an area of ongoing technical development, and is critical to establishing the clinical utility of these models. For example, cerebral spinal fluid (CSF) is highly conductive (a preferred "super highway" for current flow) such that details of CSF architecture profoundly shape current flow through adjacent brain regions (see later discussion).

Especially relevant for rehabilitative applications is the recognition that individual anatomical idiosyncrasies can result in significant distortions in current flow. This is apparent when skull defects and brain lesions occur. The final section of this review highlights the nature and degree of distortions in brain current flow produced by defects and lesions, as well as dose considerations for susceptible populations such as children.

METHODS AND PROTOCOLS IN THE GENERATION OF COMPUTATIONAL FORWARD MODELS OF tDCS

This is the first of two sections aimed at outlining the technical steps and principles of computational models for tDCS, and so aimed primarily at engineers and programmers developing these tools. Clinicians and experimentalists interested in understanding the technical challenges and limitations of modeling would also benefit from these sections, but may otherwise continue to the final four sections on using models in clinical practice and case examples.

During tDCS, current is generated in the brain. Because different electrode montages result in distinct brain current flow, researchers and clinicians can adjust the montage to target or avoid specific brain regions in an application-specific manner. Though tDCS montage design often follows basic rules of thumb (e.g., increased/decreased excitability under the anode/cathode electrode), computational forward models of brain current flow provide a more accurate insight into detailed current flow patterns, and in some cases can even challenge simplified electrode-placement assumptions. For example, clinical studies are often designed by placing the anode electrode directly over the target region desired to be excited, while the cathode electrode is placed over a region far removed from the target, to avoid unwanted reverse effects. This region could be the contralateral hemisphere or, in some cases, even extracephalic locations like the neck, shoulder, or arm. Researchers have used smaller stimulation-electrode sizes and bigger reference-electrode sizes to offset the focality limitations of tDCS. With the increased recognized value of computational forward models in informing tDCS montage design and interpretation of results, there have been recent advances in modeling tools and a greater proliferation of publications (Bikson, Datta, Rahman, & Scaturro, 2010; DaSilva et al., 2012; Datta, Elwassif, Battaglia, & Bikson, 2008, 2010, 2011; Datta, Baker, Bikson, & Fridriksson, 2011; Datta, Bikson, & Fregni, 2010; Datta, Elwassif, & Bikson, 2009; Halko et al., 2011; Mendonca et al., 2011; Miranda, Lomarev, & Hallett, 2006, Miranda, Faria, & Hallett, 2009; Oostendorp et al., 2008; Parazzini, Fiocchi, Rossi, Paglialonga, & Ravazzani, 2011; Sadlier, Vannorsdall, Schretlen, & Gordon, 2010; Salvador, Mekonnen, Ruffini, & Miranda, 2010; Suh, Kim, Lee, & Kim, 2009; Turkeltaub et al., 2011; Wagner et al., 2007).

Miranda et al. (2006) was the first numerical modeling effort specifically looking at tDCS montages and intensities. In another spherical head paper, focality of cortical electrical fields was compared across various small electrode configurations and configurations proposed to achieve targeted modulation (Datta et al., 2008). Wagner et al. (2007) was the first CAD (Computer Aided Design)-rendered head model where current density distributions were analyzed for various montages including healthy versus cortical stroke conditions. The more recent efforts have been mostly MRI derived. Oostendorp et al. (2008) was the first to consider anisotropy in the skull and the white matter; Datta et al. built the first high-resolution head model with gyri/sulci specificity (Datta, Bansal, et al., 2009); Suh et al. (2009) concluded that skull anisotropy causes a large shunting effect and may shift the stimulated areas;

Sadleir et al. (2010) compared modeling predictions of frontal tDCS montages to clinical outcomes; Datta et al. (2010) studied the effect of tDCS montages on TBI and skull defects; Parazzini et al. (2011) was the first to analyze current flow patterns across subcortical structures; and Dmochowski, Datta, Bikson, Su, and Parra (2011) showed how a multi-electrode stimulation can be optimized for focality and intensity at the target.

Recent efforts have focused on building patient-specific models and comparing modeling predictions to experimental outcomes. In considering new electrode montages, and especially in potentially vulnerable populations (e.g., skull damage, children), forward models are the main tool used to relate the externally controllable dose parameters (e.g., electrode number, position, size, shape, current) to resulting brain current flow. While the specific software applications can vary across groups, in general the approach and workflow for model generation follow a similar pattern (Fig. 4.3).

The steps for generating high-resolution (anatomically specific) forward models of non-invasive neuromodulation are adapted from extensive prior work on computational modeling. These involve the following.

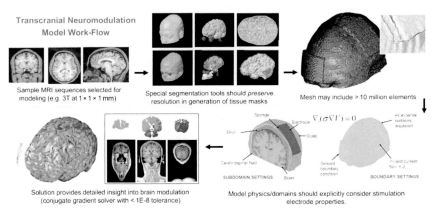

FIGURE 4.3 **Imaging and computational work-flow for the generation of high-resolution individualized models.** Though the specific processes and software packages will vary across technical groups and applications, in each case high-resolution modeling initiated with precise anatomical scans that allow demarcation of key tissues. Tissues with distinct resistivity are used to form "masks." These masks, along with the representation of the physical electrodes, are "meshed" to allow FEM calculations. The boundary conditions (generally simply reflecting how the electrodes are energized) and the governing equations (related to Ohm's law) are well established. The reproduction of the stimulation dose and the underlying anatomy thus allow for the prediction of resulting brain current. These current flow patterns are represented in a false-color map and analyzed through various post-processing tools.

1. Demarcation of individual tissue types (masks) from high-resolution anatomical data (e.g., magnetic resonance imaging slices obtained at 1-mm slice thickness) using a combination of automated and manual segmentation tools. Specifically, from the perspective of stimulating current flow, it is necessary to distinguish tissues by their resistivity. A majority of effort in the development and implementation of models has involved this step (see also next section). The number and precision of the individual masks obtained is pivotal for the generation of accurate 3D models in order to capture critical anatomical details that may influence current flow.

2. Modeling of the exact physical properties of the electrodes (e.g., shape and size) and precise placement within the segmented image data (i.e., along the skin mask outer surface).

3. Generation of accurate meshes (with a high quality factor) from the tissue/electrode masks whilst preserving resolution of subject anatomical data. The generation of meshes is a process where each mask is divided into small contiguous "elements" which allow the current flow to then be numerically computed – hence the term "finite element method" stimulations. In modern efforts, the number of elements in tDCS models can exceed 10 million.

4. Importing the resulting volumetric meshes into a commercial finite element (FE) solver.

5. Assigning resistivity to each mask (every element in each mask) and imposing boundary conditions, including the current applied to the electrodes.

6. Solving the standard Laplacian equation using the appropriate numerical solver and tolerance settings. In modern efforts the degrees of freedom can exceed 14 million.

7. Plotting the data as induced cortical electric field or current density maps (Fig. 4.3).

Though each of the above steps is required for high-resolution modeling, there remains technical expertise and hence variation in protocols across groups and publications (Bikson et al., 2010; DaSilva et al., 2012; Datta et al., 2008, 2010, 2011; Datta, Bansal, et al., 2009; Halko et al., 2011; Mendonca et al., 2011; Miranda et al., 2006, 2009; Oostendorp et al., 2008; Parazzini et al., 2011; Sadleir et al., 2010; Salvador et al., 2010; Suh et al., 2009; Turkeltaub et al., 2011; Wagner et al., 2007). These variations are relevant to clinical practice only in the sense that they change predictions in current flow that meaningfully effect dose decisions. The sources and impact of these variations are addressed in the next section.

Initial models of transcranial current flow assumed simplified geometries such as concentric spheres that could be solved analytically as well as numerically (Datta et al., 2008; Miranda et al., 2006). Such concentric sphere models are useful to address generic dose questions, such as the global role of inter-electrode distance, electrode montage, or the relationship between electrode and brain current density, precisely because they exclude regional anatomical differences. More realistic models started to include explicit representation of human anatomy (Wagner et al., 2007). Datta et al. (2009) published the first model of tDCS with gyri resolution, illustrating the importance of anatomical precision in determining complex brain current flow. Addition of diffusion tensor imaging (DTI) incorporates anisotropic properties in the skull and the white matter regions (Suh et al., 2009). Fine resolution of gyri/sulci leads to current "hotspots" in the sulci, thereby reinforcing the need for high-resolution modeling (Salvador et al., 2010). An open-source head model comprising several different tissue types was adapted to analyze current flow through cortical, subcortical, and brainstem structures (Parazzini et al., 2011). Such models help determine whether current of sufficient magnitude reaches the deeper subcortical structures.

Only a few studies have attempted to more directly link clinical outcomes and model predictions – and thus validate model utility. Clinical evaluation was combined with model predictions to investigate the effects of different montages in clinical conditions such as fibromyalgia (Mendonca et al., 2011). Patient-specific models have been used to analyze, retrospectively, the therapeutic success of a given experimental stimulation montage (Datta et al., 2011) and compare model predictions with patterns of activation revealed by functional magnetic resonance imaging (fMRI) (Halko et al., 2011). *Post-mortem* "current flow imaging" was also used to validate general model predictions (Antal et al., 2012). A focalized form of tDCS, called 4×1 High-Definition tDCS, was developed through computational models and then validated in a clinical neurophysiology trial (Kuo et al., 2012). The focal delivery of current using the 4×1 montage was further validated using supra-threshold Transcranial Electrical Stimulation (tES) pulses (Edwards et al., 2013); moreover, the models predicted individual variation in sensitivity to currents' delivery, among typical adults, of greater than two-fold. These example applications opened the door for potentially customizing tDCS on a subject to subject basis within the clinical setting (Datta, Truong, Minhas, Parra, & Bikson, 2012). Table 4.1 summarizes the various tDCS montages explored in computational modeling studies.

In a subsequent section we describe avenues for clinicians to practically access and use computational modeling tools but precisely because this is now the "standard" models approach, limitations of varied approaches need to be understood. If tDCS continues to emerge as an effective tool in clinical treatment and cognitive neuroscience, and concurrent modeling studies emphasize the need for rational (and in cases individualized) dose decisions, then it will become essential for tDCS researchers to understand

TABLE 4.1   Synopsis of Analytical and Numerical tDCS Computer Models*

Study	Masks	Electrode Montage	Additional Methods
Concentric sphere			
Miranda et al. (2006)	4	4 montages	
Datta et al. (2008)	4	6 montages	
Dmochowski, Bikson, and Parra (2012) *neuralengr.com/ spheres*	4	Arbitrary, user-specific, optimized montages	
CAD rendered			
Wagner et al. (2007)	5	Healthy and stroke models with varied montages	
MRI derived			
Oostendorp et al. (2008)	5	C3–SO montage	Anisotropic conductivities for skull and white matter. Model derived from Wolters et al. (2006)
Datta, Bansal, et al. (2009)	4	C3–SO and high-definition (HD) montages.	High resolution with gyri-sulci topography
Suh et al. (2009)	5	C3–C4 montage using point-source stimulation electrodes	Anisotropic conductivity for white matter
Datta et al. (2009)	4	Tissue temperature increases of C3–SO montage and HD montage	
Sadleir et al. (2010)	11	F3–SO and F4–SO montage and comparison to reported clinical outcomes in literature	
Datta et al. (2010)	4	Effect of skull defects and skull plates for C3–SO and O1–SO montages	
Bikson et al. (2010)	7	C3–SO and C3-contralateral mastoid	Effect of "return electrode" position and size
Salvador et al. (2010)	5	C3–SO montage	High-resolution gyri-sulci model

Continued

TABLE 4.1   Synopsis of Analytical and Numerical tDCS Computer Models—cont'd

Study	Masks	Electrode Montage	Additional Methods
Suh, Lee, Cho, Kim, and Kim (2010)	5	C3 HD-tDCS montage	Comparison of isotropy and anisotropy in white matter and skull
Parazzini et al. (2011)	26	Analysis of current flow through cortical, subcortical, and brainstem regions for C3–SO montage	Model derived from virtual family open-source database
Mendonca et al. (2011)	8	C3-extracephalic, SO-extracephalic and C3–SO montages.	Correlation of clinical effects in a fibromyalgia study with model predictions
Halko et al. (2011)	7	Oz–Cz montage	Patient-specific visual stroke model of a hemianopia patient undergoing tDCS; correlation of high-resolution current flow model predictions with fMRI
Datta et al. (2011)	8	Retrospective analysis comparing experimental outcome with model predictions; LFC-RS, LFC-contralateral mastoid, LFC-SO, and RFC-LS	Patient-specific left hemisphere stroke model of a tDCS responder
DaSilva et al. (2012)	15	C3–SO montage analysis of current flow through subcortical structures	High-resolution individualized model
Turkeltaub et al. (2011)	8	Analysis of left pTC and right pTC montage in dyslexia study	
Bonsai – Model Solution Analyzer *neuralengr.com/ bonsai*	6–8	Healthy and stroke model with varied montages	Online database of solved patient-specific head models; overlaid views of 2D MRI scans and model solutions
Dmochowski et al. (2011)	6	Healthy Head models with need-specific montages	Two distinct selections, focality-based or intensity-based
Datta et al. (2012)	8	C3–SO and HD tDCS montage	Interindividual variation across three subject-specific models

TABLE 4.1 Synopsis of Analytical and Numerical tDCS Computer Models—cont'd

Study	Masks	Electrode Montage	Additional Methods
Minhas et al. (2012)	8	C3–SO and C3 HD-tDCS montages	Pediatric Brain modeling
Truong, Magerowski, Blackburn, Bikson, and Alonso-Alonso (2013)	9	C3–SO, C3 HD-tDCS, IFG–SO montage	Comparison of five individuals of varying body mass index
Shahid, Wen, and Ahfock (2013)	9	C3–SO montage	Effect of modeling white matter anisotropy

Summary of tDCS forward head models using FEM techniques. Head models have progressed from being spherical-based to being MRI-derived. The most recent ones have employed patient-specific models. The second, third, and fourth columns list number of tissue types, the montage used, and particular model specifics, respectively.
Abbreviations: C3, C4, F3, F4, O1, Oz, Cz correspond to 10/20 EEG system; SO, contralateral supra-orbital; LFC, left frontal cortex; RFC, right frontal cortex; RS, right shoulder; LS, left shoulder; pTC, posterior temporal cortex; IFG, inferior frontal gyrus.

the applications (and limitations) of computational forward models (Borckardt et al., 2012).

PITFALLS AND CHALLENGES IN THE APPLICATION AND INTERPRETATION OF COMPUTATIONAL MODEL PREDICTIONS

Computational models of tDCS range in complexity from concentric sphere models to high-resolution models based on individuals' MRIs (as described above). The appropriate level of modeling detail depends on the clinical question being asked, as well as the available computational resources. Whereas simple geometries (e.g., spheres) may be solved analytically (Rush & Driscoll, 1968), realistic geometries employ numerical solvers, namely Finite Element Methods (FEMs). Regardless of complexity, all forward models share the goal of correctly predicting brain current flow during transcranial stimulation to guide clinical therapeutic delivery. Special effort has been recently directed towards increasing the precision of tDCS models. However, it is important to note that increased model complexity does not necessarily equate with greater accuracy or clinical value.

To meaningfully guide clinical utility, attempts to enhance model precision must rationally balance detail (i.e. complexity) and accuracy. First, beginning with high-resolution anatomical scans, the entire model workflow should preserve precision. Any human head model is limited by the precision and accuracy of tissue segmentation (i.e., "masks") and of the assigned conductivity values. One hallmark of precision is that the cortical surface used in the final FEM solver should capture realistic sulci and gyri anatomy. Models incorporating gyri-level resolution, starting with Datta et al. (Datta, Bansal, et al., 2009), clearly show that current is "clustered" in local hot spots correlated with cortical folding. Second, simultaneously, *a priori* knowledge of tissue anatomy and factors known to influence current flow should be applied to further refine segmentation. We believe that particularly critical are discontinuities not present in nature that result from limited scan resolution; notably, both unnatural perforations in planar tissues (e.g., ventricular architecture, discontinuities in CSF where brain contacts skull, misrepresented skull fissures) and microstructures (e.g., incomplete or voxelized vessels) can produce significant deviations in predicted current flow. Moreover, because of the sensitivity of current flow to any conductivity boundary, increasingly detailed segmentation (e.g., globe of the eye and related structures, glands, and deeper midbrain structures) without reliable reported human conductivity values in literature (especially at static frequency) may also lead to errors. It is worth noting that the respective contribution of the automated/manual interventions also depends on: (1) sophistication of the particular database or automated algorithm employed since they are usually not optimized for forward transcranial modeling (Datta et al., 2011), and (2) the need for identification of anomalies in suspect populations like skull defects, lesions, shunts, etc. Thus, addition of complexity without proper parameterization can evidently decrease prediction accuracy. An improper balance between these factors can introduce distortions in predicted brain current flow.

Divergent modeling methods illustrate existing outstanding issues, including:

1. Detail in physically representing the stimulation electrodes and leads, including shape and material (Datta, Bansal, et al., 2009), and energy source boundary conditions. The approach taken by our group is to model both the electrodes and electrolyte substrate, and to do so with realistic dimensions. Typical electrode/sponge sizes are either 5×5 cm (25 cm^2) or 5×7 cm (35 cm^2). Small circular high-definition (HD) electrodes and gel are also modeled to either a 1- or 2-cm radius. Anode and cathode conditions are defined as an inward current density and ground, respectively.

2. Differences between conductivity values derived from static resistivity measures and those extrapolated from 10-Hz data. The data available in literature vary from source to source in acquisition method as well as numerical value. Some data are extrapolated from low-frequency impedance rather than true DC resistance, such as that found in Gabriel, Gabriel, and Corthout (1996). The values used by our group were originally derived from averaged

values found in literature (Wagner, Zahn, Grodzinsky, & Pascual-Leone, 2004).

3. Sufficient caudal head volume representation (such that the caudal boundary condition does not affect relevant model prediction), including potential use of synthetic volumes (Datta et al., 2011; Mendonca et al., 2011).

4. Optimal imaging modalities/sequences to differentiate amongst tissue types. Typically, T1 MRIs are used to identify soft tissue such as gray and white matter, while T2 MRIs are especially usefully for fluid-filled lesions as a result of stoke, epilepsy, or traumatic brain injury. CT scans, when available, are excellent for bone and sinus cavities. As an alternative to individualized modeling, simulated MRI- and segmentation atlases-based averaged anatomical data are also available (http://brainweb.bic.mni.mcgill.ca/brainweb/).

5. Appropriate incorporation of anisotropy (from DTI) if relevant (Sadleir & Argibay, 2007; Shahid et al., 2013; Suh et al., 2009). While inclusion of anisotropy produces a numerical change in predicted current flow these changes are qualitatively far less significant than precision in anatomy and tissue conductivity; moreover, how anisotropy is implemented profoundly influences the predicted relevance of inclusion, as much as complete omission(Shahid et al., 2013).

6. Suitability of existing image segmentation algorithms (generally developed for other applications) (Smith, 2002).

7. The degree and nature of manual correction.

8. The adequacy of the numerical solver (especially when making detailed predictions at tissue boundaries). To verify precision, one can assess whether refining the mesh (e.g., doubling the number of elements) or varying the solver (either the method within one program, or comparing across program) significantly changes model predictions.

9. When modeling defects/injury, detail in segmenting true lesion borders (Datta et al., 2011) versus idealized defects.

10. The need for parametric and interindividual analysis (see below).

Optimization of the above issues remains an open question, and inevitably reflects available resources (e.g., imaging, computational, anatomical expertise) and the specific clinical question addressed in each modeling effort. Even as computational and engineering groups continue developing greater modeling sophistication, clinicians must be aware of the limitations in any modeling approach and the inevitability of technical methodology affecting the predictions made.

Having mentioned the importance of balancing increased complexity with clinical access to modeling, it is fundamental to emphasize a difference between the "value" of adding precision (complexity) as it is evaluated in engineering papers versus clinical translation. Increasingly detailed computational approaches have been proposed in recent years of varying anatomical and physiological detail (Oostendorp et al., 2008; Parazzini et al., 2011; Parazzini, Fiocchi, & Ravazzani, 2012). At the same time, computational models indicate subject-specific variability in susceptibility to the same dose (Datta et al., 2012; Shahid et al., 2013), indicating the value of individualized modeling, or at least modeling across a set of archetypes. Real clinical translational utility must therefore balance the value of increased sophistication with the cost associated with clinical scanning, computational time, and human resources/intervention (e.g., manual correction/pre- and post-processing, etc.). Thus the question is not whether "different models will yield different predictions" (as must be posed in an engineering paper), but rather does increased complexity change model predictions in a way that is clinically meaningful – that is, will complexity influence clinical decisions in study design? While this is a complex and application-specific question, a first step toward systematizing value, across a myriad of groups and efforts, is to develop a metric of change versus a simpler approach, and then apply a threshold based on perceived clinical value and added cost versus the simpler approach.

A priori, it is simplistically assumed that added detail/complexity will enhance model precision and, if done rationally, model accuracy (Bikson & Datta, 2012; Bikson, Rahman, & Datta, 2012). Though an engineering group can devote extended resources and time to a "case" modeling study, the myriad of potential electrode combinations (dose) and variation across a normal head (Datta et al., 2012) and pathological heads means that in clinical trial design the particular models will likely now be solved (e.g., 4×1 over FP3 in a female head). Moreover, while different models will yield different predictions, practical dose decision is based on a clinical study-specific criterion: "a meaningful clinical difference." Thus, two clinical applications of modeling are considered: (1) Deciding across montages – namely, which montage is expected to achieve the optimal clinical outcomes (safety/efficacy) in a given subject or on average across subjects; (2) Deciding on dose variation across subjects – namely, if and how to vary dose based on subject-specific anatomy. These aspects of using computational models in clinical practice are addressed in subsequent sections. Therefore, additional complexity and detail in model generation is only clinically meaningful if it results in a different clinical decision being made based on the model with regard to dose and/or individualization; otherwise, the additional detail is "academic" since this detail adds complexity without impacting clinical decisions.

Assuming accurate and precise representation of all tissue compartments (anatomy, resistivity, anisotropy) relevant to brain current flow, it is broadly assumed that, using modern numerical solvers, the resulting prediction is independent of the numerical technique used. Our own experience across various commercial solvers confirms this implicit assumption when meshes are of sufficient detail – precise description in methods (use of publically available programs) and representation of resulting mesh density and quality (in figures or methods), as well as tests using various solvers, provides explicit control for errors generated by the computation itself.

Literature regarding forward modeling – or, more broadly, the dissemination of modeling analysis to the clinical hands – introduces still further issues with regard to (1) interpretability, reproducibility, and accuracy (tissue masks), and (2) graphical representation of regions of influence (degree of "activation"). As there is no standard protocol for tissue imaging or segmentation, diversity in the nature of resulting tissue masks will invariably influence predicted current flow. As such, it is valuable to illustrate each 3D tissue mask in publication methods and/or classified serial sections. With regard to representation of relative activation, studies employ either maps of current density (unit of A/m^2) or electric field (unit of V/m). Because the two are related linearly by local tissue resistivity, when plotting activation in a region with uniform resistivity (for example, the cortical surface) the spatial profile is identical. When plotting activation across tissues (e.g., coronal section), current density may be advantageous to illustrate overall brain current flow. However, the electric field in the brain is directly related to neuronal activation (e.g., for varied resistivity, the electric field, but not current density, provides sufficient information to predict activation). Despite best efforts, figure preparation invariably restricts tissue mask perspectives and comprehensive display of volumetric current flow, which can be supplemented with online data publication (http://www.neuralengr.com/bonsai).

When interpreting simulation predictions, it is important to recognize that the intensity of current flow in any specific brain region does not translate in any simple (linear) manner to the degree of brain activation or modulation (even when considering current direction). Moreover, recent neurophysiological studies indicate that changes in "excitability" may not be monotonic with stimulation (Lindenberg, Zhu, & Schlaug, 2012). For example, increasing stimulation amplitude or duration can invert the direction of modulation, as can the level of neuronal background activity (Nitsche & Paulus, 2001). However, to a first approximation, it seems reasonable to predict that regions with more current flow are more likely to be "affected" by stimulation while regions with little or no current flow will be spared the direct effects of stimulation. As a first step to understanding the mechanism of action of tDCS, a relationship between model predicted regional current flow and changes in functional activation was recently demonstrated (Halko et al., 2011). The "quasi-uniform" assumption considers that if the electric field (or current density) is uniform on the scale of a region/neuron of interest, then "excitability" may be modulated with local electric field intensity (Bikson et al., 2004; see also discussion in Datta et al., 2008 and Miranda, Correia, Salvador, & Basser, 2007). Though efforts to develop suitable biophysical detailed models considering myriad neurons with distinct positions and morphologies or "continuum" approximations (Joucla & Yvert, 2009) of modulation are pending, the current state of the art requires (implicit) application of the "quasi-uniform" assumption.

Many of the theoretical and technical foundations for modeling brain stimulation were established through modeling studies on peripheral nerve stimulation (Functional Electrical Stimulation, FES) and then Spinal Cord Stimulation (SCS) and Deep Brain Stimulation (DBS) (reviewed in McIntyre, 2007; Holsheimer, 1998; Rattay, 1986). In light of the challenges to tDCS modeling cited above, we note that FES and DBS use electrodes implanted in the body such that relatively small volume of brain is needed to be modeled, and with none of the complications associated with precisely representing gross anatomy (e.g., skull, fat, CSF...). From the perspective of computational burden, the volume, number of masks, and mask complexity results in tDCS models with > 5 million elements, compared to < 200,000 elements for FES and DBS models. In addition, FES and DBS are suprathreshold, allowing modeling studies to represent simply demarcated "regions of influence" inside which action potentials are triggered. tDCS affects large areas of superficial and deep brain structures (many types of cells and processes) and is subthreshold, interacting with ongoing activity rather than driving action potentials, making it challenging to simply delineate "black-and-white" regions of influence.

Forward modeling studies and analysis are often published as "case reports" with predictions only on a single head (Mendonca et al., 2011; Parazzini et al., 2011; Salvador et al., 2010; Turkeltaub et al., 2011). The suitability of single-subject analysis reflects available (limited) resources and the clinical question being addressed. For a given electrode montage and stimulation dose, the sensitivity of global brain current to normal variation in anatomy (including across ages, gender) is unknown; however, high-resolution modeling suggests gyri-specific dispersion of current flow, which could potentially account for individual variability. More generally, gross differences in tissue dimensions, notably skull thickness and CSF architecture, are expected to influence current flow. In some cases, modeling efforts specifically address the role of individual anatomical pathology, such as skull defects (Datta et al., 2010) or brain lesions (Datta et al., 2011); it is precisely because these studies have shown the importance of specific defect/lesion details, that findings cannot be arbitrarily generalized. This in turn stresses the importance of individualized modeling, as illustrated in the next section.

Though this section has focused on the technical features of modeling, there is a broader concern in promoting effective collaboration between engineers and clinicians. For analogy, clinicians are generally aware of the challenges and pitfalls in post-processing and feature-selection of fMRI data, and indeed are thus intimately involved in data analysis rather than blindly relying on a technician. For computational "forward" models of neuromodulation, where results may inform study design and patient treatment, it is evidently as important to consider the uses and technical limitations of modeling approaches, and vigilance and skepticism on the part of clinicians will only enhance model rigor. Critically, for this reason, clinician/investigator experience and "judgment" supersedes all model predictions, even as these models form one important tool in dose design.

USE OF COMPUTATIONAL MODELS IN CLINICAL PRACTICE

Consideration for Efficacy

Before beginning our sections regarding consideration for clinical practice, we note that the ability of clinicians to leverage computational models is limited by access to modeling tools. For clinicians who are interested in using computational forward models to inform study design or interpretation but do not have the time and resources to establish an independent modeling program (e.g., hire engineers), several options are available:

1. Collaboration with a modeling group (Turkeltaub et al., 2011) or a company can allow for customized exploration of montage options.
2. Existing published reports or databases (Table 4.1; www.neuralengr.com/bonsai) can be referenced for comparable montages (with careful consideration of the role of individual variation and other caveats presented in the next section).
3. With some coding experience, a novel process where a desired brain region can be selected and the optimized electrode montage is proposed within a single step (Dmochowski et al., 2011) can be used.
4. A GUI-based program to stimulate arbitrary electrode montages in a spherical model is now available (www.neuralengr.com/spheres).

The latter solution illustrates an important trend: even as increasingly complex and resource-expensive modeling tools are being developed, parallel efforts to simplify and automate (high-throughput) model workflow are needed to facilitate clinical translation.

With regard to efficacy, it is typically the case that scientists and clinicians identify one or more brain regions that they wish to modulate (e.g., based on fMRI and prior behavioral studies (Bikson, Rahman, Datta, Fregni, & Merabet, 2012; Coffman, Trumbo, & Clark, 2012; Dmochowski et al., 2013; Medina et al., 2013; Turkeltaub et al., 2012), and typically this modulation is expressed as a desire to enhance or inhibit function in the region. While this is a starting point for rational dose optimization using computational models, several additional parameters and constraints need to be specified.

A central issue relates to the concern, if any, about current flow through other brain regions. In one extreme, current flow through other regions outside of those targeted is considered unimportant for trial outcomes; in such a case, the optimization would be for intensity at the target while ignoring details of current flow through other brain regions. Conversely, the requirement may be to minimize current flow through all other brain regions while maximizing current flow intensity in the targeted brain region; in this case, the optimization would be for focality. The reason this distinction between optimization for intensity and optimization for focality is so critical is that it produces highly divergent "best" dose solutions (Dmochowski et al., 2011). Optimization for intensity often produces a bipolar (one anode and one cathode) montage across the head; such montages typically produce broad current flow across both the target and other brain regions. Optimization for focality typically produces a "ring" montage (with one polarity surrounded by another, analogous to the HD-tDCS 4×1 [Datta, Bansal, et al., 2009]) that spares much of the brain regions outside of the target but also produces less relative current flow at the target than does optimization for intensity. Practically, though distinctions between optimization for intensity and optimization for focality must be made, the (iterative) process of dose optimization may be subtler. Certain brain regions outside of the target may be "neutral" regarding collateral stimulation, others may be "avoid" regions, and others may in fact be considered "beneficial" to the outcomes. The best montage therefore is highly dependent on both the trial design outcomes and the experimenter's opinion on how distinct brain regions are implicated.

A second critical parameter to consider in trial design is the desired electric field intensity at the target(s). As emphasized throughout this review, optimization based on the electric field at the target is expected to produce more consistent outcomes then optimization by external current intensity. Nonetheless, an experimenter may choose to select a current level (e.g., 1 mA, 2 mA) simply because of historical experience and trends. It is important to emphasize that, at least for neurophysiological measures (such as transcranial magnetic stimulation, TMS) and likely for behavioral and clinical outcomes, the relationship between current and outcomes is not linear and not necessarily monotonic (Batsikadze, Moliadze, Paulus, Kuo, & Nitsche, 2013; Weiss & Lavidor, 2012) – meaning that reversing current direction (at the level of electrodes and the brain) may not reverse the direction of change, and increasing current intensity may not increase (and can even reverse) the direction of change. The effects of stimulation may vary with the brain region (e.g., prefrontal may not respond as motor) or the state of that region (e.g., is there ongoing activity [due to a concurrent task] or pathology [due to injury or disease; Hasan et al., 2013]?) in ways that remain poorly understood. In general, more applied current does not necessarily mean more brain changes, and thus the decision regarding what current intensity is desired is a complex and critical one for outcomes. The same challenges apply to selecting a desired brain electric field where a higher electric field at a target may not produce increased neuromodulation or more of the type of change desired; moreover, increasing electric-field intensity at the target by increasing applied current will increase electric field intensity at every other brain region proportionally. Finally, the orientation of the electric field at the target may be critical, and, depending on the orientation, different montages may be considered.

Though the above paints an increasingly complex picture of dose optimization in tDCS, it may be unwise to simply ignore these issues and use "historical" montages (e.g., whatever is popular in the literature) and not leverage computational models to the extent possible to optimize dose. In the face of complexity (and risk), experimenters may wish simply to revert to using what has already been reported as successful in the literature, but such an approach seems inconsistent with broader efforts to advance the field, especially when these previous approaches did not involve optimization (and indeed a very limited set of montages are used across highly disparate indications). Nonetheless, given the complexity and unknowns, historical montages do represent a good starting point for dose optimization. Practically, we recommend that the optimization process begins by simulating previously used successful and unsuccessful montages to consider the brain current flow patterns generated in each case; it is against these standard montages that any optimized montage can be compared.

Safety parameters provide additional constraint parameters for optimization, as discussed below.

CONSIDERATION FOR SAFETY

Computational models also provide a tool to support assessment of safety. tDCS is considered a well-tolerated technique (Brunoni et al., 2012), but vigilance is always warranted with an investigational tool; moreover, given that most montages produce current flow through many brain regions, combined with the desire to explore increasing intensities and durations/repetitions of treatment, as well as stimulation in susceptible subjects (e.g., children), computational models (though only predictions) provide quantitative methods to increase confidence and identify hazards.

We distinguish effects at the skin (which relate largely to electrode design/electrochemical issues and electrode current density) from effects at the brain (which relate to electric fields in the brain) (Bikson, Datta, & Elwassif, 2009). Computational models predict current flow at both the skin and the brain. Often, dose design simply avoids crossing (or even approaching) a threshold for intensity in any given region both inside and outside the target. This threshold is often based on historical approaches. Here, the distinction between dose optimization based only on stimulation parameters (e.g., total current) versus brain electric field (with leveraged computational models) is evident. Maintaining applied current (e.g., 1 mA) but changing electrode montage and/or subject inclusion (e.g., skull defects) may profoundly change current density/electric field in the skin and brain. Computational models are thus useful to relate new montages/approaches to historically safe ones. It is often the case that even when current density/electric field is predicted, the experimenter still used the upper limit of applied current. Thus, maximum current density/electric field and maximum current intensity become constraints in the efficacy optimization process.

CONSIDERATION FOR INDIVIDUAL DOSE TITRATION

There are two general uses for computational models in designing rational experiments and clinical trials. The first is the selection of the best generic dose as discussed above. The second point to consider is whether and how to customize doses to individual subjects. Even across normal healthy adults there is a $>2\times$ difference in the electric field generated in the brain for a given applied current (Datta et al., 2012; Edwards et al., 2013). This variation is potentially profoundly significant when considering that two-fold changes in applied current can invert the direction of change (see above). Therefore, anatomical differences, even across healthy adults, may explain some of the known variation in existing tDCS studies, and normalizing for brain electric field across subjects, by leveraging computational models, may in part correct for individual differences.

When considering extremes of age (Minhas, Bikson, Woods, Rosen, & Kessler, 2012) or body mass (Truong, Magerowski, Pascual-Leone, Alonso-Alonso, & Bikson, 2012), or the presence of variable brain or skull injuries (Datta et al., 2010), the potential for individual differences to influence current flow increases (Dmochowski et al., 2013). While it is not unusual for tDCS montages to be changed based on individual disease etiology (e.g., stroke location), this is often done using basic rules of thumb (e.g., position the "active" electrode over the brain region), which may not always produce the desired brain current flow (Datta et al., 2011).

The need to normalize (wide) individual variations in response to tDCS is universally recognized (along with the desire to increase efficacy), and it is rational that normalizing the brain electric field should help to reduce variability, since the brain electric field determines outcomes. Yet the use of computational models for individual optimization is rare, and limited by accessibility to rapid modeling tools.

We note that the value of individualization is evident in TMS studies in the visual and motor domains, where it is almost unheard of to apply the same intensity across subjects. It is no less important in tDCS, but because tDCS does not produce an overt physiological response such as TMS does, computational models are valuable tools to individualize doses.

EXAMPLE RESULTS OF COMPUTATIONAL ANALYSIS IN SUSCEPTIBLE POPULATIONS

We conclude this chapter with some case studies to illustrate the application of computational models for informing clinical guidelines.

Case 1: Skull Defects

There is interest in the application of tDCS during rehabilitation of patients with brain lesions or skull defects (i.e., with or without skull plates) – for example, subjects with traumatic brain injury (TBI) or patients undergoing neurosurgery. As some of the neurological sequelae are presumably consequences of disrupted cortical activity following the traumatic event, the use of tDCS to deliver current to both damaged and compensatory regions in such circumstances can be a useful tool to reactivate and restore activity in essential neural networks associated with cognitive or motor processing. In addition, because of the reported anti-seizure effects of tDCS (Fregni et al., 2006), this technique might be useful for patients with refractory epilepsy who have undergone surgery and have skull plates or decompressive craniectomy for trauma and cerebro-vascular disease.

Despite rational incentives for investigation of tDCS in TBI or patients with other major neurological deficits and skull defects, one perceived limitation for the use of tDCS in these patients is the resulting modification of current flow by the skull defects and the presence of surgical skull plates. Modeling studies can provide insight into how skull defects and skull plates would affect current flow through the brain, and how to modify tDCS dose and/or electrode locations in such cases (Fig. 4.4, adapted from Datta et al., 2010). For example, a skull defect (craniotomy) that is filled with relatively highly conductive fluid or tissue represents a "shunt"

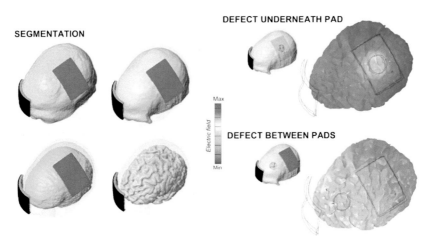

FIGURE 4.4 **Computational model of current flow in subjects with skull defects/ plates.** A defect in skull tissue, which is the most resistive tissue in the head, would hypothetically affect current flow in the underlying brain regions. Furthermore, the exact location of the defect (under/between the stimulation pads) in combination with the "material" filling up the defect with the stimulation montage employed will influence induced current flow. Sample segmentation masks are shown on the left. A small defect under the anode pad (top right) leads to current flow in the cortex restricted to directly under the defect (avoiding the intermediate regions). A similar sized defect placed between the pads (bottom right) does not significantly alter current flow patterns in comparison with a healthy head with no defects. *Figure adapted from Datta et al. (2010).*

pathway for current entering the brain, but in a manner highly dependent on defect position relative to electrode montage. In such cases, the underlying cortex would then be exposed to a higher intensity of focused current flow. This in turn might be either beneficial in targeting the underlying brain region, or hazardous if the increased current levels resulted in undesired neurophysiologic or pathological changes. Our modeling results confirm the notion that skull defects and skull plates can change the distribution of the current flow induced in cortical areas by tDCS. However, the details of current modulation depend entirely on the combination of electrode configuration and nature of the defect/ plate, thus indicating the importance of individual analysis. Based on model predictions, application of tDCS without accounting for skull defects can lead to suboptimal and undesired brain current.

Case 2: Brain Lesions (Stroke)

Transcranial DCS has been shown to modulate cognitive, linguistic, and motor performance in both healthy and neurologically impaired individuals, with results supporting the feasibility of leveraging interactions between stimulation-induced neuromodulation and task executio emphasized throughout this review, electrode montage (i.e., the position and size of electrodes) determines the resulting brain current flow and, as a result, neurophysiological effects. The ability to customize tDCS treatment through electrode montage provides clinical flexibility and the potential to individualize therapies. However, while numerous reports have been published in recent years demonstrating the effects of tDCS upon task performance, there remain fundamental questions about the optimal design of electrode configuration, especially around lesioned tissue (Datta et al., 2011; Fridriksson, 2011). Several modeling studies have predicted a profound influence of stroke-related brain lesions on resulting brain current produced by tDCS (Datta et al., 2011; Halko et al., 2011; Wagner et al., 2007).

Fig. 4.5 illustrates an example of predicted current flow during tDCS from two subjects with a lesion due to stroke located within the motor-frontal cortex (A) and occipital cortex (B) (adapted from Datta et al., 2011 and Halko et al., 2011). Computational modeling suggests that current flow pattern during tDCS may be significantly altered by the presence of the lesion as compared to intact neurological tissue. Importantly, significant changes in the resulting cortical electric fields were observed not just around peri-lesional regions but also within wider cortical regions beyond the location of the electrodes. In a sense, the lesion itself acts as a "virtual" electrode modulating the overall current flow pattern (Datta et al., 2011).

Case 3: Pediatric Populations

There is increasing interest in the use of neuromodulation in pediatric populations for a range of indications, including rehabilitation, cognitive performance, and epilepsy treatment (Krause & Cohen Kadosh, 2013; Mattai et al., 2011; Schneider & Hopp, 2011; Varga et al., 2011). However, a rational protocol/guideline for the use of tDCS on children has not been formally established. Previous modeling studies have shown that current flow behavior is dependent on *both* the tDCS dose (montage and current intensity) and the underlying brain anatomy. Because of anatomical differences (skull thickness, CSF volume, and gray/white matter volume) between a growing child and an adult, it is expected that the resulting brain current intensity in a child would be different as compared to that in an adult. Evidently, it would not be prudent to adjust the stimulation dose for children through an arbitrary rule of thumb (e.g., reduce electrode size and current intensity by the ratio of head diameter). Again, computational forward models provide direct insight into the relation between external tDCS dose and resulting brain current, and thus can

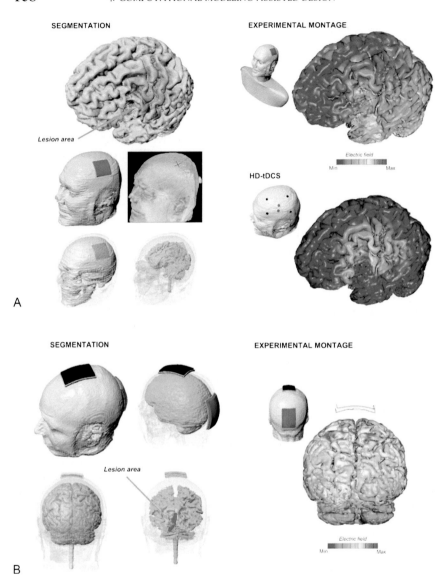

FIGURE 4.5 **Computational models predict current flow during tDCS in subjects with lesions.** Brain lesions, as occur during stroke, are considered to be largely cannibalized and replaced by CSF, which is significantly more conductive than brain. For this reason, brain current flow during tDCS is expected to be altered. (A) Patient-specific left hemisphere stroke model. Two stimulation montages are illustrated: a conventional sponge montage (top right), and a high-definition montage (bottom right). (B) Patient-specific visual stroke model. Segmentation masks (left) and induced current flow using the experimental montage (right).

M1-Supraorbital

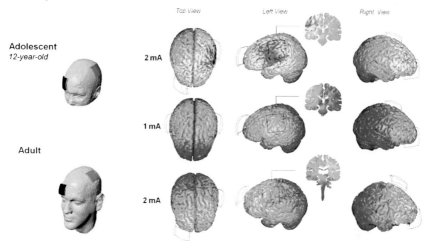

FIGURE 4.6   Individualized head model of two adolescents as compared to an adult: induced current flow for motor cortex tDCS at different intensities. 1 mA of stimulation in the adolescent is similar to 2 mA of stimulation in an adult.

inform dose design in children. Fig. 4.6 shows an example of a model of tDCS in a 12-year-old compared to a standard adult model. Both the peak and spatial distributions of current in the brain are altered compared to the typical adult case. In fact, for this particular case, the peak electric fields, at a given intensity, were nearly double in the 12-year-old as compared to the adult. Though questions remain about the impact of gross anatomical differences (e.g., as a function of age or gender) in altering generated brain current flow during neuromodulation, computational "forward" models provide direct insight into this question, and may ultimately be used to rationally adjust stimulation dose.

Case 4: Obese Populations

Montages that have been evaluated for pain, depression, or appetite suppression have been modeled in average adults, but unique challenges exist in the obese model (Fig. 4.7, adapted from Truong et al., 2012). The additional subcutaneous fat present in the obese model warranted an additional layer of complexity beyond the commonly used five-tissue model (skin, skull, CSF, gray matter, white matter). Including fat in the model of a super-obese subject led to an increase in cortical electric field magnitude of approximately 60 percent compared to the model without

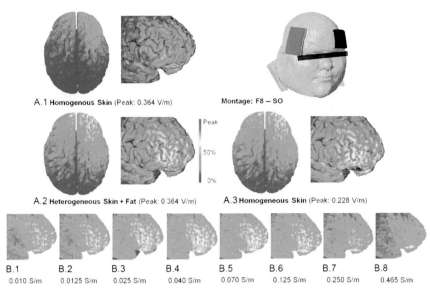

FIGURE 4.7 **Predicted cortical electric field during inferior prefrontal cortex stimulation via 5″ × 7″ pads.** Two conditions, homogenous skin (A.1) and heterogeneous skin (A.2), are contrasted on the same scale (0.364 V/m per mA peak). The homogeneous skin condition is displayed (A.3) at a lowered scale (0.228 V/m per mA peak) to compare the spatial distribution to the heterogeneous condition (A.2). The effect due to a range of varying fat conductivities (B.1–B.8) is compared on a fixed scale (0.364 V/m per mA peak). The conductivity of fat (0.025 S/m) is within an "optimum" range of influence that causes an increase in peak cortical electric field when included. *Figure adapted from Truong et al. (2012).*

fat (Fig. 4.7A.1–A.3). A shift was also seen in the spatial distribution of the cortical electric field, most noticeably on the orbito-frontal cortex.

To gain an intuition regarding how subcutaneous fat influences the cortical electric field and current density, additional models examined a range of conductivity values from the conductivity of skull (0.010 S/m, Fig. 4.7B.1) to the conductivity of skin (0.465 S/m, Figure 4.7B.8). Coincidentally, the conductivity commonly used for fat (0.025 S/m, Fig. 4.7B.4) was in the range that causes a peak increase in cortical electric field magnitude. It was postulated that more current was blocked by subcutaneous fat at an extremely low conductivity (4.7B.1), while more current was redirected at an extremely high conductivity. This, in effect, led to an "optimum" range of influence where the conductivity of fat is believed to reside.

Ultimately, the need to precisely parameterize models rests hand in hand with the intended use of the model. From an engineering perspective, the increased complexity of this model caused a noteworthy change within the subject modeled, but this change would not be clinically noteworthy if the stimulation dose were not to change from subject to subject. This clinical analysis requires an additional comparison between subjects, and consideration of the wide variation already inherent in "typical" subjects (Datta et al., 2012). What can be concluded, however, is that a comparison between models would require consistent parameterization of subcutaneous fat.

Case Design

These cases demonstrate the potentially profound influence of lesions and skull defects on resulting current flow, as well as the need to customize tDCS montages to gross individual head dimensions. If tDCS continues to become a viable option for treatment in cases such as chronic stroke, the consideration of tDCS-induced current flow through the brain is of fundamental importance for the identification of candidates, optimization of electrotherapies for specific brain targets, and interpretation of patient-specific results. Thus, the ability and value of individualized tDCS therapy must be leveraged. Whereas tDCS electrode montages are commonly designed using "gross" intuitive general rules (e.g., anode electrode positioned "over" the target region), the value of applying predictive modeling as one tool in the rational design of safe and effective electrotherapies is becoming increasingly recognized.

Electrode montage (i.e., the position and size of electrodes) determines the resulting brain current flow and, as a result, neurophysiological effects. The ability to customize tDCS treatment through electrode montage provides clinical flexibility and the potential to individualize therapies (Bikson et al., 2010; Datta et al., 2011; Mendonca et al., 2011). However, while numerous reports have been published in recent years demonstrating the effects of tDCS upon task performance, there remain fundamental questions about the optimal design of electrode configurations, with computational "forward" models playing a pivotal role.

CONCLUSION

While numerous published reports have demonstrated the beneficial effects of tDCS upon task performance, fundamental questions remain regarding the optimal electrode configuration on the scalp. Moreover, it is expected that individual anatomical differences, in the extreme case manifest as skull defects and lesioned brain tissue, will consequently influence current flow and should therefore be considered (and perhaps leveraged) in the optimization of neuromodulation therapies. Variance in clinical responses may result from many sources, but the alteration of brain current flow due to both normal and pathological causes can be elucidated through computational "forward" models, which can then be leveraged to individualized therapy.

References

Antal, A., Bikson, M., Datta, A., Lafon, B., Dechent, P., Parra, L. C., et al. (2012). Imaging artifacts induced by electrical stimulation during conventional fMRI of the brain. *NeuroImage*. http://dx.doi.org/10.1016/j.neuroimage.2012.10.026.

Ardolino, G., Bossi, B., Barbieri, S., & Priori, A. (2005). Non-synaptic mechanisms underlie the after-effects of cathodal transcutaneous direct current stimulation of the human brain. *Journal of Physiology, 568,* 653–663.

Batsikadze, G., Moliadze, V., Paulus, W., Kuo, M. F., & Nitsche, M. A. (2013). Partially nonlinear stimulation intensity-dependent effects of direct current stimulation on motor cortex excitability in humans. *The Journal of Physiology, 591*(Pt 7), 1987–2000.

Bikson, M., & Datta, A. (2012). Guidelines for precise and accurate computational models of tDCS. *Brain Stimulation, 5*(3), 430–431.

Bikson, M., Datta, A., & Elwassif, M. (2009). Establishing safety limits for transcranial direct current stimulation. *Clinical Neurophysiology, 120*(6), 1033–1034.

Bikson, M., Datta, A., Rahman, A., & Scaturro, J. (2010). Electrode montages for tDCS and weak transcranial electrical stimulation: Role of "return" electrode's position and size. *Clinical Neurophysiology, 121*(12), 1976–1978.

Bikson, M., Inoue, M., Akiyama, H., Deans, J. K., Fox, J. E., Miyakawa, H., et al. (2004). Effects of uniform extracellular DC electric fields on excitability in rat hippocampal slices *in vitro. Journal of Physiology, 557,* 175–190.

Bikson, M., Rahman, A., & Datta, A. (2012). Computational models of transcranial direct current stimulation. *Clinical EEG and Neuroscience, 43*(3), 176–183.

Bikson, M., Rahman, A., Datta, A., Fregni, F., & Merabet, L. (2012). High-resolution modeling assisted design of customized and individualized transcranial direct current stimulation protocols. *Neuromodulation, 15*(4), 306–315.

Borckardt, J., Bikson, M., Frohman, H., Reeves, S., Datta, A., Bansal, V., et al. (2012). A pilot study of the tolerability, safety and effects of high-definition transcranial direct current stimulation (HD-tDCS) on pain perception. *The Journal of Pain, 13*(2), 112–120.

Brunoni, A. R., Nitsche, M. A., Bolognini, N., Bikson, M., Wagner, T., Merabet, L., et al. (2012). Clinical research with transcranial direct current stimulation (tDCS): Challenges and future directions. *Brain Stimulation, 5*(3), 175–195.

Coffman, B. A., Trumbo, M. C., & Clark, V. P. (2012). Enhancement of object detection with transcranial direct current stimulation is associated with increased attention. *BMC Neuroscience, 13,* 108.

DaSilva, A., Zaghi, S., Lopes, M., DosSantos, M., Spierings, E., Bajwa, Z., et al. (2012). tDCS-induced analgesia and electrical fields in pain-related neural networks in chronic migraine. *Headache, 52,* 1283–1295.

Datta, A., Baker, J. M., Bikson, M., & Fridriksson, J. (2011). Individualized model predicts brain current flow during transcranial direct-current stimulation treatment in responsive stroke patient. *Brain Stimulation, 4*(3), 169–174.

Datta, A., Bansal, V., Diaz, J., Patel, J., Reato, D., & Bikson, M. (2009). Gyri-precise head model of transcranial direct current stimulation: Improved spatial focality using a ring electrode versus conventional rectangular pad. *Brain Stimulation, 2,* 201–207.

Datta, A., Bikson, M., & Fregni, F. (2010). Transcranial direct current stimulation in patients with skull defects and skull plates: High-resolution computational FEM study of factors altering cortical current flow. *NeuroImage, 52*(4), 1268–1278.

Datta, A., Elwassif, M., Battaglia, F., & Bikson, M. (2008). Transcranial current stimulation focality using disc and ring electrode configurations: FEM analysis. *Journal of Neural Engineering, 5*(2), 163–174.

Datta, A., Elwassif, M., & Bikson, M. (2009). Bio-heat transfer model of transcranial DC stimulation: Comparison of conventional pad versus ring electrode. *Conference proceedings: . . . Annual International Conference of the IEEE Engineering in Medicine and Biology, 2009,* 670–673.

Datta, A., Truong, D., Minhas, P., Parra, L. C., & Bikson, M. (2012). Inter-individual variation during transcranial direct current stimulation and normalization of dose using MRI-derived computational models. *Front in Psychiatry*, 3, 91.

Dmochowski, J. P., Bikson, M., & Parra, L. C. (2012). The point spread function of the human head and its implications for transcranial current stimulation. *Physics in Medicine and Biology*, 57(20), 6459–6477.

Dmochowski, J. P., Datta, A., Bikson, M., Su, Y., & Parra, L. C. (2011). Optimized multi-electrode stimulation increases focality and intensity at target. *Journal of Neural Engineering*, 8(4), 046011.

Dmochowski, J. P., Datta, A., Huang, Y., Richardson, J. D., Bikson, M., Fridriksson, J., et al. (2013). Targeted transcranial direct current stimulation for rehabilitation after stroke. *NeuroImage*, 75, 12–19.

Edwards, D., Cortes, M., Datta, A., Minhas, P., Wassermann, E. M., & Bikson, M. (2013). Physiological and modeling evidence for focal transcranial electrical brain stimulation in humans: A basis for high-definition tDCS. *NeuroImage*, 74, 266–275.

Edwards, D. J., Krebs, H. I., Rykman, A., Zipse, J., Thickbroom, G. W., Mastaglia, F. L., et al. (2009). Raised corticomotor excitability of M1 forearm area following anodal tDCS is sustained during robotic wrist therapy in chronic stroke. *Restorative Neurology and Neuroscience*, 27(3), 199–207.

Fregni, F., Thome-Souza, S., Nitsche, M. A., Freedman, S. D., Valente, K. D., & Pascual-Leone, A. (2006). A controlled clinical trial of cathodal DC polarization in patients with refractory epilepsy. *Epliepsia*, 47(2), 335–342.

Fridriksson, J. (2011). Measuring and inducing brain plasticity in chronic aphasia. (Research Support, N.I.H., Extramural Review). *Journal of Communication Disorders*, 44 (5), 557–563.

Gabriel, C., Gabriel, S., & Corthout, E. (1996). The dielectric properties of biological tissues: I. Literature survey. *Physics in Medicine and Biology*, 41(11), 2231–2249.

Halko, M. A., Datta, A., Plow, E. B., Scaturro, J., Bikson, M., & Merabet, L. B. (2011). Neuroplastic changes following rehabilitative training correlate with regional electrical field induced with tDCS. *NeuroImage*, 57(3), 885–891.

Hasan, A., Misewitsch, K., Nitsche, M. A., Gruber, O., Padberg, F., Falkai, P., et al. (2013). Impaired motor cortex responses in non-psychotic first-degree relatives of schizophrenia patients: A cathodal tDCS pilot study. *Brain Stimulation*, 6(5), 821–829.

Holsheimer, J. (1998). Computer modelling of spinal cord stimulation and its contribution to therapeutic efficacy. *Spinal Cord*, 36(8), 531–540.

Joucla, S., & Yvert, B. (2009). The "mirror" estimate: An intuitive predictor of membrane polarization during extracellular stimulation. (Research Support, Non-U.S. Gov't). *Biophysical Journal*, 96(9), 3495–3508.

Krause, B., & Cohen Kadosh, R. (2013). Can transcranial electrical stimulation improve learning difficulties in atypical brain development? A future possibility for cognitive training. *Developmental Cognitive Neuroscience*. http://dx.doi.org/10.1016/j.dcn.2013.04.001.

Kuo, H. I., Bikson, M., Datta, A., Minhas, P., Paulus, W., Kuo, M. F., et al. (2012). Comparing cortical plasticity induced by conventional and high-definition 4 x 1 ring tDCS: A neurophysiological study. *Brain Stimulation*, 6(4), 644–648.

Lindenberg, R., Zhu, L. L., & Schlaug, G. (2012). Combined central and peripheral stimulation to facilitate motor recovery after stroke: The effect of number of sessions on outcome. *Neurorehabilitation and Neural Repair*, 26(5), 479–483.

Mattai, A., Miller, R., Weisinger, B., Greenstein, D., Bakalar, J., Tossell, J., et al. (2011). Tolerability of transcranial direct current stimulation in childhood-onset schizophrenia. *Brain Stimulation*, 4(4), 275–280.

McIntyre, C. C., Miocinovic, S., & Butson, C. R. (2007). Computational analysis of deep brain stimulation. *Expert Review of Medical Devices*, 4(5), 615–622.

Medina, J., Beauvais, J., Datta, A., Bikson, M., Coslett, H. B., & Hamilton, R. H. (2013). Transcranial direct current stimulation accelerates allocentric target detection. *Brain Stimulation, 6*(3), 433–439.

Mendonca, M. E., Santana, M. B., Baptista, A. F., Datta, A., Bikson, M., Fregni, F., et al. (2011). Transcranial DC stimulation in fibromyalgia: Optimized cortical target supported by high-resolution computational models. *Journal of Pain, 12*(5), 610–617.

Minhas, P., Bikson, M., Woods, A. J., Rosen, A. R., & Kessler, S. K. (2012). Transcranial direct current stimulation in pediatric brain: A computational modeling study. *Conference proceedings: . . . Annual International Conference of the IEEE Engineering in Medicine and Biology, 2012,* 859–862.

Miranda, P. C., Correia, L., Salvador, R., & Basser, P. J. (2007). The role of tissue heterogeneity in neural stimulation by applied electric fields. *Conference proceedings: . . . Annual International Conference of the IEEE Engineering in Medicine and Biology, 2007,* 1715–1718.

Miranda, P. C., Faria, P., & Hallett, M. (2009). What does the ratio of injected current to electrode area tell us about current density in the brain during tDCS? *Clinical Neurophysiology, 120*(6), 1183–1187.

Miranda, P. C., Lomarev, M., & Hallett, M. (2006). Modeling the current distribution during transcranial direct current stimulation. *Clinical Neurophysiology, 117*(7), 1623–1629.

Nitsche, M. A., & Paulus, W. (2001). Sustained excitability elevations induced by transcranial DC motor cortex stimulation in humans. *Neurology, 57,* 1899–1901.

Oostendorp, T. F., Hengeveld, Y. A., Wolters, C. H., Stinstra, J., van Elswijk, G., & Stegeman, D. F. (2008). Modeling transcranial DC stimulation. *Conference proceedings: . . . Annual International Conference of the IEEE Engineering in Medicine and Biology, 2008,* 4226–4229.

Parazzini, M., Fiocchi, S., & Ravazzani, P. (2012). Electric field and current density distribution in an anatomical head model during transcranial direct current stimulation for tinnitus treatment. *Bioelectromagnetics, 33*(6), 476–487.

Parazzini, M., Fiocchi, S., Rossi, E., Paglialonga, A., & Ravazzani, P. (2011). Transcranial direct current stimulation: Estimation of the electric field and of the current density in an anatomical head model. *IEEE Transactions on Bio-Medical Engineering, 58*(6), 1773–1780.

Peterchev, A., Wagner, T., Miranda, P., Nitsche, M., Paulus, W., Lisanby, S., et al. (2011). Fundamentals of transcranial electric and magnetic stimulation dose: Definition, selection, and reporting practices. *Brain Stimulation.* http://dx.doi.org/10.1016/j.brs.2011.10.001, 1 Nov.

Rattay, F. (1986). Analysis of models for external stimulation of axons. *IEEE Transactions on Biomedical Engineering, 33*(10), 974–977.

Rush, S., & Driscoll, D. A. (1968). Current distribution in the brain from surface electrodes. *Anesthesia and Analgesia, 47*(6), 717–723.

Sadleir, R., & Argibay, A. (2007). Modeling skull electrical properties. *Annals of Biomedical Engineering, 35*(10), 1699–1712.

Sadleir, R. J., Vannorsdall, T. D., Schretlen, D. J., & Gordon, B. (2010). Transcranial direct current stimulation (tDCS) in a realistic head model. *NeuroImage, 51*(4), 1310–1318.

Salvador, R., Mekonnen, A., Ruffini, G., & Miranda, P. C. (2010). Modeling the electric field induced in a high resolution head model during transcranial current stimulation. *Conference proceedings: . . . Annual International Conference of the IEEE Engineering in Medicine and Biology, 2010,* 2073–2076.

Schneider, H. D., & Hopp, J. P. (2011). The use of the bilingual aphasia test for assessment and transcranial direct current stimulation to modulate language acquisition in minimally verbal children with autism. *Clinical Linguistics & Phonetics, 25*(6–7), 640–654.

Shahid, S., Wen, P., & Ahfock, T. (2013). Numerical investigation of white matter anisotropic conductivity in defining current distribution under tDCS. *Computer Methods and Programs in Biomedicine, 109*(1), 48–64.

Smith, S. M. (2002). Fast robust automated brain extraction. (Comparative Study Research Support, Non-US Government Review). *Human Brain Mapping, 17*(3), 143–155.

Suh, H. S., Kim, S. H., Lee, W. H., & Kim, T. S. (2009). Realistic simulation of transcranial direct current stimulation via 3-D high resolution finite element analysis: Effect of tissue anisotropy. *Conference proceedings: ... Annual International Conference of the IEEE Engineering in Medicine and Biology, 2009,* 638–641.

Suh, H. S., Lee, W. H., Cho, Y. S., Kim, J. H., & Kim, T. S. (2010). Reduced spatial focality of electrical field in tDCS with ring electrodes due to tissue anisotropy. *Conference proceedings: ... Annual International Conference of the IEEE Engineering in Medicine and Biology, 1,* 2053–2056.

Truong, D. Q., Magerowski, G., Blackburn, G. L., Bikson, M., & Alonso-Alonso, M. (2013). Computational modeling of transcranial direct current stimulation (tDCS) in obesity: Impact of head fat and dose guidelines. *NeuroImage Clinical, 2,* 759–766.

Truong, D. Q., Magerowski, G., Pascual-Leone, A., Alonso-Alonso, M., & Bikson, M. (2012). Finite element study of skin and fat delineation in an obese subject for transcranial direct current stimulation. Paper presented at the 34th Annual International Conference of the IEEE Engineering in Medicine and Biology Society, *Conference proceedings: ... Annual International Conference of the IEEE Engineering in Medicine and Biology Society, 2012,* 6587–6590.

Turkeltaub, P. E., Benson, J., Hamilton, R. H., Datta, A., Bikson, M., & Coslett, H. B. (2011). Left lateralizing transcranial direct current stimulation improves reading efficiency. *Brain Stimulation, 5,* 201–207.

Turkeltaub, P. E., Benson, J., Hamilton, R. H., Datta, A., Bikson, M., & Coslett, H. B. (2012). Left lateralizing transcranial direct current stimulation improves reading efficiency. *Brain Stimulation, 5*(3), 201–207.

Varga, E. T., Terney, D., Atkins, M. D., Nikanorova, M., Jeppesen, D. S., Uldall, P., et al. (2011). Transcranial direct current stimulation in refractory continuous spikes and waves during slow sleep: A controlled study. *Epilepsy Research, 97*(1–2), 142–145.

Wagner, T., Fregni, F., Fecteau, S., Grodzinsky, A., Zahn, M., & Pascual-Leone, A. (2007). Transcranial direct current stimulation: A computer-based human model study. *NeuroImage, 35*(3), 1113–1124.

Wagner, T. A., Zahn, M., Grodzinsky, A. J., & Pascual-Leone, A. (2004). Three-dimensional head model simulation of transcranial magnetic stimulation. *IEEE Transactions on Biomedical Engineering, 51*(9), 1586–1598.

Weiss, M., & Lavidor, M. (2012). When less is more: Evidence for a facilitative cathodal tDCS effect in attentional abilities. *Journal of Cognitive Neuroscience, 24*(9), 1826–1833.

Wolters, C. H., Anwander, A., Tricoche, X., Weinstein, D., Koch, M. A., & MacLeod, R. S. (2006). Influence of tissue conductivity anisotropy on EEG/MEG field and return current computation in a realistic head model: A simulation and visualization study using high-resolution finite element modeling. *NeuroImage, 30*(3), 813–826.

Zentner, J. (1989). Noninvasive motor evoked potential monitoring during neurosurgical operations on the spinal cord. *Neurosurgery, 24,* 709–712.

Transcranial Electrical Stimulation in Animals

Javier Márquez-Ruiz[1], Rocío Leal-Campanario[1],
Fabrice Wendling[2,3], Giulio Ruffini[4], Agnès Gruart[1],
and José María Delgado-García[1]

[1]Division of Neurosciences, University of Pablo de Olavide, Seville, Spain
[2]INSERM, Rennes, France
[3]Université de Rennes, Rennes, France
[4]Starlab Barcelona SL, Barcelona, Spain

INTRODUCTION

Although the number of publications concerning the potential use of transcranial electrical stimulation (tES) in basic human brain studies and in the treatment of human neurological disorders has increased exponentially in the past decade, little is known about the basic mechanisms underlying tES effects in cortical circuits, or its implications in complex cognitive processes. Basic knowledge is urgently needed in order to (1) establish safety limits for electrical brain stimulation, (2) design new experimental protocols aiming to optimize tES effects, (3) perform systematic studies of tES effects on neuronal pathological states, and (4) explore the potential uses of tES for computer-to-brain interactions. Although much effort has been made, mainly providing indirect evidence of the cellular and molecular mechanisms in human studies, a deep understanding of the different tES aspects requires direct electrophysiological measurements, fine pharmacological manipulation of local networks, and precise histological characterization. In this regard, the use of animal experimental models offers a unique opportunity to deepen our understanding of the basic processes underlying some of the behavioral and electrophysiological effects observed in human studies.

The study of the effects of direct current (DC) on the excitability of cerebral cortex started in the 1960s with invasive experimental studies carried out in anesthetized animals. In 1962, Creutzfeldt and colleagues used the *encéphale isolé* preparation in anesthetized cats (which consists of using artificially ventilated animals in which a transection between the brainstem and spinal cord has been performed) to demonstrate that DC administered between cortical surface and neck muscles modulates spontaneous neuronal activities and electroencephalographic (EEG) recordings in the motor and visual cortices in a polarity-dependent manner (Creutzfeldt, Fromm, & Kapp, 1962). The same animal preparation was later used by Purpura and McMurtry (1965) to demonstrate intracellular activity and evoked potential changes induced by DC application over the motor cortex. In addition, early evidence for long-lasting aftereffects in response to polarizing currents over the cortex came from Bindman and colleagues (Bindman, Lippold, & Redfearn, 1964). Bindman's work describes the immediate and aftereffects induced by DC application on unitary recordings and sensory evoked potentials in the somatosensory cortex of anesthetized rats. These studies carried out in acute animals established the electrophysiological basis of our current knowledge on DC-stimulation effects. Seminal works concerning molecular mechanisms underlying the effects of weak DC appeared in the 1990s. These studies, performed in anesthetized rats, demonstrated that anodal DC applied to a stimulating electrode placed over the sensorimotor cortex with the reference electrode placed in the midline of the nasal bone modifies adenosine-elicited accumulation of cAMP (Hattori, Moriwaki, & Hori, 1990), inducing an increase of protein kinase C and calcium levels (Islam, Moriwaki, Hattori, & Hori, 1994; Islam, Aftabuddin, Moriwaki, Hattori, & Hori, 1995).

Following these pioneering studies carried out in animal models under anesthesia, the interest in basic neuronal mechanisms of DC-stimulation effects almost disappeared in favor of more accurate invasive stimulation techniques allowing more precise control of the stimulated area in time and space. However, after the seminal work of Nitsche and Paulus in 2000 showing immediate and long-lasting changes in the excitability of motor cortex induced by transcranial DC application in humans, there was a resurgence of interest in neuronal mechanisms underlying DC effects. The increasing use of the tES technique in basic and clinical studies in humans has fostered the appearance of new animal models aiming to answer new and old questions regarding tES effects on the nervous system. Thus, during the past few years, different approaches for tES research in animals have been developed in order to mimic human experimental designs (Cambiaghi et al., 2010; Liebetanz, Klinker, et al., 2006; Liebetanz et al., 2009; Rueger et al., 2012) or to design new stimulation protocols for altering brain patterns (Berényi, Belluscio, Mao, & Buzsaki, 2012). Recently, selective animal models have been used to characterize tES effects on different fronts, including cortical excitability modulation of different brain regions, changes in sensory perception, modulation of learning and memory processes, impact on different neurological pathologies, exploration of safety protocols, and validation of computational models.

In this chapter we will review different methodological strategies used in animal models for performing tES stimulation, and summarize the main findings from animal experimental work in different topics.

EXPERIMENTAL APPROACHES FOR TRANSCRANIAL ELECTRICAL STIMULATION IN ANIMALS

The main differences in the methodological strategies used in animal models are related to the size and the relative position of stimulating electrodes over/in the head of the animal, the location of the electrodes in relation to the cerebral tissues (on the skin, on the skull, or on the dura mater), and the state (anesthetized or awake, constrained, or freely moving) of the animal during current application. Additionally, detailed information about changes in the membrane potential of neurons during and after tES application requires electrical stimulation of identified neurons in slice preparations (the *in vitro* approach). While these different strategies have provided interesting information about how weak electrical currents interact with cortical neurons, the heterogeneous nature of the experimental methods makes it difficult to interpret and to analyze comparatively the different results and, consequently, to translate these results to human studies. In the following pages, we will deal with each one of these aspects separately.

Current Delivery and Density Levels

Diverse strategies for current delivery have been used to stimulate animal brains. These differences lie in the shape and size of the active and counter (or return) electrode, the intensity and duration of the applied current, and the position of both active and counter electrodes with respect to the cerebral cortex. The size of the electrode, together with the applied intensity, determines the current density applied on the skull. Current density – which is the current intensity passing through a certain surface area – is one of the most important parameters, because it is directly related to electric field strength and has been demonstrated to be linked with the effects of DC application on neural networks, the occurrence and duration of the induced plastic changes, and potential DC-induced lesions on the cortex (Nitsche et al., 2008). Several types of active electrode have been used for animal brain stimulation, including cup-shaped; plastic tubes filled with saline solution; silver balls; and square rubber electrodes (Fig. 5.1A–D). Unlike the big active sponge electrodes used for human brain stimulation, active electrodes used in mice, rats, and rabbits are necessarily small due to the small size of their brains. The active electrode is usually placed on the head of the animal, over the brain area to be stimulated. The contact surface of these electrodes with the skull (epicranial electrodes) or the skin ranges from $1.6 \, mm^2$ (Márquez-Ruiz et al., 2012; Molaee-Ardekani et al., 2013) to $150 \, mm^2$ (Laste et al., 2012), $\sim3.5 \, mm^2$ being the most common value. With regard to the counter electrode, most of the authors use a rubber plate in a sponge wetted with saline solution, attached to the ventral thorax (Liebetanz, Klinker, et al., 2006) or the back of the animal (Dockery, Liebetanz, Birbaumer, Malinowska, & Wesierska, 2011) in the case of rats, or attached to the ear in the case of rabbits (Márquez-Ruiz et al., 2012; Molaee-Ardekani et al., 2013). Needle electrodes inserted in the neck (Kamida et al., 2011) and carbon-fiber plate electrodes placed on the neck (Takano et al., 2011) have also been used in rats (Fig. 5.1E–G). The size of this counter electrode ranges from $48 \, cm^2$ (Yoon, Oh, & Kim, 2012) to $3 \, cm^2$ (Takano et al., 2011), $\sim10 \, cm^2$ being the most common value.

The nominal current density at the electrode used in the various experiments can differ by an order of magnitude ranging from $10 \, A/m^2$ (Li, Tian, Qian, Yu, & Jiang, 2011; Takano et al., 2011) to $150 \, A/m^2$

Active electrodes

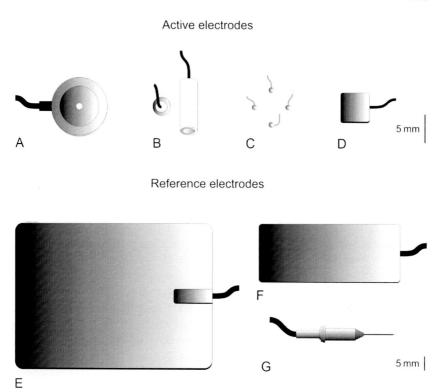

Reference electrodes

E

FIGURE 5.1 **Current delivery strategies for transcranial electrical stimulation in animals.** Differences in methodological strategies for current delivery used in animals are related to the shape and size of the active and counter electrodes used. Several kinds of active electrode have been used for animal transcranial stimulation, including cup-shaped (A), plastic tubes filled with saline solution (B), multiple silver balls (C), and square rubber electrodes (D). Reference electrodes used in animal transcranial stimulation include rubber plate electrodes of various sizes (E, F), and needle electrodes inserted in the neck of the animals (G). Scale bars for active and reference electrodes are shown at top and bottom, respectively.

(Rueger et al., 2012). The total stimulation time and the number of stimulation sessions must also be taken into account (Liebetanz et al., 2009). The charge density (expressed as C/m^2) considers the total current density value and the total stimulation time. Charge densities used in tDCS animal models range from 10,000 C/m^2 (Takano et al., 2011) to 200,000 C/m^2 (Kim et al., 2010; Liebetanz, Klinker, et al., 2006).

Finally, it is important to point out that the relative position of active and reference electrodes on the head of the animal will determine the final currents – and hence the electric fields – passing through a particular area of the cerebral cortex (see Chapter 4 for computational modeling in humans).

Acute and Chronic Experiments: The Importance of Brain State

Several findings indicate the importance of brain state in explaining the final effect of non-invasive brain stimulation techniques such as transcranial magnetic stimulation (TMS) and transcranial direct current stimulation (tDCS) (Silvanto & Pascual-Leone, 2008). In this sense, the physiological changes induced in the brain during and after tDCS must be interpreted as the result of the interaction between the imposed electrical currents and fields, and the ongoing, endogenous cortical activities. Supporting this contention, important differences have been found depending on the animal state – acute animal preparations versus non-anesthetized awake and asleep animals. For example, it has been shown that cortical neuronal populations can be entrained by transcranial electric stimulation in anesthetized and sleeping rats, whereas no effect on neuronal discharge was observed when the same electrical stimulation was applied in alert behaving animals (Ozen et al., 2010). In general terms, tES application in anesthetized animals is normally combined with electrophysiological characterization of cortical regions, whereas in awake animals it is combined with behavioral tests and histological analysis. However, some studies based on direct recording of neuronal or local field-potential activity during tES application have dealt with electrophysiological characterization of tES effects on the brain cortex of alert animals (Márquez-Ruiz et al., 2012; Molaee-Ardekani et al., 2013; Ozen et al., 2010). Accordingly, rather than being an irrelevant technical and methodological aspect, the use of acute or chronic animal preparations involves very important functional differences. The systematic use of anesthetized animals for basic tDCS experiments can make it difficult to interpret and to translate the results obtained in animal models to human basic and clinical tES studies.

The *In Vitro* Approach

Understanding tES effects on neuronal excitability of the cerebral cortex requires a deep knowledge of how subthreshold and suprathreshold electrical stimulations modify, through the electric fields created, the membrane potential of excitatory neurons (pyramidal cells) and inhibitory interneurons in the different cortical layers. Many important features, such as the effects of electric fields on each neuronal segment or the role of cell-type morphology and the orientation of the neuron in the electric field (apical-dendritic and axonal orientation) must be unraveled. The studies performed on artificially maintained brain slices allow intracellular recording of identified neurons in very well-known circuits, together with a good control of spatially uniform electric fields. In addition, this approach allows the accurate reconstruction of the morphology of recorded neurons after biocytin intracellular microinjection. For some decades, brain slices have also constituted the most widely used experimental set-up to study short- and long-term potentiation, as they allow detailed investigation of plasticity-related mechanisms in neuronal networks. For all these reasons, *in vitro* experimental studies provide a powerful tool for answering very important basic questions about tES-induced effects.

Electric field stimulation *in vitro* is normally generated by passing current between two parallel silver–silver chloride electrodes placed on the surface of the artificial cerebrospinal fluid (ACSF) in the recording chamber (Bikson et al., 2004) (Fig. 5.2A). Hippocampal, motor, and visual cortex slices from mice, rats, guinea pigs, and ferrets have been used in DC and AC stimulation *in vitro* experiments. The current intensity used in slices for stimulation ranges from 10 μA to 400 μA for both anodal and cathodal stimulation, but the most interesting parameter is the electric field created in the slice, ranging from 1 V/m to 100 V/m. The stimulation time depends on the described phenomena, ranging from a few seconds when neuronal excitability during DC stimulation is characterized (Bikson et al., 2004; Jefferys, 1981; Radman, Ramos, Brumberg & Bikson 2009) to up to 15–20 minutes when DC-stimulation effects on long-term plastic changes are being studied (Fritsch et al., 2010; Ranieri et al., 2012). The main

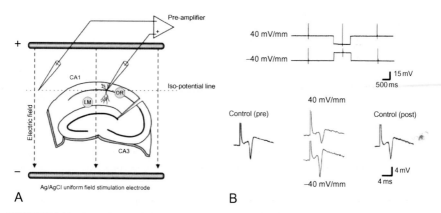

FIGURE 5.2 **Experimental design for DC stimulation in *in vitro* experiments.** (A) Uniform electric fields were generated by passing current between two large parallel silver–silver chloride wires positioned in the bath across the slice. Electrophysiological activity was monitored in the CA1 pyramidal cell layer. In some experiments, activity was evoked with a bipolar stimulating electrode positioned in either stratum lacunosum moleculare (LM) or stratum oriens (OR). (B) One-second electric fields were applied 500 ms before OR stimulation (top). Population spikes evoked before, during, and after application of 40-mV/mm uniform electric fields are shown at bottom. *Figure reproduced from Bikson et al. (2004), with permission from John Wiley & Sons.*

electrophysiological variables measured to determine DC effects on slices in the *in vitro* approach are field, intracellular, and voltage-sensitive dye recordings. Thus, population excitatory postsynaptic potentials (fEPSP) in response to orthodromic stimuli (the impulse is conducted in the usual direction), and population spikes in response to orthodromic and antidromic stimuli (the impulse is conducted in a direction opposite to the usual one), have been used to measure the DC-stimulation effect on the excitability of neurons in hippocampal (Bikson et al., 2004; Jefferys, 1981; Kabakov, Muller, Pascual-Leone, Jensen, & Rotenberg, 2012; Ranieri et al., 2012) and motor cortex slices (Fritsch et al., 2010). Intracellular and whole-cell patch clamp performed in hippocampal (Bikson et al., 2004) and motor cortex slices (Radman, Ramos, Brumberg, & Bikson, 2009) highlighted the polarity-dependent effects induced by DC stimulation on transmembrane potential of the recorded neurons (Fig. 5.2B). In addition, intracellular recordings performed in acute slices from ferret visual cortex showed that the sine-wave electric fields successfully entrain slow oscillation *in vitro* (Fröhlich & McCormick, 2010). This study also demonstrated that the application of external fields with *in vivo* amplitudes caused small changes (net membrane voltage depolarization $\sim$0.5 and $\sim$1.3 mV for 2 and 4 mV/mm, respectively) in the somatic membrane potential of individual neurons. Finally, voltage-sensitive dye imaging has also been used in slices to monitor transmembrane voltage changes in the hippocampal CA1 pyramidal layer in response to electric fields (Bikson et al., 2004).

It is important to note here that although the *in vitro* approach brings us some insights into the very basic mechanisms underlying short- and long-term effects associated with electrical stimulation, there are important functional differences between the artificial slice and the intact whole brain conditions. Despite the above-described advantages, several drawbacks should also be kept in mind, especially if the goal is to extrapolate *in vitro* results to *in vivo* situations. Indeed, although these points are very rarely discussed in papers, it should be mentioned that (1) the complex relationship between oxygen/glucose delivery and cellular energy demand is strongly altered in slice preparations; (2) the ACSF is an essential issue, as many metabolites (present in real CSF) are not included; and (3) both intrinsic and extrinsic connections are severed in the slice model, reducing the potential use in the interpretation of field effects on actual brain rhythms. A full understanding of tES effects on the human brain thus involves the integration of non-uniform electric fields interacting with neuronal networks (including deep brain structures) and its spontaneous activity associated with different brain states. These conditions are met only *in vivo* but, to date, the number of tES studies involving living animals remains limited.

TRANSCRANIAL ELECTRICAL STIMULATION EFFECTS IN ANIMALS

Modulation of Cortical Excitability

Different electrophysiological, histological, and imaging techniques have been used to measure directly the short- and long-term changes in the excitability of cortical neurons during and after tES application in the animal brain. Thus, intracellular and extracellular unitary recording of neurons, field excitatory postsynaptic potentials, population spikes, sensory and motor evoked potentials, and electroencephalographic activities have been characterized during and after weak current application in different animal preparations (e.g., in brain slices, and acute anesthetized and chronic awake animals).

As mentioned above, pioneering studies performed in anesthetized and *encéphale isolé* preparations demonstrated that weak electrical currents applied on the brain cortical surface by epidural electrodes could modify the spontaneous firing rate and the electroencephalographic activity in a polarity-dependant manner when recorded from motor, visual, and somatosensory cortices (Bindman et al., 1964; Creutzfeldt et al., 1962; Purpura & McMurtry, 1965). Interestingly, in some experiments these effects were maintained for more than 2 hours after weak DC stimulation, suggesting the induction of some plasticity-associated phenomena (Bindman et al., 1964).

The modulation of motor cortex excitability by tES is a topic that has recently been addressed in a number of studies using brain slices and *in vivo* anesthetized animals. In 2009, Radman and colleagues characterized the effects of subthreshold and suprathreshold electrical stimulation on identified cortical neurons in rat motor cortex slices. In that work, they studied the contribution of neuronal morphology in the neuronal excitability by using a whole-cell patch clamp in combination with intracellular dialysis of biocytin, allowing morphological reconstruction of the recorded cells. Using the collected results as a basis, the authors proposed that the population of pyramidal cells in layer V is the most sensitive to weak electric fields applied over the skull (Radman et al., 2009). Motor cortical slices have also been used to study molecular mechanisms underlying tDCS effects on motor-skill learning (Fritsch et al., 2010). Based on field excitatory postsynaptic potentials recorded in layer II/III in response to afferent stimulation, it has been demonstrated that 15 minutes of anodal DC application in the slice increased the amplitude of fEPSP for more than 2 hours after DC offset. Furthermore, pharmacological manipulation of the ACSF in the bath showed that adding N-methyl-D-aspartate (NMDA) receptor antagonist or incubating the slice with a brain-derived neurotrophic factor (BDNF) scavenger prior to DC stimulation abolished the induced long-term effects in the slice. These results suggest that synaptic potentiation in the motor cortex after anodal stimulation is mediated by NMDA receptor and that BDNF is a key mediator of this phenomenon. Modulation of motor cortex excitability has also been demonstrated in anesthetized mice. In an acute mouse preparation, Cambiaghi et al. (2010) showed that mean area and amplitude of motor-evoked potentials recorded in the forelimb of animals in response to transcranial electrical stimulation of the motor cortex before and after 10 minutes of epicranial DC stimulation increase or decrease depending on the polarity of the applied current (anodal or cathodal, respectively) – i.e., electric field direction. These results are consistent with those coming from human studies reporting changes in the size of motor evoked potential induced by TMS after tDCS application (Nitsche & Paulus, 2000).

The short- and long-term effects of tDCS over the somatosensory cortex have also been addressed in anesthetized (Bindman et al., 1964, Ozen et al., 2010) and awake animals (Márquez-Ruiz et al., 2012; Molaee-Ardekani et al., 2013). The combined use of four small silver-ball electrodes placed over the skull acting together as a single active electrode allows for intracortical local field potential recording in the somatosensory cortex in response to whisker stimulation during and after tDCS application (Fig. 5.3).

It has recently been demonstrated by using this model that the application of anodal and cathodal tDCS increases or decreases the amplitude and area of the recorded local field potentials in response to whisker stimulation, and that these effects are current-intensity dependent (Fig. 5.4A–C). The same effects were observed when whisker stimulation was substituted by an electrical stimulus in the ventro-posterior medial thalamus corresponding to whisker afferents to the somatosensory cortex. Interestingly, only cathodal tDCS induced long-term changes (Fig. 5.4D). Simultaneous local administration of the adenosine A1 receptor antagonist DCPCX in the recorded area prevented long-term depression induced by cathodal tDCS when the vehicle alone was injected (Fig. 5.4E). In this regard, it has been demonstrated that anodal DC stimulation applied to the rat sensorimotor cortex modifies adenosine-elicited accumulation of cAMP (Hattori et al., 1990), inducing an increase of protein kinase C and calcium levels (Islam et al., 1994, 1995). This mechanism would explain the cellular excitability increase after anodal tDCS by an increase in Ca^{2+} intracellular level. Interestingly, the adenosine A1 receptor suppresses neuronal activity by coupling with protein G_i to inhibit the adenylate cyclase–cAMP–protein kinase A signaling pathway (van Calker, Muller, & Hamprecht, 1979).

Transcranial electric stimulation by using a sinusoidal waveform (referred to as tACS, for transcranial alternating current stimulation) has also been shown to entrain neuronal activity in the somatosensory

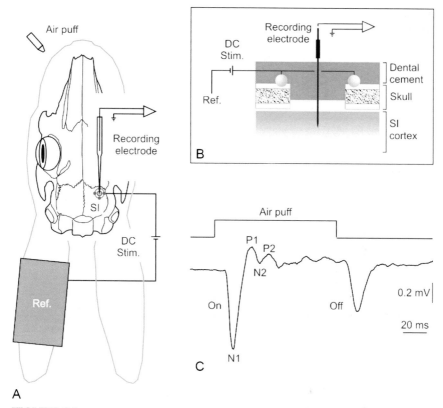

FIGURE 5.3 **Experimental design for the intracortical recording of sensory evoked potentials during simultaneous tDCS.** (A) Experimental design illustrating the electrode locations for tDCS and the recording micropipette. Both anodal and cathodal tDCS were applied between the active (red circles) and the reference (Ref.) electrodes. Air-puff stimulation of the contralateral whisker pad is also shown. (B) Schematic sagittal view of the recording site at which local field potential corresponding to vibrissae was mapped, the tungsten electrode (Rec.) was attached to the skull, and the window was cut in the parietal bone overlying the somatosensory cortex and subsequently covered with dental cement. (C) Different components of the LFP evoked in response to air-puff presentation (N1, P1, N2, and P2) and removal (off). *Figure reproduced from Márquez-Ruiz et al. (2012), with permission from the National Academy of Sciences USA.*

and prefrontal cortices of anesthetized (Ozen et al., 2010) and awake (Berényi et al., 2012) animals. The sinusoidal stimulation frequencies used in experiments range from 0.8 Hz to 1.7 Hz, mimicking the frequency of cortical slow oscillations.

Besides motor and somatosensory cortices, modulation of excitability by tES has also been studied in other animal cerebral regions, such as visual and frontal cortices and the hippocampus. Modulation of visual cortex excitability was first reported by Creutzfeldt et al. (1962), and more

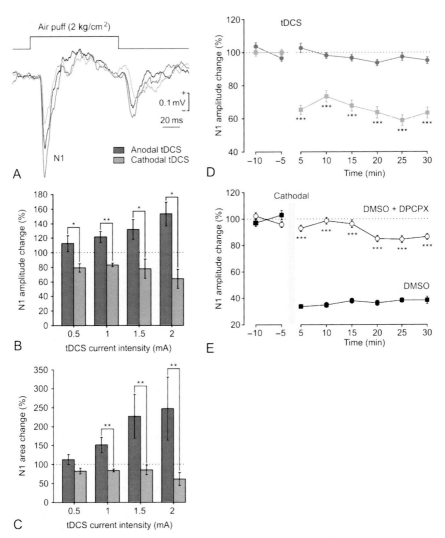

FIGURE 5.4   **Effects of anodal and cathodal tDCS on sensory evoked potentials in the vibrissal area of the somatosensory cortex of rabbits.** (A) Representative examples of sensory evoked potentials in the vibrissal somatosensory cortex by air-puff stimulation of the contralateral whisker pad in control situation (black recording) and during the application of anodal (red recording) or cathodal (blue recording) tDCS. (B, C) Changes in amplitude (B) and area (C) of the N1 component, indicated in (A), of air-puff evoked sensory potentials in the presence of anodal (red histograms) or cathodal (blue histograms) currents at increasing intensities. *, $P < 0.005$; **, $P < 0.01$. (D) Sensory evoked potential evolution after 20 min of anodal (red) and cathodal (blue) tDCS. ***, $P < 0.001$. (E) Sensory evoked potential evolution after cathodal tDCS in the presence of the selective A1 adenosine receptor antagonist DPCPX (open circles) or the injection of vehicle DMSO (squares in black). Pharmacological antagonism of the adenosine A1 receptor significantly impaired LTD. Error bars represent one standard error of mean (SEM). *Figure reproduced from Márquez-Ruiz et al. (2012), with permission from the National Academy of Sciences USA.*

recently by Cambiaghi et al. (2011). In the latter study, the amplitude of field potentials evoked in the visual cortex of anesthetized animals in response to a light flash was evaluated after 10 minutes of anodal and cathodal tDCS. Anodal tDCS increased the amplitude of visual evoked potential, whereas cathodal stimulation decreased it. Application of anodal tDCS over the frontal cortex of anesthetized animals has been shown to increase functional magnetic resonance imaging (fMRI) signal intensities in the frontal cortex and its connected brain region – the accumbens nucleus (Takano et al., 2011). The hippocampus constitutes one of the best-known circuits associated with synaptic plasticity in the brain. Many important *in vitro* studies have been carried out in the past few decades in the hippocampus slice, which today is a common experimental subject for the study of long-term potentiation and depression processes. For this reason, it is not surprising that some basic knowledge about the mechanisms underlying tES comes from hippocampal slice experiments under weak electric fields (Bikson et al., 2004; Kabakov et al., 2012; Ranieri et al., 2012). The first to apply electrical fields to hippocampal slices was Jefferys, in 1981. Jefferys observed that direct currents applied to the recording chamber modified the population discharge of granule cells during postsynaptic responses. More recently, Bikson et al. (2004) showed that DC fields parallel to the somato-dendritic axis induced polarization of CA1 pyramidal cells, whereas electric fields perpendicular to the apical-dendritic axis did not induce somatic polarization. Later *in vitro* studies performed in hippocampal slices revealed the important role of axonal orientation in the modulation of excitatory transmission (Kabakov et al., 2012), and the important role of some immediate early genes (Ranieri et al., 2012) in the induction and maintenance of the long-term plasticity processes induced by DC stimulation. Regarding neuron orientation with respect to electric field, these results are consistent with our current understanding of the effects of tES electric fields on the transmembrane potential of elongated neurons (Ruffini et al., 2012) (see also Computational Models Based on Experimental Data from Animals, below). Finally, the recording of neurons in the hippocampus/subiculum of anesthetized rats has been shown to be affected by tACS displaying different phase-locking modulation degrees depending on intensity and underlying network activity (Ozen et al., 2010).

Effects of tES on Sensory Perception

The application of tES in human brains has been demonstrated to be useful (1) for the modulation of sensory perception thresholds (Ragert, Vandermeeren, Camus, & Cohen, 2008; Rogalewski, Breitenstein, Nitsche, Paulus, & Knecht, 2004); (2) for the induction of artificial visual and tactile sensations when weak alternating currents at specific frequencies are applied (Feurra, Paulus, Walsh, & Kanai, 2011; Kanai, Chaieb, Antal, Walsh, & Paulus, 2008); and (3) for the modulation of pain perception (Antal et al., 2008) (for a detailed discussion see Chapter 7). As previously mentioned in this chapter, a change in the excitability of somatosensory and visual cortices after tDCS application has been demonstrated in different animal models. Thus, anodal DC stimulation increased the spontaneous firing rate of visual and somatosensory cortices in anesthetized animals, whereas cathodal application decreased the spontaneous neuronal discharge (Bindman et al., 1964; Creutzfeldt et al., 1962). In addition, similar modulatory effects were observed in the amplitude of sensory and visual evoked potentials when anodal and cathodal tDCS were applied to the somatosensory and visual cortices of anesthetized animals (Bindman et al., 1964; Cambiaghi et al., 2010). In these animal preparations, sensory and visual potentials were obtained in response to forepaw skin electrical stimulation and light-flash stimulation, respectively.

The effects of tDCS on sensory evoked potentials have been corroborated in alert behaving animals. It has been shown that the amplitude of the local field potentials recorded with glass electrodes in the cerebral cortex in response to air-puff stimulation of the whiskers is modulated by the simultaneous presentation of tDCS (Márquez-Ruiz et al., 2012; Molaee-Ardekani et al., 2013). The functional meaning of this result was investigated by using whisker stimulation in a well-established associative learning protocol. Márquez-Ruiz et al. (2012) demonstrated that tDCS application over the somatosensory cortex of rabbits modulated the percentage of conditioned responses when whisker stimulation was used as conditioned stimulus in a well-known classical conditioning protocol, suggesting that anodal tDCS potentiates the whisker sensation intensity, whereas cathodal tDCS diminishes it.

One of the most obvious clinical applications for tDCS in relation to sensory process modification is the possibility of modulating pain perception. Human studies have demonstrated that cathodal tDCS applied over the somatosensory cortex decreases the amplitude of pain perception-related potentials in response to laser stimulus (Antal et al., 2008). Antinociceptive effects of tES have been explored in a freely moving rat model. Nekhendzy and colleagues measured nociceptive thresholds in alert animals during and after direct- and alternating-current stimulation administered through the skin overlying the anterior pole of the frontal lobe (Nekhendzy et al., 2004). In that experiment, the authors measured the impact of DC and AC stimulation on the nociceptive threshold obtained from tail-flick and hot-plate tests. They reported a significant frequency-dependent antinociceptive effect when AC was used at frequencies ranging from 40 Hz to 60 Hz in the presence of DC offset.

Impact of tES on Learning and Memory

The effects of tES on learning acquisition and memory consolidation represent one of the most interesting possibilities of this technique as a neuromodulatory tool. Improvement of memory and learning processes in healthy people, in patients recovering deteriorated learning capabilities following pathological brain states, and in subjects with atypical development are now beginning to be explored in both basic and clinical research (see Chapters 8–9, 12, 16). Thus, tES application on prefrontal, premotor, and motor cortices has been demonstrated to improve learning capabilities (Galea & Celnik, 2009; Iuculano & Cohen Kadosh, 2013; Kincses, Antal, Nitsche, Bartfai, & Paulus, 2004; Marshall, Molle, Hallschmid, & Born, 2004; Snowball et al., 2013), working memory (Andrews, Hoy, Enticott, Daskalakis, & Fitzgerald, 2011; Fregni et al., 2005; Mulquiney, Hoy, Daskalakis, & Fitzgerald, 2011), and memory retrieval (Boggio et al., 2009; Chi, Fregni, & Snyder, 2010; Penolazzi et al., 2010). In order to understand the neuronal mechanisms underlying the interaction between weak current application and learning and memory processes, new animal models combining tES during behavioral tests are urgently needed. Addressing this important issue, some recent studies have been carried out to characterize tES effects on motor skill acquisition, associative learning, and visuospatial working memory.

Consistent with the polarity-specific effects observed in the intracortical sensory evoked potential recorded in the somatosensory cortex of alert rabbits (Márquez-Ruiz et al., 2012; Molaee-Ardekani et al., 2013), the acquisition of a classical eyeblink conditioning was potentiated or depressed by the simultaneous application of anodal or cathodal tDCS over the somatosensory cortex when stimulation of the whisker pad was used in the associative learning protocol as a conditioned stimulus (Márquez-Ruiz et al., 2012). As shown in Figure 5.5, the application of anodal tDCS during the second conditioning session (Fig. 5.5A) was associated with a significant increase in the percentage of conditioned responses, whereas cathodal tDCS applied during the eighth conditioning session, once animals had reached asymptotic values for their learning curves, was associated with a significantly lower percentage of conditioned responses compared with the control group (Fig. 5.5B, C). Intra-session analysis of classical conditioning evolution during anodal and cathodal sessions is presented in Figure 5.5D. Thus, this work demonstrates that it is possible to modulate the animal's ability to acquire a typical associative learning test using tDCS to decrease or enhance the sensory perception process.

tDCS has also been used in the prefrontal cortex of rats to study the impact of DC stimulation on visuospatial working memory and skill learning. Using a place-avoidance alternation task, Dockery et al. (2011) showed that rats treated with 30 minutes of cathodal tDCS before training

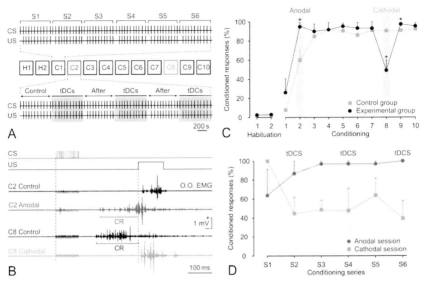

FIGURE 5.5   **Effects of tDCS on classical eyeblink conditioning in rabbits.** (A) Experimental design. Two habituation (H1 and H2) and 10 conditioning (C1–C10) sessions were carried out. Conditioning sessions consisted of 66 trials (6 series of 11 trials each) separated at random by intervals of 50–70 s. Of the 66 trials, 6 were test trials in which the CS was presented alone. Anodal tDCS was presented during series 2, 4, and 6 of C2 (in red), whilst cathodal tDCS was presented in these same series during C8 (in blue). (B) From top to bottom are illustrated the conditioning paradigm (CS and US presentations) and representative orbicularis oculi electromyographic (O.O. EMG) recordings collected from the same animal during the C2 session, from a control series (conditioning series 1, black trace) and during anodal stimulation (red trace), as well as during the C8 session from a control series (black trace) and during cathodal stimulation (blue trace). The presence of conditioned responses (CR) is indicated for the anodal-stimulated animal during the C2 session and for the control animal during the C8 session. (C) Evolution of learning curves for a control group of animals (gray squares and line) and the experimental group. The experimental group received anodal tDCS during C2 and cathodal tDCS during C8. (C) Evolution of the percentage of conditioned responses during sessions with anodal (C2, in red) and cathodal (C8, in blue) tDCS. Series during which tDCS was applied (S2, S4, and S6) are indicated by a gray bar. Error bars represent one SEM. *Figure reproduced from Márquez-Ruiz et al. (2012), with permission from the National Academy of Sciences USA.*

improved place-avoidance and skill-retention efficiency in comparison with untreated control animals.

In addition, the recovery of deteriorated learning capabilities under pathological brain states has been addressed in rat models associated with epilepsy (Kamida et al., 2011), Parkinson's disease (PD) (Li et al., 2011), and cerebral ischemia (Yoon et al., 2012) (see Exploring tES Effects on Animal Models of Human Pathologies, below, for tES effects on animal models of human pathologies).

In summary, in spite of obvious difficulties in translating these animal learning studies into complex human processes and therapies, animal models have demonstrated that tES is a useful tool for improving learning capabilities in healthy animals or in animal models resembling human brain disorders, such as epilepsy, stroke, or PD.

Experimental Evidence for Safety Limits

One of the most interesting possibilities associated with the use of tES in animals is the systematic characterization of tES-associated deleterious effects on the nervous system. Although the use of tES is becoming extensive as a neuromodulatory tool for basic and clinical purposes, the safety limits of DC stimulation at higher current densities and long stimulation treatments is still a matter of discussion. Thus, stimulation safety limits in animals, for subsequent human applications, need to be considered.

In a pioneering study, Liebetanz et al. (2009) addressed the effects of single sessions of cathodal tDCS applied through epicranial electrodes over the rat skull. The study covered DC stimulation at intensities ranging from 1 μA to 1000 μA and for up to 270 minutes. Histological evaluation of brain tissues showed that cathodal nominal electrode current densities higher than 142.9 A/m^2 for durations greater than 10 minutes are needed to produce DC-induced lesions in the cortex – that is, charge densities higher than 52,400 C/m^2 (Fig. 5.6). This value is at least two orders of

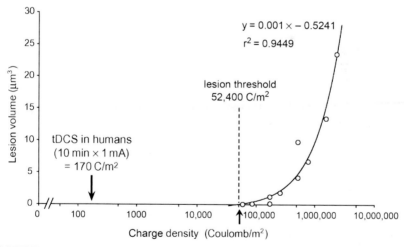

FIGURE 5.6   Safety limits of cathodal tDCS in rats. Threshold estimation from the relation of charge density and lesion size at current intensities of 500–1000 μA. The results are depicted with respect to the charge density (C/m^2) and the size of the DC-induced brain lesion (μm^3). For better overview, the charge density is scaled logarithmically. The regression analysis indicates a linear relation of charge density and lesion size (r^2 = 0.945, F = 171.33, P < 0.001). The intercept point, at which the lesion size is theoretically zero, corresponds to 52,400 C/m^2. The upwards-directed arrow indicates the daily charge density of the group that received repetitive tDCS over 5 days without inducing tissue damage. *Figure reproduced from Liebetanz et al. (2009), with permission from Elsevier.*

magnitude higher than the charge density that is normally applied in clinical studies (171–480 C/m^2) (Nitsche et al., 2008).

More recently, the effect of multisession tDCS in the rat brain has been explored. Inflammatory and regenerative processes associated with tDCS have been demonstrated to occur in the absence of cortical lesion after 5 and 10 consecutive days of transcranial DC stimulation (Rueger et al., 2012). Both anodal and cathodal tDCS induced immune response with microglial activation, whereas only cathodal tDCS increased the number of endogenous neural stem cells in the stimulated cortex. Thus, cathodal tDCS attracts neural stem cells implicated in reparative and regenerative responses in the stimulated site, suggesting a mechanism for its beneficial use in human stroke patients. These results show that tDCS modulates neuroinflammation and neural stem cell activation at higher charge densities ([current × time]/electrode area) than those used in humans (128,571 C/m^2 used in the experiment compared to 480 C/m^2 usually applied in humans).

Furthermore, multisite anodal and cathodal tDCS through equidistant epicranial electrodes in rabbits has been shown not to induce cortical lesions (Fig. 5.7A–D) (Márquez-Ruiz et al., 2012). The current density applied in this latter multisite stimulation experiment was 39.8 A/m^2 through each of the electrodes, and the distance between opposite stimulating electrodes was 6 mm (Fig. 5.1C).

Exploring tES Effects on Animal Models of Human Pathologies

During the past decade, tDCS has been used in many different pathologies in order to explore the benefits of its neuromodulatory properties (Nitsche et al., 2008). For this reason, it is not surprising that tES has started to be applied in animal models resembling human pathologies related to cortical excitability. In this direction, animal models offer a unique opportunity to show how DC and AC stimulation interact with different elements related to the pathophysiology of well-characterized neuronal disorders such as epilepsy or stroke.

Since cathodal tDCS has been demonstrated to decrease cortical excitability in some regions of the brain, its potential anticonvulsant effects have been evaluated in various animal models. Liebetanz, Klinker, et al. (2006) used the rat cortical ramp model to test whether the threshold for localized seizure activity changes after cathodal tDCS. The authors demonstrated that 60 minutes of cathodal tDCS increased the threshold for localized seizure activity, and that this effect lasted for more than 2 hours. Interestingly, anodal stimulation did not induce any threshold change. Following the same rationale, cathodal tDCS has been applied in an epileptic lithium–pilocarpine rat model in immature animals

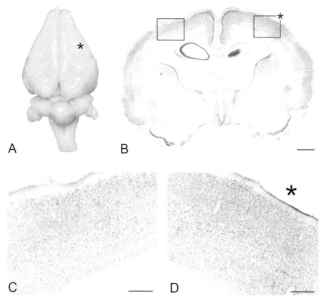

FIGURE 5.7   **Histological analysis of the stimulated cortical regions in the rabbit.**
(A) Macroscopic illustration showing the brain of a rabbit after the application of tDCS during a classical eyelid conditioning paradigm. The asterisk indicates the location of the stimulated somatosensory cortex, where no evidence of brain lesion was found. (B) Low-magnification photomicrograph of a coronal section, stained with toluidine blue, showing the stimulated (asterisk) somatosensory cortex. (C, D) Higher-magnification microphotographs corresponding to the two squared regions indicated in (B). No histopathological alterations were observed when comparing the non-stimulated control side (C) with the stimulated region (D, asterisk). Scale bars: 2 mm in (B); 500 μm in (C) and (D). *Figure reproduced from Márquez-Ruiz et al. (2012), with permission from the National Academy of Sciences USA.*

(Kamida et al., 2011). Long-term cathodal tDCS treatment, based on 30 minutes of daily tDCS for 2 weeks, reduced convulsions, hippocampal cell loss, and supragranular and CA3 mossy fiber sprouting associated with the status epilepticus over 2 weeks. In addition to the application of cathodal DC for several minutes to reduce cortical excitability, the possibility of using tES with higher amplitude currents based on feedback brain control has also been explored. Thus, it has been shown that seizure-triggered feedback tES reduced spike-and-wave episodes in a rat model of generalized epilepsy (Berényi et al., 2012).

The recovery of deteriorated learning capabilities under pathological brain states has been addressed in rat models associated with epilepsy, PD, and cerebral ischemia. Clinical studies with patients have demonstrated that anodal tDCS over the injured motor cortex benefits motor recovery when applied after stroke (Baker, Rorden, & Fridriksson, 2010; Lindenberg, Renga, Zhu, Nair, & Schlaug, 2010; see also Chapter 12). The middle cerebral artery occlusion model developed in rats has been combined with anodal tDCS in some studies in order to validate and support the results seen in humans. Kim et al. (2010) observed that applying 30 minutes of daily anodal tDCS over the motor cortex for 2 weeks after ischemia improved the animal's motor performance, while no significant change of the infarct volume was observed after either anodal or cathodal tDCS. Supporting this result, it has been reported with the same rat model that anodal tDCS applied 1 day after occlusion and reperfusion of the middle cerebral artery for 5 days resulted in improved spatial memory and motor behavior with respect to the sham-stimulation group (Yoon et al., 2012). Moreover, anodal tDCS applied for 5 days, 1 week after ischemia, resulted in improved spatial memory, motor behavior, and balance ability with respect to the sham-stimulation group (Yoon et al., 2012). These results suggest that anodal tDCS applied over the ischemic region modulates neural plasticity around the ischemic penumbra. In addition to motor function improvement, anodal tDCS after stroke increased the density of dendritic spines in comparison with sham-lesion animals, and downregulated the elevated hemichannel pannexin-1 mRNA expression associated with stroke (Jiang et al., 2012).

Besides epilepsy and stroke, the effects of tDCS on some other pathological states have been studied in animal models. Thus, tDCS effects on cortical spreading depression – a phenomenon associated with abnormal cortical excitability in migraine – have been studied in anesthetized rats (Liebetanz, Fregni, et al., 2006). In that study, it was shown that 20 minutes of anodal DC induced an increase of propagation velocity, whereas no changes were observed with cathodal or sham stimulation. The results suggest that anodal tDCS may increase the probability of migraine attacks in these patients.

The rat model of PD based on the unilateral injection of 6-hydroxydopamine into the medial forebrain bundle has also been used to explore the impact of tDCS in the modulation of unilateral neglect associated with this model. It has been reported that the ipsilateral bias observed in the orientation to food stimuli reported in this rat model is reduced when anodal tDCS is applied over the motor cortex of the lesioned side (Li et al., 2011). This result suggests that modulation of motor cortex excitability may induce some compensatory mechanisms that allow partial recovery of lost function associated with the pathological state.

Finally, the analgesic effects of multisession tDCS have been evaluated in a rat model of chronic inflammation (Laste et al., 2012). In that experiment, 20 minutes of cathodal tDCS per day for 8 days resulted in antinociceptive effects when tested immediately or 24 hours after tDCS application.

In summary, animal models of human pathologies have been used successfully to determine tDCS effects in some important diseases. The use of animals for tDCS studies offers significant potential for exploring the neuromodulatory benefits of tDCS in many pathological states, allowing for testing and optimizing of protocols that could be used subsequently in future clinical applications.

Computational Models Based on Experimental Data from Animals

Computational models are currently being developed in order to provide insights into the mechanisms involved in the interaction between neurons and externally applied electric fields. The basic mechanism for interaction in tES is today thought to be through the coupling of electric fields to elongated form-factor neurons such as pyramidal cells (Ruffini et al., 2012). The role of other types of neuron (e.g., interneurons such as basket cells) or other brain cells such as glia is not well understood, since they are in principle less sensitive to such fields due to their more isotropic structures. Physically, the external electric field forces the displacement of intracellular ions (which mobilize to cancel the intracellular field), altering the neuron's internal charge distribution and modifying the transmembrane potential difference (Fig. 5.8A). For a long, straight finite

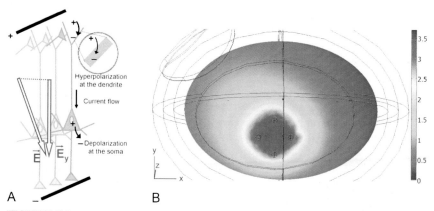

FIGURE 5.8   Current distribution models based on experimental data from animals. (A) The variation of the average membrane potential of a given subpopulation is proportional to the intensity of the component of the electric field oriented along the main axis of the cells (E_y). A field aligned with the orthodromic direction (dendritic tuft to axon) will result in a positive (depolarizing or excitatory) perturbation of the soma membrane potential. The opposite effect is observed on the dendritic tuft. *Figure reproduced from Molaee-Ardekani et al. (2013), with permission from Elsevier.* (B) Plot of the magnitude of current density on the cortical surface of a rabbit head model, showing the four spherical stimulation electrodes on the skull surface. A large high-current density region covers the brain area directly under the ring of electrodes with a maximum value of $3.7\,A/m^2$, for a total injected current of $1000\,\mu A$ ($250\,\mu A$ through each spherical electrode). The return electrode is the circular section at the top left, which represents the root of the ear. The model consists of four concentric ellipsoids representing the scalp, skull, CSF, and brain. The large elliptical region surrounding the electrodes represents the part of the scalp that was removed and replaced with dental cement. *Figure reproduced from Márquez-Ruiz et al. (2012), with permission from the National Academy of Sciences USA.*

fiber with space constant λ in a homogeneous electric field, the transmembrane potential difference is largest at the fiber termination, with a value that can be approximated by $\lambda \vec{E} \cdot \vec{n}$, where $\vec{n}$ is the unit vector defining the fiber axis. This is an expected first-order result from the biophysical point of view, with a spatial scale provided by the membrane space constant λ, and directions by field and fiber orientation. According to this model, a necessary first step in understanding the effects of tES is to determine the spatial distribution of the generated electric field in the brain. Such electric fields are described by vector fields (with units of V/m).

Realistic current distribution models, which provide such electric field distributions, have recently been developed based on experimental data from animals (Márquez-Ruiz et al., 2012). Figure 5.8A displays the magnitude of current density on the cortical surface of a simple rabbit head model, showing the four spherical stimulation electrodes on the skull surface. This simple model consists of four concentric ellipsoids representing the scalp, skull, cerebrospinal fluid (CSF), and brain. A large high-current density region covers the brain area directly under the ring of electrodes with a maximum value of 3.7 A/m^2, for a total injected current of 1 mA (0.25 mA through each spherical electrode). Realistic head models in the human highlight the strong interplay between currents, fields, and cortical and other anatomic geometric structures (Miranda, Mekonnen, Salvador, & Ruffini, 2013), and, in particular, the significant role of sulci and gyri in the human cortex.

Different functional scales may be addressed by computational models, from single-neuron interaction with external electrical fields to networks of neurons and macroscopic computational models of the cerebral cortex (Ruffini et al., 2012). In this sense, tES studies performed in animals offer a good opportunity for validating existing computational models and enabling the development of new ones. Regarding the understanding of small-scale (single-neuron) interactions with external electric fields, as mentioned previously, *in vitro* preparations provide a proper approach to characterize the response of physiologically and anatomically characterized neurons in the presence of well-controlled external electrical fields. Different studies performed in hippocampal (Bikson et al., 2004; Kabakov et al., 2012; Ozen et al., 2010; Ranieri et al., 2012) and motor cortex (Fritsch et al., 2010; Radman et al., 2009) slices from mice and rats have significantly contributed to our current knowledge of the mechanisms underlying tES effects. Thanks to these experiments, basic models regarding the local effects of electric fields on distinct neural compartments have been proposed (Radman et al., 2009). Concerning the macroscopic approach, computational neural-mass models have also been used to investigate the immediate effects of anodal and cathodal tDCS on sensory evoked potentials recorded in the somatosensory cortex of alert rabbits (Molaee-Ardekani et al., 2013). Results from the latter study revealed that

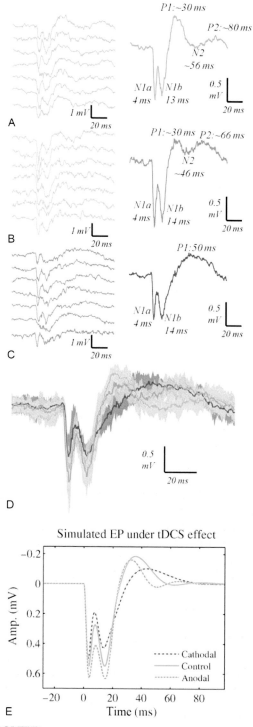

FIGURE 5.9—CONT'D

externally applied fields are likely to affect not only pyramidal cells but also cortical interneurons. When interneuron polarization is included in the model, the characteristics of simulated sensory evoked potentials match more closely those of real evoked potentials recorded in alert rabbits (Fig. 5.9).

CONCLUSIONS

As with other clinically relevant techniques, the use of animal models is essential for the correct understanding of the neuronal mechanisms underlying tES-associated effects. Although this basic knowledge may appear to be unnecessary for the development of general clinical purposes, the future success of the tES technique depends partially on a comprehensive understanding of neuronal network responses to externally applied electrical fields. As emphasized throughout this chapter, animal models have proved to be useful in studying the basic mechanisms underlying short- and long-term tDCS-associated effects, in exploring potentially deleterious effects on the nervous system and establishing safety limits for human applications, in testing tES effects in different animal models resembling human pathologies related with abnormal cortical excitability, and in validating and generating new computational models. However, important differences between animal and human brains make it difficult to translate accurately results from animal studies to humans. One of the major problems is the simple geometry of animals' brains as compared with the complex anatomy of the human cortex. The animal's brain size and the absence of cortical circumvolutions in rodents are clear examples of this limitation. Actually, the small brain size constitutes a technical problem that has forced the use of various alternative technical approaches, thereby generating some experimental heterogeneity, as reflected in the literature.

FIGURE 5.9—CONT'D **Computational model of tDCS effects on cortical activity based on experimental data obtained in rabbits.** (A) Some typical sensory evoked potentials in response to air puffs (left) under control condition where no tDCS is applied, and averaged somatosensory evoked potential ($n=10$) (right). (B, C) The same quantities as in (A) under anodal and cathodal tDCS conditions, respectively. (D) Superimposition of sensory evoked potentials under control condition (green) as well as under anodal (red) and cathodal (dark blue) tDCS conditions. Color-coded patches show the interval between 15% and 85% percentiles of evoked potential values for each tDCS condition. (E) Simulated sensory evoked potentials under control (green), anodal (light red), and cathodal (dark blue) tDCS. Simulated sensory evoked potentials do reproduce the observed modifications of peak amplitudes and latencies, as measured in the real sensory evoked potentials in rabbits. *Figure from Molaee-Ardekani et al. (2013), reproduced with permission from Elsevier.*

In conclusion, animal models provide a useful contribution to the growing knowledge of tES-associated neural mechanisms and to the evaluation of the potential use of tES in human pathologies related to abnormal cortical excitability. Moreover, to make these results truly useful for clinical applications, further efforts are needed in order to mimic more closely the current density values and electrode locations in human protocols.

References

Andrews, S. C., Hoy, K. E., Enticott, P. G., Daskalakis, Z. J., & Fitzgerald, P. B. (2011). Improving working memory: The effect of combining cognitive activity and anodal transcranial direct current stimulation to the left dorsolateral prefrontal cortex. *Brain Stimulation, 4*, 84–89.

Antal, A., Brepohl, N., Poreisz, C., Boros, K., Csifcsak, G., & Paulus, W. (2008). Transcranial direct current stimulation over somatosensory cortex decreases experimentally induced acute pain perception. *The Clinical Journal of Pain, 24*, 56–63.

Baker, J. M., Rorden, C., & Fridriksson, J. (2010). Using transcranial direct-current stimulation to treat stroke patients with aphasia. *Stroke, 41*, 1229–1236.

Berényi, A., Belluscio, M., Mao, D., & Buzsaki, G. (2012). Closed-loop control of epilepsy by transcranial electrical stimulation. *Science, 337*, 735–737.

Bikson, M., Inoue, M., Akiyama, H., Deans, J. K., Fox, J. E., Miyakawa, H., et al. (2004). Effects of uniform extracellular DC electric fields on excitability in rat hippocampal slices *in vitro*. *The Journal of Physiology, 557*, 175–190.

Bindman, L. J., Lippold, O. C., & Redfearn, J. W. (1964). The action of brief polarizing currents on the cerebral cortex of the rat (1) during current flow and (2) in the production of long-lasting after-effects. *The Journal of Physiology, 172*, 369–382.

Boggio, P. S., Fregni, F., Valasek, C., Ellwood, S., Chi, R., Gallate, J., et al. (2009). Temporal lobe cortical electrical stimulation during the encoding and retrieval phase reduces false memories. *PloS One, 4*, e4959.

Cambiaghi, M., Teneud, L., Velikova, S., Gonzalez-Rosa, J. J., Cursi, M., Comi, G., et al. (2011). Flash visual evoked potentials in mice can be modulated by transcranial direct current stimulation. *Neuroscience, 185*, 161–165.

Cambiaghi, M., Velikova, S., Gonzalez-Rosa, J. J., Cursi, M., Comi, G., & Leocani, L. (2010). Brain transcranial direct current stimulation modulates motor excitability in mice. *The European Journal of Neuroscience, 31*, 704–709.

Chi, R. P., Fregni, F., & Snyder, A. W. (2010). Visual memory improved by non-invasive brain stimulation. *Brain Research, 1353*, 168–175.

Creutzfeldt, O. D., Fromm, G. H., & Kapp, H. (1962). Influence of transcortical d-c currents on cortical neuronal activity. *Experimental Neurology, 5*, 436–452.

Dockery, C. A., Liebetanz, D., Birbaumer, N., Malinowska, M., & Wesierska, M. J. (2011). Cumulative benefits of frontal transcranial direct current stimulation on visuospatial working memory training and skill learning in rats. *Neurobiology of Learning and Memory, 96*, 452–460.

Feurra, M., Paulus, W., Walsh, V., & Kanai, R. (2011). Frequency specific modulation of human somatosensory cortex. *Frontiers in Psychology, 2*, 13.

Fregni, F., Boggio, P. S., Nitsche, M., Bermpohl, F., Antal, A., Feredoes, E., et al. (2005). Anodal transcranial direct current stimulation of prefrontal cortex enhances working memory. *Experimental Brain Research, 166*, 23–30.

Fritsch, B., Reis, J., Martinowich, K., Schambra, H. M., Ji, Y., Cohen, L. G., et al. (2010). Direct current stimulation promotes BDNF-dependent synaptic plasticity: Potential implications for motor learning. *Neuron, 66*, 198–204.

Fröhlich, F., & McCormick, D. A. (2010). Endogenous electric fields may guide neocortical network activity. *Neuron, 67*, 129–143.

Galea, J. M., & Celnik, P. (2009). Brain polarization enhances the formation and retention of motor memories. *Journal of Neurophysiology, 102*, 294–301.

Hattori, Y., Moriwaki, A., & Hori, Y. (1990). Biphasic effects of polarizing current on adenosine-sensitive generation of cyclic AMP in rat cerebral cortex. *Neuroscience Letters, 116*, 320–324.

Islam, N., Aftabuddin, M., Moriwaki, A., Hattori, Y., & Hori, Y. (1995). Increase in the calcium level following anodal polarization in the rat brain. *Brain Research, 684*, 206–208.

Islam, N., Moriwaki, A., Hattori, Y., & Hori, Y. (1994). Anodal polarization induces protein kinase C gamma (PKC gamma)-like immunoreactivity in the rat cerebral cortex. *Neuroscience Research, 21*, 169–172.

Iuculano, T., & Cohen Kadosh, R. (2013). The mental cost of cognitive enhancement. *The Journal of Neuroscience, 33*, 4482–4486.

Jefferys, J. G. (1981). Influence of electric fields on the excitability of granule cells in guinea-pig hippocampal slices. *The Journal of Physiology, 319*, 143–152.

Jiang, T., Xu, R. X., Zhang, A. W., Di, W., Xiao, Z. J., Miao, J. Y., et al. (2012). Effects of transcranial direct current stimulation on hemichannel pannexin-1 and neural plasticity in rat model of cerebral infarction. *Neuroscience, 226*, 421–426.

Kabakov, A. Y., Muller, P. A., Pascual-Leone, A., Jensen, F. E., & Rotenberg, A. (2012). Contribution of axonal orientation to pathway-dependent modulation of excitatory transmission by direct current stimulation in isolated rat hippocampus. *Journal of Neurophysiology, 107*, 1881–1889.

Kamida, T., Kong, S., Eshima, N., Abe, T., Fujiki, M., & Kobayashi, H. (2011). Transcranial direct current stimulation decreases convulsions and spatial memory deficits following pilocarpine-induced status epilepticus in immature rats. *Behavioural Brain Research, 217*, 99–103.

Kanai, R., Chaieb, L., Antal, A., Walsh, V., & Paulus, W. (2008). Frequency-dependent electrical stimulation of the visual cortex. *Current Biology, 18*, 1839–1843.

Kim, S. J., Kim, B. K., Ko, Y. J., Bang, M. S., Kim, M. H., & Han, T. R. (2010). Functional and histologic changes after repeated transcranial direct current stimulation in rat stroke model. *Journal of Korean Medical Science, 25*, 1499–1505.

Kincses, T. Z., Antal, A., Nitsche, M. A., Bartfai, O., & Paulus, W. (2004). Facilitation of probabilistic classification learning by transcranial direct current stimulation of the prefrontal cortex in the human. *Neuropsychologia, 42*, 113–117.

Laste, G., Caumo, W., Adachi, L. N., Rozisky, J. R., de Macedo, I. C., Filho, P. R., et al. (2012). After-effects of consecutive sessions of transcranial direct current stimulation (tDCS) in a rat model of chronic inflammation. *Experimental Brain Research, 221*, 75–83.

Li, Y., Tian, X., Qian, L., Yu, X., & Jiang, W. (2011). Anodal transcranial direct current stimulation relieves the unilateral bias of a rat model of Parkinson's disease. *Conference Proceedings: 33rd Annual International Conference of the IEEE Engineering in Medicine and Biology Society*, 765–768.

Liebetanz, D., Fregni, F., Monte-Silva, K. K., Oliveira, M. B., Amancio-dos-Santos, A., Nitsche, M. A., et al. (2006). After-effects of transcranial direct current stimulation (tDCS) on cortical spreading depression. *Neuroscience Letters, 398*, 85–90.

Liebetanz, D., Klinker, F., Hering, D., Koch, R., Nitsche, M. A., Potschka, H., et al. (2006). Anticonvulsant effects of transcranial direct-current stimulation (tDCS) in the rat cortical ramp model of focal epilepsy. *Epilepsia, 47*, 1216–1224.

Liebetanz, D., Koch, R., Mayenfels, S., Konig, F., Paulus, W., & Nitsche, M. A. (2009). Safety limits of cathodal transcranial direct current stimulation in rats. *Clinical Neurophysiology, 120*, 1161–1167.

Lindenberg, R., Renga, V., Zhu, L. L., Nair, D., & Schlaug, G. (2010). Bihemispheric brain stimulation facilitates motor recovery in chronic stroke patients. *Neurology, 75,* 2176–2184.

Márquez-Ruiz, J., Leal-Campanario, R., Sánchez-Campusano, R., Molaee-Ardekani, B., Wendling, F., Miranda, P. C., et al. (2012). Transcranial direct-current stimulation modulates synaptic mechanisms involved in associative learning in behaving rabbits. *Proceedings of the National Academy of Sciences of the United States of America, 109,* 6710–6715.

Marshall, L., Molle, M., Hallschmid, M., & Born, J. (2004). Transcranial direct current stimulation during sleep improves declarative memory. *The Journal of Neuroscience, 24,* 9985–9992.

Miranda, P. C., Mekonnen, A., Salvador, R., & Ruffini, G. (2013). The electric field in the cortex during transcranial current stimulation. *NeuroImage, 70,* 48–58.

Molaee-Ardekani, B., Márquez-Ruiz, J., Merlet, I., Leal-Campanario, R., Gruart, A., Sanchez-Campusano, R., et al. (2013). Effects of transcranial direct current stimulation (tDCS) on cortical activity: A computational modeling study. *Brain Stimulation, 6,* 25–39.

Mulquiney, P. G., Hoy, K. E., Daskalakis, Z. J., & Fitzgerald, P. B. (2011). Improving working memory: Exploring the effect of transcranial random noise stimulation and transcranial direct current stimulation on the dorsolateral prefrontal cortex. *Clinical Neurophysiology, 122,* 2384–2389.

Nekhendzy, V., Fender, C. P., Davies, M. F., Lemmens, H. J., Kim, M. S., Bouley, D. M., et al. (2004). The antinociceptive effect of transcranial electrostimulation with combined direct and alternating current in freely moving rats. *Anesthesia and Analgesia, 98,* 730–737.

Nitsche, M. A., Cohen, L. G., Wassermann, E. M., Priori, A., Lang, N., Antal, A., et al. (2008). Transcranial direct current stimulation: State of the art 2008. *Brain Stimulation, 1,* 206–223.

Nitsche, M. A., & Paulus, W. (2000). Excitability changes induced in the human motor cortex by weak transcranial direct current stimulation. *The Journal of Physiology, 527,* 633–639.

Ozen, S., Sirota, A., Belluscio, M. A., Anastassiou, C. A., Stark, E., Koch, C., et al. (2010). Transcranial electric stimulation entrains cortical neuronal populations in rats. *The Journal of Neuroscience, 30,* 11476–11485.

Penolazzi, B., Di Domenico, A., Marzoli, D., Mammarella, N., Fairfield, B., Franciotti, R., et al. (2010). Effects of transcranial direct current stimulation on episodic memory related to emotional visual stimuli. *PloS One, 5,* e10623.

Purpura, D. P., & McMurtry, J. G. (1965). Intracellular activities and evoked potential changes during polarization of motor cortex. *Journal of Neurophysiology, 28,* 166–185.

Radman, T., Ramos, R. L., Brumberg, J. C., & Bikson, M. (2009). Role of cortical cell type and morphology in subthreshold and suprathreshold uniform electric field stimulation *in vitro. Brain Stimulation, 2,* 215–228.

Ragert, P., Vandermeeren, Y., Camus, M., & Cohen, L. G. (2008). Improvement of spatial tactile acuity by transcranial direct current stimulation. *Clinical Neurophysiology, 119,* 805–811.

Ranieri, F., Podda, M. V., Riccardi, E., Frisullo, G., Dileone, M., Profice, P., et al. (2012). Modulation of LTP at rat hippocampal CA3-CA1 synapses by direct current stimulation. *Journal of Neurophysiology, 107,* 1868–1880.

Rogalewski, A., Breitenstein, C., Nitsche, M. A., Paulus, W., & Knecht, S. (2004). Transcranial direct current stimulation disrupts tactile perception. *The European Journal of Neuroscience, 20,* 313–316.

Rueger, M. A., Keuters, M. H., Walberer, M., Braun, R., Klein, R., Sparing, R., et al. (2012). Multi-session transcranial direct current stimulation (tDCS) elicits inflammatory and regenerative processes in the rat brain. *PloS One, 7,* e43776.

Ruffini, G., Wendling, F., Merlet, I., Molaee-Ardekani, B., Mekkonen, A., Salvador, R., et al. (2012). Transcranial current brain stimulation (tCS): Models and technologies. *IEEE Transactions on Neural Systems and Rehabilitation Engineering, 21,* 333–345.

Silvanto, J., & Pascual-Leone, A. (2008). State-dependency of transcranial magnetic stimulation. *Brain Topography, 21*, 1–10.

Snowball, A., Tachtsidis, I., Popescu, T., Thompson, J., Delazer, M., Zamarian, L., et al. (2013). Long-term enhancement of brain function and cognition using cognitive training and brain stimulation. *Current Biology, 23*, 987–992.

Takano, Y., Yokawa, T., Masuda, A., Niimi, J., Tanaka, S., & Hironaka, N. (2011). A rat model for measuring the effectiveness of transcranial direct current stimulation using fMRI. *Neuroscience Letters, 491*, 40–43.

van Calker, D., Muller, M., & Hamprecht, B. (1979). Adenosine regulates via two different types of receptors, the accumulation of cyclic AMP in cultured brain cells. *Journal of Neurochemistry, 33*, 999–1005.

Yoon, K. J., Oh, B. M., & Kim, D. Y. (2012). Functional improvement and neuroplastic effects of anodal transcranial direct current stimulation (tDCS) delivered 1 day vs 1 week after cerebral ischemia in rats. *Brain Research, 1452*, 61–72.

The Physiological Basis of Brain Stimulation

Charlotte J. Stagg

Oxford Centre for Functional MRI of the Brain (FMRIB), Department of
Clinical Neurosciences, University of Oxford, Oxford, UK

OUTLINE

INTRODUCTION

Background

Since the advent of transcranial magnetic stimulation (TMS) over 25 years ago (Barker & Jalinous, 1985), transcranial stimulation techniques have attracted ever-increasing attention both as tools for neuroscience applications and as putative treatments of neurological and psychiatric disorders. This attention has grown particularly as evidence suggesting that they may be capable of inducing Long Term Potentiation (LTP)-like plasticity increases (Stagg & Nitsche, 2011).

In particular, transcranial direct current stimulation (tDCS) has become increasingly studied as it is relatively cheap, easy to use, and, in the main, well-tolerated. Understanding the physiological mechanisms underpinning the effects of tDCS and related techniques is therefore of prime importance for interpreting the behavioral effects of stimulation, and predicting the likely response to treatment in clinical populations. This chapter aims to summarize the literature describing the known effects of tDCS and related techniques in terms of the underlying physiology, and discuss the implications of these findings for future studies.

Neuroplasticity

Neuroplasticity can be defined as the reorganization of the brain's structure and function in response to intrinsic or environmental challenges. A profusion of physiological mechanisms underlie plasticity, which occur over a range of anatomical and temporal scales, including the modulation of synaptic strength (synaptic plasticity), remodeling of motor cortical representations, and formation of new synapses and dendrites. Understanding these processes and how interventions such as transcranial stimulation protocols may interact with endogenous processes to underpin behavioral improvements is of vital importance both to our understanding of the effects of transcranial stimulation techniques on behavior (e.g., motor learning) in humans, and to our understanding of how we can aid behavioral recovery after a brain injury such as a stroke.

One of the earliest and key responses of the brain to novel challenges is synaptic plasticity or changes in synaptic strength, which form the focus of this review. The modulation of synaptic strength was perhaps most memorably predicted by Hebb in 1949: *"When an axon of cell A is near enough to excite a cell B and repeatedly or persistently takes part in firing it, some growth process or metabolic change takes place in one or both cells such that A's efficiency, as one of the cells firing B, is increased"* (Hebb, 1949). First demonstrated experimentally in 1973 by Bliss and Lømo, long-term potentiation (LTP) and related LTP-like processes have now been described across the brain in response to a number of environmental and exogenous stimulation protocols in a variety of animal models (Bliss & Lømo, 1973). LTP-like plasticity refers to the well-described strengthening of synapses, due to synchronous stimulation of the presynaptic and postsynaptic cell, and classically has been described at glutamatergic synapses (Bliss, Collingridge, & Morris, 2003). The corollary of LTP, long-term depression (LTD), refers to a *decrease* in synaptic strength in response to stimulation (Kirkwood & Bear, 1994).

LTP-like processes are of particular interest for neuroscientists and clinicians as they are thought to be the physiological substrate of learning and memory formation, both in healthy subjects and in the functional recovery of various neurological and psychiatric conditions (Cooke, 2006).

LTP- and LTD-like phenomena depend on a vast number of individual signaling pathways, and the relative importance of many of the molecules involved is only slowly being understood. However, one molecule in particular, Brain Derived Neurotrophic Factor (BDNF), has aroused particular interest in studies of plasticity. BDNF is intimately involved in LTP-like plasticity (Akaneya, Tsumoto, Kinoshita, & Hatanaka, 1997; Lu, 2003), and a common polymorphism in humans (val66met) has a significant impact on a subject's ability to learn a motor task (Kleim et al., 2006; McHughen et al., 2010).

Early Electrical Stimulation Techniques

Low-level electrical currents have been used for millennia in the treatment of a variety of neurological and psychiatric conditions (see also Chapter 1). Torpedo electric fish were in common use in ancient Egypt and ancient Greece for the treatment of migraine and epilepsy (Kellaway, 1946). The effects of electrical, or galvanic, currents were subsequently studied in greater depth by eminent 17th-century scientists such as Aldini, Galvani, and Volta (Priori, 2003), from whom the use of electrical currents in the form of electric convulsive therapy (ECT) was derived. Subsequent studies using low-level electrical currents continued alongside those using ECT, although the relatively small and variable results of low-level currents meant that research into this area was somewhat limited (for a full review, see Stagg & Nitsche, 2011).

Transcranial Direct Current Stimulation

Transcranial direct current stimulation (tDCS) in its modern form was first described around the turn of the new millennium and involves passing a small electric current, in the range of 1–2mA, through the brain via one or more electrodes placed on the scalp. Anodal stimulation is facilitatory to the cortex underlying the active electrode, and cathodal stimulation, where the current direction is reversed, is inhibitory to the cortex (Nitsche & Paulus, 2000). Current may be passed for up to 30 minutes and, if applied for approximately 10 minutes or longer, has effects on cortical excitability which outlast the stimulation period by up to 90 minutes (Nitsche & Paulus, 2001). The duration of these tDCS aftereffects can be increased by concurrent pharmacological modulation, as discussed in more detail later in this chapter. In addition, repeated sessions of tDCS have been shown to lead to long-lasting neurophysiological (Monte-Silva et al., 2012) and behavioral improvements (Cohen Kadosh, Soskic, Iuculano, Kanai, & Walsh, 2010; Reis et al., 2009), making it a potentially important adjunct therapy in rehabilitation.

tDCS is commonly referred to as both a "subthreshold" and a "neuromodulatory" stimulation technique. These terms refer to the fact that tDCS, unlike TMS (discussed in detail later in the chapter) and transcranial electric stimulation (tES; Merton, Hill, Morton, & Marsden, 1982), does not induce action potential volleys in the descending motor pathways, as it does not cause sufficient depolarization of the underlying neurons. Rather, tDCS acts to modulate the rate of naturally occurring firing of neurons within the stimulated tissue.

Related Electrical Stimulation Techniques

Recently, more complex stimulation paradigms have been developed from tDCS that rely on modulating current intensity rather than utilizing a constant current. The most widely used of these are commonly referred to as transcranial alternating current stimulation (tACS) and random noise stimulation (tRNS) (see also Chapter 2).

tACS involves the application of sinusoidally-varying currents at a range of frequencies, and it seems likely, although has yet to be definitively demonstrated, that the behavioral effects of tACS are driven by the entrainment of neuronal networks to the tACS stimulation (Marshall, Helgadóttir, Mölle, & Born, 2006; Ozen et al., 2010). tRNS uses a random noise frequency pattern which is thought to desynchronize natural cortical oscillatory rhythms (Terney, Chaieb, Moliadze, Antal, & Paulus, 2008), and therefore has potential in situations where pathological overactivity within certain oscillatory frequencies occurs. In its standard protocol, tRNS utilizes a normally distributed random level of current, changing in amplitude with a rate of up to 640 Hz, with no overall DC offset (Terney et al., 2008). In the frequency spectrum, all coefficients have a similar size, giving a "white noise" characteristic. However, the physiological underpinnings of tACS and tRNS have yet to be explored in detail, and therefore are not discussed here. For a review of these techniques, as well as what is known about their physiological and behavioral effects, see Paulus (2011).

Transcranial Magnetic Stimulation

TMS is a technique that induces localized, relatively small amplitude currents in cortical tissue via the principles of electromagnetic induction. The passage of a brief current (in the order few milliseconds) through a figure-of-eight current placed on the scalp generates a rapidly changing magnetic field, which in turn induces currents in the underlying brain tissue. TMS can be targeted to the primary motor cortex (M1) via placement of the coil over the motor "hotspot" of a specific muscle – most commonly the first dorsal interosseous (FDI), one of the intrinsic muscles of the hand. The motor hotspot is defined as the scalp position at which the lowest intensity TMS pulse evokes a just noticeable response within the target muscle. The muscle response can be recorded using electromyography (EMG), and the resulting activity within the muscle after a TMS pulse is known as the motor evoked potential (MEP).

TMS can be used to study brain activity both as a tool for modulating cortical excitability and as a method for probing neurophysiology within the primary motor cortex (M1). There is a large and increasing number of TMS protocols that allow modulation of cortical excitability. A full review of the use of TMS as a neuromodulatory technique is beyond the scope of this chapter, but readers are referred to Nitsche, Muller-Dahlhaus, Paulus, and Ziemann (2012) for a review.

METHODS TO MEASURE THE PHYSIOLOGICAL MECHANISMS UNDERLYING TRANSCRANIAL STIMULATION IN HUMANS

A number of indirect methods can be used to determine the neurophysiological mechanisms underpinning transcranial stimulation. Historically, the majority of physiology studies have been performed in M1 due to the relative ease with which accurate readout measures can be obtained via TMS/EMG. More recently, technical advances have enabled the combination of TMS with electroencephalography (EEG). Although technically challenging to perform and somewhat complex to interpret, this approach has the potential to allow the effects of tDCS on brain regions outside M1 to be studied in some depth. However, to date, physiological studies using this technique are limited, and therefore this chapter will concentrate mainly on studies of the primary motor cortex.

It is important to note, however, that although it is likely that the majority of the information acquired from M1 can inform studies in other cortical regions, inter-regional differences, particularly in gyral anatomy, may significantly alter the direction of current flow and therefore make a direct comparison difficult (Miranda, Lomarev, & Hallett, 2006). Indeed, a recent study of the effects of tDCS on the diaphragm showed that tDCS was inhibitory regardless of stimulation polarity (Azabou et al., 2013), suggesting that direct translation even within M1 must be approached with caution.

It is also important to note that physiological studies have, in the main, been performed in young, healthy adults, and it is difficult to know to what extent these findings can inform our understanding of the effects of transcranial stimulation parameters in the context of cortical damage or potentially disordered regulation, such as in patients after a stroke.

Pharmacological Agents

A number of pharmacological agents have been used to determine the neurochemical basis of transcranial stimulation approaches. The major pharmacological agents used are summarized in Table 6.1. Although pharmacological studies give unparalleled information in humans about the physiological effects of transcranial stimulation, it should be noted that none of the agents listed in Table 6.1 are truly specific for a given receptor. In addition, as pharmacological agents are given systemically they will all have actions across the whole brain, which may complicate the interpretation of the effects of stimulation on a localized region of tissue.

TMS Protocols

Single-Pulse TMS

Single TMS pulses can be used in a number of ways to assess neurophysiology. In its most simple form, a single pulse can be applied at a given intensity. The amplitude of the resulting MEP gives an index of the ease with which action potentials can pass from the pyramidal neurons within the cortex to the effector muscle. Unlike the paired-pulse protocols described below, single-pulse TMS approaches cannot distinguish between changes in cortical, subcortical, or spinal excitability (Chen, 2000).

The simplest TMS approach for assessing underlying physiology is via quantification of the motor threshold (MT). The MT can be defined in a number of ways, but the resting motor threshold is normally defined as

TABLE 6.1 Summary of Common Pharmacological Agents That Have Been Used to Explore the Effects of tDCS

Name	Role	Effects on tDCS-induced Excitability Changes				Notes
		Anodal		Cathodal		
		During	After	During	After	
NON-SYNAPTIC CHANGES						
Carbamazepine	Sodium channel blocker	0	0	↕	↕	Also increases Acetylcholine release (Mizuno et al., 2000) and raises dopamine levels (Okada et al., 1997)
Flunarizine	Calcium channel blocker	↓	0	↕	↕	
NEUROTRANSMITTERS						
Dextromethorphan	NMDA receptor antagonist	↕	0	↕	0	Also blocks sodium, potassium, and calcium channels at higher concentrations (Netzer, Pflimlin, & Trube, 1993)
D-cycloserine	Partial NMDA receptor agonist	NT	↑D	NT	↕	Binds to the glycine binding site, leading to upregulation of NMDA receptor function (Thomas, Hood, Monahan, Contreras, & O'Donohue, 1988)
Lorazepam	GABA$_A$ receptor agonist	↕	↑	↕	↕	
NEUROMODULATORS						
Amphetamine	Non-specific NA and DA agonist	↕	↑D	↕	↓	Also decreases extracellular GABA concentration (Bourdelais & Kalivas, 1990) and stimulates the glutamatergic system (Karler, Calder, Thai, & Bedingfield, 1995)

Continued

TABLE 6.1 Summary of Common Pharmacological Agents That Have Been Used to Explore the Effects of tDCS—cont'd

Name	Role	Effects on tDCS-induced Excitability				Notes
		Changes				
Citalopram	Selective serotonin reuptake inhibitor (SSRI)	NT	↑,↑D	NT	↺	Shows higher affinity for D_2 than D_1 receptors, but is less specific to D_2 than PGL
L-DOPA	DA agonist Low (25 mg)	NT	0	NT	0	
	Medium (100 mg)	NT	↺,↑D	NT	↑D	
	High (200 mg)	NT	0	NT	0	
Pergolide	DA agonist	NT	↕	NT	↕	Shows much higher affinity for D_2 than D_1 receptors (Fici, Wu, Voigtlander Von, & Sethy, 1997; Kvernmo, Härtter, & Burger, 2006)
Sulpiride	D_2 agonist	NT	0	NT	0	
Ropinerole	D_2 agonist Low (0.125 mg)	NT	0	NT	0	
	Medium (0.5 mg)	NT	↕	NT	↕, ↑D	
	High (1 mg)	NT	0	NT	↺	
Propranolol	β receptor antagonist	NT	↓D	NT	↓D	
Rivastigmine	ACh esterase inhibitor	NT	0	NT	↓, then ↑	Increases ACh by reducing the rate of its catabolism

NT, not tested; ↑, increased size of effect; ↓, decreased size of effect; 0, abolished effect; ↺, reversed effect (i.e., anodal tDCS leading to inhibition or cathodal tDCS leading to facilitation); ↑D, increased duration of effect; ↓D, decreased duration of effect.

the minimum stimulus intensity that elicits a peak-to-peak MEP amplitude of 50 μV or more in resting muscle, in at least 5 out of 10 measurements. The MT reflects the activity of a small region of pyramidal neurons, and is not thought to be influenced by activity within GABAergic or glutamatergic interneurons (Ziemann, 2008).

Another approach to assessing physiology using single TMS pulses is via the input/output curve (I/O curve, also known as a recruitment curve). An I/O curve can be acquired by measuring MEP amplitude at a set range of TMS intensities, calculated on a subject-by-subject basis as a percentage of the MT (Ridding & Rothwell, 1997). The slope of the I/O curve reflects the excitability of cortico-spinal neurons across a relatively wide area of the cortex (Nitsche et al., 2005), and is modulated by GABAergic and adrenergic activity, and possibly by glutamatergic activity (Boroojerdi, Battaglia, Muellbacher, & Cohen, 2001; Di Lazzaro et al., 2003).

Paired-Pulse TMS

TMS can be used as a tool to probe cortical physiology, using paired-pulse TMS (ppTMS) approaches. ppTMS paradigms involve the application of two TMS pulses to the same region of cortex with a very short interstimulus interval (ISI). Depending on the length of the ISI, ppTMS techniques are sensitive to GABAergic or glutamatergic transmission. Short interval intracortical inhibition (SICI) and related protocols are ppTMS approaches which utilize a subthreshold conditioning stimulus (CS) followed a few milliseconds later by a suprathreshold test stimulus (TS) which elicits an MEP. The ratio of the amplitude of the conditioned TS-evoked MEP to the unconditioned TS-evoked MEP is then calculated. Depending on the ISI, inhibition or facilitation of the MEP can be induced by the application of the conditioning stimulus (see Table 6.2). This modulation of MEP amplitude can be attributed to glutamatergic or GABAergic function with varying degrees of specificity (for a full review, see Ziemann, 2008).

Two distinct phases of inhibition can be observed using SICI; one at an ISI of 1 ms and one at an ISI of 2–4 ms (Kujirai et al., 1993). The SICI seen at an ISI of 2–4 ms has been demonstrated to reflect activity at $GABA_A$ synapses (Di Lazzaro et al., 2006; Ilić et al., 2002; Ziemann, Lönnecker, Steinhoff and Paulus, 1996). Less is understood about the 1-ms ISI SICI, but it is also a GABAergic phenomenon (Ni, Gunraj, & Chen, 2007) with a distinct mechanism from that of the 2- to 4-ms ISI SICI (Fisher, Nakamura, Bestmann, Rothwell, & Bostock, 2002; Roshan, Paradiso, & Chen, 2003), and has recently been proposed to represent non-synaptic GABAergic tone (Stagg, Bestmann et al., 2011).

$GABA_B$ synaptic activity can be assessed using a related ppTMS approach, that of long interval intracortical inhibition (LICI), which is

TABLE 6.2   Summary of Single- (spTMS) and Paired-Pulse TMS (ppTMS) Protocols

TMS Protocol	Abbreviation	Protocol Details	Neurons Stimulated	Notes
Motor threshold	MT	Single pulse	Corticospinal tract (CST) neurons and closely associated interneurons	No clear involvement for glutamate or GABA
Input/output curve	I/O curve	Single pulse at multiple intensities	CST neurons and intracortical neurons over a wider area than M1	Glutamatergic involvement (Boroojerdi et al., 2001) and some GABAergic involvement at higher intensities (Boroojerdi et al., 2001; Schönle et al., 1989)
Short-interval intracortical inhibition	SICI	Paired pulse, subthreshold then suprathreshold pulse, ISI 1–5 ms (Kujirai et al., 1993)	$GABA_A$ergic interneurons (Di Lazzaro et al., 2000, 2005; Ilić et al., 2002; Ziemann, Lönnecker, Steinhoff, & Paulus, 1996)	Also increased by glutamate antagonists
Intracortical facilitation	ICF	Subthreshold CS, suprathreshold TS, ISI 7–20 ms (Kujirai et al., 1993; Ziemann, Rothwell, & Ridding, 1996)	Primarily glutamatergic interneurons, with some GABAergic effects	Modulated by GABA (Inghilleri, Berardelli, Marchetti, & Manfredi, 1996; Schwenkreis et al., 1999, 2000; Ziemann, Lönnecker, Steinhoff and Paulus, 1996, Ziemann, Chen, Cohen, & Hallett, 1998); increased by DA (Korchounov, Ilić, & Ziemann, 2007; Ziemann, Bruns, & Paulus, 1996); decreased by NA (Korchounov, Ilić, & Ziemann, 2003) and ACh (Korchounov, Ilić, Schwinge, & Ziemann, 2005)

Reproduced from Stagg and Nitsche (2011), with permission.

studied using a suprathreshold CS with an ISI of 100–200 ms (McDonnell, Orekhov, & Ziemann, 2006; Werhahn, Kunesch, Noachtar, Benecke, & Classen, 1999).

Facilitation of the MEP by the conditioning stimulus can be achieved using intracortical facilitation (ICF), a paired-pulse technique related to SICI, but with an ISI of between 10 and 15 ms (Kujirai et al., 1993; Ziemann, Rothwell & Ridding, 1996). The neurochemical underpinning of ICF is somewhat complex, but is thought to be related to a combination of both GABA$_A$ergic and glutamatergic activity (Ziemann, 2008).

Electroencephalography and Magnetoencephalography

Electroencephalography (EEG) and magnetoencephalography (MEG) allow for the study of endogenous oscillatory brain activity, and its modulation by tDCS. Although there are technical considerations when combining tDCS and EEG/MEG concurrently, the frequency and temporal resolution of EEG and MEG allow for subtle stimulation-induced changes in network properties to be determined (Schestatsky, Morales-Quezada, & Fregni, 2013; Soekadar et al., 2013).

In addition, EEG can be used in combination with TMS to further prove the connectivity of a given brain region, where the readout from a TMS pulse is a TMS-evoked potential (TEP) rather than an MEP from EMG. There are significant technical challenges to combining these techniques that need to be overcome, but both single-pulse TMS and paired-pulse TMS have been combined with EEG to study connectivity between brain regions other than M1. Although at the time of writing this approach has not been used to study the effects of tDCS, it is a promising research avenue that undoubtedly will be utilized for the study of stimulation (for a review of the technique, including technical considerations, see Rogasch & Fitzgerald, 2012).

Magnetic Resonance Spectroscopy

Magnetic resonance spectroscopy (MRS) is a non-invasive method of quantifying the concentration of neurochemicals within a specific region of interest in the brain. Depending on the details of the protocol used, MRS allows accurate quantification of various neurochemicals, including GABA and glutamate, within a predefined region of tissue (Fig. 6.1A). For studies of transcranial stimulation in the motor system, a $2 \times 2 \times 2$-cm voxel has most commonly been used, which is normally centered on the hand knob of the primary motor cortex (Fig. 6.1B). Values acquired from this voxel therefore reflect the concentration of neurotransmitters within both M1 and the primary sensorimotor cortex.

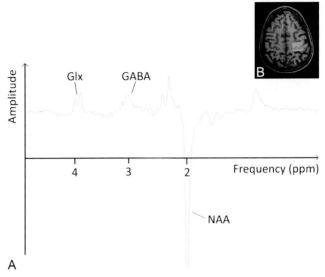

FIGURE 6.1   (A) Typical GABA-edited spectrum from a 2 × 2 × 2-cm voxel sited in the left primary motor cortex. Peaks for GABA, Glx (a composite measure of glutamate and gluta-mine), and N-Acetylaspartate, a common reference molecule, can clearly be seen. (B) A representative location for the M1 voxel placed over the hand region of the primary motor cortex.

It is important to note that measurements acquired using MRS reflect the total concentration of a given neurochemical within the region of interest, and do not necessarily directly reflect synaptic activity. Both GABA and glutamate have important roles within the brain other than as neurotransmitters and these pools will be reflected as much, if not more, than the proportion involved in neurotransmission. However, a recent study demonstrated a close positive relationship between the MRS-derived measure of glutamate and TMS measures of cortical excitability (Stagg, Bestmann et al., 2011), suggesting that at baseline, at least, MRS-assessed glutamate may provide a good index of glutamatergic synaptic activity. Conversely, at baseline, the MRS-assessed measure of GABA has been shown to be unrelated to $GABA_A$ or $GABA_B$ synaptic activity, but rather shows a relationship with 1-ms ISI SICI, which has been suggested to reflect extrasynaptic GABAergic tone (Stagg, Bestmann et al., 2011) – a finding in line with studies in animal models (Mason et al., 2001).

Despite this baseline finding, it should not be inferred that the *change* in GABA in response to plasticity induction protocols such as an ischemic nerve block (Levy, Ziemann, Chen, & Cohen, 2002) or motor learning (Floyer-Lea, Wylezinska, Kincses, & Matthews, 2006) solely reflects changes in extrasynaptic GABA tone. Although it is not yet clear precisely how the MRS-assessed GABA decreases relates to changes in the individual GABAergic pools, it most likely reflects decreases in more than one pool. For a detailed review of the utility and limitations of MRS for the study of motor cortical plasticity, see Stagg (2013).

Animal Models

A number of tDCS animal models have been described which aim to recreate the current densities seen in human cortex as closely as possible. These models have undoubted utility for studying the safety of applied currents, but the differences in current flow through animal and human brain may make utilizing the model for human studies more difficult. More details on these aspects can be found in Chapter 3 in this volume; however, a brief discussion of the important findings is essential for a full understanding of the physiological effects of tDCS.

The first studies of the modern era to investigate the effects of low-level electrical stimulation demonstrated direct increases in spontaneous firing rates of neurons when the anode was placed directly in or above the cortex, whereas reversal of polarity led to a decrease in spontaneous neuronal firing (Bindman, Lippold, & Redfearn, 1964; Creutzfeldt, Fromm, & Kapp, 1962; Purpura & McMurtry, 1965; see also Fig. 6.2A).

Two important findings arose from these early studies. The effects of tDCS were not found to be consistent across the cortical layers – neurons in deep cortical layers were often deactivated by anodal stimulation and activated by cathodal stimulation (Purpura & McMurtry, 1965). In addition, non-pyramidal neurons were stimulated at lower total charges than pyramidal neurons, which were modulated only at higher charge densities, suggesting that interneuronal populations are more sensitive than pyramidal neurons to the effects of tDCS.

The direction of the applied current has been subsequently studied in greater depth and demonstrated to be of prime importance in terms of the overall effects of tDCS. In pioneering work, Jefferys studied the effects of pulsed electrical currents on the granule cell layer of the hippocampus *in vitro* (Jefferys, 1981). Jefferys demonstrated that conventional current passed parallel to the somato-dendritic axis (i.e., from the dendrites to the cell bodies) increased excitability (effects that were reversed when the current direction was reversed), but when current was passed perpendicular to the somato-dendritic axis no effects on cortical excitability were observed.

In a subsequent study of rat hippocampal slices, small electric fields of $< |40|$ mV/mm were applied parallel to the somato-dendritic axis, and the relationship between the applied field and the response was linear (Bikson et al., 2004). DC fields applied perpendicular to the somato-dendritic axis did not induce somatic polarization but did modulate orthodromic responses.

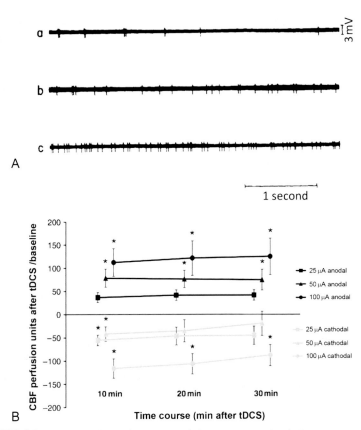

FIGURE 6.2   (A) The effects of transcortical direct current stimulation on spontaneous neuronal firing in the optic cortex of the cat during (a) 500-μA cathodal stimulation, (b) control condition, and (c) 500-μA anodal stimulation. *Figure adapted from Creutzfeldt et al. (1962), with permission from Elsevier.* (B) Cerebral blood flow changes induced in the cortex underlying the stimulating electrode after 15 minutes of 25-μA, 50-μA, and 100-μA tDCS applied to the rat. *Figure reproduced from Wachter et al. (2011), with permission from Elsevier.*

It is important to note, however, that both these studies were performed using relatively strong electric fields, although Bikson and colleagues did suggest that weaker fields might have an influence. More recently, a series of experiments has been performed investigating the effects of the application of direct currents on slice preparations with field strengths more similar to those seen *in vivo* with tDCS. Currents were applied parallel to the somato-dendritic axis and were able to cause small changes in somatic membrane potential of individual neurons, resulting from polarization of the somato-dendritic axis (Fröhlich & McCormick, 2010). Further, weak, surface-positive, constant currents accelerated neocortical slow oscillations *in vivo*, but were shown to modulate rather than override "natural" network dynamics (Fröhlich & McCormick, 2010).

Other recent work used *in vitro* slice preparations of mouse M1 to study the effects of tDCS-like currents (Fritsch et al., 2010). The authors showed that anodal stimulation led to LTP-like plasticity, and that this phenomenon was dependent on BDNF (Fritsch et al., 2010). The authors did not study cathodal stimulation, but a human study suggests that the val66met polymorphism in BDNF has no effect on a subject's response to cathodal tDCS (Cheeran et al., 2008).

Local Perfusion Changes Induced by tDCS

In addition to studies investigating local changes in neuronal firing and synaptic strength, there has also been interest in studying the perfusion changes associated with transcranial stimulation. A recent study in the rat has suggested that anodal tDCS increases cortical perfusion under the stimulating electrode, whereas cathodal stimulation decreased cortical perfusion in a dose-dependent manner (Wachter et al., 2011; see also Fig. 6.2B). A study in humans using near infrared spectroscopy (NIRS) showed a similar increase in perfusion during anodal tDCS, though cathodal tDCS was not studied (Merzagora et al., 2010). Similar results, using the MR technique arterial spin labeling (ASL), have been described in humans both in M1 (Zheng, Alsop, & Schlaug, 2011) and in the dorsolateral prefrontal cortex (DLPFC) (Stagg et al., 2013). ASL, unlike other functional MRI techniques, directly quantifies cerebral blood flow, and therefore these findings in humans can be directly compared with those demonstrated in animals by Wachter and colleagues.

Effects on Oscillatory Activity

There is a small but rapidly increasing literature on the effects of tDCS on cortical oscillatory activity.

A recent MEG study demonstrated that both anodal and cathodal tDCS decreased oscillatory activity within the alpha frequency, and increased gamma-frequency oscillations (Venkatakrishnan, Contreras-Vidal, Sandrini, & Cohen, 2011). An earlier EEG study showed a significant increase in oscillation synchrony within the beta frequency at rest, and a significant increase in oscillation synchrony within the high gamma (60–90 Hz) range during voluntary hand movements after anodal tDCS (Polanía, Nitsche, & Paulus, 2011). Cathodal tDCS was not studied. Although the neurochemical basis of oscillations within particular frequencies is complex and not currently well understood, these finding would be in line with a decrease in GABAergic activity after both anodal and cathodal tDCS, as has been seen in MRS studies (Stagg et al., 2009).

MEG and EEG studies are even more limited outside the hand region of M1. A study of the effects of tDCS on swallowing showed an anodal tDCS-induced decrease in task-related theta (4–8 Hz) activity within the motor network (Suntrup et al., 2010). In another study, anodal tDCS to the right inferior frontal gyrus *decreased* local activity within the theta band at rest (Jacobson, Ezra, Berger, & Lavidor, 2012). There is not, as yet, sufficient evidence from the literature to know how to bring these findings together into a coherent narrative of the effects of tDCS, but further studies will hopefully inform our understanding of the effects of tDCS on oscillatory activity within the brain.

NEURONAL AND SYNAPTIC EFFECTS INDUCED BY tDCS

The majority of physiological studies into the effects of tDCS have been performed using the "classic" montage, where one 5 × 7-cm electrode is placed over M1 and the reference placed over the contralateral supraorbital ridge, and the current is run for up to 20 minutes (Nitsche & Paulus, 2000). The effects of tDCS are determined by current direction as well as duration and current density.

It is important to note that current direction is determined not only by which direction the current is run within the circuit, but also by the location of the reference electrode. The facilitatory effects of anodal tDCS described using the classic montage (Nitsche & Paulus, 2000) are not seen when the reference electrode is placed on the chin; indeed using this montage, anodal stimulation led to a significant *decrease* in cortical excitability (Priori, Berardelli, Rona, Accornero, & Manfredi, 1998).

The duration and current density applied may also have highly significant effects on the direction of tDCS-induced cortical excitability changes. It has repeatedly been shown that a single application of 13 minutes of anodal tDCS leads to a significant *increase* of motor cortical excitability (Monte-Silva et al., 2012; Nitsche & Paulus, 2001). However, 13 minutes of anodal tDCS followed immediately by another 13-minute period of anodal tDCS (i.e., a total stimulation period of 26 minutes) led to a significant *decrease* of motor cortical excitability (Monte-Silva et al., 2012; see also Fig. 6.3). This finding, which was reversed by the application of the calcium channel blocker flumazenil, suggests that cortical regulatory mechanisms that exist to prevent over-excitability are activated with longer stimulation durations. The precise mechanisms underlying this reversal in excitability effects are unclear, but, as the authors suggest, probably involve the activation of hyper-polarizing potassium channels, which are dependent on the levels of intracellular calcium (Monte-Silva et al., 2012).

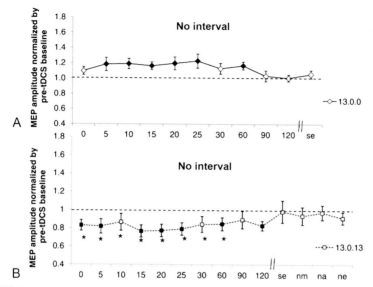

FIGURE 6.3   **The effects of current duration on cortical excitability changes induced by tDCS.** (A) 13 minutes of 1-mA anodal tDCS induced an increase in cortical excitability that lasted for 60 minutes after stimulation. (B) 26 minutes of 1-mA tDCS induced a significant *decrease* in cortical excitability that outlasted the stimulation period for 120 minutes. Filled symbols indicate significant difference from baseline; *, a significant difference from the effects of 13 minutes of anodal tDCS demonstrated in A ($P < 0.05$); se, same evening; nm, next morning; na, next afternoon; ne, next evening. *Figure reproduced from Monte-Silva et al. (2012), with permission from Elsevier.*

Effects During Stimulation

The effects of tDCS during stimulation have been studied using both pharmacological and TMS approaches, and, in the main, the results from these two approaches have been in line. During stimulation it appears that tDCS predominantly modulates interneurons. Although this conclusion is somewhat speculative, it is supported by the finding that the motor threshold (MT), usually considered a relatively specific measure of pyramidal neuron excitability, is unaltered by both anodal and cathodal stimulation (Nitsche et al., 2005).

Anodal tDCS

The effects of anodal tDCS during stimulation appear to be solely dependent on the modulation of membrane potential. The increase in cortical excitability typically induced by anodal tDCS (Nitsche & Paulus, 2000) is reduced by the calcium channel blocker flunarizine, and abolished by the sodium channel blocker carbamezipine (Nitsche, Fricke et al., 2003).

Neither GABAergic nor glutamatergic modulation appears to have a role in the increase of cortical excitability during anodal tDCS. Anodal tDCS had no effect on TMS measures of either glutamatergic activity (ICF) or GABAergic interneuronal function (SICI) (Table 6.2; see also Nitsche et al., 2005), suggesting that no significant modulation of the glutamatergic or GABAergic interneuronal pools occurred during stimulation (Nitsche et al., 2005). In line with these findings, neither the NMDA receptor antagonist dextromethorphan (Nitsche, Fricke et al., 2003) nor lorazepam, a $GABA_A$ receptor agonist (Nitsche, Liebetanz et al., 2004), modulated the magnitude of the intrastimulation response to anodal tDCS.

Cathodal tDCS

Likewise, excitability changes during cathodal stimulation are also probably due to modulation of membrane potential, although, unlike anodal stimulation, blockade of neither voltage-dependent calcium nor sodium channels had any effect on excitability shifts (Nitsche, Fricke et al., 2003). This initially counterintuitive finding is in accordance with the hypothesis that tDCS-generated hyper-polarization of the neuron leads to inactivation of the relevant voltage gated channels and therefore negation of any drug effect.

GABA antagonists do not modulate the effects of intrastimulation cathodal tDCS (Nitsche, Fricke et al., 2003; Nitsche, Liebetanz et al., 2004). However, evidence for the role of glutamate in cathodal tDCS-induced intrastimulation decreases in cortical excitability is somewhat contradictory. The NMDA antagonist dextromethorphan has no effect on intrastimulation effects of cathodal tDCS (Nitsche, Fricke et al., 2003). However, cathodal tDCS did lead to a decrease in ICF during stimulation, suggesting that there may be some involvement of glutamatergic interneurons (Nitsche et al., 2005). These two initially contradictory findings may be reconciled by the finding that cathodal tDCS also modulated the input/output curve (I/O) (Nitsche et al., 2005). I/O curves are probably influenced by excitability within the interneuronal pool to a greater extent than is the motor threshold, and therefore a change in the I/O curve is usually taken to represent a modulation of interneuronal activity. In the light of this finding, and taking the TMS and pharmacological evidence together, it would appear that the change in ICF and the I/O curve during cathodal tDCS is most probably due to a direct influence in resting membrane potential of the glutamatergic interneurons, rather than modulation of the glutamatergic synapses.

Aftereffects of tDCS

In contrast to the effects of tDCS during stimulation, the aftereffects of tDCS appear to be largely driven by changes in synaptic strength. The duration of the aftereffects depend to a great extent on the length of application of the stimulation. Stimulation periods of up to 7 minutes only induce aftereffects for a few minutes, while those of more than 9 minutes (for cathodal stimulation) or 13 minutes (for anodal stimulation) induce neurophysiological aftereffects that last for over 1 hour. The nature of these aftereffects induced by short-term and long-term stimulation, however, seems to be similar.

Anodal tDCS

1-mA STIMULATION

The induction of the aftereffects of anodal tDCS, at least, is dependent on membrane depolarization. If changes in membrane potential are prevented by either the calcium channel blocker flumazenil or the sodium channel blocker carbamezepine then no aftereffects of stimulation are observed (Liebetanz, Nitsche, Tergau, & Paulus, 2002; Nitsche, Fricke et al., 2003). It would appear that the aftereffects of anodal stimulation arise from modulation of the intracortical interneurons rather than the pyramidal output neurons in the main, as evidenced by the lack of modulation of the MT but an increase in the slope of the I/O curve (Nitsche et al., 2005). However, unlike the effects of tDCS during stimulation, the aftereffects *do* appear to be dependent on changes in neurotransmitter and neuromodulator activity, as will be described in the next section.

MODULATION OF GLUTAMATERGIC ACTIVITY

The increase in cortical excitability seen after anodal tDCS is, at least in part, driven by modulation of glutamatergic synapses. Cortical excitability increases were blocked by the addition of dextromethorphan (Liebetanz et al., 2002; Nitsche, Fricke et al., 2003), and anodal tDCS was observed to increase ICF (Nitsche et al., 2005). An MRS study performed in the parietal lobe showed a significant increase in glutamate concentration after 30 minutes of 2-mA anodal stimulation (Clark, Coffman, Trumbo, & Gasparovic, 2011). Within the primary motor cortex, a non-significant trend towards an increase in Glx (a composite measure of glutamate and glutamine) has also been observed after 10 minutes of 1-mA anodal tDCS (Stagg et al., 2009). Indeed, it may be that modulation of glutamatergic synapses reaches a ceiling after anodal tDCS, as further increasing glutamatergic activity using the NMDA receptor agonist d-cycloserine increases the duration but not the magnitude of the aftereffects of anodal tDCS (Nitsche, Jaussi et al., 2004).

MODULATION OF GABAERGIC INHIBITION

In addition to the effects on glutamatergic processing, the aftereffects of anodal tDCS are, at least in part, driven by decreases in GABAergic inhibition. TMS studies show that anodal tDCS leads to a reduction in SICI

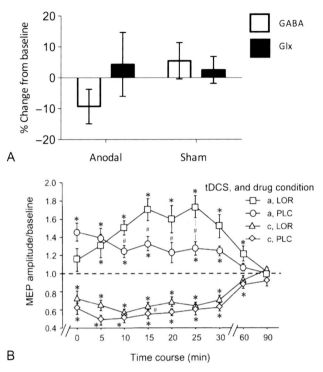

FIGURE 6.4 Modulation of GABAergic activity by tDCS. (A) MRS-assessed GABA levels within the stimulated primary motor cortex are decreased after 10 minutes of 1-mA anodal tDCS. No significant change in Glx (a composite of glutamate and glutamine) was demonstrated *Figure adapted from Stagg et al. (2009).* (B) Lorazepam (LOR), a GABA$_A$ agonist, led to a significant *increase* in cortical excitability after anodal tDCS compared with placebo (PLC). No modulation on the aftereffects of cathodal tDCS was demonstrated. *, a significant difference from baseline; #, a significant difference between the lorazepam and placebo conditions ($P < 0.05$). *Figure reproduced from Nitsche, Liebetanz et al. (2004), with permission.*

(Nitsche et al., 2005), and MRS studies have demonstrated a significant decrease in GABA concentration within M1 after anodal tDCS (Stagg et al., 2009, Stagg, Bachtiar, & Johansen-Berg, 2011; see also Fig. 6.4A). The evidence from pharmacological studies, however, is somewhat counterintuitive. The GABA$_A$ agonist lorazepam led to an initial decrease in excitability during the first 10 minutes, after which a significant *increase* in excitability was seen (Fig. 6.4B; see also Nitsche, Liebetanz et al., 2004). The interpretation of this finding from a pharmacological study is not clear, but has been postulated to reflect an increase in local GABAergic inhibition in sites distant to the stimulated M1, thereby reducing inhibition from these regions to the stimulated region (Stagg & Nitsche, 2011).

THE ROLE OF NEUROMODULATORS

Anodal tDCS aftereffects have been demonstrated to be significantly modulated by drugs acting on the noradrenergic, cholinergic, dopaminergic, and serotinergic systems. The duration, but not the magnitude, of the aftereffects of anodal tDCS was significantly decreased by the β-adrenoreceptor antagonist propranolol (Nitsche, Grundey et al., 2004). Likewise, the duration, but not the magnitude, of the aftereffects was enhanced by the addition of amphetamine, but only when given in the absence of dextromethorphan. This finding suggests that the catecholaminergic system specifically modulates plasticity occurring at the glutamatergic synapses (Nitsche, Grundey et al., 2004).

Dopaminergic activity improves learning and memory formation, and is thought to have an important role in focusing of synaptic plasticity *in vivo* (Foote & Morrison, 1987; Seamans & Yang, 2004). Therefore, it should act to decrease non-specific plasticity induction, such as that seen with tDCS. In line with this hypothesis, simply increasing overall dopaminergic tone via application of L-DOPA abolishes the excitability increases seen after anodal tDCS, in an inverted U-shaped response. Low and high doses of L-DOPA abolish all aftereffects, whereas an intermediate dose leads to a *decrease* in excitability, resulting in aftereffects of anodal tDCS that were statistically indistinguishable in magnitude but longer in duration than those elicited by cathodal tDCS alone (Kuo, Paulus, & Nitsche, 2008; Monte-Silva, Liebetanz, Grundey, Paulus, & Nitsche, 2010; see also Fig. 6.5).

Further studies have suggested that the interaction of effects at D_1 and D_2 receptors may be important in this reversal of the aftereffects of tDCS. The specific enhancement of D_1 or D_2 receptors does not, alone, replicate this conversion of the aftereffects of anodal tDCS to inhibition. An intervention aimed at specifically increasing D_1 activity led to no modulation of the aftereffects of tDCS (Nitsche et al., 2009), whereas both low and high doses of the selective D_2 agonist ropinerole abolished the aftereffects of anodal tDCS but did not convert them into inhibition. Interestingly, an intermediate dose of ropinerole (1 mg) had no effect on the tDCS aftereffects, thereby demonstrating an inverted U-shaped response curve (Monte-Silva et al., 2009).

Increasing cholinergic tone via the administration of rivistigmine abolished the aftereffects of anodal tDCS (Kuo, Grosch, Fregni, Paulus, & Nitsche, 2007). By contrast, increasing serotonergic tone via the administration of the selective serotonin reuptake inhibitor (SSRI) citalopram increased both the duration and magnitude of the aftereffects of anodal tDCS.

2-mA STIMULATION

The after effects of 2-mA stimulation have been studied less thoroughly than those of 1-mA tDCS, but there do not appear to be important differences between the two stimulation paradigms. Like 1-mA stimulation,

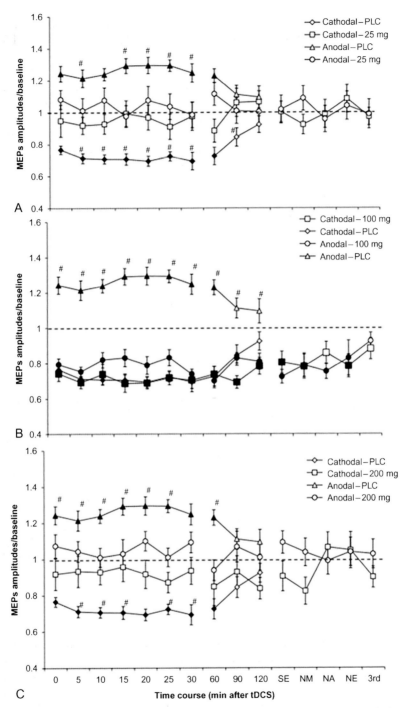

FIGURE 6.5 Dopaminergic influences on the aftereffects of tDCS. Low (25 mg [A]) and high (200 mg [C]) doses of L-DOPA abolish the aftereffects of both anodal and cathodal tDCS. An intermediate dose (100 mg [B])of L-DOPA led to a reversal of the expected increase in cortical excitability after anodal tDCS. No effect on the magnitude or direction of the cathodal tDCS aftereffects was observed. However, the duration of the aftereffects of both anodal and cathodal tDCS are increased by 100-mg L-DOPA, until the next evening (NE, [B]). Filled symbols indicate significant deviations from baseline; #, a significant difference between the L-DOPA and placebo conditions. *Figure reproduced from Monte-Silva et al. (2010), with permission.*

2-mA anodal tDCS leads to an overall increase in excitability, although, unlike 1-mA stimulation, no change in the I/O curve was observed. In terms of the effects of 2-mA anodal tDCS on GABA and glutamatergic signaling, as assessed by SICI and ICF, 2-mA stimulation led to a significant increase in ICF and a decrease in the level of GABAergic inhibition (Batsikadze, Moliadze, Paulus, Kuo, & Nitsche, 2013). These findings are very similar to those seen after 1-mA tDCS.

Cathodal tDCS

1-mA STIMULATION

It is more difficult to know to what degree the aftereffects of cathodal tDCS are dependent on membrane polarization changes than those of anodal tDCS. The aftereffects of cathodal tDCS are not modulated by flunarizine or carbamazepine. However, as discussed in "Effects during stimulation", above, this may be for technical reasons rather than actually reflecting a lack of membrane polarization changes in cathodal tDCS (Nitsche, Fricke et al., 2003). MT was not altered by cathodal tDCS but the I/O curve was, possibly suggesting a relatively widespread effect on intracortical neurons (Nitsche et al., 2005; Stagg & Nitsche, 2011).

MODULATION OF GLUTAMATERGIC ACTIVITY The aftereffects of cathodal tDCS are dependent on the modulation of glutamatergic activity. They are blocked by the administration of dextromethorphan (Nitsche, Fricke et al., 2003); cathodal tDCS led to a significant decrease in ICF (Nitsche et al., 2005), and an MRS study demonstrated a significant decrease in glutamate concentration within the stimulated voxel after cathodal tDCS (Stagg et al., 2009). Although another study suggested that the application of the NMDA receptor agonist d-cycloserine did not increase the aftereffects of tDCS (Nitsche, Jaussi et al., 2004), this may be explained via tDCS-induced hyperpolarization of the postsynaptic cell leading to modification of the d-cycloserine binding site (Stagg & Nitsche, 2011).

THE ROLE OF GABAERGIC INHIBITION IN THE EFFECTS OF CATHODAL tDCS

The role of GABAergic inhibition in cathodal tDCS is less clear than with anodal tDCS. The results from TMS, pharmacological studies, and MRS studies give conflicting results. SICI has been shown to be enhanced after cathodal tDCS (Nitsche et al., 2005), but the GABA agonist lorazepam does not modulate the aftereffects of cathodal tDCS (Nitsche, Liebetanz et al., 2004). A significant reduction in MRS-assessed GABA concentration was observed after cathodal tDCS (Stagg et al., 2009). These conflicting results may be accounted for by the different sensitivities and specificities of the techniques involved, but to date no clear consensus has been reached as to the importance of GABAergic modulation in the aftereffects of cathodal tDCS.

THE ROLE OF NEUROMODULATORS

The aftereffects of cathodal tDCS are not increased by increased catecholaminergic tone – amphetamine did not alter either the magnitude or the duration of the aftereffects – but the duration of the aftereffects was decreased by propranolol (Nitsche, Grundey et al., 2004). Similarly to anodal tDCS, the effects of dopaminergic modulation on the aftereffects of cathodal stimulation are somewhat complex. An intermediate dose of L-DOPA led to an increased duration (though not magnitude) of the aftereffects of cathodal tDCS (Kuo, Paulus, & Nitsche, 2008; Monte-Silva et al., 2010), although low or high doses of L-DOPA led to an abolishment of the aftereffects (Monte-Silva et al., 2010). Selective enhancement of D_1 receptor activity had no effect on the aftereffects of cathodal tDCS (Nitsche et al., 2009). An intermediate dose of the selective D_2 agonist ropinerole led to an increase in the duration (but not the magnitude) of the aftereffects of tDCS (Monte-Silva et al., 2009). The D_2 antagonist sulpiride abolished the aftereffects of cathodal tDCS (Nitsche et al., 2006), and this effect was not reversed by the addition of pergolide to give a selective D_1 enhancement. Therefore, the D_2 receptor seems to be important in the aftereffects of cathodal tDCS, but these responses are not linear. Rather, they appear to have an inverted U-shaped response such that both high and low doses of ropinerole led to an abolition of the aftereffects of cathodal tDCS.

Increasing cholinergic tone via application of rivistigmine led to an increase in the duration (but not the magnitude) of the aftereffects of cathodal tDCS (Kuo et al., 2007). Conversely, the application of the SSRI citalopram led to an *increase* in cortical excitability after cathodal tDCS, in line with the known significant pro-facilitatory effects of serotonin on plasticity induction.

2-mA STIMULATION

Unlike 1-mA stimulation, 2-mA cathodal tDCS applied for 20 minutes led to a significant *increase* in cortical excitability, as demonstrated by an increase in MEP amplitude after stimulation (Batsikadze et al., 2013). There was no change in the I/O curve, but both a decrease in inhibition, as assessed via SICI, and an increase in ICF were observed. This finding suggests that this increase in cortical excitability was driven by changes in both GABAergic and glutamatergic processing (Batsikadze et al., 2013).

The physiological mechanism by which a higher current intensity can lead to a reversal to the previously well-described decrease in excitability is not well understood. The authors suggest that an increase in calcium flux may be responsible, with the animal literature suggesting that a low postsynaptic calcium enhancement leads to LTD-like plasticity whereas a high postsynaptic calcium influx leads to LTP-like plasticity (Lisman, 2001). Whatever the mechanism, this finding is of vital importance when interpreting behavioral results from studies using current intensities of more than 1 mA.

EFFECTS OF tDCS ON OSCILLATORY ACTIVITY

A number of studies have been performed studying the physiological effects of tDCS applied to brain regions other than the primary motor cortex.

A recent study investigated the effects of tDCS to the right posterior parietal cortex on endogenous oscillatory activity. Anodal tDCS significantly increased oscillatory activity within the alpha band (8–13 Hz) but had no significant effects on activity in other frequency bands. Cathodal tDCS did not modulate oscillatory activity significantly in any frequency band studied. Alpha activity has been linked to cortical inhibition and network connectivity (Palva & Palva, 2007), making this a somewhat counterintuitive result, but one that at the least highlights the potential of this approach.

RELATIONSHIP BETWEEN tDCS AND MOTOR LEARNING

Intuitively, tDCS might be thought to have few similarities in terms of its cortical effects to other plasticity induction protocols, such as motor learning, which are more anatomically specific. However, there is growing evidence that anodal tDCS in particular modulates the cortex in a manner at least similar to endogenous plasticity, such as motor learning (see also Chapter 8).

There is increasing evidence that anodal tDCS and motor learning modulate similar intracortical mechanisms. This interaction has been studied by investigating whether simultaneous application of anodal tDCS and motor learning results in an improvement in behavior. However, it is possible that any improvement seen using this experimental protocol may be a result of a non-specific increase in cortical excitability rather than a specific facilitation at a synaptic level. If tDCS and motor learning are applied consecutively rather than concurrently, then their interaction at a more specific synaptic level might be investigated.

The response of a synapse to a given stimulation is modulated by prior experience. Homeostatic, or metaplastic, mechanisms have been proposed to maintain neural activity within a useful dynamic range. At their simplest, homeostatic mechanisms mean that at a synapse where LTP-like plasticity has been induced, the subsequent application of a stimulus that would normally induce LTP-like effects will instead lead to LTD-like downregulation (Bienenstock, Cooper, & Munro, 1982). Homeostatic mechanisms have been shown to operate both at the same synapse (homosynaptic metaplasticity) and at functionally related synapses (heterosynaptic metaplasticity). Therefore, although the demonstration of a homeostatic interaction cannot necessarily be taken to mean that two stimuli act at the same synapse, it may more reasonably be taken as an indication that they at least affect functionally related synapses, and therefore functionally related interneuronal circuits.

Anodal tDCS, when applied simultaneously with a motor learning task, leads to enhancement of motor learning (Nitsche, Schauenburg et al., 2003; Reis et al., 2009; Stagg, Jayaram et al., 2011). Further, the two interventions appear to interact in a homeostatic manner, suggesting that they affect closely related, if not identical, synapses (Kuo, Unger et al., 2008; Stagg, Jayaram et al., 2011). Both anodal tDCS and motor learning lead to a decrease in MRS-assessed GABA levels within M1 (Floyer-Lea et al., 2006; Stagg et al., 2009; Stagg, Bachtiar, & Johansen-Berg, 2011), and, importantly, the magnitude of the GABA decrease induced by tDCS correlates with the subject's ability to learn a motor sequence performed on a separate day (Stagg, Bachtiar, & Johansen-Berg, 2011).

Whether or not tDCS is able to interact at a synaptic level with endogenous plasticity-induction protocols is not only an interesting academic question but also has important implications for the use of tDCS as an adjunctive therapy in recovery of function after brain injury, such as a stroke. A single session of anodal tDCS applied to the motor cortex within the ipsilesional hemisphere has been demonstrated to improve function in the chronic stages of stroke recovery for short periods of time (Hummel et al., 2005, 2006; Stagg et al., 2012). Additionally, daily applications of tDCS with the anode placed over the M1 in the ipsilesional hemisphere and the cathode placed over M1 in the contralesional hemisphere appear to induce longer-lasting behavioral improvements (Lindenberg, Renga, Zhu, Nair, & Schlaug, 2010). However, optimizing tDCS as a therapeutic tool on a patient-by-patient basis will rely on an in-depth understanding of the physiological underpinnings of both tDCS and natural recovery processes after a stroke (see also Chapter 12).

CONCLUSIONS

There is increasing evidence that the "classical" tDCS montage is capable of inducing either glutamatergic LTP-like or LTD-like plasticity, depending on the polarity of the current applied. This evidence gives a strong rationale for the use of concurrent tDCS with motor learning protocols to improve behavior. Some questions remain, however, as to the role of GABA and the neuromodulators such as dopamine, serotonin, and acetylcholine. Results from pharmacological studies in healthy controls suggest that these interventions may lead to greatly increased cortical excitability aftereffects. These effects may potentially increase the utility of these techniques to induce long-lasting behavioral improvements in clinical situations, such as in patients in the chronic stages of stroke recovery. However, the role of these agents in combination with tDCS has yet to be tested in subjects other than young healthy controls, and should therefore be applied with caution. In addition, although the effects of the "classical" tDCS approach are increasingly well understood, recent studies strongly suggest that these may be modulated by current duration, current density, and direction. This has important implications for studies using very long-lasting stimulation protocols, or those outside the primary motor cortex where gyral anatomy and selection of an appropriate reference placement may reduce or even reverse the cortical excitability effects induced by "classical" tDCS.

However, although significant questions remain about the use of tDCS, evidence to date strongly suggests tDCS may have significant potential utility as an adjunctive therapy in stroke recovery. As more is understood about the effects of tDCS in other clinical conditions, its increasing use in diverse neurological and psychiatric conditions may be optimized.

References

Akaneya, Y. Y., Tsumoto, T. T., Kinoshita, S. S., & Hatanaka, H. H. (1997). Brain-derived neurotrophic factor enhances long-term potentiation in rat visual cortex. *The Journal of Neuroscience: The Official Journal of the Society for Neuroscience, 17*(17), 6707–6716.

Azabou, E., Roche, N., Sharshar, T., Bussel, B., Lofaso, F., & Petitjean, M. (2013). Transcranial direct-current stimulation reduced the excitability of diaphragmatic corticospinal pathways whatever the polarity used. *Respiratory Physiology & Neurobiology, 189*(1), 183–187. http://dx.doi.org/10.1016/j.resp.2013.07.02.

Barker, A. T., & Jalinous, R. (1985). Non-invasive magnetic stimulation of human motor cortex. *Lancet, 325*(8437), 1106–1107.

Batsikadze, G., Moliadze, V., Paulus, W., Kuo, M. F., & Nitsche, M. A. (2013). Partially non-linear stimulation intensity-dependent effects of direct current stimulation on motor cortex excitability in humans. *The Journal of Physiology, 591*(Pt 7), 1987–2000.

Bienenstock, E., Cooper, L., & Munro, P. (1982). Theory for the development of neuron selectivity: Orientation specificity and binocular interaction in visual cortex. *The Journal of Neuroscience, 2*(1), 32–48.

Bikson, M., Inoue, M., Akiyama, H., Deans, J. K., Fox, J. E., Miyakawa, H., et al. (2004). Effects of uniform extracellular DC electric fields on excitability in rat hippocampal slices *in vitro*. *The Journal of Physiology, 557*(1), 175–190.

Bindman, L., Lippold, O. C., & Redfearn, J. W. (1964). The action of brief polarizing currents on the cerebral cortex of the rat (1) during current flow and (2) in the production of long-lasting aftereffects. *The Journal of Physiology, 172*, 369–382.

Bliss, T., Collingridge, G., & Morris, R. (2003). LTP: Long term potentiation; Enhancing neuroscience for 30 years. *Philosophical Transactions of the Royal Society, B: Biological Sciences, 358*, 607–842.

Bliss, T., & Lømo, T. (1973). Long-lasting potentiation of synaptic transmission in the dentate area of the anaesthetized rabbit following stimulation of the perforant path. *The Journal of Physiology, 232*(2), 331–356.

Boroojerdi, B., Battaglia, F., Muellbacher, W., & Cohen, L. G. (2001). Mechanisms influencing stimulus-response properties of the human corticospinal system. *Clinical Neurophysiology, 112*(5), 931–937.

Bourdelais, A., & Kalivas, P. W. (1990). Amphetamine lowers extracellular GABA concentration in the ventral pallidum. *Brain Research, 516*(1), 132–136.

Cheeran, B., Talelli, P., Mori, F., Koch, G., Suppa, A., Edwards, M., et al. (2008). A common polymorphism in the brain-derived neurotrophic factor gene (BDNF) modulates human cortical plasticity and the response to rTMS. *The Journal of Physiology, 586*(Pt 23), 5717–5725.

Chen, R. (2000). Studies of human motor physiology with transcranial magnetic stimulation. *Muscle & Nerve, 23*(S9), S26–S32.

Clark, V. P., Coffman, B. A., Trumbo, M. C., & Gasparovic, C. (2011). Transcranial direct current stimulation (tDCS) produces localized and specific alterations in neurochemistry: A 1H magnetic resonance spectroscopy study. *Neuroscience Letters, 500*(1), 67–71.

Cohen Kadosh, R., Soskic, S., Iuculano, T., Kanai, R., & Walsh, V. (2010). Modulating neuronal activity produces specific and long-lasting changes in numerical competence. *Current Biology, 20*(22), 2016–2020.

Cooke, S. F. (2006). Plasticity in the human central nervous system. *Brain, 129*(7), 1659–1673.

Creutzfeldt, O. D., Fromm, G. H., & Kapp, H. (1962). Influence of transcortical d-c currents on cortical neuronal activity. *Experimental Neurology, 5*, 436–452.

Di Lazzaro, V., Oliviero, A., Meglio, M., Cioni, B., Tamburrini, G., Tonali, P., et al. (2000). Direct demonstration of the effect of lorazepam on the excitability of the human motor cortex. *Clinical Neurophysiology, 111*(5), 794–799.

Di Lazzaro, V., Oliviero, A., Profice, P., Pennisi, M. A., Pilato, F., Zito, G., et al. (2003). Ketamine increases human motor cortex excitability to transcranial magnetic stimulation. *The Journal of Physiology, 547*(Pt 2), 485–496.

Di Lazzaro, V., Oliviero, A., Saturno, E., Dileone, M., Pilato, F., Nardone, R., et al. (2005). Effects of lorazepam on short latency afferent inhibition and short latency intracortical inhibition in humans. *The Journal of Physiology, 564*(Pt 2), 661–668.

Di Lazzaro, V., Pilato, F., Dileone, M., Ranieri, F., Ricci, V., Profice, P., et al. (2006). GABAA receptor subtype specific enhancement of inhibition in human motor cortex. *The Journal of Physiology, 575*(Pt 3), 721–726.

Fici, G. J., Wu, H., Voigtlander Von, P. F., & Sethy, V. H. (1997). D1 dopamine receptor activity of anti-parkinsonian drugs. *Life Sciences, 60*(18), 1597–1603.

Fisher, R. J., Nakamura, Y., Bestmann, S., Rothwell, J. C., & Bostock, H. (2002). Two phases of intracortical inhibition revealed by transcranial magnetic threshold tracking. *Experimental Brain Research, 143*(2), 240–248.

Floyer-Lea, A., Wylezinska, M., Kincses, T., & Matthews, P. M. (2006). Rapid modulation of GABA concentration in human sensorimotor cortex during motor learning. *Journal of Neurophysiology, 95*(3), 1639–1644.

Foote, S. L., & Morrison, J. H. (1987). Extrathalamic modulation of cortical function. *Annual Review of Neuroscience, 10*, 67–95.

Fritsch, B., Reis, J., Martinowich, K., Schambra, H. M., Ji, Y., Cohen, L. G., et al. (2010). Direct current stimulation promotes BDNF-dependent synaptic plasticity: Potential implications for motor learning. *Neuron, 66*(2), 198–204.

Fröhlich, F., & McCormick, D. A. (2010). Endogenous electric fields may guide neocortical network activity. *Neuron, 67*(1), 129–143.

Hebb, D. (1949). *The organization of behaviour*. New York, NY: Wiley.

Hummel, F., Celnik, P., Giraux, P., Floel, A., Wu, W. -H., Gerloff, C., et al. (2005). Effects of non-invasive cortical stimulation on skilled motor function in chronic stroke. *Brain*, 128(Pt 3), 490–499.

Hummel, F. C., Voller, B., Celnik, P., Floel, A., Giraux, P., Gerloff, C., et al. (2006). Effects of brain polarization on reaction times and pinch force in chronic stroke. *BMC Neuroscience*, 7, 73.

Ilić, T. V., Meintzschel, F., Cleff, U., Ruge, D., Kessler, K. R., & Ziemann, U. (2002). Short-interval paired-pulse inhibition and facilitation of human motor cortex: The dimension of stimulus intensity. *The Journal of Physiology*, 545(Pt 1), 153–167.

Inghilleri, M., Berardelli, A., Marchetti, P., & Manfredi, M. (1996). Effects of diazepam, baclofen and thiopental on the silent period evoked by transcranial magnetic stimulation in humans. *Experimental Brain Research*, 109(3), 467–472.

Jacobson, L., Ezra, A., Berger, U., & Lavidor, M. (2012). Modulating oscillatory brain activity correlates of behavioral inhibition using transcranial direct current stimulation. *Clinical Neurophysiology*, 123(5), 979–984.

Jefferys, J. G. (1981). Influence of electric fields on the excitability of granule cells in guinea-pig hippocampal slices. *The Journal of Physiology*, 319, 143–152.

Karler, R., Calder, L. D., Thai, L. H., & Bedingfield, J. B. (1995). The dopaminergic, glutamatergic, GABAergic bases for the action of amphetamine and cocaine. *Brain Research*, 671(1), 100–104.

Kellaway, P. (1946). The part played by electric fish in the early history of bioelectricity and electrotherapy. *Bulletin of the History of Medicine*, 20, 112–137.

Kirkwood, A., & Bear, M. F. (1994). Homosynaptic long-term depression in the visual cortex. *The Journal of Neuroscience*, 14(5 Pt 2), 3404–3412.

Kleim, J. A., Chan, S., Pringle, E., Schallert, K., Procaccio, V., Jimenez, R., et al. (2006). BDNF val66met polymorphism is associated with modified experience-dependent plasticity in human motor cortex. *Nature Neuroscience*, 9(6), 735–737.

Korchounov, A., Ilić, T. V., Schwinge, T., & Ziemann, U. (2005). Modification of motor cortical excitability by an acetylcholinesterase inhibitor. *Experimental Brain Research*, 164(3), 399–405.

Korchounov, A., Ilić, T. V., & Ziemann, U. (2003). The α2-adrenergic agonist guanfacine reduces excitability of human motor cortex through disfacilitation and increase of inhibition. *Clinical Neurophysiology*, 114(10), 1834–1840.

Korchounov, A., Ilić, T. V., & Ziemann, U. (2007). TMS-assisted neurophysiological profiling of the dopamine receptor agonist cabergoline in human motor cortex. *Journal of Neural Transmission*, 114(2), 223–229.

Kujirai, T., Caramia, M. D., Rothwell, J. C., Day, B. L., Thompson, P. D., Ferbert, A., et al. (1993). Corticocortical inhibition in human motor cortex. *The Journal of Physiology*, 471, 501–519.

Kuo, M. -F., Grosch, J., Fregni, F., Paulus, W., & Nitsche, M. A. (2007). Focusing effect of acetylcholine on neuroplasticity in the human motor cortex. *Journal of Neuroscience*, 27(52), 14442–14447.

Kuo, M. -F., Paulus, W., & Nitsche, M. A. (2008). Boosting focally-induced brain plasticity by dopamine. *Cerebral Cortex*, 18(3), 648–651.

Kuo, M. -F., Unger, M., Liebetanz, D., Lang, N., Tergau, F., Paulus, W., et al. (2008). Limited impact of homeostatic plasticity on motor learning in humans. *Neuropsychologia*, 46(8), 2122–2128.

Kvernmo, T., Härtter, S., & Burger, E. (2006). A review of the receptor-binding and pharmacokinetic properties of dopamine agonists. *Clinical Therapeutics*, 28(8), 1065–1078.

Levy, L. M., Ziemann, U., Chen, R., & Cohen, L. G. (2002). Rapid modulation of GABA in sensorimotor cortex induced by acute deafferentation. *Annals of Neurology*, 52(6), 755–761.

Liebetanz, D., Nitsche, M., Tergau, F., & Paulus, W. (2002). Pharmacological approach to the mechanisms of transcranial DC-stimulation-induced aftereffects of human motor cortex excitability. *Brain: A Journal of Neurology, 125*(Pt 10), 2238–2247.

Lindenberg, R., Renga, V., Zhu, L. L., Nair, D., & Schlaug, G. (2010). Bihemispheric brain stimulation facilitates motor recovery in chronic stroke patients. *Neurology, 75*(24), 2176–2184.

Lisman, J. E. (2001). Three Ca^{2+} levels affect plasticity differently: The LTP zone, the LTD zone and no man's land. *The Journal of Physiology, 532*(Pt 2), 285.

Lu, B. (2003). Pro-region of neurotrophins: Role in synaptic modulation. *Neuron, 39*(5), 735–738.

Marshall, L., Helgadóttir, H., Mölle, M., & Born, J. (2006). Boosting slow oscillations during sleep potentiates memory. *Nature, 444*(7119), 610–613.

Mason, G. F., Martin, D. L., Martin, S. B., Manor, D., Sibson, N. R., Patel, A., et al. (2001). Decrease in GABA synthesis rate in rat cortex following GABA-transaminase inhibition correlates with the decrease in GAD (67) protein. *Brain Research, 914*(1–2), 81–91.

McDonnell, M. N., Orekhov, Y., & Ziemann, U. (2006). The role of GABA (B) receptors in intracortical inhibition in the human motor cortex. *Experimental Brain Research, 173*(1), 86–93.

McHughen, S., Rodriguez, P. F., Kleim, J. A., Kleim, E. D., Crespo, L. M., Procaccio, V., et al. (2010). BDNF val66met polymorphism influences motor system function in the human brain. *Cerebral Cortex, 20*(5), 1254–1262.

Merton, P. A., Hill, D. K., Morton, H. B., & Marsden, C. D. (1982). Scope of a technique for electrical stimulation of human brain, spinal cord, and muscle. *The Lancet, 2*(8298), 597–600.

Merzagora, A. C., Foffani, G., Panyavin, I., Mordillo-Mateos, L., Aguilar, J., Onaral, B., et al. (2010). Prefrontal hemodynamic changes produced by anodal direct current stimulation. *NeuroImage, 49*(3), 2304–2310.

Miranda, P., Lomarev, M., & Hallett, M. (2006). Modeling the current distribution during transcranial direct current stimulation. *Clinical Neurophysiology, 117*(7), 1623–1629.

Mizuno, K., Okada, M., Murakami, T., Kamata, A., Zhu, G., Kawata, Y., et al. (2000). Effects of carbamazepine on acetylcholine release and metabolism. *Epilepsy Research, 40*(2–3), 187–195.

Monte-Silva, K., Kuo, M. -F., Hessenthaler, S., Fresnoza, S., Liebetanz, D., Paulus, W., et al. (2012). Induction of late LTP-like plasticity in the human motor cortex by repeated non-invasive brain stimulation. *Brain Stimulation*, 1–9.

Monte-Silva, K., Kuo, M. -F., Thirugnanasambandam, N., Liebetanz, D., Paulus, W., & Nitsche, M. A. (2009). Dose-dependent inverted U-shaped effect of dopamine (D2-like) receptor activation on focal and nonfocal plasticity in humans. *The Journal of Neuroscience, 29*(19), 6124–6131.

Monte-Silva, K., Liebetanz, D., Grundey, J., Paulus, W., & Nitsche, M. A. (2010). Dosage-dependent non-linear effect of L-dopa on human motor cortex plasticity. *The Journal of Physiology, 588*(18), 3415–3424.

Netzer, R., Pflimlin, P., & Trube, G. (1993). Dextromethorphan blocks N-methyl-D-aspartate-induced currents and voltage-operated inward currents in cultured cortical neurons. *European Journal of Pharmacology, 238*(2–3), 209–216.

Ni, Z., Gunraj, C., & Chen, R. (2007). Short interval intracortical inhibition and facilitation during the silent period in human. *The Journal of Physiology, 583*(3), 971–982.

Nitsche, M., Fricke, K., Henschke, U., Schlitterlau, A., Liebetanz, D., Lang, N., et al. (2003). Pharmacological modulation of cortical excitability shifts induced by transcranial direct current stimulation in humans. *The Journal of Physiology, 553*(Pt 1), 293–301.

Nitsche, M., Grundey, J., Liebetanz, D., Lang, N., Tergau, F., & Paulus, W. (2004). Catecholaminergic consolidation of motor cortical neuroplasticity in humans. *Cerebral Cortex, 14* (11), 1240–1245.

Nitsche, M. A., Jaussi, W., Liebetanz, D., Lang, N., Tergau, F., & Paulus, W. (2004). Consolidation of human motor cortical neuroplasticity by D-cycloserine. *Neuropsychopharmacology, 29*(8), 1573–1578.

Nitsche, M. A., Kuo, M. -F., Grosch, J., Bergner, C., Monte-Silva, K., & Paulus, W. (2009). D1-receptor impact on neuroplasticity in humans. *The Journal of Neuroscience, 29*(8), 2648–2653.

Nitsche, M. A., Lampe, C., Antal, A., Liebetanz, D., Lang, N., Tergau, F., et al. (2006). Dopaminergic modulation of long-lasting direct current-induced cortical excitability changes in the human motor cortex. *The European Journal of Neuroscience, 23*(6), 1651–1657.

Nitsche, M. A., Liebetanz, D., Schlitterlau, A., Henschke, U., Fricke, K., Frommann, K., et al. (2004). GABAergic modulation of DC stimulation-induced motor cortex excitability shifts in humans. *The European Journal of Neuroscience, 19*(10), 2720–2726.

Nitsche, M. A., Muller-Dahlhaus, F., Paulus, W., & Ziemann, U. (2012). The pharmacology of neuroplasticity induced by non-invasive brain stimulation: Building models for the clinical use of CNS active drugs. *The Journal of Physiology, 590*(19), 4641–4662.

Nitsche, M., & Paulus, W. (2000). Excitability changes induced in the human motor cortex by weak transcranial direct current stimulation. *Journal of Physiology, 527*(3), 633–639.

Nitsche, M. A., & Paulus, W. (2001). Sustained excitability elevations induced by transcranial DC motor cortex stimulation in humans. *Neurology, 57*(10), 1899–1901.

Nitsche, M., Schauenburg, A., Lang, N., Liebetanz, D., Exner, C., Paulus, W., et al. (2003). Facilitation of implicit motor learning by weak transcranial direct current stimulation of the primary motor cortex in the human. *Journal of Cognitive Neuroscience, 15*(4), 619–626.

Nitsche, M. A., Seeber, A., Frommann, K., Klein, C. C., Rochford, C., Nitsche, M. S., et al. (2005). Modulating parameters of excitability during and after transcranial direct current stimulation of the human motor cortex. *The Journal of Physiology, 568*(Pt 1), 291–303.

Okada, M., Kiryu, K., Kawata, Y., Mizuno, K., Wada, K., Tasaki, H., et al. (1997). Determination of the effects of caffeine and carbamazepine on striatal dopamine release by *in vivo* microdialysis. *European Journal of Pharmacology, 321*(2), 181–188.

Ozen, S., Sirota, A., Belluscio, M. A., Anastassiou, C. A., Stark, E., Koch, C., et al. (2010). Transcranial electric stimulation entrains cortical neuronal populations in rats. *The Journal of Neuroscience, 30*(34), 11476–11485.

Palva, S., & Palva, J. M. (2007). New vistas for α-frequency band oscillations. *Trends in Neurosciences, 30*(4), 150–158.

Paulus, W. (2011). Transcranial electrical stimulation (tES–tDCS; tRNS, tACS) methods. *Neuropsychological Rehabilitation, 21*(5), 602–617.

Polanía, R., Nitsche, M. A., & Paulus, W. (2011). Modulating functional connectivity patterns and topological functional organization of the human brain with transcranial direct current stimulation. *Human Brain Mapping, 32*(8), 1236–1249.

Priori, A. (2003). Brain polarization in humans: A reappraisal of an old tool for prolonged non-invasive modulation of brain excitability. *Clinical Neurophysiology, 114*(4), 589–595.

Priori, A., Berardelli, A., Rona, S., Accornero, N., & Manfredi, M. (1998). Polarization of the human motor cortex through the scalp. *Neuroreport, 9*(10), 2257–2260.

Purpura, D. P., & McMurtry, J. G. (1965). Intracellular activities and evoked potential changes during polarization of motor cortex. *Journal of Neurophysiology, 28*, 166–185.

Reis, J., Schambra, H., Cohen, L. G., Buch, E. R., Fritsch, B., Zarahn, E., et al. (2009). Non-invasive cortical stimulation enhances motor skill acquisition over multiple days through an effect on consolidation. *Proceedings of the National Academy of Sciences, 106*(5), 1590–1595.

Ridding, M. C. M., & Rothwell, J. C. J. (1997). Stimulus/response curves as a method of measuring motor cortical excitability in man. *Electroencephalography and Clinical Neurophysiology, 105*(5), 340–344.

Rogasch, N. C., & Fitzgerald, P. B. (2012). Assessing cortical network properties using TMS-EEG. *Human Brain Mapping, 34*(7), 1652–1669.

Roshan, L., Paradiso, G. O., & Chen, R. (2003). Two phases of short-interval intracortical inhibition. *Experimental Brain Research*, *151*(3), 330–337.

Schestatsky, P., Morales-Quezada, L., & Fregni, F. (2013). Simultaneous EEG monitoring during transcranial direct current stimulation. *Journal of Visualized Experiments*,(76).

Schönle, P. W., Isenberg, C., Crozier, T. A., Dressler, D., Machetanz, J., & Conrad, B. (1989). Changes of transcranially evoked motor responses in man by midazolam, a short acting benzodiazepine. *Neuroscience Letters*, *101*(3), 321–324.

Schwenkreis, P., Liepert, J., Witscher, K., Fischer, W., Weiller, C., Malin, J. -P., et al. (2000). Riluzole suppresses motor cortex facilitation in correlation to its plasma level. *Experimental Brain Research*, *135*(3), 293–299.

Schwenkreis, P., Witscher, K., Janssen, F., Addo, A., Dertwinkel, R., Zenz, M., et al. (1999). Influence of the N-methyl-D-aspartate antagonist memantine on human motor cortex excitability. *Neuroscience Letters*, *270*(3), 137–140.

Seamans, J. K., & Yang, C. R. (2004). The principal features and mechanisms of dopamine modulation in the prefrontal cortex. *Progress in Neurobiology*, *74*(1), 1–58.

Soekadar, S. R., Witkowski, M., Cossio, E. G., Birbaumer, N., Robinson, S. E., & Cohen, L. G. (2013). *In vivo* assessment of human brain oscillationsduring application of transcranial electric currents. *Nature Communications*, *4*, 1–10.

Stagg, C. J. (2013). Magnetic resonance spectroscopy as a tool to study the role of GABA in motor-cortical plasticity. *NeuroImage*. http://dx.doi.org/10.1016/j.neuroimage.2013.01.009 (epub ahead of print).

Stagg, C. J., Bachtiar, V., & Johansen-Berg, H. (2011). The role of GABA in human motor learning. *Current Biology*, 1–5, .

Stagg, C. J. C., Bachtiar, V. V., O'Shea, J. J., Allman, C. C., Bosnell, R. A. R., Kischka, U. U., et al. (2012). Cortical activation changes underlying stimulation-induced behavioural gains in chronic stroke. *Brain: A Journal of Neurology*, *135*(Pt 1), 276–284.

Stagg, C. J., Best, J. G., Stephenson, M. C., O'Shea, J., Wylezinska, M., Kincses, Z. T., et al. (2009). Polarity-sensitive modulation of cortical neurotransmitters by transcranial stimulation. *The Journal of Neuroscience: The Official Journal of the Society for Neuroscience*, *29*(16), 5202–5206.

Stagg, C. J., Bestmann, S., Constantinescu, A. O., Moreno, L. M., Allman, C., Mekle, R., et al. (2011). Relationship between physiological measures of excitability and levels of glutamate and GABA in the human motor cortex. *The Journal of Physiology*, *589*(Pt 23), 5845–5855.

Stagg, C. J., Jayaram, G., Pastor, D., Kincses, Z. T., Matthews, P. M., & Johansen-Berg, H. (2011). Polarity and timing-dependent effects of transcranial direct current stimulation in explicit motor learning. *Neuropsychologia*, *49*(5), 800–804.

Stagg, C. J., Lin, R. L., Mezue, M., Segerdahl, A., Kong, Y., Xie, J., et al. (2013). Widespread modulation of cerebral perfusion induced during and after transcranial direct current stimulation applied to the left dorsolateral prefrontal cortex. *The Journal of Neuroscience: The Official Journal of the Society for Neuroscience*, *33*(28), 11425–11431.

Stagg, C. J., & Nitsche, M. A. (2011). Physiological basis of transcranial direct current stimulation. *The Neuroscientist*, *17*(1), 37–53.

Suntrup, S., Teismann, I., Wollbrink, A., Winkels, M., Warnecke, T., Floel, A., et al. (2010). Magnetoencephalographic evidence for the modulation of cortical swallowing processing by transcranial direct current stimulation. *NeuroImage*, *83*, 346–354.

Terney, D., Chaieb, L., Moliadze, V., Antal, A., & Paulus, W. (2008). Increasing human brain excitability by transcranial high-frequency random noise stimulation. *The Journal of Neuroscience: The Official Journal of the Society for Neuroscience*, *28*(52), 14147–14155.

Thomas, J. W., Hood, W. F., Monahan, J. B., Contreras, P. C., & O'Donohue, T. L. (1988). Glycine modulation of the phencyclidine binding site in mammalian brain. *Brain Research*, *442*(2), 396–398.

Venkatakrishnan, A., Contreras-Vidal, J. L., Sandrini, M., & Cohen, L. G. (2011). *Independent component analysis of resting brain activity reveals transient modulation of local cortical processing by transcranial direct current stimulation* (pp. 8102–8105). Proceedings of the 33rd Annual International IEEE EMBS Conference.

Wachter, D., Wrede, A., Schulz-Schaeffer, W., Taghizadeh-Waghefi, A., Nitsche, M. A., Kutschenko, A., et al. (2011). Transcranial direct current stimulation induces polarity-specific changes of cortical blood perfusion in the rat. *Experimental Neurology, 227*(2), 322–327.

Werhahn, K. J., Kunesch, E., Noachtar, S., Benecke, R., & Classen, J. (1999). Differential effects on motorcortical inhibition induced by blockade of GABA uptake in humans. *The Journal of Physiology, 517*(Pt 2), 591–597.

Zheng, X., Alsop, D. C., & Schlaug, G. (2011). Effects of transcranial direct current stimulation (tDCS) on human regional cerebral blood flow. *NeuroImage, 58*(1), 26–33.

Ziemann, U. (2008). Pharmacology of TMS measures. In E. Wasserman, C. Epstein, U. Ziemann, V. Walsh, T. Paus, & S. Lisanby (Eds.), *The oxford handbook of transcranial stimulation*. Oxford, UK: Oxford University Press.

Ziemann, U., Bruns, D., & Paulus, W. (1996). Enhancement of human motor cortex inhibition by the dopamine receptor agonist pergolide: Evidence from transcranial magnetic stimulation. *Neuroscience Letters, 208*(3), 187–190.

Ziemann, U., Chen, R., Cohen, L. G., & Hallett, M. (1998). Dextromethorphan decreases the excitability of the human motor cortex. *Neurology, 51*(5), 1320–1324.

Ziemann, U., Lönnecker, S., Steinhoff, B. J., & Paulus, W. (1996). The effect of lorazepam on the motor cortical excitability in man. *Experimental Brain Research, 109*(1), 127–135.

Ziemann, U., Rothwell, J. C., & Ridding, M. C. (1996). Interaction between intracortical inhibition and facilitation in human motor cortex. *The Journal of Physiology, 496*(Pt 3), 873–881.

PART II

IMPROVING FUNCTIONS IN THE TYPICAL BRAIN

Effects of Transcranial Electrical Stimulation on Sensory Functions

Leila Chaieb[1], Catarina Saiote[2], Walter Paulus[2], and Andrea Antal[2]

[1]Clinic for Epileptology, University Clinic of Bonn, Bonn, Germany
[2]Georg-August-University, Department of Clinical Neurophysiology, Göttingen, Germany

INTRODUCTION

Sensory processes take place on the basis of physiological changes of cerebral excitability and activity. Over the past 20 years, non-invasive magnetic and electrical brain stimulation techniques have been developed in order to reflect, induce, and modify these excitability modulations, at least to a certain extent. Transcranial direct current stimulation (tDCS) is one of these methods. The primary mechanism of tDCS is thought to be a modulation of the resting membrane potential of targeted neurons (Bindman, Lippold, & Redfearn, 1964; see also Chapter 5 in this volume). It induces polarity-dependent cortical activity and excitability increases or reductions, which emerge during the stimulation, but – depending on the duration and the intensity of the application – can remain for longer than 1 hour after the end of the stimulation (Nitsche & Paulus, 2000, 2001; Nitsche, Nitsche et al., 2003; Nitsche et al., 2008). The stimulation-induced changes resemble neuroplastic alterations in the brain, which are thought to be the basis of many sensory processes. The aftereffects of stimulation are dependent upon the normal functioning of the glutamatergic system and calcium channels (Liebetanz, Nitsche, Tergau, & Paulus, 2002; Nitsche et al., 2003, 2004). During the past 10 years, several studies have explored the impact of tDCS on sensory processing in the visual, somatosensory, auditory, and multisensory domains. In this review we will gather the knowledge obtained so far about the impact of electrical brain stimulation techniques on mainly visual processes in healthy humans, and give an outlook on future research directions.

PERCEPTION AND ATTENTION

In humans, the effects of tDCS were first explored in the primary motor cortex (M1). It was demonstrated that such stimulation induces prolonged polarity-dependent cortical excitability alterations (Nitsche & Paulus, 2000, 2001; Nitsche, Nitsche et al., 2003). It has been known for a long time that the visual cortex, similarly to M1, can also undergo spontaneous and induced neuroplastic changes, leading to both short- and long-term alterations of synaptic strength (Sherman & Spear, 1982). However, in early animal experiments the DC effect on the visual cortex was less pronounced than on M1, possibly due to the different cytoarchitecture of the cortices and different spatial orientations of the neurons (Creutzfeldt, Fromm, & Kapp, 1962). Later human studies confirmed these results, demonstrating that the tDCS aftereffects are relatively short-lasting in the visual areas compared to those of the motor cortex, using the same stimulation intensity and durations. Indeed, the visual and motor cortices vary with regard to factors influencing excitatory/inhibitory circuitries. Differences in cortical connections and neuronal membrane properties, including receptor expression, between M1 and the visual cortices may also account for the altered responses to the application of tDCS. Furthermore, results also indicate that gender differences exist within the visual cortex of humans, and may be subject to the influences of modulatory neurotransmitters, which affect neuroplasticity (Chaieb, Antal, & Paulus, 2008).

In human investigations, in a first study exploring the effects of tDCS on visual perception, the effectiveness of relatively short-lasting (7-minute) stimulation of the primary visual cortex (V1) on contrast perception was proven (Antal, Nitsche, & Paulus, 2001; see also Table 7.1). Excitability-diminishing cathodal tDCS reduced contrast perception, while excitability-increasing anodal tDCS did not exert any effect. In a later study, longer stimulation duration (15 min) of V1 showed enhanced contrast sensitivity of central visual regions via anodal tDCS (Kraft, Kehrer, Hagendorf, & Brandt, 2011). Using a contrast discrimination task, anodal stimulation enhanced performance (Olma, Kraft, Roehmel, Irlbacher, & Brandt, 2011), whilst cathodal stimulation had no effect. The differences between the results reported in these studies might be attributed to the differences between the stimulation protocols as well as by the more detailed analysis of contrast perception in the second study.

The effectiveness of tDCS over visual areas can also be demonstrated by measuring phosphene thresholds (PTs). Transcranial magnetic stimulation (TMS) pulses delivered to the visual areas can elicit visual sensations, called phosphenes (Meyer, Diehl, Steinmetz, Britton, & Benecke, 1991). The mean TMS intensity required to elicit phosphenes is defined as the PT. The PT is stable within subjects across time, and can be used as a representation of visual cortex excitability (Boroojerdi, Prager, Muellbacher, & Cohen, 2000). Antal and colleagues elicited phosphenes by applying short trains of 5-Hz rTMS delivered over V1 (Antal, Kincses, Nitsche, & Paulus, 2003a). They found that cathodal stimulation over V1 significantly increased PTs, probably due to diminished cortical excitability. Anodal stimulation resulted in the opposite effect, probably via induction of cortical hyperexcitability.

Studying the electrophysiological evidence for the efficacy of tDCS to alter excitability of the human V1, the first work examining these potential effects was published in 2004 (Antal, Kincses, Nitsche, Bartfai, & Paulus, 2004). In this study, the amplitude and latency of the N70 and P100 visual evoked potentials (VEPs) were measured. Significant aftereffects of the stimulation were observed only on the VEP amplitudes using low-contrast stimuli; when high-contrast stimuli were presented, tDCS did not modify VEP amplitudes. Using a V1–Cz montage, anodal tDCS significantly enhanced, while cathodal stimulation diminished, the amplitude of the N70 component. Cathodal tDCS slightly (but not significantly)

TABLE 7.1　Summarizing the Stimulation Protocols, Paradigms and Main Outcomes of Studies Examining the Effects of tDCS Over the Primary Visual areas

Stimulation (polarity/ intensity/ duration)	Site of Stimulation/ Montage/Current Density Under Electrodes	Measurements	Task	Outcomes	Participant Population	Reference
Anodal and cathodal tDCS/1 mA/ 7 min	Oz–Cz montage; 5 × 7-cm sponges, current density 0.029 mA/cm^2	Gabor patches, Binocular static and dynamic contrast sensitivity (sCS, dCS) at 4 cycles/degree and at 4 Hz, before, during, immediately after and 10-min post-tDCS	Gabor patches were adjusted according to participant feedback until just barely visible; after 10 trials minimal contrast level (contrast threshold) was determined	Using 4-cycles/ degree spatial and 4-Hz temporal frequencies significant sCS and dCS loss was found during and 0 min after 7-min cathodal stimulation, while anodal stimulation had no effect	Healthy; $n = 15$	Antal et al., 2001
Anodal and cathodal tDCS/1 mA/ 10 min	Oz–Cz montage; 5 × 7-cm sponges, current density 0.029 mA/cm^2	Phosphene thresholds: five trains of five pulses (5 Hz) were applied 2–4 cm above the inion, 0, 10 and 20 min post-tDCS	Subjects were asked to describe the shape, the color, and the position of phosphenes	Reduction on PTs 0 and 10 min post-anodal tDCS; increase in PTs after cathodal tDCS	Healthy; $n = 16$	Antal, Kincses, Nitsche, & Paulus, 2003a
Anodal and cathodal tDCS/1 mA/ 10 min	Oz–Cz; 5 × 7-cm sponges, current density 0.029 mA/cm^2.	Moving and stationary PTs were measured before, immediately after and 10, 20 and 30 min post-tDCS over V1 and V5	Participants were asked to rate TMS-elicited phosphenes in visual field	Reduced PTs were recorded immediately and 10 min after the end of anodal tDCS, cathodal stimulation showed opposite effect	Healthy; $n = 9$	Antal, Kincses, Nitsche, & Paulus, 2003b

Anodal and cathodal tDCS/1 mA/5, 10 or 15 min	5 × 7-cm sponges; three experimental designs: (1) Oz–Cz montage; (2) O1–O2 montage; (3) Oz–left mastoid. Current density 0.029 mA/cm².	VEPs measured using scalp electrodes; at 0, 10, 20, 30 min, and 40 min after end of 15-min tDCS	Visual stimuli (sinusoidal luminance grating in an on/off mode)	Cathodal tDCS decreased amplitude of N70 component and increased amplitude of P100; anodal tDCS had opposite effect and did not affect P100	Healthy; n = 20	Antal, Kincses, Nitsche, Bartfai, & Paulus, 2004
Anodal and cathodal tDCS/1 mA/10 min	Oz–Cz; 5 × 7-cm sponges, current density 0.029 mA/cm²	VEPs recorded using sinusoidal luminance gratings in an on/off mode 0, 10, 20, and 30 min post-tDCS.	VEP recording before stimulation at 0, 10, 20 and 30 min after the end of the stimulation	Cathodal stimulation decreased while anodal stimulation slightly increased the normalized beta and gamma frequency powers	Healthy; n = 13	Antal, Varga, Kincses, Nitsche, & Paulus, 2004
Anodal and cathodal tDCS/1 mA/10 min	Oz–Cz montage; 5 × 7-cm sponges, current density 0.029 mA/cm²	Phosphene thresholds after priming cortex with tDCS and then stimulating over Oz using 5-Hz rTMS	Participants asked to rate phosphene sensations after cortex was primed using tDCS	Anodal tDCS led to decrease in PT, and subsequent 5-Hz rTMS induced return of PT back to baseline Cathodal tDCS induced short-lasting increase in PT, but 5-Hz rTMS did not influence the tDCS-induced increase in PT	Healthy; n = 9 (4 in control study)	Lang et al., 2007

Continued

II. IMPROVING FUNCTIONS IN THE TYPICAL BRAIN

TABLE 7.1　Summarizing the Stimulation Protocols, Paradigms and Main Outcomes of Studies Examining the Effects of tDCS Over the Primary Visual areas—cont'd

Stimulation (polarity/ intensity/ duration)	Site of Stimulation/ Montage/Current Density Under Electrodes	Measurements	Task	Outcomes	Participant Population	Reference
Anodal and cathodal tDCS/1 mA/3 and 10 min	Oz and anterior neck base or the back over C7; 5 × 8-cm sponges, current density 0.025 mA/cm²	VEP recordings using checkerboards (2 cycles/degree), at two levels of contrast: 100 cd/m², 50 cd/m²	P100 latencies and amplitudes were assessed before, during, and after tDCS	Anodal tDCS reduced P100 amplitude whereas cathodal polarization significantly increased it; both polarities left latency unchanged	Healthy; $n = 20$	Accornero et al., 2007
Anodal and cathodal tDCS/1 mA/7 or 10 min	Oz–Cz montage; 5 × 7-cm sponges, current density 0.029 mA/cm²	PT, CS, and VEPs, prior to, immediately after, and 10 min after cathodal and anodal tDCS stimulation	No active task for participants: retrospective study	No effect of cathodal stimulation; anodal stimulation heightened cortical excitability significantly in women when compared to the age-matched male subject group	Healthy; $n = 46$	Chaieb et al., 2008

Continued

Stimulation	Montage	Task	Description	Results	Population	Reference
Anodal and cathodal tDCS/1 mA/ 15 min	O1/O2–Cz montage; 5 × 5-cm to 7 × 10-cm sponges, current density 0.04–0.014 mA/cm²	Threshold perimetry before and after stimulation	Threshold perimetry was measured for both eyes using Humphrey perimetry with 68 visual field positions within 10 degrees of the visual field	Anodal stimulation yielded a significant increase in contrast sensitivity within 8° of the visual field A significant increase in contrast sensitivity between the conditions "pre" and "post" anodal stimulation was obtained for the central positions (smaller than 2°)	Healthy; n = 12	Kraft et al., 2010
Anodal and cathodal tDCS/1 mA/ 30 min	2 cm above inion–supraorbital region; 5 × 5-cm sponges, current density 0.04 mA/cm²	Magnitude of synesthetic interference: performance of congruent vs incongruent targets in digit-priming task	Achromatic digit primes evoking color photisms were followed by color targets; color targets were congruent/ incongruent with evoked photisms; participants had to identify the color of the target Stroop task	Cathodal tDCS enhanced synesthesia, anodal tDCS decreased synesthesia; Stroop task not affected	Six synesthetes cathodal, five synesthetes anodal	Terhune, Tai, Cowey, Popescu, & Cohen Kadosh, 2011
Anodal and cathodal tDCS/2 mA/ 8–17 min	Oz–Cz montage; 7.2 × 6.0-cm to 11.5 × 9.5-cm sponges, current density 0.046–0.018 mA/cm²	Contrast detection threshold, suppressive effect of masks on contrast detection	Detecting the target stimulus above or below the fixation point in three conditions: target alone, surround suppression and overlay suppression	Anodal stimulation reduced the psychophysical surround suppression and had no effect on overlay suppression; cathodal stimulation had no effect	Healthy; n = 10	Spiegel, Hansen, Byblow, & Thompson, 2012

TABLE 7.1   Summarizing the Stimulation Protocols, Paradigms and Main Outcomes of Studies Examining the Effects of tDCS Over the Primary Visual areas—cont'd

Stimulation (polarity/ intensity/ duration)	Site of Stimulation/ Montage/Current Density Under Electrodes	Measurements	Task	Outcomes	Participant Population	Reference
Anodal and cathodal tDCS/2 mA/ 10 min	Occipital montage: between O2 and PO8–supraorbital region; centro-parietal montage, between CP4 and C4–supraorbital region; 35-cm² sponges, current density 0.057 mA/cm²	Verbally reported pain ratings before and after stimulation.	Subjects received a 500-ms train of high- or low-intensity electrical shocks at 10 Hz over the digital nerve path of the left hand; they had to rate the pain between 0 and 100	Anodal tDCS over the occipital cortex enhanced the analgesic effect of viewing the body	Healthy; $n=24$	Mancini, Bolognini, Haggard, & Vallar, 2012
Anodal and cathodal tDCS/1.5 mA/ 22 min	Oz–Cz montage; 5 × 5-cm sponges, current density: 0.06 mA/cm²	Chromaticity values for discrimination threshold for protan, deutan and tritan color vectors; area and ratio of major and minor axes of the ellipse determined by the ellipse protocol Chromaticity value for threshold of contrast detection	Cambridge color test, spatial chromatic contrast sensitivity task	Anodal and cathodal tDCS increased tritan sensitivity; cathodal tDCS decreased deutan sensitivity	Healthy; $n=15$	Costa, Nagy, Barboni, Boggio, & Ventura, 2012

increased the amplitude of P100. No significant effects were detected for the latency of the VEP components.

However, another study using pattern-reversal checkerboard stimuli and a different electrode montage (reference electrode over the anterior or posterior neck-base versus Cz position in the previous study) reported that anodal tDCS reduced the P100 amplitude, whereas cathodal stimulation significantly increased it (Accornero, Li Voti, La Riccia, & Gregori, 2007). In this study the duration of the aftereffect was about 10 minutes with regard to cathodal stimulation and about 2–3 minutes with regard to anodal tDCS, when low contrast stimuli were presented. The discrepancy concerning the results of the two studies is probably due to the different visual stimulation paradigms and different electrode positions applied. The spatial arrangement of cortical neurons was different in the two studies with regard to the current direction. Nevertheless, in both studies the effect of tDCS depended on the contrast level of the visual stimuli: cathodal and anodal tDCS seemed to have a greater effect on VEP amplitudes elicited by low-contrast stimuli than on high-contrast stimuli. Low-contrast visual stimuli recruit cortical neurons submaximally, thus allowing a more pronounced decrease or increase of neuronal recruitment by locally induced electrical stimulation.

In summary, these results show that anodal and cathodal stimulation can change the excitability of the visual cortex. Furthermore, tDCS-induced neuroplastic changes in healthy subjects are in line with the observation of improved visual functions in patients after application of phosphene-generating current impulses (see following paragraphs).

Stimulation of Higher-Order Visual Areas

The number of studies with regard to tDCS of higher-order visual areas is limited. Stimulation of the motion-sensitive area MT (or V5) had distinct effects on motion perception, dependent upon the specific kind of task: using a moving dot paradigm without distractors, anodal stimulation improved performance while cathodal stimulation impaired it (Antal, Nitsche, Kruse, Kincses et al., 2004; see also Table 7.2). However, with visual distractors the effects of tDCS were reversed. These results were explained by a noise-reducing effect of excitability-diminishing cathodal tDCS in the condition in which visual distracters were introduced, whereas anodal stimulation was suggested to enhance performance by increased neuronal activation in the condition without distractors.

Stimulation of the same area using a different type of paradigm (measuring the duration of motion aftereffect) resulted in a reduction of the duration of aftereffects under both stimulation conditions (Antal, Nitsche, Kruse, Kincses et al., 2004). This might be caused by a reduction

TABLE 7.2   Summarizing the Stimulation Protocols, Paradigms and Main Outcomes of Studies Examining the Effects of tDCS Over the Higher-Order Visual Areas

Stimulation (polarity/ intensity/ duration)	Site of Stimulation/ Montage/Current Density Under Electrodes	Measurements	Task	Outcomes	Participant Population	Reference
Anodal and cathodal tDCS/1 mA/ 10 min	V5/M1 stimulation: 5 × 7-cm sponges; current density 0.029 mA/cm² V5 stimulation: electrode was placed approximately 4 cm above the mastoid–inion line and 7 cm left of the midline in the sagittal plane Return electrode: Cz	Movements of the hand on a horizontal plane were recorded using a 2D manipulandum and visual feedback from a cue onscreen	Visually guided tracking task/ visuomotor co-ordination task	Percentage of correct tracking movements increased during early learning phase during anodal tDCS when left V5 or M1 was stimulated; no effect of cathodal tDCS	Healthy; $n = 42$	Antal, Nitsche, Kincses, Kruse et al., 2004
Anodal and cathodal tDCS/ 1 mA/7 min	MT+/V5, M1, V1: left V5 stimulation: the electrode was placed 3–4 cm above the mastoid–inion line and 6–7 cm left of the midline in the sagittal plane; V1 stimulation: Oz–Cz montage, current density 0.029 mA/cm²	Visuomotor co-ordination task; random dot kinetograms to investigate role of MT +/V5 in visuomotor co-ordination	(1) Tracking the movement of a target using a manipulandum, (2) reporting the direction of coherent motion in a random dot stimulus Performance was measured at 0, 10 and 20 min poststimulation	Cathodal tDCS applied to the left V5 improved performance in visuomotor co-ordination Stimulation of V1 and the left M1 did not result in significant changes in performance, or reaction times in the random dot kinetogram task Percentage of correct tracking movements increased during and immediately after cathodal stimulation	Healthy; $n = 12$ (visuomotor coordination task) and 10 (random dot kinetogram)	Antal, Nitsche, Kruse, Kincses et al., 2004

Anodal and cathodal tDCS/1 mA/ 10 min	V5/M1 stimulation: 5 × 7-cm sponges; current density 0.029 mA/cm²; V5 stimulation: electrode was placed approximately 4 cm above the mastoid–inior line and 7 cm left of the midline in the sagittal plane. Return electrode: Cz	Number of correct tracking movements × time × site of stimulation; 0 min and 24 h poststimulation	Visuomotor co-ordination task	Percentage of correct tracking movements increased significantly in the early phase of practice after both anodal and cathodal stimulations over both cortical areas	Healthy; $n = 78$	Antal, Begemeier, Nitsche, & Paulus, 2008

in activation of task-related neurons via cathodal stimulation, and increased activation of interfering visual stimuli-representing neurons after the end of the presentation of the moving stimuli via anodal tDCS. tDCS has also been shown to modify perception of more complex visual stimuli: Varga and colleagues described a reduced facial adaptation after-effect induced by cathodal tDCS of right lateral parieto-temporal areas, known to be involved in face perception (Varga et al., 2007).

It was also demonstrated that tDCS over V5 is able to improve visually guided tracking movements (Antal, Nitsche, Kincses, Kruse et al., 2004). Interestingly, the use of this task showed that the effect of stimulation was learning-phase specific: when tDCS was applied during the learning phase, performance increased significantly after the beginning of anodal stimulation of V5 or M1, whereas cathodal stimulation had no significant effect. It might be speculated that excitability-enhancing anodal tDCS improved task-related synaptic connectivity. In an overlearned state of the task, the percentage of correct tracking movements increased significantly during and immediately after cathodal tDCS of V5, whilst anodal stimulation had no effect (Antal, Nitsche, Kincses, Kruse et al., 2004). This effect is not yet clarified. It has been suggested that cathodal stimulation, by decreasing the global excitation level and diminishing the amount of activation of concurrent neuronal patterns below threshold, may increase the signal-to-noise ratio and improve performance. The results of these studies show that a beneficial effect of tDCS critically depends on task characteristics and related physiological mechanisms.

STIMULATION OF TEMPORAL AND PARIETAL AREAS COMBINED WITH VISUAL STIMULATION

Transcranial direct current stimulation seems to be an efficient tool for altering visual working memory performance in healthy humans. The effects have been most extensively tested for parietal and temporal cortex stimulation. However, the results of different studies are not completely consistent. Berryhill and colleagues explored the effects of tDCS over right inferior parietal regions on an object recognition and recall working memory task (Berryhill, Wencil, Branch Coslett, & Olson, 2010). tDCS was applied before task performance. In this study, cathodal stimulation impaired task performance. Clark and colleagues explored the impact of tDCS on identification of concealed objects, stimulating the right inferior frontal and right parietal areas. Here, anodal stimulation resulted in improved performance (Clark et al., 2012). Furthermore, this effect was dosage dependent, and its size was larger for naïve subjects as compared to experienced subjects (Bullard et al., 2011). Bolognini and colleagues explored the effects of anodal tDCS applied to the posterior parietal cortex on multisensory field exploration (Bolognini, Fregni, Casati, Olgiati, & Vallar, 2010). Stimulation of the right parietal cortex improved visual exploration and orienting, when compared to sham stimulation, supporting the causal involvement of this area in visual attentional processes. Recently, Flöel and co-workers demonstrated that anodal tDCS over the right temporo-parietal cortex improved memory consolidation in a task involving memorizing an object's location in a natural surrounding (Flöel et al., 2012). Chi and colleagues conducted a study which involved bilateral stimulation of the anterior temporal lobes during encoding and retrieval of a visual memory task (Chi, Fregni, & Snyder, 2010). They found an improvement in visual memory using right anodal–left cathodal stimulation, but not under reversed polarity or sham stimulation conditions. Penolazzi and colleagues studied the impact of bilateral fronto-temporal stimulation on encoding of emotionally valenced pictures (Penolazzi et al., 2010). Right anodal–left cathodal tDCS resulted in improved memory for emotionally pleasant pictures, while left anodal–right cathodal stimulation increased recall of emotionally unpleasant pictures.

Taken together, many studies have been conducted in recent years in which the impact of tDCS on visual memory formation was explored. The results of these studies show that tDCS can be used in the evaluation of the contribution of specific areas to task performance, and that stimulation can have a positive effect on performance. However, the effects of stimulation show some heterogeneity, and it will be important for future studies to reproduce previous results and to explore the factors influencing the beneficial effects of stimulation to a larger degree.

EFFECTS OF ALTERNATING CURRENT STIMULATION ON SENSORY FUNCTIONS

Transcranial alternating current stimulation (tACS) and random noise stimulation (tRNS) are newly developed stimulation techniques which modulate cortical excitability and activity non-invasively (Antal, Boros et al., 2008; Terney, Chaieb, Moliadze, Antal, & Paulus, 2008). tACS and tRNS are thought to affect neuronal membrane potentials by oscillatory electrical stimulation with specific or random frequencies, and believed to interact with ongoing rhythmic cortical activities during sensory processing or cognitive processes. While tACS is applied using a specific frequency, tRNS is applied within a broad frequency spectrum (0.1–640 Hz) with a random noise distribution (Terney et al., 2008). It is suggested that this kind of stimulation possibly induces LTP-like cortical plasticity via augmenting the activity of neuronal sodium channels.

For visual perception, tACS of the visual cortex affected phosphene perception in a frequency-dependent manner (Kanai, Chaieb, Antal,

Walsh, & Paulus, 2008): phosphene perception was more effective when tACS was applied in the beta frequency range in an illuminated condition, whereas tACS at alpha frequencies improved phosphene perception in a dark surrounding. However, according to later results, this effect might be due not to direct cortical but to more retinal stimulation (Schwiedrzik, 2009). In a recent study, tACS applied at a frequency of 60 Hz over V1 enhanced contrast perception, whereas no influence on spatial attention was observed (Laczo, Antal, Niebergall, Treue, & Paulus, 2011). The direct electrophysiological evidence of tACS effects has recently been reported by Zaehle, Rach, and Herrmann, (2010). tACS was delivered over V1 of healthy participants to entrain the neuronal oscillatory activity in their individual alpha frequency range. This kind of stimulation elevated the endogenous alpha power in parieto-central electrodes of the EEG. These results suggest that tACS might evolve as an elegant tool to alter visual functions in a non-invasive and painless way.

Fertonani and colleagues reported a facilitation of perceptual learning using tRNS applied over V1. They found that the accuracy of an orientation discrimination task was significantly increased by high-frequency tRNS (100–640 Hz) (Fertonani, Pirulli, & Miniussi, 2011).

With regard to other modalities, it was recently suggested that tACS might be suited not only to modulate but also to induce perceptions: tactile sensations could be induced when the primary somatosensory cortex (S1) was stimulated using tACS, most effectively by stimulation within the alpha range frequency, followed by high gamma and beta stimulation (Feurra, Paulus, Walsh, & Kanai, 2011).

These results reveal that tACS and tRNS could influence sensory, including visual, functions mainly when applied within certain task-related frequency ranges. This might make tACS and tRNS important tools not only for altering sensory processes but also for exploring the causal relevance of cortical oscillations for sensory interaction.

CLINICAL APPLICATIONS WITH REGARD TO THE STIMULATION OF THE VISUAL CORTEX

The goal of the clinical investigations concerning stimulation of the visual pathway (optic nerve or V1) is to replace or augment lost visual input by artificial electrical signals. The idea of using electrical currents over V1 in order to treat diseases is relatively old. In 1755 Charles Le Roy generated light sensations, called phosphenes, probably attributed to the stimulation of the occipital cortex, in an attempt to cure a blind man. He wound conducting wires around the patient's head and tied one wire to his leg. The electrodes were connected to a Leyden jar, which discharged electric shocks to the patient. The patient underwent several treatments but unfortunately remained blind. Foerster stimulated the visual cortex in order to induce phosphene perceptions (Foerster, 1929), and observed that there was a correlation between the position of phosphenes in the visual field and the stimulated cortical area. Nevertheless, the first systematic clinical studies were carried out almost 10 years later by intra-cranial electrical stimulation of the brain during neurosurgery (Penfield & Boldrey, 1937; Penfield & Rasmussen, 1950). At that time it was clearly demonstrated that occipital stimulation produced phosphenes whose position, color, and shape varied according to the location of the electrodes. Brindley and Lewin, (1968) stimulated the occipital cortex of a blind subject with implanted electrodes and reported the properties of elicited phosphenes in detail. Since these electrical treatments did not prove useful to patients, clinical research with regard to this direction remained in its infancy (Brindley & Lewin, 1968). Similarly, two decades later the application of a non-invasive stimulation method, called tran-scranial electrical stimulation (tES), over the visual cortex attracted only minimal attention because the high-voltage electrical current caused pain and contraction of the scalp muscles (Merton & Morton, 1980). A few years later transcranial magnetic stimulation (TMS), which also induces a current flow in the brain but (in contrast to tES) without pain, was developed as a non-invasive method for changing the activity of cortical neurons. In their first report on TMS in humans, Barker and colleagues mentioned that light sensations were evoked by magnetic stimulation of the occipital cortex (Barker, Jalinous, & Freeston, 1985).

Low-current microstimulation was already being applied successfully invasively over the visual cortex to test whether visually perceived phos-phenes would be useful in creating spatial patterns of sufficiently high res-olution such that subjects would recognize objects in the environment, and also to determine if a blind person could respond to electrical stimulation (Bak et al., 1990; Schmidt et al., 1996).

Whether tDCS has a positive impact on vision restoration in patients with damaged visual pathways is still an open question. Recent studies have shown that the combination of occipital anodal tDCS with visual field rehabilitation appears to enhance visual functional outcomes com-pared with visual rehabilitation alone (Plow et al., 2011; Plow, Obretenova, Fregni, Pascual-Leone, & Merabet, 2012; see also Table 7.3). Recently, a case study was presented reporting on a patient with hemia-nopia due to stroke who benefited from a combined visual rehabilitation training and tDCS treatment program (Halko et al., 2011). Functional magnetic resonance imaging (fMRI) activation associated with a visual motion perception task was used to characterize local changes in brain activity at baseline and after training. Significant correlations between the electrical field and change in fMRI signal were region-specific,

TABLE 7.3 Summarizing the Stimulation Protocols, Paradigms and Main Outcomes of Studies Examining the Effects of tDCS Over the Visual Areas in Different Patient Populations

Stimulation (polarity/ intensity/ duration)	Site of Stimulation/ Montage/ Current Density Under Electrodes	Measurements	Task	Outcomes	Participant population	Reference
	Oz–Cz montage; 5×7-cm sponges, current density 0.029 mA/cm^2	TMS-elicited phosphene thresholds	Participants were asked to rate and state location of phosphene sensations in visual field	Migraine patients showed lower baseline PT values Anodal stimulation decreased PTs in migraineurs similarly to controls, having a larger effect in migraineurs with aura; cathodal stimulation had no effect in patients	Patient; $n = 16$; healthy; $n = 9$	Chadaide et al., 2007
Cathodal tDCS/1 mA/ 15 min plus sham for 6 weeks, ($3 \times$/week)	Oz–Cz montage; 5×7-cm sponges, positioned using 10/20 system, current density 0.029 mA/cm^2	Detailed report on migraine attack and characteristics; 6-week treatment period; 8-week follow-up period	Patients must maintain a 6-week pain diary and undergo tDCS and complete questionnaires pertaining to tDCS	Patients treated by cathodal tDCS showed a significant reduction in the duration of attacks, the intensity of pain and the number of migraine-related days post-treatment	Patient; $n = 26$	Antal, Kriener, Lang, Boros, & Paulus, 2011

| Anodal tDCS/2 mA/ 30 min | Oz–Cz; 5 × 7-cm sponges, current density 0.029 mA/cm^2 | Visual field border; subjective characterization of visual deficit; surveys on performance of daily living activities VRT training: detecting peripheral stimuli presented with variable luminance (performed twice 3 days/week for 3 months) | Patients were asked to fixate on a central target on a screen and report detection of a periphery target with suprathreshold intensity | Anodal tDCS caused a greater shift in visual field borders and increased recovery in activities of daily living | Patients with right hemianopia after occ. stroke damage; $n = 2$. | Plow et al., 2011 |
| Anodal and cathodal tDCS/1 mA/ 30 min | 2 cm above in-on–supraorbital region; 5 × 5-cm sponges, current density 0.04 mA/cm^2 | Magnitude of synesthetic interference: performance of congruent vs incongruent targets in digit-priming task Stroop task (control) | Achromatic digit primes evoking color photisms were followed by color targets; color targets were congruent/ incongruent with evoked photisms; participants had to identify the color of the target. | Cathodal tDCS enhanced synesthesia, anodal tDCS decreased synesthesia; Stroop task not affected | Six synesthetes cathodal, five synesthetes anodal | Terhune et al., 2011 |

Continued

TABLE 7.3 Summarizing the Stimulation Protocols, Paradigms and Main Outcomes of Studies Examining the Effects of tDCS Over the Visual Areas in Different Patient Populations—cont'd

Stimulation (polarity/ intensity/ duration)	Site of Stimulation/ Montage/ Current Density Under Electrodes	Measurements	Task	Outcomes	Participant population	Reference
Anodal and cathodal tDCS/1 mA/ 10 min	Oz–Cz montage; 5 × 7-cm sponges, current density: 0.029 mA/cm²	8-week pain diary; VEPs recorded using EEG and MRI in addition to MRS (magnetic resonance spectroscopy)	Anodal or cathodal tDCS to the V1; in each session 2 × MRS measurements for glutamate/creatine rations without photic stimulation (PS) and then MRS during PS (unpatterned and achromatic flashes of light) at 2 Hz 600 VEP trials were recorded	Increased lactate and decreased N-acetylaspartate (NAA) signals under PS in migraine patients with aura At baseline, migraine patients showed increased Glx/Cr ratios and higher glutamate/ creatine ratios (Glx/Cr) In healthy subjects, anodal tDCS increased and cathodal tDCS decreased the Glx/Cr ratio; subsequent PS returned Glx/Cr ratios back to baseline In migraine patients, both anodal and cathodal tDCS decreased the Glx/Cr ratio, which did not return to baseline after PS Healthy subjects showed an increase in VEP amplitude under anodal and a reduction under cathodal tDCS The ability to modify VEP under tDCS was reduced in migraineurs	Patient; n = 10 (migraine with aura), +10 healthy aged/gender-matched controls	Siniatchkin et al., 2012

Stimulation	Montage	Measures	Task	Results	Population	Reference
Anodal tDCS/2 mA/ 30 min	Oz–Cz montage; 5 × 7 cm sponges, current density 0.057 mA/cm²	Visual field border; subjective characterization of visual deficit; surveys on performance of daily living activities VRT training: detecting peripheral stimuli presented with variable luminance (performed twice 3 days/week for 3 months	Patients were asked to fixate on a central target on a screen and report detection of a periphery target with suprathreshold intensity	Anodal tDCS led to greater expansion in visual field and improvement on activities of daily living, compared to the sham group	Patients with hemianopia or quadrantanopia; $n = 8$	Plow, Obretenova, Fregni, Pascual-Leone, & Merabet, 2012
Anodal tDCS/2 mA/ 30 min	Oz–Cz montage; 5 × 7-cm sponges, current density: 0.057 mA/cm²	Visual field border; VRT was performed twice 3 days per week for 3 months and post-test contrast sensitivity; Reading performance	High-resolution perimetry, Pelli-Robson letter chart, Minnesota reading test	Anodal tDCS caused faster recovery of stimulus detection and higher visual field gain at post-test.	Patients with hemianopia or quadrantanopia; $n = 12$	Plow, Obretenova, Jackson, & Merabet, 2012

including cortical areas under the anodal electrode and peri-lesional visual areas. These patterns were consistent with effective tDCS facilitating rehabilitation.

Non-invasive transorbital AC stimulation has also been shown to possess therapeutic efficacy in diminishing functional deficits of visual perception in patients with optic nerve disease (Gall et al., 2011). However, in these studies it should be considered that there are continuous intra-individual changes in vision after the lesion occurred. It has been suggested that the likelihood of achieving vision restoration seems to be a function of the residual visual capacities of the damaged system (Sabel, Henrich-Noack, Fedorov, & Gall, 2011). Future clinical studies are required to explore the mechanisms of stimulation in vision restoration, to reach the highest degree of vision recovery possible.

tDCS AND OTHER SENSORY MODALITIES

Most of the studies discussed here focused on the visual domain. However, there is increasing evidence that tDCS modifies perception with regard to other sensory modalities. With regard to somatosensory perception, Rogalewski and colleagues explored the effect of tDCS applied to C4 on the ability of healthy humans to discriminate between vibratory stimuli of different frequencies applied to the left ring finger (Rogalewski, Breitenstein, Nitsche, Paulus, & Knecht, 2004). They reported reduced performance during and after cathodal tDCS, while anodal tDCS had no effect. However, in another study anodal tDCS applied to S1 resulted in improved spatial acuity of the contralateral index finger (Ragert, Vandermeeren, Camus, & Cohen, 2008). Generally, the studies conducted in the field of somatosensory perception show heterogeneous results, and the effects of stimulation depend on the kind of task under investigation.

Regarding the effects of tDCS on auditory perception, Loui and colleagues found reduced auditory pitch-matching ability when cathodal tDCS was applied over the inferior frontal and superior temporal areas (Loui, Hohmann, & Schlaug, 2010). In another study, anodal tDCS over the auditory cortex improved temporal processing while cathodal stimulation resulted in reversed effects (Ladeira et al., 2011).

It has recently been demonstrated that tDCS of occipital and temporal areas alters multisensory perception in a sound-induced flash illusion task (Bolognini, Rossetti, Casati, Mancini, & Vallar, 2011). The perceptual fission of a single flash due to multiple beeps was enhanced by anodal tDCS of the temporal cortex and reduced by anodal tDCS of the occipital cortex. Cathodal tDCS of the same areas resulted in opposite effects.

In summary, the studies conducted in the field of "other" sensory perception show heterogeneous results, and that the direction of the effects is strongly task-dependent.

SUMMARY

This review has summarized prominent effects of transcranial electrical stimulation on elementary and complex sensory processes. Taken together, tDCS has been demonstrated to alter visual performance bidirectionally. However, the effects are determined by stimulation polarity, area of stimulation, and, most importantly, the type of task. The number of currently available studies assessing the effects of stimulation in this area is still limited; in the future more efforts should be made to enhance our understanding of the reasons behind the reported heterogeneous effects. Further studies systematically probing stimulation parameters might be needed to explore the reasons for the inconsistencies among studies.

Due to the small number of experiments conducted so far using tACS and tRNS on sensory processing, the underlying mechanisms are not yet sufficiently clear. Future studies should make more effort to provide further information to improve our understanding of the neurophysiological basis of these new stimulation tools. Beyond basic neuroscience research, these efforts will be relevant for the application of these stimulation techniques to neurological diseases accompanied by visual disturbances (Antal, Paulus, & Nitsche, 2011).

References

Accornero, N., Li Voti, P., La Riccia, M., & Gregori, B. (2007). Visual evoked potentials modulation during direct current cortical polarization. *Experimental Brain Research, 178,* 261–266.

Antal, A., Begemeier, S., Nitsche, M. A., & Paulus, W. (2008). Prior state of cortical activity influences subsequent practicing of a visuomotor coordination task. *Neuropsychologia, 46,* 3157–3161.

Antal, A., Boros, K., Poreisz, C., Chaieb, L., Terney, D., & Paulus, W. (2008). Comparatively weak aftereffects of transcranial alternating current stimulation (tACS) on cortical excitability in humans. *Brain Stimulation, 1,* 97–105.

Antal, A., Kincses, T. Z., Nitsche, M. A., Bartfai, O., & Paulus, W. (2004). Excitability changes induced in the human primary visual cortex by transcranial direct current stimulation: Direct electrophysiological evidence. *Investigative Ophthalmology & Visual Science, 45,* 702 707.

Antal, A., Kincses, T., Nitsche, M., & Paulus, W. (2003a). Manipulation of phosphene thresholds by transcranial direct current stimulation in man. *Experimental Brain Research, 150,* 375–378.

Antal, A., Kincses, T. Z., Nitsche, M. A., & Paulus, W. (2003b). Modulation of moving phosphene thresholds by transcranial direct current stimulation of V1 in human. *Neuropsychologia, 41,* 1802–1807.

Antal, A., Kriener, N., Lang, N., Boros, K., & Paulus, W. (2011). Cathodal transcranial direct current stimulation of the visual cortex in the prophylactic treatment of migraine. *Cephalalgia, 31,* 820–828.

Antal, A., Nitsche, M., Kincses, T., Kruse, W., Hoffmann, K., & Paulus, W. (2004). Facilitation of visuo-motor learning by transcranial direct current stimulation of the motor and extrastriate visual areas in humans. *The European Journal of Neuroscience, 19,* 2888–2892.

Antal, A., Nitsche, M., Kruse, W., Kincses, T., Hoffmann, K., & Paulus, W. (2004). Direct current stimulation over V5 enhances visuomotor coordination by improving motion perception in humans. *Journal of Cognitive Neuroscience, 16,* 521–527.

Antal, A., Nitsche, M., & Paulus, W. (2001). External modulation of visual perception in humans. *Neuroreport, 12,* 3553–3555.

Antal, A., Paulus, W., & Nitsche, M. A. (2011). Electrical stimulation and visual network plasticity. *Restorative Neurology and Neuroscience, 29,* 365–374.

Antal, A., Varga, E., Kincses, T., Nitsche, M., & Paulus, W. (2004). Oscillatory brain activity and transcranial direct current stimulation in humans. *Neuroreport, 15,* 1307–1310.

Bak, M., Girvin, J. P., Hambrecht, F. T., Kufta, C. V., Loeb, G. E., & Schmidt, E. M. (1990). Visual sensations produced by intracortical microstimulation of the human occipital cortex. *Medical and Biological Engineering and Computing, 28,* 257–259.

Barker, A. T., Jalinous, R., & Freeston, I. L. (1985). Non-invasive magnetic stimulation of human motor cortex. *Lancet, 1,* 1106–1107.

Berryhill, M. E., Wencil, E. B., Branch Coslett, H., & Olson, I. R. (2010). A selective working memory impairment after transcranial direct current stimulation to the right parietal lobe. *Neuroscience Letters, 479,* 312–316.

Bindman, L. J., Lippold, O. C., & Redfearn, J. W. (1964). The action of brief polarizing currents on the cerebral cortex of the rat (1) during current flow and (2) in the production of longlasting aftereffects. *The Journal of Physiology, 172,* 369–382.

Bolognini, N., Fregni, F., Casati, C., Olgiati, E., & Vallar, G. (2010). Brain polarization of parietal cortex augments training-induced improvement of visual exploratory and attentional skills. *Brain Research, 1349,* 76–89.

Bolognini, N., Rossetti, A., Casati, C., Mancini, F., & Vallar, G. (2011). Neuromodulation of multisensory perception: A tDCS study of the sound-induced flash illusion. *Neuropsychologia, 49,* 231–237.

Boroojerdi, B., Prager, A., Muellbacher, W., & Cohen, L. G. (2000). Reduction of human visual cortex excitability using 1-Hz transcranial magnetic stimulation. *Neurology, 54,* 1529–1531.

Brindley, G. S., & Lewin, W. S. (1968). The sensations produced by electrical stimulation of the visual cortex. *The Journal of Physiology, 196,* 479–493.

Bullard, L. M., Browning, E. S., Clark, V. P., Coffman, B. A., Garcia, C. M., Jung, R. E., et al. (2011). Transcranial direct current stimulation's effect on novice versus experienced learning. *Experimental Brain Research, 213,* 9–14.

Chadaide, Z., Arlt, S., Antal, A., Nitsche, M. A., Lang, N., & Paulus, W. (2007). Transcranial direct current stimulation reveals inhibitory deficiency in migraine. *Cephalalgia, 27,* 833–839.

Chaieb, L., Antal, A., & Paulus, W. (2008). Gender-specific modulation of short-term neuroplasticity in the visual cortex induced by transcranial direct current stimulation. *Visual Neuroscience, 25,* 77–81.

Chi, R. P., Fregni, F., & Snyder, A. W. (2010). Visual memory improved by non-invasive brain stimulation. *Brain Research, 1353,* 168–175.

Clark, V. P., Coffman, B. A., Mayer, A. R., Weisend, M. P., Lane, T. D., Calhoun, V. D., et al. (2012). TDCS guided using fMRI significantly accelerates learning to identify concealed objects. *NeuroImage, 59,* 117–128.

Costa, T. L., Nagy, B. V., Barboni, M. T., Boggio, P. S., & Ventura, D. F. (2012). Transcranial direct current stimulation modulates human color discrimination in a pathway-specific manner. *Frontiers in Psychiatry*, *3*, 78.

Creutzfeldt, O. D., Fromm, G. H., & Kapp, H. (1962). Influence of transcortical d-c currents on cortical neuronal activity. *Experimental Neurology*, *5*, 436–452.

Fertonani, A., Pirulli, C., & Miniussi, C. (2011). Random noise stimulation improves neuroplasticity in perceptual learning. *Journal of Neuroscience: The Official Journal of the Society for Neuroscience*, *31*, 15416–15423.

Feurra, M., Paulus, W., Walsh, V., & Kanai, R. (2011). Frequency specific modulation of human somatosensory cortex. *Frontiers in Psychology*, *2*, 13.

Floel, A., Suttorp, W., Kohl, O., Kurten, J., Lohmann, H., Breitenstein, C., et al. (2012). Noninvasive brain stimulation improves object-location learning in the elderly. *Neurobiology of Aging*, *33*, 1682–1689.

Foerster, O. (1929). Beitrage zur Pathophysiologie der Sehbahn und der Sehsphare. *Journal für Psychologie und Neurologie*, *39*, 463–485.

Gall, C., Sgorzaly, S., Schmidt, S., Brandt, S., Fedorov, A., & Sabel, B. A. (2011). Noninvasive transorbital alternating current stimulation improves subjective visual functioning and vision-related quality of life in optic neuropathy. *Brain Stimulation*, *4*, 175–188.

Halko, M. A., Datta, A., Plow, E. B., Scaturro, J., Bikson, M., & Merabet, L. B. (2011). Neuroplastic changes following rehabilitative training correlate with regional electrical field induced with tDCS. *NeuroImage*, *57*, 885–891.

Kanai, R., Chaieb, L., Antal, A., Walsh, V., & Paulus, W. (2008). Frequency-dependent electrical stimulation of the visual cortex. *Current Biology*, *18*, 1839–1843.

Kraft, A., Kehrer, S., Hagendorf, H., & Brandt, S. A. (2011). Hemifield effects of spatial attention in early human visual cortex. *The European Journal of Neuroscience*, *33*, 2349–2358.

Kraft, A., Roehmel, J., Olma, M. C., Schmidt, S., Irlbacher, K., & Brandt, S. A. (2010). Transcranial direct current stimulation affects visual perception measured by threshold perimetry. *Experimental Brain Research*, *207*, 283–290.

Laczo, B., Antal, A., Niebergall, R., Treue, S., & Paulus, W. (2011). Transcranial alternating stimulation in a high gamma frequency range applied over V1 improves contrast perception but does not modulate spatial attention. *Brain Stimulation*.

Ladeira, A., Fregni, F., Campanha, C., Valasek, C. A., De Ridder, D., Brunoni, A. R., et al. (2011). Polarity-dependent transcranial direct current stimulation effects on central auditory processing. *PLoS One*, *6*, e25399.

Lang, N., Siebner, H. R., Chadaide, Z., Boros, K., Nitsche, M. A., Rothwell, J. C., et al. (2007). Bidirectional modulation of primary visual cortex excitability: A combined tDCS and rTMS study. *Investigative Ophthalmology & Visual Science*, *48*, 5782–5787.

Liebetanz, D., Nitsche, M., Tergau, F., & Paulus, W. (2002). Pharmacological approach to the mechanisms of transcranial DC-stimulation-induced aftereffects of human motor cortex excitability. *Brain*, *125*, 2238–2247.

Loui, P., Hohmann, A., & Schlaug, G. (2010). Inducing disorders in pitch perception and production: A reverse-engineering approach. *Proceedings of Meetings on Acoustics*, *9*, 50002.

Mancini, F., Bolognini, N., Haggard, P., & Vallar, G. (2012). tDCS modulation of visually-induced analgesia. *Journal of Cognitive Neuroscience*.

Merton, P. A., & Morton, H. B. (1980). Stimulation of the cerebral cortex in the intact human subject. *Nature*, *285*, 227.

Meyer, B. U., Diehl, R., Steinmetz, H., Britton, T. C., & Benecke, R. (1991). Magnetic stimuli applied over motor and visual cortex: Influence of coil position and field polarity on motor responses, phosphenes, and eye movements. *Electroencephalography and Clinical Neurophysiology Supplement*, *43*, 121–134.

Nitsche, M. A., Cohen, L. G., Wassermann, E. M., Priori, A., Lang, N., Antal, A., et al. (2008). Transcranial direct current stimulation: State of the art 2008. *Brain Stimulation*, *1*, 206–223.

Nitsche, M., Fricke, K., Henschke, U., Schlitterlau, A., Liebetanz, D., Lang, N., et al. (2003). Pharmacological modulation of cortical excitability shifts induced by transcranial direct current stimulation in humans. *The Journal of Physiology, 553,* 293–301.

Nitsche, M., Jaussi, W., Liebetanz, D., Lang, N., Tergau, F., & Paulus, W. (2004). Consolidation of human motor cortical neuroplasticity by D-cycloserine. *Neuropsychopharmacology, 29,* 1573–1578.

Nitsche, M., Nitsche, M., Klein, C., Tergau, F., Rothwell, J., & Paulus, W. (2003). Level of action of cathodal DC polarisation induced inhibition of the human motor cortex. *Clinical Neurophysiology, 114,* 600–604.

Nitsche, M., & Paulus, W. (2000). Excitability changes induced in the human motor cortex by weak transcranial direct current stimulation. *The Journal of Physiology, 527*(Pt 3), 633–639.

Nitsche, M., & Paulus, W. (2001). Sustained excitability elevations induced by transcranial DC motor cortex stimulation in humans. *Neurology, 57,* 1899–1901.

Olma, M. C., Kraft, A., Roehmel, J., Irlbacher, K., & Brandt, S. A. (2011). Excitability changes in the visual cortex quantified with signal detection analysis. *Restorative Neurology and Neuroscience, 29,* 453–461.

Penfield, W., & Boldrey, E. (1937). Somatic motor and sensory representation in the cerebral cortex of man as studied by electrical stimulation. *Brain, 60,* 389–443.

Penfield, W., & Rasmussen, T. L. (1950). *The cerebral cortex of man: A clinical study of localization of function.* London: Macmillan.

Penolazzi, B., Di Domenico, A., Marzoli, D., Mammarella, N., Fairfield, B., Franciotti, R., et al. (2010). Effects of transcranial direct current stimulation on episodic memory related to emotional visual stimuli. *PLoS One, 5,* e10623.

Plow, E. B., Obretenova, S. N., Fregni, F., Pascual-Leone, A., & Merabet, L. B. (2012). Comparison of visual field training for hemianopia with active versus sham transcranial direct cortical stimulation. *Neurorehabilitation and Neural Repair, 26,* 616–626.

Plow, E. B., Obretenova, S. N., Halko, M. A., Kenkel, S., Jackson, M. L., Pascual-Leone, A., et al. (2011). Combining visual rehabilitative training and noninvasive brain stimulation to enhance visual function in patients with hemianopia: A comparative case study. *PM&R, 3,* 825–835.

Plow, E. B., Obretenova, S. N., Jackson, M. L., & Merabet, L. B. (2012). Temporal profile of functional visual rehabilitative outcomes modulated by transcranial direct current stimulation. *Neuromodulation, 15,* 367–373.

Ragert, P., Vandermeeren, Y., Camus, M., & Cohen, L. G. (2008). Improvement of spatial tactile acuity by transcranial direct current stimulation. *Clinical Neurophysiology, 119,* 805–811.

Rogalewski, A., Breitenstein, C., Nitsche, M., Paulus, W., & Knecht, S. (2004). Transcranial direct current stimulation disrupts tactile perception. *The European Journal of Neuroscience, 20,* 313–316.

Sabel, B. A., Henrich-Noack, P., Fedorov, A., & Gall, C. (2011). Vision restoration after brain and retina damage: The "residual vision activation theory". *Progress in Brain Research, 192,* 199–262.

Schmidt, E. M., Bak, M. J., Hambrecht, F. T., Kufta, C. V., O'Rourke, D. K., & Vallabhanath, P. (1996). Feasibility of a visual prosthesis for the blind based on intracortical microstimulation of the visual cortex. *Brain, 119*(Pt 2), 507–522.

Schwiedrzik, C. M. (2009). Retina or visual cortex? The site of phosphene induction by transcranial alternating current stimulation. *Frontiers in Integrative Neuroscience, 3,* 6.

Sherman, S. M., & Spear, P. D. (1982). Organization of visual pathways in normal and visually deprived cats. *Physiological Reviews, 62,* 738–855.

Siniatchkin, M., Sendacki, M., Moeller, F., Wolff, S., Jansen, O., Siebner, H., et al. (2012). Abnormal changes of synaptic excitability in migraine with aura. *Cerebral Cortex, 22,* 2207–2216.

Spiegel, D. P., Hansen, B. C., Byblow, W. D., & Thompson, B. (2012). Anodal transcranial direct current stimulation reduces psychophysically measured surround suppression in the human visual cortex. *PLoS One, 7,* e36220.

Terhune, D. B., Tai, S., Cowey, A., Popescu, T., & Cohen Kadosh, R. (2011). Enhanced cortical excitability in grapheme-color synesthesia and its modulation. *Current Biology, 21,* 2006–2009.

Terney, D., Chaieb, L., Moliadze, V., Antal, A., & Paulus, W. (2008). Increasing human brain excitability by transcranial high-frequency random noise stimulation. *Journal of Neuroscience: The Official Journal of the Society for Neuroscience, 28,* 14147–14155.

Varga, E. T., Elif, K., Antal, A., Zimmer, M., Harza, I., Paulus, W., et al. (2007). Cathodal transcranial direct current stimulation over the parietal cortex modifies facial gender adaptation. *Ideggyógyászati Szemle, 60,* 474–479.

Zaehle, T., Rach, S., & Herrmann, C. S. (2010). Transcranial alternating current stimulation enhances individual alpha activity in human EEG. *PLoS One, 5,* e13766.

Motor System

Janine Reis[1], George Prichard[1,2], and Brita Fritsch[1]

[1]Albert-Ludwigs-University Freiburg, Department of Neurology,
Freiburg, Germany
[2]Institute of Cognitive Neuroscience, UCL, London, UK

THE MOTOR SYSTEM

The human motor system involves a number of anatomically and functionally connected brain areas. These areas are not solely responsible for motor execution; they also coordinate higher-order associative functions, integration of sensory information, and decision-making (Rowe & Siebner, 2012; Shadmehr & Krakauer, 2008). Such functions are organized by cortico-spinal, cortico-cerebello-thalamo-cortical, and cortico-striato-pallido-thalamo-cortical networks (Ungerleider, Doyon, & Karni, 2002). Hence, the motor system is not one uniform system; it comprises many subsystems with different task-related involvement, though co-activation of subsystems is common. The structure and function of these subsystems are inter-individually variable (Klöppel et al., 2008). The primary, pre- and supplementary motor cortices, cerebellum, thalamus, and striatum are key players involved in the control of motor output (Fig. 8.1). These areas are also relevant for motor learning, with their relative contribution changing over the time course of training (Doyon & Benali, 2005; Halsband & Lange, 2006; Karni et al., 1998; Muellbacher et al., 2002; Ungerleider et al., 2002) (Fig. 8.2). Most of the areas of the motor system can be exogenously modulated by non-invasive brain stimulation, either directly if the area is close to the cortical surface or via remote network effects (Baudewig, Nitsche, Paulus, & Frahm, 2001; Venkatakrishnan & Sandrini, 2012). Since there is close proximity of some areas, such as the premotor cortex and primary motor cortex, it should be noted that often several areas may be stimulated simultaneously, depending on the electrode size or montage utilized (see Chapter 4). For the purpose of this chapter, we will particularly focus on the electrophysiological and behavioral studies exploring the

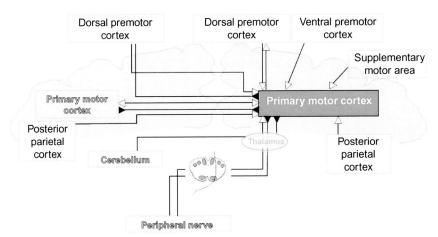

FIGURE 8.1   **Influence of different areas of the motor network on excitability and output of the left primary motor cortex (M1, blue box).** While the opposite primary motor cortex, the cerebellum, and the peripheral nervous system exert a net inhibitory effect on M1 (indicated by the black arrows and bold font), the other areas act primarily as excitatory (white arrows). These cortical areas are susceptible to non-invasive brain stimulation methods. *Figure modified from Reis et al. (2008).*

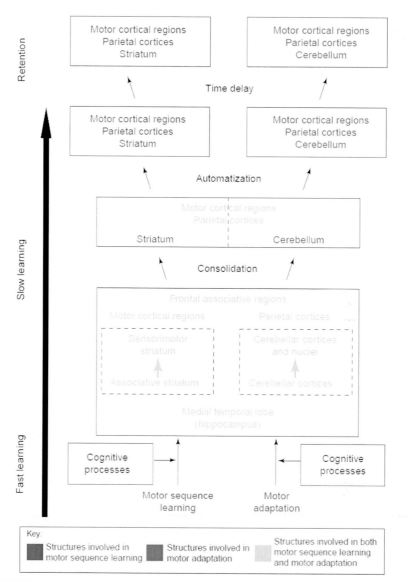

FIGURE 8.2 Schematic illustration of changes within the cortico-striatal and cortico-cerebellar systems during learning of a new sequence of movements (motor sequence learning) or adaptation to environmental perturbations (motor adaptation). Motor sequence learning and motor adaptation initially recruit similar cortical areas during the early learning phase, namely striatum, cerebellum, motor cortex, prefrontal, parietal, and limbic areas. For the establishment of the motor routines required for skill acquisition, dynamic interaction between these structures seems to be relevant. A shift of motor representation from the associative to the sensorimotor striatal territory can be seen during sequence learning, whereas additional representation of the skill can be observed in the cerebellar nuclei after practice on a motor adaptation task. When consolidation has occurred and performance is automatized, the neural representation of a new motor skill is likely located in a cortical network that involves either a cortico-striatal or a cortico-cerebellar circuit, depending on the type of skill acquired. For motor adaptation, the striatum is no longer relevant for the retention and execution of the acquired skill. Instead, the cerebellum and related parietal and motor cortical regions are involved. By contrast, in motor sequence learning, the cerebellum is less essential at later stages of learning, and the long-lasting retention of the skill is thought to involve representational changes in the striatum and associated motor cortical regions. *Figure reproduced from Doyon and Benali (2005), with permission from Elsevier.*

effects of transcranial electrical stimulation (tES), and, more specifically, transcranial direct current stimulation (tDCS), alternating current stimulation (tACS), and random noise stimulation (tRNS), in the motor domain.

tES AND MOTOR CORTICAL EXCITABILITY

To study the effects of non-invasive electrical brain stimulation on the motor system it is important to consider how the effects can be measured. One advantage of the motor system is the ability to assess the cortical parts of the system by electrophysiological and imaging methods. A frequently used measure of motor cortical excitability is the size of the motor evoked potential (MEP): MEPs result from the application of a suprathreshold magnetic stimulus to the motor cortex (using transcranial magnetic stimulation, TMS) to elicit neuronal action potentials. In turn, these cause muscle potentials, which can be recorded a few milliseconds later using surface EMG electrodes (Hallett, 2007). By means of double-pulse paradigms the amplitude of the MEP can be modulated by a preceding conditioning pulse delivered to M1 or to a remote cortical area, enabling further assessment of intra- and interhemispheric interactions (for a detailed review on the technique see Reis et al., 2008).

There is accumulating evidence that non-invasive electrical brain stimulation, in the form of tDCS, tRNS, and tACS, modifies motor cortical excitability (see also Chapter 2) in a time-, dose-, and, in the case of tDCS, polarity-specific manner. Early *in vivo* animal studies in the 1960s had already described polarity-specific alteration of neuronal firing rates after several minutes of direct current stimulation (Bindman & Lippold, 1964; Bindman, Lippold, & Redfearn, 1962; see also Chapter 5 in this volume). In humans, cortical excitability changes after short durations (seconds) of weak direct currents applied to the motor cortex were first described in 1998 (Priori, Berardelli, Rona, Accornero, & Manfredi, 1998). However, it was not until 2000 that Nitsche and Paulus first demonstrated robust and outlasting changes in motor cortical excitability after application of several minutes of tDCS in healthy humans (Nitsche & Paulus, 2000): after approximately 5 minutes of anodal tDCS applied to the motor cortex MEP amplitudes were increased, while they were decreased after cathodal tDCS. Moreover, effects outlasting the stimulation duration of anodal tDCS on excitability were found. Stimulation durations of less than 5 minutes induced transient effects for 5–10 minutes after stimulation offset. However, with stimulation durations of 9 minutes or longer, remarkable aftereffects for up to 90 minutes were found (Batsikadze,

Moliadze, Paulus, Kuo, & Nitsche, 2013; Nitsche & Paulus, 2001). The magnitude and endurance of aftereffects also depends on stimulation intensity, with $0.017\,\mathrm{mA/cm^2}$ ($0.6\,\mathrm{mA}/35\,\mathrm{cm^2}$ electrode size) needed to induce any aftereffect at all (Nitsche & Paulus, 2000). For cathodal tDCS a clear dose–response relationship has been found in the range of 0–$0.028\,\mathrm{mA/cm^2}$ with a decrease in excitability; however $0.057\,\mathrm{mA/cm^2}$ seems to have excitatory effects (Batsikadze et al., 2013). Interestingly, a prolongation of the aftereffect is only found when stimulation is repeated within the first 20 minutes after a first stimulation, but not when the second stimulation is applied 3 hours later (Monte-Silva et al., 2012). For a detailed review on the physiological basis of these excitability modifications, readers are referred to Chapter 6.

While the effects of tDCS on motor cortical excitability have been explored in great detail, information on such effects induced by tACS and tRNS is relatively sparse. In 2008 it was first demonstrated that these stimulations, which use alternating currents at fixed or random frequencies (tACS and tRNS, respectively), can be safely applied to humans. The advantage of using non-direct currents is the lack of polarity-specific effects. Clear excitability enhancing effects were found for tRNS, depending on the noise spectrum, with high frequencies (100–640 Hz) showing more robust effects than low frequencies (<100 Hz) (Terney, Chaieb, Moliadze, Antal, & Paulus, 2008). tACS effects also seem to depend on the applied frequency, but the picture evolving with regard to frequency is less clear and results are in some cases contradictory. In other words, lower frequencies (1–45 Hz) did not reproducibly alter excitability in one study (Antal, Boros et al., 2008), but another study showed a decreasing effect of 15 Hz (Zaghi et al., 2010). Wach et al., (2012) showed an enhancing effect of 10 Hz and decreasing effect at 20 Hz. Higher frequencies of tACS (140 and 250 Hz) increase excitability, with 140 Hz having a robust effect (Moliadze, Antal, & Paulus, 2010). Even higher frequencies in the kHz range (1, 2, 5 kHz) all increase MEPs after stimulation durations of 10 minutes (Chaieb, Antal, & Paulus, 2011).

tES, MOTOR PERFORMANCE AND SIMPLE MOTOR MEMORY

The finding of an excitability modulating effect of tES soon raised the question of whether such interventions could also be behaviorally relevant – i.e., capable of altering motor performance. Improvement in motor performance is usually determined by a shorter time to complete a task, or higher accuracy of an executed movement. Indeed, in several early studies, in which a pre–post stimulation study design was chosen (i.e., tDCS was applied *in the absence of motor practice*), small positive effects of anodal tDCS applied to the right motor cortex on simple motor functions of the non-dominant left hand have been described, for example in finger coordination tasks or gross motor activities like the Jebsen-Taylor Test (Boggio et al., 2006; Sohn, Kim, & Song, 2012; Vines, Cerruti, & Schlaug, 2008). In contrast, anodal tDCS applied to the left motor cortex did not significantly affect subsequent performance of the dominant right hand, at least in healthy young participants (Boggio et al., 2006; see also supplementary material in Fritsch et al., 2010). In elderly subjects, however, a clear positive effect of anodal tDCS applied to the left motor cortex on motor performance of the Jebsen-Taylor Test was observed, which was even more pronounced the older the subjects were (Hummel et al., 2010). Altogether, these data suggest that the more non-proficient the motor system is at baseline (either hand-specific or brain-specific – for example, due to aging), the greater the room for improvement by tDCS. It is unknown whether this also applies to other body parts, such as the lower extremity. Nevertheless, there is some evidence that motor cortical excitability of the leg representation can be enhanced by anodal tDCS (Madhavan & Stinear, 2010), as well as simple motor performance of the foot (e.g., toe pinch force) (Tanaka, Hanakawa, Honda, & Watanabe, 2009). Due to the observation of greater behavioral effects when tDCS is directly combined with performance/training (see sections on serial reaction time paradigms, motor adaptation, and fine motor skills and visuomotor learning, below), studies using a simple pre–post stimulation design and the novel stimulation techniques, tACS and tRNS are sparse. In fact, only a single study reported higher variability in movement speed and accuracy after 10-Hz tACS, and a reduced movement speed after 20-Hz tACS, suggesting an interfering effect of tACS at these frequencies (Wach et al., 2012).

The cortical representation of a simple movement can undergo rapid changes induced by short amounts of practice. This phenomenon is observable as the directional change of TMS-induced thumb movements: the direction of movement elicited by TMS is measured at baseline, then practiced in the opposite direction. After a short practice session (15–30 minutes), TMS-induced movements are in the opposite direction (Classen, Liepert, Wise, Hallett, & Cohen, 1998; see also Fig. 8.3). This form of use-dependent plasticity is usually short-lasting (return of the TMS-induced movement direction towards that induced before training within approximately 20–25 minutes). When anodal tDCS was applied to the motor cortex during the practice period, more TMS-evoked movements are found in the trained direction compared to sham. Furthermore, the practiced movement direction was elicited for a longer period of time afterwards (return to baseline direction after

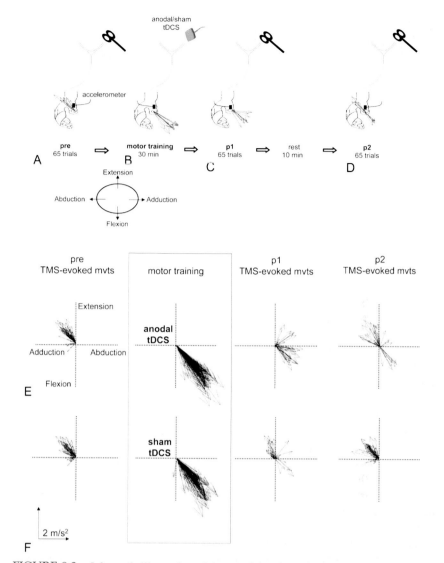

FIGURE 8.3 **Schematic illustration of the use-dependent plasticity experiment in the presence of tDCS.** (A) Before training (pre) TMS-evoked movement directions were derived from the first-peak acceleration of the thumb in the two major axes of the movement (extension/flexion and abduction/adduction). Black arrows indicate the direction of individual TMS-evoked thumb movements (in this case extension and abduction). (B) Motor training with either sham or anodal tDCS applied to the left primary motor cortex. Voluntary thumb movements were performed in a direction opposite to the baseline TMS-evoked movement direction (in this case: flexion and adduction). (C) post 1 (p1). The direction of TMS-evoked thumb movements was determined as previously measured in pre. (D) post 2 (p2). The direction of TMS-evoked thumb movements was again determined after 10 min of rest. (E) Intervention-dependent changes in TMS-evoked thumb movement directions in a representative subject. Each line represents the first-peak acceleration direction vector of a single thumb movement. The pre block is characterized by predominantly extension/adduction movement directions in both sessions. After motor training with anodal tDCS, the direction of TMS-evoked thumb movements (p1 and partially p2) changed to a direction similar to training (flexion/abduction). (F) After training with sham tDCS the direction of TMS-evoked thumb movements immediately changed back to baseline direction within p1. At p2 all movements were in the direction similar to the baseline block. *Figure reproduced from Galea and Celnik (2009), with permission from the American Physiological Society.*

about 50 minutes). This effect was not found for cathodal tDCS, suggesting that anodal tDCS but not cathodal tDCS enhances the formation of the simple motor memory induced by simple repeated movements (Galea & Celnik, 2009; see also Fig. 8.3). This result was not found in an earlier study using the same paradigm when tDCS was applied for only 5 minutes during the latter 10 minutes of the training period (Rosenkranz, Nitsche, Tergau, & Paulus, 2000), supporting the view that the timing of tDCS relative to training onset as well as the stimulation duration of tDCS (>5 min needed to alter excitability; Nitsche & Paulus, 2001) play important roles for the behavioral outcome.

tES AND MOTOR LEARNING: SERIAL REACTION TIME PARADIGMS

In the motor learning domain, tasks testing changes in movement execution speed (i.e., reaction time paradigms which account for the strategic selection of goals) can be grossly separated from tasks testing changes in movement accuracy/quality and speed (kinematic control of movement effectors). A classical task utilized to assess implicit motor sequence learning is the serial reaction time task (SRTT; Nissen & Bullemer, 1987). In this task, a visual cue is presented to the subject on a computer screen in any of four different positions. Each of the four positions corresponds to a button on a response pad. When a visual cue is presented, subjects have to press the corresponding button. With training, an underlying 12-item sequence is repeated over and over again, usually without the explicit knowledge of the subject. Response time in a repeated sequence block is compared to response times of a block in which visual cues are presented at random. This task can be considered a motor learning paradigm, because the subject learns a visuo-spatial mapping (cue position and corresponding response position) and a prediction of the sequential order of movements to execute, allowing subjects to respond faster (Robertson, 2007). In a laboratory setting, the SRTT has frequently been used to explore the effects of tES on motor learning. Anodal tDCS as well as tACS (10 Hz) and tRNS – applied during training – have been shown to improve the implicit learning of the underlying sequence, expressed as faster reaction times in the blocks containing the sequence compared to random blocks (Antal, Boros et al., 2008; Kantak, Mummidisetty, & Stinear, 2012; Nitsche, Schauenburg et al., 2003; Terney et al., 2008). Such behavioral effects are relatively short-lived (less than 1 hour). Longer performance changes were only found in a recent study by Kantak and colleagues, who used a slightly longer stimulation duration (15 min instead of

10 min) and higher stimulation intensity than previous studies (Kantak et al., 2012). Cathodal tDCS did not significantly affect learning of the SRTT (Nitsche, Fricke et al., 2003), suggesting that the inhibitory effect on excitability introduced by cathodal stimulation may not be strong enough to interfere with the activating (usually excitability enhancing) effect of motor practice. However, when a bihemispheric montage is utilized (anode over M1 contralateral to the training hand and cathode ipsilateral to the training hand), the inhibitory cathodal influence applied to the ipsilateral M1 could further augment the facilitatory effect of stimulation applied to the contralateral M1 (e.g., by a reduced interhemispheric inhibition) and then improve learning of the SRTT (Kang & Paik, 2011). When tACS frequency was increased to the ripple range (80–250 Hz) no effect of stimulation on implicit motor learning was observed, despite a clear enhancing effect on cortical excitability (Moliadze et al., 2010). This is in contrast to the above-mentioned study using 10 Hz (Antal, Boros et al., 2008), hence frequency-dependency appears to be a crucial factor for tACS to alter behavior.

As well as polarity or frequency (of alternating stimulation) specificity, a third factor that may need consideration is the timing relative to training: in above-mentioned studies stimulation was applied directly during performance of the SRTT. In a recent study with an explicit version of the SRTT (subjects are informed of the repeating practice sequence), tDCS applied during training had a polarity-specific effect (anodal enhancing performance, cathodal decreasing it). In contrast, anodal and cathodal tDCS applied before training both had a negative effect on motor learning of this task, pointing to a potentially homeostatic influence (Stagg, Jayaram et al., 2011). However, this effect was not observed using the implicit version of the SRTT with stimulation applied before training (Kuo et al., 2008). In addition, no negative effects of tDCS were found when anodal tDCS was applied to M1 immediately after training using a similar nine-digit explicit finger sequence learning task. Instead, execution time of correct sequences was even faster, a finding interpreted as a positive effect of anodal tDCS on early motor memory consolidation (Tecchio et al., 2010). Yet, to clearly make this point, a delayed retest of performance would have been needed to differentiate between an immediate effect of tDCS on motor performance (positive effect of tDCS applied before retest) or on consolidation *per se*.

Finally, stimulation of other cortical areas of the motor system can also result in beneficial effects on motor learning. An example is given in a recent study by Kantak and colleagues. They directly compared the effects of anodal tDCS applied to the primary motor cortex or the dorsal premotor cortex (PMd) when learning the SRTT. Interestingly, PMd stimulation also improved sequence-specific learning, but in contrast to M1 stimulation had no effect on consolidation of the implicit motor memory, since behavioral effects were no longer present 24 hours later in the PMd group (Kantak et al., 2012). Nevertheless, while the lack of effect on consolidation may be true for PMd-stimulation during training, PMd-tDCS applied during REM sleep after learning the SRTT may actually affect consolidation, resulting in improved performance on the SRTT in subsequent tests (Nitsche et al., 2010).

It should be noted that comparative studies on motor learning of the SRTT under the influence of tDCS, tACS, and tRNS are so far lacking. Hence, it is not known whether these mechanistically different types of stimulation have similar effect sizes when applied during training (though visible inspection of the results in above-mentioned studies suggests so) and whether timing relative to training plays a crucial role for tACS and tRNS as well. Moreover, the SRTT is typically mastered within a single session – there is little performance benefit from multiple sessions of training. Hence, this paradigm is not sufficient to address the effects of tES on prolonged learning – for example, when acquiring a novel motor skill from scratch. We will comment on the differences between sequence learning and (visuomotor) skill learning in the following sections.

tES AND MOTOR LEARNING: MOTOR ADAPTATION

Motor adaptation is a primarily error-based learning process by which a person learns to account for predictable perturbations in the environment, such as the correction for directional errors in visually guided reaching movement when wearing prism glasses. After a drop in performance is introduced by the perturbation, the adaptation process leads to a trial-by-trial adjustment of performance until reaching previous levels. Since this process operates relatively fast (within minutes), adaptation is a model to study short-term motor learning. However, it should be noted that repeated practice of adaptation tasks could also lead to performance improvements beyond pre-existing levels – e.g., in the form of faster readaptation to external perturbations relative to the initial rate of adaptation ("savings"; Huang, Haith, Mazzoni, & Krakauer, 2011; Landi, Baguear, & Della-Maggiore, 2011).

To date, information regarding the effects of tDCS on motor adaptation is limited. Hunter and colleagues applied anodal tDCS to M1 during force-field adaptation of the contralateral arm (Hunter, Sacco, Nitsche, & Turner, 2009). In another study, participants were exposed to an unfamiliar visuomotor transformation while anodal tDCS was applied to M1

(Galea, Vazquez, Pasricha, Orban de Xivry, & Celnik, 2011). In both experiments, the anodal tDCS group showed a similar amount of adaptation to the introduced perturbation as the sham tDCS group. Yet, during de-adaptation in the force-field study and in the visuomotor study, anodal tDCS resulted in a significantly stronger retention of the internal model of the new task condition generated during adaptation. Both studies suggest that the primary motor cortex plays an essential role in the retention of the newly acquired internal model. In accordance, it was demonstrated that neither anodal nor cathodal tDCS applied to M1 affected force-field adaptation to a single target, but both types of stimulation positively affected the generalization to intrinsic coordinates (same joint movement), suggesting that the activity in M1 is crucial for specific aspects of generalization to occur (Orban de Xivry et al., 2011). This effect was also site-specific, since it was not found after stimulation of the posterior parietal cortex.

In contrast to M1 stimulation, anodal tDCS applied to the ipsilateral cerebellum resulted in faster correction of reaching errors during adaptation without an effect on retention, supporting two independent functions of these cortical regions in motor adaptation, both susceptible to tDCS (Galea et al., 2011). In accordance, anodal tDCS over the cerebellum also positively influenced adaptation to a new walking pattern on a split-belt treadmill, while cathodal tDCS slowed down the locomotor adaptation rate (Jayaram et al., 2012). Taken together, the primary motor cortex and the cerebellum appear to be key structures in motor adaptation, and tDCS can positively modulate the formation and likely early retention of the internal model acquired during training. To our knowledge, the effects of tACS and tRNS on aspects of motor adaptation are unknown at present.

tES AND MOTOR LEARNING: FINE MOTOR SKILLS, VISUOMOTOR LEARNING

As opposed to motor adaptation, acquisition of a novel motor skill includes the development of new muscle synergies and movement qualities (in terms of speed or accuracy) which increase the level of performance beyond naïve levels. Acquiring a skill is often time-consuming and requires days to weeks to years of training before reaching proficiency (for example, learning to play the piano, or tennis).

Since the development of a skill takes time, it is also of great interest and a matter of ongoing research whether and how tES interacts with the different stages of motor skill learning. It has been proposed that motor skill learning and electrical brain stimulation share some mechanisms of action with regard to the excitability enhancing effect; this raises the important question of whether they can substitute or complement each other to achieve better skills, condense training courses, or even cure patients with lost motor skills due to neurological disease (see also Chapter 12). This question can only be answered in multisession studies, with higher demands for accomplishment in an experimental setting.

However, a few tES studies have focused on particular aspects of motor skill learning. First, as an indicator of better skill acquisition (within a single session), movement accuracy (measured as the percentage of correctly tracked movements) was enhanced in the early learning phase of a visuo-motor tracking task when 10 min of anodal tDCS was applied either to the motor cortex or to the mediotemporal cortex V5 during training; cathodal tDCS did not alter performance (Antal et al., 2004). When tDCS was applied before training, there was a polarity-independent positive effect on subsequent learning success – i.e., subjects made less tracking errors in the first 5–10 minutes of the training (Antal, Begemeier, Nitsche, & Paulus, 2008) – suggesting that the prior state of cortical excitability may play a role for subsequent plastic processes (see comments regarding homeostatic effects of tDCS in reaction time paradigms, above). However, it could also well be that a simple performance improvement is obtained by preceding stimulation, while learning itself is unaffected. This is suggested by the same level of performance achieved by participants at the end of training.

In elderly subjects, practice of a sequential finger tapping task was significantly improved in a single session when anodal tDCS was applied to the motor cortex contralateral to the tapping hand. This improvement was maintained 24 hours later. This positive effect was not observed in young subjects, which could be due to greater overall learning in young people in the absence of stimulation (Zimerman, Nitsch et al., 2012). What is also important to consider is the relevance of the ipsilateral motor cortex in older subjects, since cathodal tDCS applied over this region during training resulted in an inhibitory effect on motor skill acquisition and retention (Zimerman, Heise, Gerloff, Cohen, & Hummel, 2012). It is currently unknown whether this finding does also apply to young subjects.

In 2009 we introduced a novel sequential visual isometric pinch force task, difficult enough for participants to learn a visually guided fine force modulation over multiple days (Reis et al., 2009). Using this task and a 5-day training schedule allowed us to investigate the effects of anodal tDCS applied to the motor cortex contralateral to the trained hand on different temporal subcomponents of motor skill learning: acquisition within session, consolidation between days, and long-term retention for a period of 3 months. Similar to other single-session

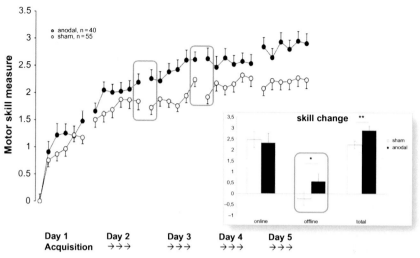

FIGURE 8.4   Learning curve of healthy subjects practicing the sequential visual isometric pinch force task under the influence of sham tDCS (white circles) or anodal tDCS (black circles) applied to the motor cortex contralateral to the trained right hand. Shown is the skill measure, an index based on the bivariate observation of movement time and error rate of the subject (mathematical approach in Reis et al., 2009). Note that over 5 days motor skill increases faster and to higher levels in anodal tDCS-stimulated subjects. When subcomponents of learning are analyzed, the greatest effect of tDCS is found in the consolidation period between sessions, which contributes to the significantly greater total learning (inlay). *Figure modified and extended from Reis et al. (2009).*

studies, we found a non-significant positive effect of anodal tDCS within the first session. However, over the course of 5 days, significant differences between sham and anodal tDCS-stimulated subjects evolved during the consolidation period between sessions. While a loss in skill was present with sham tDCS, positive offline skill gains were found with anodal tDCS, suggesting that the co-application of tDCS and training strengthened consolidation of the acquired motor memory (Reis et al., 2009; see also Fig. 8.4). Since the sequential motor task used in our study is consolidated in a time-dependent fashion (independent of sleep) and positive offline skill gains also occur in a critical time window after the end of training, it is conceivable that tDCS and training share some physiological mechanisms which interact with each other (J. Reis, unpublished data). Because tDCS did not affect the slope of forgetting after the end of training in the previous study, the larger skill present at the end of training also resulted in greater skill present even 3 months later, a finding that holds promise for clinical aspects of tDCS application.

Focusing on the role of hemispheric specialization, Schambra and colleagues trained subjects for 3 consecutive days on the same task, either with their left or their right hand, with anodal tDCS or sham stimulation applied to the left or the right M1 (Schambra et al., 2011). They reported two important findings: first, in right-handed subjects the left motor cortex may be more susceptible to tDCS than the right motor cortex in the context of skill learning (contrary to the studies testing motor performance; see above). Second, an extracephalic cathode position led to much weaker effects on learning in this study compared to a previous study using the same current density but a M1–contralateral forehead montage (Reis et al., 2009). Thus, electrode montage (current intensity and/or direction of current flow) seems to be important for the positive effect on motor skill learning (for further discussion, see Chapter 4). Aside from M1, it has also been shown that anodal tDCS over the supplementary motor area can improve motor skill learning on a similar task, at least during a single training session (Vollmann et al., 2012). This is not surprising, given that the SMA is critically involved – like M1– in learning this task (J. Reis, unpublished data) and the close proximity of the SMA and M1 could lead to co-stimulation.

Again, with regard to the newer stimulation protocols, we can only refer to preliminary unpublished work, presented at the 2012 Neuroscience meeting (G. Prichard, unpublished data). In our most recent study we examined, over 3 days, the effects of unihemispheric anodal or bihemispheric tDCS (anodal stimulation over M1 contralateral to the training hand–cathodal stimulation over the ipsilateral M1) tRNS and sham stimulation applied to the motor cortex on motor skill learning in a word and figure tracing task. Strikingly, all types of stimulation enhanced learning compared to sham, but we did not observe differences between the active stimulation modes. This is surprising, given the likely differences in the mechanism of action of a constant current and changing currents applied to the cortex. However, since all of these interventions targeted the motor cortex, it is also plausible that any excitability increase within the motor cortex in combination with training leads to a beneficial effect on motor skill. This is supported by the finding that tRNS over a control region (right temporal lobe) did not significantly improve total learning (Prichard et al., unpublished data).

Finally, it should be noted that individual genetic predispositions could play a role in the rate of skill acquisition, and this could also be true for the response to brain stimulation. Brain-derived neurotrophic factor (BDNF) belongs to a class of proteins regulating neuronal survival and differentiation in the developing and adult brain, but also synaptic development and plasticity (Lessmann, Gottmann, & Malcangio, 2003; Lu, Christian, & Lu, 2008; Schuman, 1999). A single nucleotide polymorphism in the gene coding for the protein BDNF (val66met polymorphism), associated with reduced activity-dependent secretion of BDNF, hampers motor skill learning (Fritsch et al., 2010; McHughen, Pearson-Fuhrhop, Ngo, & Cramer, 2011). This likely lowers the impact of anodal tDCS on the learning process, since anodal tDCS operates at least partially through BDNF-dependent mechanisms (see next section) (Fritsch et al., 2010).

MECHANISTIC CONSIDERATIONS

While much of this review has exclusively focused on behavior, we would like to highlight again some aspects of the mechanisms of tDCS-enhanced motor learning. This is particularly important to consider before advancing from motor learning studies in healthy participants to treatment after brain injury (see Chapter 12). On the neurotransmitter level, both an increase of the excitatory and a decrease of the inhibitory drive within or towards M1 could result in an increase in excitability. Suppression of the inhibitory system after anodal tDCS has been demonstrated with different methods: in a paired-pulse TMS paradigm, short interval intracortical inhibition (SICI) decreased after anodal tDCS, suggestive of a locally reduced activity of the gamma-aminobutyric acid (GABA)ergic system (Nitsche et al., 2005). In accordance with this, a study using *in vivo* proton (H^1)magnetic resonance spectroscopy (MRS) revealed decreased contents of GABA in the resting human M1 after anodal tDCS, with the magnitude of GABA reduction predicting performance improvements achieved by training on an explicit sequential motor sequence task (Stagg, Bachtiar, & Johansen-Berg, 2011). Of note, tDCS was not applied concurrently with training in this study. In a different MRS study, Floyer-Lea and colleagues showed a significant reduction in GABA concentration in M1 after 30 minutes of training on an isometric motor sequence learning task (Floyer-Lea, Wylezinska, Kincses, & Matthews, 2006). Therefore, it is conceivable that tDCS modulates the motor cortical transmitter system in a way similar to motor training (see also Chapter 6). To date, a direct investigation of neurotransmitter levels by MRS after combined tDCS and motor training has not been performed. Such a study would be valuable to gain mechanistic insight into the beneficial effects observed in behavioral studies, as it could help disentangle to what degree tDCS and training can substitute or complement each other.

Using a motor cortical brain slice model of DCS, with electrical field strength, stimulation duration, and current flow direction chosen to resemble that of human studies, we investigated the cellular mechanisms by which tDCS alters synaptic transmission. Application of DCS alone to M1 slices did not result in changes of synaptic strength as measured by field excitatory postsynaptic potentials. In contrast, the combination of DCS and a second weak synaptic input (low-frequency stimulation, LFS), as a model of training, was sufficient to increase the synaptic efficacy of the thalamo-cortical pathway (DCS-induced long-term potentiation, DCS-LTP; Fritsch et al., 2010). Furthermore, it was shown that DCS-LTP depends on N-methyl-D-aspartate receptor activation as well as on the secretion of BDNF. Since BDNF is critically involved in human motor learning, an increase of BDNF by external stimulation could help restore the neuroplastic potential when BDNF is lacking.

In summary, these data clearly emphasize the need to combine tDCS with a concomitant synaptic activation. This is in accordance with the lack of behavioral effects in individuals undergoing anodal tDCS alone without training in several studies (see section on motor performance and simple motor memory, above). While the sole increase in excitability induced by anodal tDCS (e.g., increased neuronal firing rates, which is likely chaotic) may not be sufficient to induce long-term changes, an additional synaptic activation (by co-stimulation or motor training) may lead to synapse specificity as a source for changes in synaptic strength.

SUMMARY AND FUTURE DIRECTIONS

There is accumulating evidence that tES is effective in promoting motor function and learning. The alteration of cortical excitability is one likely mechanistic key player promoting long-term behavioral changes, when increased excitability and changes in synaptic efficacy induced by training co-occur. To assess and optimize the therapeutic potential of non-invasive brain stimulation techniques in clinical applications (see, for example, Chapters 12 and 13), more studies in healthy people and in animals are clearly needed. This is particularly important because of the limited comparability of tES studies (see Table 8.1): motor task, performance/skill measures, training schedule, stimulation type, duration, intensity, and electrode montage regularly differ dramatically between studies. Moreover, sample sizes are often small, between 6 and 10 subjects per experimental group, leaving results and their discussion in some cases open to suspicion. Ideally, stimulation types and motor tasks should be directly compared in well-controlled larger studies (Table 8.2) to gain further insight into the mechanisms underlying the alteration of physiological learning processes.

TABLE 8.1 Overview of Cited Studies

Reference	Field of Study	Execution	Brain Area/ Montage	Stimulation Type	Intensity	Duration	Electrode Size	Co-application	Effect	Key Findings
MOTOR PERFORMANCE (PRE–POST STIMULATION DESIGNS AND UDP)										
Boggio et al., 2006	Jebsen-Taylor Test	Non-dom hand	M1 (non-dom or dom)–SO	tDCS (anodal, sham)	1 mA ($=29\ \mu A/cm^2$)	20 min	35 cm^2	No	+	Test completed faster after atDCS compared to sham
Sohn et al., 2012	Jebsen-Taylor Test	Non-dom hand	M1 (non-dom) –SO	tDCS (anodal, sham)	1 mA ($=40\ \mu A/cm^2$)	15 min	25 cm^2	No	+	Test completed faster after atDCS compared to sham
Vines et al., 2008	Finger sequence task	Non-dom hand	M1 (non-dom) –SO; M1–M1 (anode nondom)	tDCS (anodal, sham)	1 mA ($=61\ \mu A/cm^2$ anode, 33 $\mu A/cm^2$ SO)	20 min	16.3-cm^2 anode, 30-cm^2 cathode	No	+	No. of correct sequences greater than sham with unilateral atDCS, even greater with dual-hemisphere tDCS
Hummel et al., 2010	Jebsen-Taylor Test	Dom hand	M1 (dom) – SO	tDCS (anodal, sham)	1 mA ($=40\ \mu A/cm^2$)	20 min	25 cm^2	Yes	+	Test completed faster after atDCS compared to sham in *elderly* subjects

Continued

II. IMPROVING FUNCTIONS IN THE TYPICAL BRAIN

TABLE 8.1 Overview of Cited Studies—cont'd

Reference	Field of Study	Execution	Brain Area/ Montage	Stimulation Type	Intensity	Duration	Electrode Size	Co-application	Effect	Key Findings
Tanaka et al., 2009	Pinch force	Leg	M1–SO	tDCS (anodal, cathodal, sham)	2 mA (=57 μA/cm^2)	10 min	35 cm^2	Yes	+	Improvement in pinch force greater with anodal tDCS compared to sham
Galea et al., 2009	UDP paradigm (thumb abduction)	Dom hand	M1–SO	tDCS (anodal, cathodal, sham)	1 mA (=40 μA/cm^2)	30 min	25 cm^2	Yes	+	Practiced movement direction was maintained longer with anodal tDCS. Cathodal tDCS had no effect
Rosenkranz et al., 2000	UDP paradigm (thumb abduction)	Dom hand	M1–SO	tDCS (anodal, cathodal, sham)	1 mA (=29 μA/cm^2)	5 min	35 cm^2	Yes	−	Practiced movement direction was maintained shorter both with anodal and cathodal tDCS
Wach et al., 2012	Fast finger-tapping	Dom hand	M1–SO	tACS 10+20 Hz, sham	1 mA (=29 μA/cm^2)	10 min	35 cm^2	No	−	Higher movement variability (10 Hz), slower movement speed (20 Hz)

SERIAL REACTION TIME PARADIGMS

Nitsche, Schauenburg et al., 2003	SRTT	Dom hand (R)	M1–SO PMd–SO Prefrontal–C4	tDCS (anodal, cathodal, sham)	1 mA (=29 µA/cm²)	15 min	35 cm²	Yes	M1 +, PMd ∅, Prefrontal ∅	M1 atDCS improved implicit learning on the SRTT; M1 cathodal tDCS had no effect; PMd or prefrontal anodal stimulation had no effect
Kantak et al., 2012	SRTT	Non-dom hand (L)	M1–SO PMd–SO	tDCS (anodal, sham)	1 mA (=125 µA/cm² anode, 21 µA/cm² left SO)	15 min	8-cm² anode, 48-cm² cathode	Yes	M1 +, PMd +	Both M1 and PMd atDCS improved implicit learning on the SRTT; only M1 tDCS improved retention of the learned sequence on day 2
Nitsche et al., 2010	SRTT	Dom hand (R)	PMd–SO	tDCS (anodal, cathodal, sham)	1 mA (=29 µA/cm²)	15 min	35 cm²	No	+	atDCS applied *during REM sleep* enhanced consolidation of previously learned implicit memory

Continued

TABLE 8.1 Overview of Cited Studies—cont'd

Reference	Field of Study	Execution	Brain Area/ Montage	Stimulation Type	Intensity	Duration	Electrode Size	Co-application	Effect	Key Findings
Kang & Paik, 2011	SRTT	Dom hand (R)	M1–SO M1–M1 (anode dom)	tDCS (anodal, sham)	1 mA (=40 μA/ cm^2)	20 min	25 cm^2	Yes	(+)	No tDCS effect on sequence specific learning; marginally positive effect of bihemispheric tDCS on retention of the learned sequence on day 2
Kuo et al., 2008	SRTT	Right hand (left- and right-handers)	M1–SO	tDCS (anodal, cathodal, sham)	1 mA (=29 μA/ cm^2)	10 min	35 cm^2	No	$\varnothing$	No effect of tDCS when applied *before* training
Stagg, Jayaram et al., 2011	SRTT explicit	Dom hand (R)	M1–SO	tDCS (anodal, cathodal, sham)	1 mA (=29 μA/ cm^2)	10 min	35 cm^2	Exp. 1, yes; Exp. 2, no	+/− (Exp. 1), − (Exp. 2)	Polarity-specific effect when applied during training (Exp. 1), negative effect of both anodal and cathodal tDCS when applied *before* training

Study	Task	Hand	Montage	Stimulation	Current	Duration	Electrode size		Effect	Notes
Tecchio et al., 2010	Explicit 9-digit sequence learning	Non-dom hand (L)	M1-extracephalic (ipsilateral arm)	tDCS (anodal, sham)	1 mA (=29 µA/cm²)	15 min	35 cm²	No	+	tDCS applied *after* training enhanced performance
Antal et al., 2008	SRTT	Dom hand (R)	M1-SO	tACS 1, 10, 45 Hz, sham	0.8 mA (=25 µA/cm² anode, 8 µA/cm² left SO)	7–10 min	16-cm² anode, 50-cm² cathode	Yes	+	10-Hz tACS improved implicit learning on the SRTT
Moliadze et al., 2010	SRTT	Dom hand (R)	M1-SO	tACS (80, 140, 250 Hz, sham)	1 mA (=62.5 µA/cm² M1, 12 µA/cm² left SO)	7 min	16 cm² M1, 84 cm² SO	Yes	∅	Only effect on cortical excitability
Terney et al., 2008	SRTT	Dom hand (R)	M1-SO	tRNS (0.1–640 Hz, sham)	1 mA (=62.5 µA/cm² M1, 12 µA/cm² rSO)	7 min	16 cm² M1, 84 cm² SO	Yes	+	M1-SO tRNS improved implicit learning on the SRTT
MOTOR ADAPTATION PARADIGMS										
Hunter et al., 2009	Force field adaptation	Dom hand (R)	M1-SO	tDCS (anodal, sham)	1 mA (=29 µA/cm²)	17 min	35 cm²	Yes	+	atDCS resulted in stronger retention of the internal model generated during adaptation (slower de-adaptation compared to sham)

Continued

TABLE 8.1 Overview of Cited Studies—cont'd

Reference	Field of Study	Execution	Brain Area/ Montage	Stimulation Type	Intensity	Duration	Electrode Size	Co-application	Effect	Key Findings
Galea et al., 2011	Visuomotor adaptation	Dom hand (R)	M1-SO rCBL-rbucc	tDCS (anodal, sham)	2 mA (=80 μA/cm²)	15 min	25 cm²	Yes	M1 +, CBL +	M1 atDCS resulted in stronger retention of the internal model (slower de-adaptation), CBL atDCS resulted in faster adaptation
Orban de Xivry et al., 2011	Force field adaptation	Dom hand (R)	M1-SO PPC-SO	tDCS (anodal, cathodal, sham)	1 mA (=40 μA/cm²)	20 min	25 cm²	Yes	M1 +, PPC Ø	No effect of tDCS on adaptation, but greater generalization to intrinsic coordinates both after anodal and cathodal tDCS applied to M1
Jayaram et al., 2012	Locomotor adaptation	Split belt walking, step symmetry	CBL-rbucc	tDCS (anodal, cathodal, sham)	2 mA (=80 μA/cm²)	15 min	25 m²	Yes	+/-	Polarity-specific effect on adaptation rate of spatial components of walking

FINE MOTOR SKILLS; VISUOMOTOR LEARNING

Study	Task	Hand	Montage	Type	Current	Duration	Electrode			Results
Antal et al., 2004	Visuomotor tracking	Dom hand (R)	M1-SO V5-Cz	tDCS (anodal, cathodal, sham)	1 mA (=29 μA/cm^2)	10 min	35 cm^2	Yes	+/Ø	Higher tracking accuracy with anodal tDCS, no effect of cathodal tDCS
Antal et al., 2008	Visuomotor tracking	Dom hand (R)	M1-SO V5-Cz	tDCS (anodal, cathodal, sham)	1 mA (=29 μA/cm^2)	10 min	35 cm^2	No	+	Anodal or cathodal tDCS applied *before* training led to higher tracking accuracy for first 5–10 min
Zimerman, Nitsch et al., 2012	Sequential finger tapping	Dom hand (R)	M1-SO	tDCS (anodal, cathodal, sham)	1 mA (=40 μA/cm^2)	20 min	25 cm^2	Yes	+/Ø	atDCS improved tapping performance in *elderly* subjects, cathodal had no effect
Zimerman et al., 2012	Sequential finger tapping	Dom hand (R)	*M1ipsi-SO*	tDCS (cathodal, sham)	1 mA (=40 μA/cm^2)	20 min	25 cm^2	Yes	−	Cathodal tDCS over *ipsilateral* M1 reduces tapping performance in *elderly* subjects

Continued

TABLE 8.1 Overview of Cited Studies—cont'd

Reference	Field of Study	Execution	Brain Area/Montage	Stimulation Type	Intensity	Duration	Electrode Size	Co-application	Effect	Key Findings
Reis et al., 2009	SVIPT	Dom hand (R)	M1–SO	tDCS (anodal, cathodal, sham)	1 mA (=40 μA/cm^2)	20 min	25 cm^2	Yes	+	atDCS improved motor skill acquisition over *5 days of training* through an effect on consolidation; lasting effect for 3 months
Schambra et al., 2011	SVIPT	Dom hand (R); non-dom hand (L)	M1–extracephalic (ipsilateral deltoid)	tDCS (anodal, sham)	1 mA (=40 μA/cm^2)	20 min	25 cm^2	Yes	+	Left M1 tDCS induced significantly greater skill learning than sham on either hand
Vollmann et al., 2012	Visuomotor pinch task	Dom hand (R)	M1–SO SMA–SO pre-SMA–SO	tDCS (anodal, sham)	0.75 mA (=70 μA/cm^2 anode, 1 μA/cm^2 SO)	20 min	10.7-cm^2 anode, 100-cm^2 cathode	Yes	M1 +, SMA +, Pre-MA ∅	Left M1 or SMA atDCS induced significantly greater skill learning than sham or pre-SMA stimulation

| Fritsch et al., 2010 | SVIPT | Dom hand (R) | M1–SO | tDCS (anodal, sham) | 1 mA (=40 µA/cm²) | 20 min | 25 cm² | Yes | + | atDCS improved motor skill acquisition over 5 days of training; learning hampered by BDNFval66met genotype |

Co-application: tDCS applied simultaneously with motor performance test or motor training. Overall direction of effect: +, positive effect of stimulation; −, negative effect of stimulation; ∅, no effect of stimulation.

Abbreviations: M1, motor cortex; SO, supraorbital area; CBL, cerebellum; PPC, posterior parietal cortex; V5, mediotemporal cortex; Cz, vertex; bucc, buccinator muscle; dom, dominant; non-dom, non-dominant; R, right; L, left; UDP, use-dependent plasticity; SRTT, serial reaction time task; SVIPT, sequential visual isometric pinch force task.

TABLE 8.2   Factors to be Considered in tES Studies on Motor (Skill) Learning

Subjects/general	Technical Aspects
Age	Stimulation type (DC, AC, RN)
Genetic predispositions (e.g., BDNF polymorphism)	Stimulation • duration • intensity • polarity/frequency • location
Handedness	Timing of stimulation relative to training
Task	Filter function of the skull (frequency spectrum alteration in case of tACS and tRNS)
Measure of motor performance or skill	
Training duration	
Psychophysical aspects (sleep, attention)	

References

Antal, A., Begemeier, S., Nitsche, M. A., & Paulus, W. (2008). Prior state of cortical activity influences subsequent practicing of a visuomotor coordination task. *Neuropsychologia, 46*(13), 3157–3161.

Antal, A., Boros, K., Poreisz, C., Chaieb, L., Terney, D., & Paulus, W. (2008). Comparatively weak after-effects of transcranial alternating current stimulation (tACS) on cortical excitability in humans. *Brain Stimulation, 1*(2), 97–105.

Antal, A., Nitsche, M. A., Kincses, T. Z., Kruse, W., Hoffmann, K. P., & Paulus, W. (2004). Facilitation of visuo-motor learning by transcranial direct current stimulation of the motor and extrastriate visual areas in humans. *The European Journal of Neuroscience, 19*(10), 2888–2892.

Batsikadze, G., Moliadze, V., Paulus, W., Kuo, M. -F., & Nitsche, M. A. (2013). Partially non-linear stimulation intensity-dependent effects of direct current stimulation on motor cortex excitability in humans. *The Journal of Physiology, 591*(Pt 7), 1987–2000.

Baudewig, J., Nitsche, M. A., Paulus, W., & Frahm, J. (2001). Regional modulation of BOLD MRI responses to human sensorimotor activation by transcranial direct current stimulation. *Magnetic Resonance in Medicine, 45*(2), 196–201.

Bindman, L. J., & Lippold, O. C. J. (1964). The action of brief polarizing currents on the cerebral cortex of the rat (1) during current flow and (2) in the production of long-lasting after-effects. *The Journal of Physiology, 172*(1), 369–382.

Bindman, L. J., Lippold, O. C., & Redfearn, J. W. (1962). Long-lasting changes in the level of the electrical activity of the cerebral cortex produced bypolarizing currents. *Nature, 196*, 584–585.

Boggio, P. S., Castro, L. O., Savagim, E. A., Braite, R., Cruz, V. C., Rocha, R. R., et al. (2006). Enhancement of non-dominant hand motor function by anodal transcranial direct current stimulation. *Neuroscience Letters, 404*(1–2), 232–236.

Chaieb, L., Antal, A., & Paulus, W. (2011). Transcranial alternating current stimulation in the low kHz range increases motor cortex excitability. *Restorative Neurology and Neuroscience, 29*(3), 167–175.

Classen, J., Liepert, J., Wise, S. P., Hallett, M., & Cohen, L. G. (1998). Rapid plasticity of human cortical movement representation induced by practice. *Journal of Neurophysiology, 79*(2), 1117–1123.

Doyon, J., & Benali, H. (2005). Reorganization and plasticity in the adult brain during learning of motor skills. *Current Opinion in Neurobiology, 15*(2), 161–167.

Floyer-Lea, A., Wylezinska, M., Kincses, T., & Matthews, P. M. (2006). Rapid modulation of GABA concentration in human sensorimotor cortex during motor learning. *Journal of Neurophysiology, 95*(3), 1639–1644.

Fritsch, B., Reis, J., Martinowich, K., Schambra, H. M., Ji, Y., Cohen, L. G., et al. (2010). Direct current stimulation promotes BDNF-dependent synaptic plasticity: Potential implications for motor learning. *Neuron, 66*(2), 198–204.

Galea, J. M., & Celnik, P. A. (2009). Brain polarization enhances the formation and retention of motor memories. *Journal of Neurophysiology, 102*(1), 294–301. http://dx.doi.org/10.1152/jn.00184.2009. Epub 2009 Apr 22.

Galea, J. M., Vazquez, A., Pasricha, N., Orban de Xivry, J. J., & Celnik, P. (2011). Dissociating the roles of the cerebellum and motor cortex during adaptive learning: The motor cortex retains what the cerebellum learns. *Cerebral Cortex, 21*(8), 1761–1770.

Hallett, M. (2007). Transcranial magnetic stimulation: A primer. *Neuron, 55*(2), 187–199.

Halsband, U., & Lange, R. K. (2006). Motor learning in man: A review of functional and clinical studies. *Journal of Physiology, Paris, 99*(4–6), 414–424.

Huang, V. S., Haith, A., Mazzoni, P., & Krakauer, J. W. (2011). Rethinking motor learning and savings in adaptation paradigms: Model-free memory for successful actions combines with internal models. *Neuron, 70*(4), 787–801.

Hummel, F. C., Heise, K., Celnik, P., Floel, A., Gerloff, C., & Cohen, L. G. (2010). Facilitating skilled right hand motor function in older subjects by anodal polarization over the left primary motor cortex. *Neurobiology of Aging, 31*(12), 2160–2168.

Hunter, T., Sacco, P., Nitsche, M. A., & Turner, D. L. (2009). Modulation of internal model formation during force field-induced motor learning by anodal transcranial direct current stimulation of primary motor cortex. *The Journal of Physiology, 587*(Pt 12), 2949–2961.

Jayaram, G., Tang, B., Pallegadda, R., Vasudevan, E. V. L., Celnik, P., & Bastian, A. (2012). Modulating locomotor adaptation with cerebellar stimulation. *Journal of Neurophysiology, 107*(11), 2950–2957.

Kang, E. K., & Paik, N. J. (2011). Effect of a tDCS electrode montage on implicit motor sequence learning in healthy subjects. *Experimental & Translational Stroke Medicine, 3*(1), 4.

Kantak, S. S., Mummidisetty, C. K., & Stinear, J. W. (2012). Primary motor and premotor cortex in implicit sequence learning – Evidence for competition between implicit and explicit human motor memory systems. *The European Journal of Neuroscience, 36*(5), 2710–2715.

Karni, A., Meyer, G., Rey-Hipolito, C., Jezzard, P., Adams, M. M., Turner, R., et al. (1998). The acquisition of skilled motor performance: Fast and slow experience-driven changes in primary motor cortex. *Proceedings of the National Academy of Sciences of the United States of America, 95*(3), 861–868.

Klöppel, S., Bäumer, T., Kroeger, J., Koch, M. A., Büchel, C., Münchau, A., et al. (2008). The cortical motor threshold reflects microstructural properties of cerebral white matter. *NeuroImage, 40*(4), 1782–1791.

Kuo, M.-F., Unger, M., Liebetanz, D., Lang, N., Tergau, F., Paulus, W., et al. (2008). Limited impact of homeostatic plasticity on motor learning in humans. *Neuropsychologia, 46*(8), 2122–2128.

Landi, S. M., Baguear, F., & Della-Maggiore, V. (2011). One week of motor adaptation induces structural changes in primary motor cortex that predict long-term memory one year later. *The Journal of Neuroscience: The Official Journal of the Society for Neuroscience, 31*(33), 11808–11813.

Lessmann, V., Gottmann, K., & Malcangio, M. (2003). Neurotrophin secretion: Current facts and future prospects. *Progress in Neurobiology, 69*(5), 341–374.

Lu, Y., Christian, K., & Lu, B. (2008). BDNF: A key regulator for protein synthesis-dependent LTP and long-term memory? *Neurobiology of Learning and Memory, 89*(3), 312–323.

Madhavan, S., & Stinear, J. W. (2010). Focal and bi-directional modulation of lower limb motor cortex using anodal transcranial direct current stimulation. *Brain Stimulation, 3*(1), 42.

McHughen, S. A., Pearson-Fuhrhop, K., Ngo, V. K., & Cramer, S. C. (2011). Intense training overcomes effects of the Val66Met BDNF polymorphism on short-term plasticity. *Experimental Brain Research, 213*(4), 415–422.

Moliadze, V., Antal, A., & Paulus, W. (2010). Boosting brain excitability by transcranial high frequency stimulation in the ripple range. *The Journal of Physiology, 588*(Pt 24), 4891–4904.

Monte-Silva, K., Kuo, M. -F., Hessenthaler, S., Fresnoza, S., Liebetanz, D., Paulus, W., et al. (2012). Induction of late LTP-like plasticity in the human motor cortex by repeated non-invasive brain stimulation. *Brain Stimulation.*

Muellbacher, W., Ziemann, U., Wissel, J., Dang, N., Kofler, M., Facchini, S., et al. (2002). Early consolidation in human primary motor cortex. *Nature, 415*(6872), 640–644.

Nissen, M. J., & Bullemer, P. (1987). Attentional requirements of learning: Evidence from performance measures. *Cognitive Psychology, 19*(1), 1–32.

Nitsche, M. A., Fricke, K., Henschke, U., Schlitterlau, A., Liebetanz, D., Lang, N., et al. (2003). Pharmacological modulation of cortical excitability shifts induced by transcranial direct current stimulation in humans. *Journal of Physiology, 553*(Pt 1), 293–301.

Nitsche, M. A., Jakoubkova, M., Thirugnanasambandam, N., Schmalfuss, L., Hullemann, S., Sonka, K., et al. (2010). Contribution of the premotor cortex to consolidation of motor sequence learning in humans during sleep. *Journal of Neurophysiology, 104*(5), 2603–2614.

Nitsche, M., & Paulus, W. (2000). Excitability changes induced in the human motor cortex by weak transcranial direct current stimulation. *The Journal of Physiology, 527*(Pt 3), 633–639.

Nitsche, M. A., & Paulus, W. (2001). Sustained excitability elevations induced by transcranial DC motor cortex stimulation in humans. *Neurology, 57*(10), 1899–1901.

Nitsche, M. A., Schauenburg, A., Lang, N., Liebetanz, D., Exner, C., Paulus, W., et al. (2003). Facilitation of implicit motor learning by weak transcranial direct current stimulation of the primary motor cortex in the human. *Journal of Cognitive Neuroscience, 15*(4), 619–626.

Nitsche, M. A., Seeber, A., Frommann, K., Klein, C. C., Rochford, C., Fricke, K., et al. (2005). Modulating parameters of excitability during and after transcranial direct current stimulation of the human motor cortex. *The Journal of Physiology, 568*(Pt 1), 291–303.

Orban de Xivry, J. J., Marko, M. K., Pekny, S. E., Pastor, D., Izawa, J., Celnik, P., et al. (2011). Stimulation of the human motor cortex alters generalization patterns of motor learning. *Journal of Neuroscience: The Official Journal of the Society for Neuroscience, 31*(19), 7102–7110.

Priori, A., Berardelli, A., Rona, S., Accornero, N., & Manfredi, M. (1998). Polarization of the human motor cortex through the scalp. *Neuroreport, 9*(10), 2257–2260.

Reis, J., Schambra, H. M., Cohen, L. G., Buch, E. R., Fritsch, B., Zarahn, E., et al. (2009). Noninvasive cortical stimulation enhances motor skill acquisition over multiple days through an effect on consolidation. *Proceedings of the National Academy of Sciences of the United States of America, 106*(5), 1590–1595.

Reis, J., Swayne, O. B., Vandermeeren, Y., Camus, M., Dimyan, M. A., Harris-Love, M., et al. (2008). Contribution of transcranial magnetic stimulation to the understanding of cortical mechanisms involved in motor control. *The Journal of Physiology, 586*(Pt 2), 325–351.

Robertson, E. M. (2007). The serial reaction time task: Implicit motor skill learning? *Journal of Neuroscience: The Official Journal of the Society for Neuroscience, 27*(38), 10073–10075.

Rosenkranz, K., Nitsche, M. A., Tergau, F., & Paulus, W. (2000). Diminution of training-induced transient motor cortex plasticity by weak transcranial direct current stimulation in the human. *Neuroscience Letters, 296*(1), 61–63.

Rowe, J. B., & Siebner, H. R. (2012). The motor system and its disorders. *NeuroImage, 61*(2), 464–477.

Schambra, H. M., Abe, M., Luckenbaugh, D. A., Reis, J., Krakauer, J. W., & Cohen, L. G. (2011). Probing for hemispheric specialization for motor skill learning: A transcranial direct current stimulation study. *Journal of Neurophysiology, 106*(2), 652–661.

Schuman, E. M. (1999). Neurotrophin regulation of synaptic transmission. *Current Opinion in Neurobiology, 9*(1), 105–109.

Shadmehr, R., & Krakauer, J. W. (2008). A computational neuroanatomy for motor control. *Experimental Brain Research, 185*(3), 359–381.

Sohn, M. K., Kim, B. O., & Song, H. T. (2012). Effect of stimulation polarity of transcranial direct current stimulation on non-dominant hand function. *Annals of Rehabilitation Medicine, 36*(1), 1–7.

Stagg, C. J., Bachtiar, V., & Johansen-Berg, H. (2011). The role of GABA in human motor learning. *Current Biology, 21*(6), 480–484.

Stagg, C. J., Jayaram, G., Pastor, D., Kincses, Z. T., Matthews, P. M., & Johansen-Berg, H. (2011). Polarity and timing-dependent effects of transcranial direct current stimulation in explicit motor learning. *Neuropsychologia, 49*(5), 800–804.

Tanaka, S., Hanakawa, T., Honda, M., & Watanabe, K. (2009). Enhancement of pinch force in the lower leg by anodal transcranial direct current stimulation. *Experimental Brain Research, 196*(3), 459–465.

Tecchio, F., Zappasodi, F., Assenza, G., Tombini, M., Vollaro, S., Barbati, G., et al. (2010). Anodal transcranial direct current stimulation enhances procedural consolidation. *Journal of Neurophysiology, 104*(2), 1134–1140.

Terney, D., Chaieb, L., Moliadze, V., Antal, A., & Paulus, W. (2008). Increasing human brain excitability by transcranial high-frequency random noise stimulation. *The Journal of Neuroscience: The Official Journal of the Society for Neuroscience, 28*(52), 14147–14155.

Ungerleider, L. G., Doyon, J., & Karni, A. (2002). Imaging brain plasticity during motor skill learning. *Neurobiology of Learning and Memory, 78*(3), 553–564.

Venkatakrishnan, A., & Sandrini, M. (2012). Combining transcranial direct current stimulation and neuroimaging: Novel insights in understanding neuroplasticity. *Journal of Neurophysiology, 107*(1), 1–4.

Vines, B. W., Cerruti, C., & Schlaug, G. (2008). Dual-hemisphere tDCS facilitates greater improvements for healthy subjects' non-dominant hand compared to uni-hemisphere stimulation. *BMC Neuroscience, 9*, 103.

Vollmann, H., Conde, V., Sewerin, S., Taubert, M., Sehm, B., Witte, O. W., et al. (2012). Anodal transcranial direct current stimulation (tDCS) over supplementary motor area (SMA) but not pre-SMA promotes short-term visuomotor learning. *Brain Stimulation.* http://dx.doi.org/10.1016/j.brs.2012.03.018.

Wach, C., Krause, V., Moliadze, V., Paulus, W., Schnitzler, A., & Pollok, B. (2012). Effects of 10Hz and 20Hz transcranial alternating current stimulation (tACS) on motor functions and motor cortical excitability. *Behavioural Brain Research, 241C*, 1–6.

Zaghi, S., De Freitas Rezende, L., De Oliveira, L. M., El-Nazer, R., Menning, S., Tadini, L., et al. (2010). Inhibition of motor cortex excitability with 15Hz transcranial alternating current stimulation (tACS). *Neuroscience Letters, 479*(3), 211–214.

Zimerman, M., Heise, K. -F., Gerloff, C., Cohen, L. G., & Hummel, F. C. (2012). Disrupting the ipsilateral motor cortex interferes with training of a complex motor task in older adults. *Cerebral Cortex.* http://dx.doi.org/10.1093/cercor/bhs385.

Zimerman, M., Nitsch, M., Giraux, P., Gerloff, C., Cohen, L. G., & Hummel, F. C. (2012). Neuroenhancement of the aging brain: Restoring skill acquisition in old subjects. *Annals of Neurology, 73*(1), 10–15, n/a–n/a.

Effects of Brain Stimulation on Declarative and Procedural Memories

Marco Sandrini[1,2] *and Leonardo G. Cohen*[1]

[1]Human Cortical Physiology and Stroke Neurorehabilitation Section,
National Institute of Neurological Disorders and Stroke, National Institutes of
Health, Bethesda, MD, USA
[2]Center for Neuroscience and Regenerative Medicine at Uniformed Services
University of Health Sciences, Bethesda, MD, USA

OUTLINE

INTRODUCTION

Memory plays a crucial role in our life. It allows us to recall an event that occurred in the past, retrieve knowledge that is stored in the brain, or remember skills that we have learned.

From a cognitive perspective, memories are acquired (encoding), maintained (storage), and later retrieved (retrieval). Short-term memory refers to the ability to maintain information in mind for a short period of time (i.e., 20–30 seconds). The amount of information one can keep is quite limited and the information itself is very unstable – a sudden distraction and the information is lost. This memory can help us to solve a problem or perform a task, such as mental calculations, using a phone number, or following a set of directions. Long-term memory refers to the ability to retain information over longer periods of time (Baddeley, Eysenck, & Anderson, 2009).

Memory can make the transition over time from short term (unstable) to long term (stable) as a result of consolidation, defined as the progressive stabilization of a recently acquired memory (Dudai, 2004). Sleep has been identified as a state that optimizes the consolidation of newly acquired information in memory (Diekelmann & Born, 2010).Consolidation theory assumes that memories are labile during a limited window after encoding, but, as time passes, memories are consolidated and become resistant to modifications (Müller & Pilzecher, 1900; McGaugh, 2000). However, recent evidence has shown that memory consolidation is a dynamic process. Retrieval or reactivation returns the consolidated memories to unstable forms, once more requiring consolidation, or "reconsolidation" – a time-limited period during which memories can be modified (Censor, Dimyan, & Cohen, 2010; Hardt, Einarsson, & Nader, 2010; Schiller & Phelps, 2011). Once memories are acquired (encoded) and consolidated, they can be retained over an extended period of time (Romano, Howard, & Howard, 2010) or forgotten. Forgetting can be caused by a failure to encode the initial experience, or by an interference from subsequent learning on prior experiences, either by disrupting the consolidation of those traces into durable memories or by interfering with the ability to retrieve them (Levy, Kuhl, & Wagner, 2010).

Five important developments have occurred in the area of memory in the past three decades:

1. Recognition that there is more than one type of long-term memory (Cohen, 1984; Squire, 1992; Tulving, 1985). This stage of memory can be divided into two main types: declarative memory (explicit) and procedural memory (implicit). Declarative memory refers to the conscious recollection of events (episodic memory) or facts (semantic memory). Procedural memory refers to situations in which some form

of learning has occurred, but is reflected in performance rather than through overt recollection (e.g., motor skills, classical conditioning, priming) (Squire, 1992; see also Fig. 9.1).

2. Establishment of a model of human amnesia in the monkey (Mishkin, 1982; Squire & Zola-Morgan, 1983). In the 1950s, Scoville and Milner (1957) described the severe amnesia that followed bilateral surgical removal of the medial temporal lobe in patient H.M. Subsequently, surgical lesions of the medial temporal lobe (MTL) in monkeys, resembling the damage sustained by patient H.M., were shown to reproduce many features of the human memory impairments reported in this patient. In particular, both monkeys and humans were impaired in tasks of declarative memory but fully intact at procedural memory tasks. Thus, declarative memory was thought to be processed within a set of neural circuits that were independent from a set of circuits responsible for procedural memory.

3. The emergence of technologies for studying anatomy and function in living subjects. Functional imaging techniques (positron emission tomography [PET], functional magnetic resonance imaging [fMRI], electroencephalography [EEG], and magnetoencephalography [MEG]) contributed experimental flexibility and temporal and spatial resolution to the study of the functional neuroanatomy of memory processes in intact humans (Cabeza & Nyberg, 2000). Studies using these tools provided unique information on the activity of various brain regions and networks associated mainly with encoding and retrieval of memories. From this information, the functional relationship between brain activity and the investigated memory functions has been inferred (Raichle, 1998).

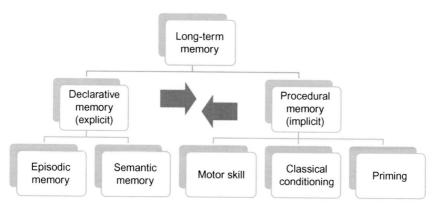

FIGURE 9.1   Components of long-term memory. The red arrows indicate that declarative and procedural memories can interact.

4. The emergence of non-invasive brain stimulation techniques (NIBS) such as transcranial magnetic stimulation (TMS; Barker, Jalinous, & Freeston, 1985; Cohen et al., 1997; Hallett, 2000; Sandrini, Umiltà, & Rusconi, 2011) and, more recently, transcranial electrical stimulation (tES) – i.e., trancranial direct current stimulation (tDCS), transcranial alternating current stimulation (tACS) and transcranial random noise stimulation (tRNS) (Kuo & Nitsche, 2012; Nitsche et al., 2008; Paulus, 2011; Priori et al., 2003). For the first time, these tools made it possible to test novel hypotheses on memory function emerging from basic science studies and neuroimaging protocols in humans with and without brain lesions. These techniques have been used for two fundamental purposes in the study of memory function: first, to test to what extent inferences or hypotheses linking activity in specific cortical regions and memory function are correct – NIBS can be used to establish a causal link between cortical brain regions and memory function; and second, to test the general hypothesis that NIBS could modulate memory and learning, an issue of obvious relevance in neurorehabilitation and cognitive neuroscience.

5. The emergence of evidence challenging the concept of independent memory systems. Although neuropsychological, functional imaging and NIBS studies have shown that anatomically distinct neural circuits are involved in the processing of declarative and procedural memories (Willingham, 1997), over the past 10 years the situation has become more complex. For example, fMRI has shown that activation within the MTL, a brain area associated with the processing of declarative memories, can be correlated with activation within the striatum, which is associated with the processing of procedural memories. Thus, rather than being independent, there may be a functional connection between different memory processes (Poldrack et al., 2001). A functional connection between memory systems makes it at least conceivable that declarative and procedural memories can interact, and interference between these memories, which has been seen in a number of recent behavioral (Brown & Robertson, 2007a, 2007b; Keisler & Shadmehr, 2010) and NIBS studies (Cohen & Robertson, 2011; Galea, Albert, Ditye, & Miall, 2010; Kantak, Mummidisetty, & Stinear, 2012), demonstrates that these memories do interact (Robertson, 2012).

The aim of this chapter is to critically review studies that have shown enhancement of declarative and procedural memory in healthy humans by means of tES.

DECLARATIVE (EXPLICIT) MEMORY

Declarative memory refers to the conscious recollection of facts and events, and is easily verbalized. Due to the fact that it is more language-based than procedural memory, declarative memory is also more easily forgotten unless it is consistently used. There are two basic subtypes of declarative memory: episodic and semantic (Tulving, 1983). Episodic memory refers to our ability to remember specific past events, regarding what happened where and when. Semantic memory refers to general factual knowledge that is independent of personal experience. For example, each of us remembers what happened when we last went to London (episodic memory), whereas although we know that London is the capital of England we do not remember when this fact was learned (semantic memory).

How are semantic and episodic memory related? One possibility is that semantic memory is simply the residue of many episodes. Consistent with this view is the fact that most amnesic patients have difficulties in building up new semantic knowledge. They typically would not know what year it is, or which teams were doing well in their favorite sport. This suggests that although semantic and episodic memory might possibly involve separate systems, they clearly interact (Tulving, 2002).

Most experiments on declarative memory consist of two phases: a study phase (encoding), in which multiple stimuli are presented, and a test phase (retrieval), during which these stimuli must be recalled or recognized from among other stimuli after an interval of time (i.e., from minutes to months). However, in some experiments on semantic memory stimuli must be named (naming task) or recalled from a specific semantic category (fluency/word generation task). Operationally, the memory performance is generally measured by a change in reaction time and/or accuracy.

The hippocampus and surrounding anatomical regions (i.e., MTL) play an important role in episodic memory (Frankland & Bontempi, 2005; Simons & Spiers, 2003). Neuroimaging techniques have confirmed the role of the MTL, together with that of the prefrontal cortex (PFC) and posterior parietal cortex (PPC) (Cabeza, Ciaramelli, Olson, & Moscovitch, 2008; Fletcher & Henson, 2001; Simons & Spiers, 2003; Tulving, Kapur, Craik, Moscovitch, & Houle, 1994; Wagner, Shannon, Kahn, & Buckner, 2005). There is evidence that both the material (verbal vs visual) and the type of memory process (encoding vs retrieval) may affect the lateralization of PFC during episodic memory tasks (Fletcher & Henson, 2001; Flöel et al., 2005; Manenti et al., 2012; Rossi et al., 2001; Sandrini, Cappa, Rossi, Rossini, & Miniussi, 2003). Finally, there is evidence for physical change occurring in the adult brain as a result of learning. This is illustrated by the case of London taxi drivers, whose many years of acquiring spatial knowledge have resulted in a change in their hippocampal structure (Maguire et al., 2000, Maguire, Woollett, & Spiers, 2006).

Regarding semantic memory, the left inferior PFC and the temporal cortex (TC) have been frequently reported as being critical to the processing of semantic information (Binder, Desai, Graves, & Conant, 2009; Patterson, Nestor, & Rogers, 2007).

In the following sections we will discuss studies that have successfully applied tES to cortical regions to enhance episodic and semantic memory in healthy humans. The MLT, a critical node in the network mediating declarative memories, has been less studied in the context of tES because it is hard to directly modulate this region due to its distance from the scalp. However, there is evidence that tES affects not only the targeted local region but also activity in remote interconnected regions (Dayan, Censor, Buch, Sandrini, & Cohen, 2013; Venkatakrishnan & Sandrini, 2012).

Episodic Memory

Several studies have shown that tDCS of cortical regions can improve encoding, consolidation, and retrieval of verbal and visual episodic memory.

Regarding verbal materials, Javadi and Walsh (2012) evaluated the role of the dorsolateral PFC (DLPFC) during encoding and retrieval. The authors applied anodal, cathodal, or sham tDCS over the left DLPFC during the encoding or recognition of words. With respect to encoding, only anodal stimulation over the left DLPFC enhanced memory. Regarding recognition, cathodal stimulation of the left DLPFC impaired recognition, whereas anodal stimulation was associated with a trend towards improving. These data essentially support the role of the left DLPFC during both encoding and retrieval of words, emphasizing the importance of the material used in the task. Jacobson, Goren, Lavidor, and Levy (2012) investigated the role of the posterior parietal cortex (PPC) during encoding. Effective encoding requires that attention be focused on target information and withheld from irrelevant events. This requires engagement of the brain substrates of selective attention, and the concurrent disengagement of brain substrates of orienting toward changes in the environment. The authors applied anodal stimulation over the left intraparietal sulcus/superior parietal cortex (IPS/SPL; a substrate of selective attention) and cathodal stimulation over the right inferior parietal cortex (IPL; a substrate of orienting). Such stimulation during study of verbal materials led to superior subsequent recognition memory relative to the opposite polarity of stimulation. These results may have implications for the development of interventions to benefit learning in individuals with attentional deficits.

There is compelling evidence that sleep contributes to consolidation of new memories (Diekelmann & Born, 2010). This function of sleep in memory consolidation has been linked to slow (<1 Hz) potential oscillations, which predominantly arise from the PFC and characterize slow-wave sleep (Huber, Ghilardi, Massimini, & Tononi, 2004; Steriade & Timofeev, 2003). Moreover, periods rich in slow-wave sleep (SWS) not only facilitate the consolidation of episodic memories (Plihal & Born, 1997, 1999) but are also accompanied by a pronounced endogenous transcortical direct current (DC) potential shift of negative polarity over PFC areas (Marshall, Mölle, & Born, 2003). To experimentally induce widespread extracellular negative DC potentials, Marshall, Mölle, Hallschmid, and Born (2004) applied anodal tDCS bilaterally over DLPFCs during a retention period rich in SWS. Compared to placebo stimulation (i.e., same locations of anodal stimulation but the stimulator remaining off), anodal tDCS increased the retention of word pairs. When applied during the wake retention interval, tDCS did not affect declarative memory. The authors suggested that tDCS enhances generation of slow oscillatory EEG activity considered to facilitate processes of neuronal plasticity. Moreover, the same authors (Marshall, Helgadóttir, Mölle, & Born, 2006) showed that slow oscillation-like potential fields induced by bilateral DLPFC-transcranial applications of oscillating potentials (0.75 Hz) during early nocturnal non-rapid eye movements, a period of emerging slow-wave sleep, enhanced the retention of declarative memories (word pairs). These findings indicate that endogenous slow potential oscillations have a causal role in sleep-associated memory consolidation.

Regarding visual materials, a recent study investigated the effects of bilateral tDCS (i.e., left cathodal and right anodal, left anodal and right cathodal, or sham) over fronto-temporal cortical areas during the encoding of images characterized by different levels of affective arousal and valence (Penolazzi et al., 2010). The results indicated that left cathodal and right anodal stimulation facilitated the recall of pleasant images, whereas the opposite pattern of stimulation facilitated the recall of unpleasant images. These findings may have implications for the rehabilitation of patients (i.e., amnesic or depressed people) with altered emotional processing. Clark et al. (2012) explored the impact of tDCS on the identification of obscured and concealed objects in a naturalistic environment via stimulation of the right inferior PFC and right PPC, identified in an fMRI task performed before training. Two-milliampere anodal tDCS performed over these regions resulted in significant improvements in learning and performance compared with 0.1-mA tDCS. Importantly, this effect was due to enhancement of alerting attention, and its size was larger for novices as compared to experienced participants, as shown in different studies of this group (Bullard et al., 2011; Coffman, Trumbo, & Clark, 2012). These tDCS results provided critical new information on the brain networks involved in learning to identify concealed objects – an issue of relevance for research fields interested in augmenting human performance in the real world. The idea of applying neuroscience tools and techniques to aid the human operator in performance of his or her work/duties was originally discussed by Parasurman and Rizzo (2008). Known as "neuroergonomics," this research area involves examination of the neural bases of such functions as seeing, hearing, attending, remembering, deciding, and planning in relation to technologies and their functioning in the real world.

Finally, Flöel et al. (2012) showed that in a group of elderly subjects, anodal tDCS over the right temporo-parietal cortex during an object location task did not alter the learning rate and the immediate free recall but significantly enhanced the delayed (1 week) recall compared to sham. Better delayed recall suggests either more efficient encoding, although this did not manifest directly during learning, or, more likely, less forgetting of learned information. These findings support the hypothesis (Reis et al., 2009) that there is a consolidation mechanism that is susceptible to anodal tDCS, and that contributes to offline effects more than to on-line effects. In conclusion, retention of object location learning in the elderly may be modulated by anodal tDCS, a finding of potential relevance not only for normal aging but also for memory deficits in pathological aging.

In conclusion, all these studies further support the critical role of fronto-temporo-parietal areas in episodic memory (Fig. 9.2), with the left hemisphere more involved in verbal information and the right hemisphere in visual information. Within this network, the PFC seems to be the area more sensitive to anodal stimulation. Indeed, functional interactions between the PFC and medial temporal lobe are vital for successful episodic memory (Simons & Spiers, 2003). Importantly, these results have implications for tDCS interventions in individuals with memory deficits

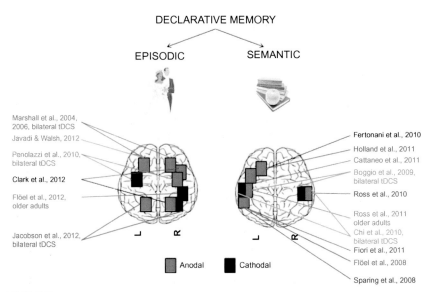

FIGURE 9.2   Illustration of tDCS polarity (anodal or cathodal) and stimulation sites in episodic and semantic memory studies.

(e.g., developmental anomia, aging, amnesic mild cognitive impairment, traumatic brain injury, stroke, and dementia), and for the development of effective new training technologies for work-related training in healthy individuals.

Semantic Memory

Many studies have shown that tDCS over left PFC or TC can improve semantic memory.

Regarding the left PFC, Fertonani, Rosini, Cotelli, Rossini, and Miniussi (2010) investigated semantic memory using a picture-naming task (i.e., objects and actions) as used in a previous facilitatory TMS study (Cappa, Sandrini, Rossini, Sosta, & Miniussi, 2002). They found that anodal stimulation on the left DLPFC improved naming reaction time whereas cathodal stimulation had no effect. Cattaneo, Pisoni, and Papagno (2011) investigated whether tDCS of Broca's area can be used to increase performance in a semantic fluency task. The authors showed that anodal tDCS applied over Broca's area enhanced verbal fluency compared to sham stimulation.

Holland et al. (2011) tested the effects of anodal tDCS over the left inferior PFC on picture-naming performance. The researchers combined tDCS during an overt picture naming with fMRI. Anodal tDCS over the left inferior PFC induced a significant improvement in naming response times compared to sham, and also reduced fMRI blood oxygen-level dependent signals in the left PFC, including Broca's area. Similar to Holland's study, Meinzer et al. (2012) used fMRI to investigate neurofunctional correlates of enhanced semantic memory induced by anodal tDCS over the left inferior frontal gyrus (IFG). Compared to sham, enhanced word generation during anodal tDCS was paralleled by selectively reduced task-related activation in the left ventral IFG, an area specifically implicated in semantic retrieval processes (Thompson-Schill, D'Esposito, Aguirre, & Farah, 1997). Under anodal tDCS, resting-state fMRI revealed increased connectivity of the left IFG and additional major hubs overlapping with the language network. In conclusion, anodal tDCS modulates endogenous low-frequency oscillations in a distributed set of functionally connected brain areas, possibly inducing more efficient processing in critical task-relevant areas and enhanced behavioral performance. The results of these tDCS-fMRI studies are in line with previous findings. For example, reduced activity in circumscribed task-related areas or more focal processing has been associated with superior memory performance (Gonsalves, Kahn, Curran, Norman, & Wagner, 2005). Moreover, increased bilateral IFG activity has been associated with reduced semantic word-generation performance in the healthy aging (Meinzer et al., 2009) and even in young adults when task demands were increased (Thompson-Schill et al., 1997).

In a combined EEG–tDCS study, Wirth et al. (2011) tested the effects of anodal tDCS, compared to sham, over the left DLPFC using electrophysiological and behavioral correlates during overt picture naming. Online effects were examined by employing the semantic interference (SI) effect, a marker that denotes the functional integrity of the language system. The SI effect is robustly evoked in semantic blocking paradigms in which lexical–semantic competition increases when subjects have to name pictures of objects displayed in a semantically homogeneous context (e.g., cherries among grapes, pears, and oranges) and decreases when the target object appears in a semantically heterogeneous context (e.g., cherries among flies, a cocktail, and a bed). So, the SI effect refers to the difference in the dependent variables (i.e., verbal RTs and event-related potentials) evoked by overt picture naming in semantically homogenous and heterogeneous contexts. During anodal tDCS the behavioral SI effect was reduced, whereas the electrophysiological SI effect was enhanced over the left compared to the right temporal sites. This modulation is suggested to reflect a superior tuning of neural responses within language-related generators. Offline effects of anodal tDCS were detected in the delta frequency band, a marker of neural inhibition. After anodal tDCS there was a reduction in delta activity during picture naming and the resting state, interpreted to indicate neural disinhibition. Together, the results demonstrate that these electrophysiological markers could prove to be useful add-on biomarkers to trace and explain facilitatory effects of PFC anodal-tDCS on language production.

Regarding the TC, Fiori et al. (2011) examined whether anodal tDCS over the left Wernicke's area, together with concomitant language training, would induce improvement in novel word learning. Subjects were asked to learn novel words (i.e., non-words) associated with pictures. They found that left anodal tDCS, compared to sham and a control site (i.e., the occipital-parietal area), led to a significantly enhanced accuracy and verbal response time on the picture-naming task. These results are in good accordance with those of previous TMS (Sparing et al., 2001) and tDCS (Flöel, Rösser, Michka, Knecht, & Breitenstein, 2008; Sparing, Dafotakis, Meister, Thirugnanasambandam, & Fink, 2008) studies. Sparing et al. (2008) found faster naming latencies only after anodal tDCS of the left perisylvian region, including Wernicke's area. Flöel et al. (2008) reported similar results. They found that anodal tDCS over the left Wernicke's area induced faster and better novel word learning compared to cathodal and sham stimulation.

Our memories are not literal representations of the past. Instead, "facts" are unconsciously constructed to fit our schemata – existing mental representations of the world (Schacter & Addis, 2007). Consequently, our visual memories are susceptible to errors (i.e., false memories), but are less so in people who have a more literal cognitive style, such as people with autism.

(Happé & Frith, 2009). Boggio et al. (2009) compared three conditions during a false word memory task: bilateral stimulation over the anterior temporal lobes (ATLs) (i.e., anode over the left ATL and cathode over the right ATL), unilateral stimulation (anode over the left ATL), and sham stimulation. The data showed that there was a reduction in false memories following both the unilateral and bilateral stimulation treatments compared with the sham stimulation. These data suggest a role of the left ATL during verbal learning in reducing false memories while maintaining veridical (literal) memory performance unchanged. Similar to Boggio et al. (2009), Chi, Fregni, and Snyder (2010) applied bilateral tDCS to the ATLs in three groups of participants during the encoding and subsequent retrieval of a set of pictures. The data showed that there was a selective improvement of visual memory during left cathodal and right anodal stimulation compared to the opposite pattern of stimulation and sham. Together, these findings are consistent with TMS evidence that stimulation of the left ATL can paradoxically lead to autistic-like skills in healthy individuals in domains such as numerical processing (Snyder, 2009) and memory (Gallate, Chi, Ellwood, & Snyder, 2009). Finally, Ross, McCoy, Wolk, Coslett, and Olson (2010) applied anodal tDCS over the left ATL, right ATL, and sham while participants were naming pictures of famous individuals and landmarks, and found that application over the right ATL significantly enhanced naming for people but not landmarks. Considering that proper names are difficult to learn and prone to loss in memory decline (James, Fogler, & Tauber, 2008), the same paradigm was applied to older adults (Ross, McCoy, Coslett, Olson, & Wolk, 2011). The results showed improvement in face naming only after anodal stimulation of the left ATL. The magnitude of the enhancing effect was similar in older and younger adults, but the lateralization of the effect differed depending on age.

In conclusion, all these findings support the critical role of left perisylvian areas in semantic memory, in particular for object naming after anodal stimulation (Fig. 9.2). These findings have important implications for tDCS interventions in individuals with memory deficits (aging, stroke, and dementia) such as anomia.

PROCEDURAL (IMPLICIT) MEMORY

Procedural (implicit) memory refers to situations in which some form of learning has occurred, but this is reflected in performance rather than through overt recollection (e.g., motor skills, classical conditioning, priming) (Baddeley et al., 2009).

Classical conditioning (also Pavlovian conditioning) is a form of learning in which one stimulus, the conditioned stimulus (CS), comes to signal the occurrence of a second stimulus, the unconditioned stimulus (US). The US is usually a biologically significant stimulus, such as food or pain, that elicits a response from the start (unconditioned response or UR). The CS usually produces no particular response at first, but after conditioning it elicits the conditioned response (CR) (Bouton, 2007). For example, a bell (CS) that is paired repeatedly with meat powder (US) – a stimulus that elicits salivation – will come to evoke the same response (salivation) (CR).

Priming is an effect in which exposure to a stimulus influences a response to a later stimulus. It can occur following perceptual, semantic, or conceptual stimulus repetition (Kolb & Whishaw, 2003). For example, if a person reads a list of words including the word *table*, and is later asked to complete a word starting with *tab*, the probability that that individual will answer *table* is greater than if he or she had not been primed.

Motor skill learning refers to the process by which movements are executed more quickly and accurately with practice (Willingham, 1998).

Since this research topic has been studied extensively, in the following sections we will focus on motor skills.

Motor Skills

The acquisition and long-term retention of motor skills plays a fundamental role in our daily lives. Skills such as writing, playing golf, or riding a bicycle are all acquired through repetitive practice. Motor skill learning has been experimentally studied using tasks designed to measure the incremental acquisition of sequential movements into a well-articulated behavior (motor sequence learning), or to test our capacity to compensate for environmental changes (sensorimotor adaptation) (Doyon et al., 2009).

Motor sequence learning involves the ability to perform new movement qualities and/or muscle synergies that enhance performance beyond pre-existing levels. On the other hand, sensorimotor adaptation has been defined as the reduction in errors introduced by altered conditions in order to return to a pre-existent level of performance (see also Chapter 8). Sensorimotor adaptation, unlike motor sequence learning, does not require new patterns of muscle activations (i.e., a new capability), but rather a new mapping between well-learned movements and spatial goals (Krakauer, 2009). For example, when learning a sequence of movements, individuals combine isolated movements into one smooth, concatenated, and coherent action, such as when practicing a perfect tennis serve. In sensorimotor adaptation, participants modify movements in response to changes in sensory inputs or motor outputs, such as when adapting the motor commands for arm movements in response to the altered limb dynamics associated with holding a tennis racket (Bo, Langan, & Seidler, 2008).

Operationally, the acquisition of such motor abilities is generally measured by a reduction in reaction time and number of errors, and/or by a change in movement synergy and kinematics (Doyon et al., 2009).

Motor sequence learning paradigms may involve implicit or explicit learning. Implicit sequence learning refers to improvement in performance of the sequence without overt information about the elements of a sequence. In contrast, explicit sequence learning is accompanied by explicit conscious recollection of each element and its order in the sequence (Robertson, 2009).

It should be kept in mind, however, that explicit memory and explicit control processes are not synonymous. While explicit awareness of sequential order enhances execution of sequence elements (Crump & Logan, 2010; Ghilardi, Moisello, Silvestri, Ghez, & Krakauer, 2009), adaptation can proceed entirely implicitly (Mazzoni & Krakauer, 2006) without precluding the possibility that it could benefit from explicit control processes such as strategies (Taylor & Ivry, 2012).

There is evidence that motor sequence learning can continue over prolonged time periods, as in musicians (Brashers-Krug, Shadmehr, & Bizzi, 1996; Dudai, 2004; McGaugh, 2000). Within-session performance improvements (online effects) occur during initial stages of a learning session. However, the effects of motor learning can also continue after the end of practice (offline effects) (Krakauer & Shadmehr, 2006; Robertson, Pascual-Leone, & Miall, 2004; Walker, Brakefield, Morgan, Hobson, & Stickgold, 2002). In relation to motor skill learning, the term "consolidation" has been used in the literature to describe two different, but not mutually exclusive, phenomena: the offline behavioral skill improvements that occur at the end of a practice session (Robertson et al., 2004), and the reduction in fragility of a memory trace that follows encoding (Robertson, 2009; Robertson et al., 2004). Online and offline skill gains can be maintained over time, resulting in long-term retention (Romano et al., 2010). Moreover, various task attributes, such as reward (Abe et al., 2011) and practice structure (Song et al., 2012; Tanaka, Honda, Hanakawa, & Cohen, 2010) can have a profound influence on long-term retention. The contextual interference effect refers to the benefits of training under interleaved or random-order conditions as opposed to blocked practice schedules (Shea & Morgan, 1979).

In sensorimotor adaptation paradigms, subjects experience a systematic perturbation, either as a deviation of the visual representation of their movements (visuomotor adaptation) or as a deflecting force on the arm (dynamic adaptation), both of which induce reaching errors. Subjects initially make a large error, but over subsequent trials they are able to adapt to the perturbation and gradually reduce the error in their movement. This error reduction process has been interpreted as the acquisition of a new mapping between well-learned movements and spatial goals (Miall, Weir, Wolpert, & Stein, 1993). If the participant is then reintroduced to a condition where the perturbation is removed, an error in the opposite direction to the perturbation is observed (aftereffect), with this fading over subsequent trials. This 'aftereffect" is thought to represent the retention of the acquired visuomotor transformation (Bock, Worringham, & Thomas, 2005; Hadipour-Niktarash, Lee, Desmond, & Shadmehr, 2007).

Motor skill learning is typically characterized by increased functional connectivity in a distributed network that involves the primary motor cortex (M1), premotor cortex (PM), supplementary motor area (SMA), somatosensory cortex (S1), DLPFC, PPC, cerebellum, thalamic nuclei, and striatum (Doyon et al., 2009; Seidler, 2010; Song et al., 2012).

At the neural level, motor skill learning is accompanied by changes in neuronal activity, excitability and synaptic plasticity (Dayan & Cohen, 2011).

The interaction between the two M1s appears to play an important role in motor control in general, and in motor learning in particular (Duque et al., 2008; Kobayashi, Hutchinson, Theoret, Schlaug, & Pascual-Leone, 2004; Perez & Cohen, 2008). However, the specific ways in which these interactions operate during motor learning remain to be determined. According to this principle, it would be theoretically possible to facilitate motor learning by enhancing excitability (anodal tDCS) in M1 contralateral to the practicing hand, or by decreasing excitability (cathodal tDCS) in M1 ipsilateral to the training hand (Kinsbourne, 1977; Ward & Cohen, 2004).

In the following sections we will discuss studies that have successfully applied tES to improve motor skill learning in healthy humans.

Motor Sequence Learning

Several studies have shown that anodal tDCS over M1 contralateral to the training hand can improve online learning of sequential finger movement tasks.

Nitsche et al. (2003) showed that anodal tDCS applied over M1 during practice led to improvement in reaction times on the serial reaction time task (SRTT), a task in which a sequence order can be learned implicitly because onset times (reaction time plus movement time) are gradually reduced when subjects make sequential movements without explicit awareness that a sequence is present (Nissen & Bullemer, 1987; Robertson, 2007). Remarkably, the improvement was restricted to M1, because stimulation of PM and PFC had no effect (Nitsche et al., 2003). Similarly, anodal tDCS over M1 enhanced finger sequence movements (Kang & Paik, 2011; Vines, Nair, & Schlaug, 2006) and performance on a visuomotor coordination task (Antal et al., 2004). Improvement of initial performance on a SRTT was also observed when 10-Hz alternating current stimulation (tACS) was applied over M1 (Antal, Boros et al., 2008). tACS consists of an alternating current delivered to the cortex in a frequency-specific fashion (Kuo & Nitsche, 2012; Paulus, 2011; see also Chapter 2). High-frequency tACS over M1 at 80, 140, and 250 Hz seemed to be less effective than low-frequency tACS with 10 Hz, regarding SRTT learning (Moliadze, Antal, & Paulus, 2010). tRNS consists of an alternating current delivered to the cortex at random frequencies (Terney, Chaieb, Moliadze, Antal, & Paulus, 2008). Currently, the noise signal can contain all of the frequencies from 0.1 Hz to 640 Hz (Kuo & Nitsche, 2012; Paulus, 2011). tRNS of M1 induced an increase of the cortical excitability and enhanced performance on the SRTT (Terney et al., 2008).

Recently, Stagg et al. (2011) examined the effects of tDCS over the M1 during an explicit motor learning task consisting of sequential finger presses. Similar to previous motor learning studies on implicit behavior, tDCS modulated learning rates in a polarity-specific manner; anodal tDCS increased the rate of motor sequence learning while cathodal stimulation decreased the rate of learning. Similar results were obtained on finger sequence movements with unilateral cathodal tDCS ipsilateral to the practicing hand (Vines et al., 2006) or bi-hemispheric tDCS (anodal to the contralateral M1 and cathodal to the ipsilateral M1 of the performing hand) (Kang & Paik, 2011; Vines, Cerruti, & Schlaug, 2008).

It should be kept in mind that while anodal tDCS over the M1 during rest generally results in an increase in motor evoked potential (MEP) amplitudes (Nitsche & Paulus, 2000), under some circumstances it may worsen subsequent learning (Antal, Begemeier, Nitsche, & Paulus, 2008; Kuo et al., 2008) – an effect that could be explained by homeostatic plasticity rules (Bienenstock, Cooper, & Munro, 1982). Thus, this dissociation between effects of tDCS on MEP amplitudes and on learning raises caution when trying to use MEP amplitudes as the sole biomarker of cortical plasticity or of likelihood of impact on behavior.

Previous work using TMS provided evidence of the functional relevance of M1 in offline learning of simple ballistic movements as well as sequential movements (Baraduc, Lang, Rothwell, & Wolpert, 2004; Muellbacher et al., 2002; Robertson, Press, & Pascual-Leone, 2005). So far, only a few studies have investigated whether tES over M1 could facilitate off-line effects of motor sequence learning.

In one study (Reis et al., 2009), subjects practiced the sequential visual isometric pinch task (SVIPT) over 5 consecutive days while receiving anodal tDCS over contralateral M1 during the training period. There was no difference of within-day improvements (online effects when considering on average the 5 training days) between anodal tDCS and sham stimulation, while anodal tDCS largely enhanced between-day improvement (offline effect) compared to sham. Anodal tDCS did not change the rate of forgetting compared to sham stimulation across the 3-month follow-up period, and consequently the skill measure of subjects who received anodal tDCS remained greater at 3 months. These findings, showing that anodal tDCS enhances offline improvement of the motor skill but did not overwhelmingly affect online learning or rate of forgetting, support the view that motor skill learning has temporally distinct stages. Furthermore, the documentation of lasting beneficial effects (3 months after training and stimulation) of anodal tDCS may have promising implications for the design of protocols in neurorehabilitation of motor deficits following brain lesions. Further, using the same paradigm, Schambra et al. (2011) showed that anodal tDCS of left M1 is more beneficial than stimulation of right M1 regarding motor learning, irrespective of the hand that is trained – a result consistent not only with the hypothesized left hemisphere specialization for motor skill learning but also with possible increased left M1 responsiveness to tDCS.

Depending on the task, offline improvement of motor skill may or may not require sleep (Robertson, Pascual-Leone, & Press, 2004). Tecchio et al. (2010) showed that anodal tDCS over M1 applied immediately after the training of a serial finger tapping task enhanced early consolidation, as assessed by the performance difference between the first block after and the last block before stimulation, compared to sham stimulation. No stimulation effect was found on online learning. These findings suggest that anodal tDCS applied immediately after training may influence early consolidation in a task-dependent manner.

In conclusion, all these studies show the critical role of M1 (Fig. 9.3) during online and offline motor sequence learning, and the possibility of improving motor skill learning with anodal tDCS, low-frequency tACS, and tRNS – an issue of critical importance for NIBS interventions in individuals with memory deficits (e.g., stroke, Parkinson's or Huntington's disease), and for the development of effective new training technologies to support work-related learning in healthy individuals.

Sensorimotor Adaptation

There is evidence that, after exposure to adaptation paradigms, the M1 is involved in the retention of the newly learnt visuomotor transformation (Hadipour-Niktarash et al., 2007; Hunter, Sacco, Nitsche, & Turner, 2009; Richardson et al., 2006). For instance, Hadipour-Niktarash et al. (2007) disrupted M1 with TMS, and found impaired retention but not acquisition of a novel visuomotor transformation. Regarding the possibility of enhancing motor learning, Orban de Xivry et al. (2011) demonstrated that anodal tDCS of the M1 also has the capacity to enhance generalization of learning. In this study, subjects adapted to a force field by reaching a single target in one trained direction, and were later tested for generalization in another workspace. Interestingly, stimulation of the M1 (and not the adjacent PPC) enhanced the generalization process in the intrinsic coordinates of the joints and muscles but did not affect the extrinsic coordinates (environment) – a finding highly relevant to rehabilitation.

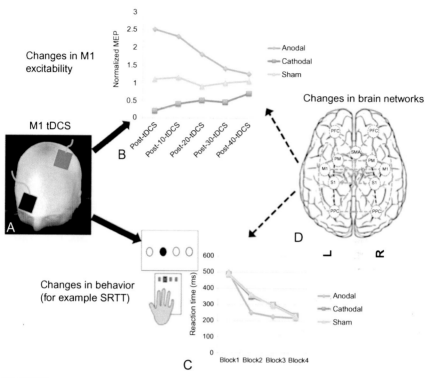

FIGURE 9.3 (A) Schematic summary of tDCS effects over M1 (bipolar electrode montage with one electrode over M1, and other over contralateral supraorbital region). (B) M1 tDCS mediates polarity-specific changes in cortical excitability (shown as motor evoked potentials, i.e., MEPs expressed as a ratio to baseline) that outlasts duration of stimulation up to 40 minutes. (C) M1 tDCS also leads to changes in behavior such as motor learning on a SRTT. Anodal tDCS over M1 improves motor performance on SRTT more than cathodal and sham tDCS (i.e., greater decrease in reaction time in the early blocks). (D) Representative cortical brain networks with interacting regional nodes that are likely modulated by tDCS over M1. PFC, prefrontal cortex; SMA, supplementary motor area; PM, premotor cortex; S1, primary somatosensory cortex; M1, primary motor cortex; PPC, posterior parietal cortex. Complex brain network dynamics recorded through neuroimaging could help identify and quantify widespread changes in brain activity and functional connectivity within brain networks to provide more novel insights into neuroplastic mechanisms modulated by tDCS. Note: data shown in graphs are representative of previously published results (Nitsche et al., 2008). *From Venkatakrishnan and Sandrini (2012).*

A few recent studies have applied tDCS over the cerebellum, a critical brain structure involved in movement control. Galea, Jayaram, Ajagbe, and Celnik (2009) showed that tDCS is capable of modifying cerebellar excitability. Cathodal tDCS decreased and anodal tDCS increased cerebellar inhibition of M1. This change in excitability lasted for 30 minutes after stimulation, and did not affect the excitability of the brainstem or corticomotor system. The same authors (Galea, Vazquez, Pasricha, de Xivry, & Celnik, 2011) dissociated the roles of the cerebellum and M1 during adaptive motor learning to a novel visuomotor transformation. They found that anodal cerebellar tDCS specifically enhanced acquisition, as shown by a faster reduction of movement error, without influencing retention. Conversely, anodal M1 tDCS increased retention (i.e., reduced forgetting) but did not affect acquisition. These results demonstrate that the cerebellum and M1 have distinct functional roles.

Interactions Between Declarative (Explicit) and Procedural (Implicit) Memory

When learned in quick succession, declarative and procedural memory tasks interfere with one another and subsequent recall is impaired(Brown & Robertson, 2007b; Keisler & Shadmehr, 2010). Interference may arise from a direct competition between different memory systems. For example, learning an explicit declarative memory task immediately after practice of an implicit motor sequences task blocked offline improvement of these procedural memories. Furthermore, the forgetting of the implicit motor skill over the retention interval was proportional to the amount of declarative learning. This suggests that offline mechanisms that support implicit motor memory stabilization may be blocked by an explicit memory (Brown & Robertson, 2007b).

To elucidate the neural substrates underlying the interactions between implicit and explicit memory, Kantak et al. (2012) applied anodal tDCS over M1, dorsal PM (PMd), or sham stimulation during SRTT practice. Implicit sequence learning is primarily associated with activity in the contralateral primary somatosensory cortex and M1. In contrast, when learners developed explicit knowledge of the practiced sequence, activation in the PMd and DLPFC correlated strongly with conscious recall of the sequence (Honda et al., 1998; Vidoni & Boyd, 2007; Robertson, 2009). Implicit sequence knowledge was assessed at baseline, at the end of acquisition (EoA), and 24 hours after practice (retention test, RET). Anodal tDCS over M1 during practice significantly enhanced practice performance and supported offline stabilization compared with sham tDCS. Performance change from EoA to RET revealed that anodal tDCS over PMd during practice attenuated offline stabilization compared to anodal tDCS over M1 and sham stimulation. The results support the role of M1 in implementing online performance gains and offline stabilization for implicit motor sequence learning. In contrast, enhancing the activity within explicit motor memory network nodes such as the PMd during practice may be detrimental to offline stabilization of the learned implicit motor sequence. These results support the notion of competition between the procedural (implicit) and declarative (explicit) memory systems, in accordance with a previous TMS study (Galea et al., 2010). Galea and colleagues demonstrated that inhibitory TMS to the DLPFC enhanced motor memory consolidation by disrupting the explicit memory system, providing the first evidence for competitive interaction at the level of neural substrates (Galea et al., 2010). Kantak et al.'s study (2012) extends the understanding of the neural structures that underlie this competition between the implicit and explicit motor memory systems, and provides evidence for differential involvement of M1 and PMd in implicit sequence learning.

Alternatively, recent TMS evidence has begun to suggest that memory interference may arise from brain areas generating a coupling or bridge between otherwise independent declarative and procedural processing, and this coupling, not the competition, causes the interference between the memories (Cohen & Robertson, 2011; Robertson, 2012).

CONCLUSIONS

Many studies have explored the impact of tES on motor skill learning, episodic, and semantic memory. The results show that tES is a safe method not only to evaluate the contribution of specific areas to memory function but also to enhance learning and memory in healthy subjects – an issue of critical importance for possible applications of tES in the clinical arena and in the work setting (i.e., neuroergonomics). A neuroergonomics approach could lead to a neuroscience-based technique that would increase the effectiveness of training and reduce the time required to achieve a specific level of expertise. Learning to interpret perceptual information quickly and accurately in a complex natural environment is essential for acquiring many forms of expertise.

Since the effects of stimulation still show some heterogeneity, it will be important for future studies to explore the determinants of the effects of stimulation to a larger degree. Future studies are needed to systematically investigate the polarity-specific changes in brain network dynamics (Buch et al., 2012; Sporns, 2010) induced by tES to provide a plausible mechanistic account of neuroplasticity and explain behavioral neurophysiological changes that are modulated by tES as well as the relatively large interindividual variability in the effects (Antal, Polanía, Schmidt-Samoa, Dechent, & Paulus, 2011; Polanía, Paulus, & Nitsche, 2012; Thut & Miniussi, 2009; Venkatakrishnan & Sandrini, 2012; see also Fig. 9.3). Finally, it will be crucial to optimize stimulation protocols in order to enhance long-term retention of newly acquired memories, and to transfer what has been learned to new conditions and task variants.

Acknowledgments

This work was supported by the Intramural Research Program of the NINDS, NIH (US), and by funding from US Department of Defense in the Center for Neuroscience and Regenerative Medicine to MS.

References

Abe, M., Schambra, H. M., Wassermann, E. M., Luckenbaugh, D., Schweighofer, N., & Cohen, L. G. (2011). Reward improves long-term retention of a motor memory through induction of off-line memory gains. *Current Biology, 21,* 557–562.

Antal, A., Begemeier, S., Nitsche, M. A., & Paulus, W. (2008). Prior state of cortical activity influences subsequent practicing of a visuomotor coordination task. *Neuropsychologia, 46*(13), 3157–3161.

Antal, A., Boros, K., Poreisz, C., Chaieb, L., Terney, D., & Paulus, W. (2008). Comparatively weak after-effects of transcranial alternating current stimulation (tACS) on cortical excitability in humans. *Brain Stimulation, 1*(2), 97–105.

Antal, A., Nitsche, M. A., Kincses, T. Z., Kruse, W., Hoffmann, K. P., & Paulus, W. (2004). Facilitation of visuo-motor learning by transcranial direct current stimulation of the motor and extrastriate visual areas in humans. *European Journal of Neuroscience, 19*(10), 2888–2892.

Antal, A., Polanía, R., Schmidt-Samoa, C., Dechent, P., & Paulus, W. (2011). Transcranial direct current stimulation over the primary motor cortex during fMRI. *NeuroImage, 55* (2), 590–596.

Baddeley, A., Eysenck, M. W., & Anderson, M. (2009). *Memory.* Hove, UK: Psychology Press.

Baraduc, P., Lang, N., Rothwell, J. C., & Wolpert, D. M. (2004). Consolidation of dynamic motor learning is not disrupted by rTMS of primary motor cortex. *Current Biology, 14* (3), 252–256.

Barker, A. T., Jalinous, R., & Freeston, I. L. (1985). Non-invasive magnetic stimulation of the human motor cortex. *Lancet, 1*(8437), 1106–1107.

Bienenstock, E. L., Cooper, L. N., & Munro, P. W. (1982). Theory for the development of neuron selectivity: Orientation specificity and binocular interaction in visual cortex. *Journal of Neuroscience, 2*(1), 32–48.

Binder, J. R., Desai, R. H., Graves, W. W., & Conant, L. L. (2009). Where is the semantic system? A critical review and meta-analysis of 120 functional neuroimaging studies. *Cerebral Cortex, 19*(12), 2767–2796.

Bo, J., Langan, J., & Seidler, R. D. (2008). Cognitive neuroscience of skill acquisition. *Advances in Psychology, 139,* 101–112.

Bock, O., Worringham, C., & Thomas, M. (2005). Concurrent adaptations of left and right arms to opposite visual distortions. *Experimental Brain Research, 162,* 513–519.

Boggio, P. S., Fregni, F., Valasek, C., Ellwood, S., Chi, R., Gallate, J., et al. (2009). Temporal lobe cortical electrical stimulation during the encoding and retrieval phase reduces false memories. *PLoS One, 4*(3), e4959.

Bouton, M. E. (2007). *Learning and behavior: A contemporary synthesis.* Sunderland, MA: Sinauer.

Brashers-Krug, T., Shadmehr, R., & Bizzi, E. (1996). Consolidation in human motor memory. *Nature, 382*(6588), 252–255.

Brown, R. M., & Robertson, E. M. (2007a). Inducing motor skill improvements with a declarative task. *Nature Neuroscience, 10,* 148–149.

Brown, R. M., & Robertson, E. M. (2007b). Off-line processing: Reciprocal interactions between declarative and procedural memories. *Journal of Neuroscience, 27*(39), 10468–10475.

Buch, E. R., Modir Shanechi, A., Fourkas, A. D., Weber, C., Birbaumer, N., & Cohen, L. G. (2012). Parietofrontal integrity determines neural modulation associated with grasping imagery after stroke. *Brain, 135*(Pt 2), 596–614.

Bullard, L. M., Browning, E. S., Clark, V. P., Coffman, B. A., Garcia, C. M., Jung, R. E., et al. (2011). Transcranial direct current stimulation's effect on novice versus experienced learning. *Experimental Brain Research, 213*(1), 9–14.

Cabeza, R., Ciaramelli, E., Olson, I. R., & Moscovitch, M. (2008). The parietal cortex and episodic memory: An attentional account. *Nature Reviews. Neuroscience*, *9*(8), 613–625.

Cabeza, R., & Nyberg, L. (2000). Neural bases of learning and memory: Functional neuroimaging evidence. *Current Opinion in Neurology*, *13*(4), 415–421.

Cappa, S. F., Sandrini, M., Rossini, P. M., Sosta, K., & Miniussi, C. (2002). The role of the left frontal lobe in action naming: rTMS evidence. *Neurology*, *59*, 720–723.

Cattaneo, Z., Pisoni, A., & Papagno, C. (2011). Transcranial direct current stimulation over Broca's region improves phonemic and semantic fluency in healthy individuals. *Neuroscience*, *183*, 64–70.

Censor, N., Dimyan, M. A., & Cohen, L. G. (2010). Modification of existing human motor memories is enabled by primary cortical processing during memory reactivation. *Current Biology*, *20*(17), 1545–1549.

Chi, R. P., Fregni, F., & Snyder, A. W. (2010). Visual memory improved by non-invasive brain stimulation. *Brain Research*, *1353*, 168–175.

Clark, V. P., Coffman, B. A., Mayer, A. R., Weisend, M. P., Lane, T. D., Calhoun, V. D., et al. (2012). TDCS guided using fMRI significantly accelerates learning to identify concealed objects. *NeuroImage*, *59*(1), 117–128.

Coffman, B. A., Trumbo, M. C., & Clark, V. P. (2012). Enhancement of object detection with transcranial direct current stimulation is associated with increased attention. *BMC Neuroscience*, *13*, 108.

Cohen, N. S. (1984). Preserved learning capacity in amnesia: Evidence for multiple memory systems. In L. R. Squire & N. Butters (Eds.), *Neuropsychology of memory* (pp. 83–103). New York, NY: Guilford.

Cohen, L. G., Celnik, P., Pascual-Leone, A., Corwell, B., Falz, L., Dambrosia, J., et al. (1997). Functional relevance of cross-modal plasticity in blind humans. *Nature*, *389*(6647), 180–183.

Cohen, D. A., & Robertson, E. M. (2011). Preventing interference between different memory tasks. *Nature Neuroscience*, *14*, 953–955.

Crump, M. J., & Logan, G. D. (2010). Episodic contributions to sequential control: Learning from a typist's touch. *Journal of Experimental Psychology. Human Perception and Performance*, *36*, 662–672.

Dayan, E., Censor, N., Buch, E. R., Sandrini, M., & Cohen, L. G. (2013). Noninvasive brain stimulation: From physiology to network dynamics and back. *Nature Neuroscience*, *16* (7), 838–844.

Dayan, E., & Cohen, L. G. (2011). Neuroplasticity subserving motor skill learning. *Neuron*, *72* (3), 443–454.

Diekelmann, S., & Born, J. (2010). The memory function of sleep. *Nature Reviews. Neuroscience*, *11*(2), 114–126.

Doyon, J., Bellec, P., Amsel, R., Penhune, V., Monchi, O., Carrier, J., et al. (2009). Contributions of the basal ganglia and functionally related brain structures to motor learning. *Behavioral Brain Research*, *199*(1), 61–75.

Dudai, Y. (2004). The neurobiology of consolidations, or, how stable is the engram? *Annual Review of Psychology*, *55*, 51–86.

Duque, J., Mazzocchio, R., Stefan, K., Hummel, F., Olivier, E., & Cohen, L. G. (2008). Memory formation in the motor cortex ipsilateral to a training hand. *Cerebral Cortex*, *18*(6), 1395–1406.

Fertonani, A., Rosini, S., Cotelli, M., Rossini, P. M., & Miniussi, C. (2010). Naming facilitation induced by transcranial direct current stimulation. *Behavioural Brain Research*, *208*, 311–318.

Fiori, V., Coccia, M., Marinelli, C. V., Vecchi, V., Bonifazi, S., Ceravolo, M. G., et al. (2011). Transcranial direct current stimulation improves word retrieval in healthy and nonfluent aphasic subjects. *Journal of Cognitive Neuroscience*, *23*, 2309–2323.

Fletcher, P. C., & Henson, R. N. (2001). Frontal lobes and human memory: Insights from functional neuroimaging. *Brain, 124*(Pt 5), 849–881.

Flöel, A., Poeppel, D., Buffalo, E. A., Braun, A., Wu, C. W., Seo, H. J., et al. (2005). Prefrontal cortex asymmetry for memory encoding of words and abstract shapes. *Cerebral Cortex, 14* (4), 404–409.

Flöel, A., Rösser, N., Michka, O., Knecht, S., & Breitenstein, C. (2008). Noninvasive brain stimulation improves language learning. *Journal of Cognitive Neuroscience, 20*(8), 1415–1422.

Flöel, A., Suttorp, W., Kohl, O., Kürten, J., Lohmann, H., Bretenstein, C., et al. (2012). Noninvasive brain stimulation improves object-location learning in the elderly. *Neurobiology of Aging, 33*(8), 1682–1689.

Frankland, P. W., & Bontempi, B. (2005). The organization of recent and remote memories. *Nature Reviews. Neuroscience, 6*(2), 119–130.

Galea, J. M., Albert, N. B., Ditye, T., & Miall, R. C. (2010). Disruption of the dorsolateral prefrontal cortex facilitates the consolidation of procedural skills. *Journal of Cognitive Neuroscience, 22*(6), 1158–1164.

Galea, J. M., Jayaram, G., Ajagbe, L., & Celnik, P. (2009). Modulation of cerebellar excitability by polarity-specific noninvasive direct current stimulation. *Journal of Neuroscience, 29*(28), 9115–9122.

Galea, J. M., Vazquez, A., Pasricha, N., de Xivry, J. J., & Celnik, P. (2011). Dissociating the roles of the cerebellum and motor cortex during adaptive learning: The motor cortex retains what the cerebellum learns. *Cerebral Cortex, 21*(8), 1761–1770.

Gallate, J., Chi, R., Ellwood, S., & Snyder, A. (2009). Reducing false memories by magnetic pulse stimulation. *Neuroscience Letter, 449*, 151–154.

Ghilardi, M. F., Moisello, C., Silvestri, G., Ghez, C., & Krakauer, J. W. (2009). Learning of a sequential motor skill comprises explicit and implicit components that consolidate differently. *Journal of Neurophysiology, 101*, 2218–2229.

Gonsalves, B. D., Kahn, I., Curran, T., Norman, K. A., & Wagner, A. D. (2005). Memory strength and repetition suppression: Multimodal imaging of medial temporal cortical contributions to recognition. *Neuron, 47*, 751–761.

Hadipour-Niktarash, A., Lee, C. K., Desmond, J. E., & Shadmehr, R. (2007). Impairment of retention but not acquisition of a visuomotor skill through time-dependent disruption of primary motor cortex. *Journal of Neuroscience, 27*(49), 13413–13419.

Hallett, M. (2000). Transcranial magnetic stimulation and the human brain. *Nature, 406*(6792), 147–150.

Happé, F., & Frith, U. (2009). The beautiful otherness of the autistic mind. *Philosophical Transactions of the Royal Society of London B: Biological Sciences, 364*(1522), 1346–1350.

Hardt, O., Einarsson, E. O., & Nader, K. (2010). A bridge over troubled water: Reconsolidation as a link between cognitive and neuroscientific memory research traditions. *Annual Review of Psychology, 61*, 141–167.

Holland, R., Leff, A. P., Josephs, O., Galea, J. M., Desikan, M., Price, C. J., et al. (2011). Speech facilitation by left inferior frontal cortex stimulation. *Current Biology, 21*(16), 1403–1407.

Honda, M., Deiber, M. P., Ibanez, V., Pascual-Leone, A., Zhuang, P., & Hallett, M. (1998). Dynamic cortical involvement in implicit and explicit motor sequence learning. A PET study. *Brain, 121*, 2159–2173.

Huber, R., Ghilardi, M. F., Massimini, M., & Tononi, G. (2004). Local sleep and learning. *Nature, 430*(6995), 78–81.

Hunter, T., Sacco, P., Nitsche, M. A., & Turner, D. L. (2009). Modulation of internal model formation during force field-induced motor learning by anodal transcranial direct current stimulation of primary motor cortex. *Journal of Physiology, 587*(12), 2949–2961.

Jacobson, L., Goren, N., Lavidor, M., & Levy, D. A. (2012). Oppositional transcranial direct current stimulation (tDCS) of parietal substrates of attention during encoding modulates episodic memory. *Brain Research, 1439*, 66–72.

James, L. E., Fogler, K. A., & Tauber, S. K. (2008). Recognition memory measures yield disproportionate effects of aging on learning face-name associations. *Psychology and Aging, 23* (3), 657–664.

Javadi, A. H., & Walsh, V. (2012). Transcranial direct current stimulation (tDCS) of the left dorsolateral prefrontal cortex modulates declarative memory. *Brain Stimulation, 5*(3), 231–241.

Kang, E. K., & Paik, N. J. (2011). Effect of a tDCS electrode montage on implicit motor sequence learning in healthy subjects. *Experimental & Translational Stroke Medicine, 3*(1), 4.

Kantak, S. S., Mummidisetty, C. K., & Stinear, J. W. (2012). Primary motor and premotor cortex in implicit sequence learning–Evidence for competition between implicit and explicit human motor memory systems. *European Journal of Neuroscience, 36*(5), 2710–2715.

Keisler, A., & Shadmehr, R. (2010). A shared resource between declarative memory and motor memory. *Journal of Neuroscience, 30*(44), 14817–14823.

Kinsbourne, M. (1977). Hemi-neglect and hemisphere rivalry. *Advances in Neurology, 18,* 41–49.

Kobayashi, M., Hutchinson, S., Theoret, H., Schlaug, G., & Pascual-Leone, A. (2004). Repetitive TMS of the motor cortex improves ipsilateral sequential simple finger movements. *Neurology, 62*(1), 91–98.

Kolb, B., & Whishaw, I. (2003). *Fundamentals of human neuropsychology.* New York, NY: Freeman.

Krakauer, J. W. (2009). Motor learning and consolidation: The case of visuomotor rotation. *Advances in Experimental Medicine and Biology, 629,* 405–421.

Krakauer, J. W., & Shadmehr, R. (2006). Consolidation of motor memory. *Trends in Neuroscience, 29*(1), 58–64.

Kuo, M. F., & Nitsche, M. A. (2012). Effects of transcranial electrical stimulation on cognition. *Clinical EEG and Neuroscience, 43*(3), 192–199.

Kuo, M. F., Unger, M., Liebetanz, D., Lang, N., Tergau, F., Paulus, W., et al. (2008). Limited impact of homeostatic plasticity on motor learning in humans. *Neuropsychologia, 46*(8), 2122–2128.

Levy, B. J., Kuhl, B. A., & Wagner, A. D. (2010). The functional neuroimaging of forgetting. In S. Della Sala (Ed.), *Forgetting* (pp. 135–163). Hove, UK: Psychology Press.

Maguire, E. A., Gadian, D. G., Johnsrude, I. S., Good, C. D., Ashburner, J., Frackowiak, R. S., et al. (2000). Navigation-related structural change in the hippocampi of taxi drivers. *Proceedings of the National Academy of Sciences of the United States of America, 97*(8), 4398–4403.

Maguire, E. A., Woollett, K., & Spiers, H. J. (2006). London taxi drivers and bus drivers: A structural MRI and neuropsychological analysis. *Hippocampus, 16*(12), 1091–1101.

Manenti, R., Cotelli, M., Robertson, I. H., & Miniussi, C. (2012). Transcranial brain stimulation studies of episodic memory in young adults, elderly adults and individuals with memory dysfunction: A review. *Brain Stimulation, 5*(2), 103–109.

Marshall, L., Helgadóttir, H., Mölle, M., & Born, J. (2006). Boosting slow oscillations during sleep potentiates memory. *Nature, 444*(7119), 610–613.

Marshall, L., Mölle, M., & Born, J. (2003). Spindle and slow wave rhythms at slow wave sleep transitions are linked to strong shifts in the cortical direct current potential. *Neuroscience, 121,* 1047–1053.

Marshall, L., Mölle, M., Hallschmid, M., & Born, J. (2004). Transcranial direct current stimulation during sleep improves declarative memory. *Journal of Neuroscience, 24*(44), 9985–9992.

Mazzoni, P., & Krakauer, J. W. (2006). An implicit plan overrides an explicit strategy during visuomotor adaptation. *Journal of Neuroscience, 26*(14), 3642–3645.

McGaugh, J. L. (2000). Memory–A century of consolidation. *Science, 287*(5451), 248–251.

Meinzer, M., Antonenko, D., Lindenberg, R., Hetzer, S., Ulm, L., Avirame, K., et al. (2012). Electrical brain stimulation improves cognitive performance by modulating functional connectivity and task-specific activation. *Journal of Neuroscience, 32*(5), 1859–1866.

Meinzer, M., Flaisch, T., Wilser, L., Eulitz, C., Rockstroh, B., Conway, T., et al. (2009). Neural signatures of semantic and phonemic fluency in young and old adults. *Journal of Cognitive Neuroscience, 21,* 2007–2018.

Miall, R. C., Weir, D. J., Wolpert, D. M., & Stein, J. F. (1993). Is the cerebellum a smith predictor? *Journal of Motor Behavior, 25,* 203–216.

Mishkin, M. (1982). A memory system in the monkey. *Philosophical Transactions of the Royal Society, B: Biological Sciences, 298,* 85–92.

Moliadze, V., Antal, A., & Paulus, W. (2010). Boosting brain excitability by transcranial high frequency stimulation in the ripple range. *Journal of Physiology, 588*(24), 4891–4904.

Muellbacher, W., Ziemann, U., Wissel, J., Dang, N., Kofler, M., Facchini, S., et al. (2002). Early consolidation in human primarymotorcortex. *Nature, 415*(6872), 640–644.

Müller, G. E., & Pilzecher, A. (1900). Experimentelle Beiträge zur Lehre vom Gedächtniss. *Zeitschrift für Psychologie. Ergänzungsband, 1,* 1–300.

Nissen, M., & Bullemer, P. (1987). Attentional requirements of learning: Evidence from performance measures. *Cognitive Psychology, 19,* 1–32.

Nitsche, M. A., Cohen, L. G., Wassermann, E. M., Priori, A., Lang, N., Antal, A., et al. (2008). Transcranial direct current stimulation: State of the art. *Brain Stimulation, 1*(3), 206–223.

Nitsche, M. A., & Paulus, W. (2000). Excitability changes induced in the human motor cortex by weak transcranial direct current stimulation. *Journal of Physiology, 3,* 633–639.

Nitsche, M. A., Schauenburg, A., Lang, N., Liebetanz, D., Exner, C., Paulus, W., et al. (2003). Facilitation of implicit motor learning by weak transcranial direct current stimulation of the primary motor cortex in the human. *Journal of Cognitive Neuroscience, 15*(4), 619–626.

Orban de Xivry, J. J., Marko, M. K., Pekny, S. E., Pastor, D., Izawa, J., Celnik, P., et al. (2011). Stimulation of the human motor cortex alters generalization patterns of motor learning. *Journal of Neuroscience, 31*(19), 7102–7110.

Parasuraman, R., & Rizzo, M. (2008). *Neuroergonomics: The Brain at Work.* New York, NY: Oxford University Press.

Patterson, K., Nestor, P. J., & Rogers, T. T. (2007). Where do you know what you know? The representation of semantic knowledge in the human brain. *Nature Reviews. Neuroscience, 8* (12), 976–987.

Paulus, W. (2011). Transcranial electrical stimulation (TES–tDCS; tRNS, tACS) methods. *Neuropsychological Rehabilitation, 5,* 602–617.

Penolazzi, B., Di Domenico, A., Marzoli, D., Mammarella, N., Fairfield, B., Franciotti, R., et al. (2010). Effects of transcranial direct current stimulation on episodic memory related to emotional visual stimuli. *PLoS One, 5*(5), e10623.

Perez, M. A., & Cohen, L. G. (2008). Mechanisms underlying functional changes in the primary motor cortex ipsilateral to an active hand. *Journal of Neuroscience, 28*(22), 5631–5640.

Plihal, W., & Born, J. (1997). Effects of early and late nocturnal sleep on declarative and procedural memory. *Journal of Cognitive Neuroscience, 9,* 534–547.

Plihal, W., & Born, J. (1999). Effects of early and late nocturnal sleep on priming and spatial memory. *Psychophysiology, 36,* 571–582.

Polanía, R., Paulus, W., & Nitsche, M. A. (2012). Modulating cortico-striatal and thalamo-cortical functional connectivity with transcranial direct current stimulation. *Human Brain Mapping, 33*(10), 2499–2508.

Poldrack, R. A., Clark, J., Pare-Blagoev, E. J., Shohamy, D., CresoMoyano, J., Myers, C., et al. (2001). Interactive memory systems in the human brain. *Nature, 414,* 546–550.

Priori, A. (2003). Brain polarization in humans: A reappraisal of an old tool for prolonged non-invasive modulation of brain excitability. *Clinical Neurophysiology, 114*(4), 589–595.

Raichle, M. E. (1998). Imaging the mind. *Seminars in Nuclear Medicine, 28*(4), 278–289.

Reis, J., Schambra, H. M., Cohen, L. G., Buch, E. R., Fritsch, B., Zarahn, E., et al. (2009). Noninvasive cortical stimulation enhances motor skill acquisition over multiple days through an effect on consolidation. *Proceedings of the National Academy of Sciences of the United States of America, 106*(5), 1590–1595.

Richardson, A. G., Overduin, S. A., Valero-Cabre, A., Padoa-Schioppa, C., Pascual-Leone, A., Bizzi, E., et al. (2006). Disruption of primary motor cortex before learning impairs memory of movement dynamics. *Journal of Neuroscience, 26*(48), 12466–12470.

Robertson, E. M. (2007). The serial reaction time task: Implicit motor skill learning? *Journal of Neuroscience, 27*(38), 10073–10075.

Robertson, E. M. (2009). From creation to consolidation: A novel framework for memory processing. *PLoS Biology, 7*, e19.

Robertson, E. M. (2012). New insights in human memory interference and consolidation. *Current Biology, 22*(2), R66–R71.

Robertson, E. M., Pascual-Leone, A., & Miall, R. C. (2004). Current concepts in procedural consolidation. *Nature Reviews. Neuroscience, 5*(7), 576–582.

Robertson, E. M., Pascual-Leone, A., & Press, D. Z. (2004). Awareness modifies the skill-learning benefits of sleep. *Current Biology, 14*(3), 208–212.

Robertson, E. M., Press, D. Z., & Pascual-Leone, A. (2005). Off-line learning and the primary motor cortex. *Journal of Neuroscience, 25*(27), 6372–6378.

Romano, J. C., Howard, J. H., Jr., & Howard, D. V. (2010). One-year retention of general and sequence-specific skills in a probabilistic, serial reaction time task. *Memory, 18*(4), 427–441.

Ross, L. A., McCoy, D., Coslett, H. B., Olson, I. R., & Wolk, D. A. (2011). Improved proper name recall in aging after electrical stimulation of the anterior temporal lobes. *Frontiers in Aging Neuroscience, 3*, 16.

Ross, L. A., McCoy, D., Wolk, D. A., Coslett, H. B., & Olson, I. R. (2010). Improved proper name recall by electrical stimulation of the anterior temporal lobes. *Neuropsychologia, 48* (12), 3671–3674.

Rossi, S., Cappa, S. F., Babiloni, C., Pasqualetti, P., Miniussi, C., Carducci, F., et al. (2001). Prefrontal [correction of Prefontal] cortex in long-term memory: An "interference" approach using magnetic stimulation. *Nature Neuroscience, 4*(9), 948–952.

Sandrini, M., Cappa, S. F., Rossi, S., Rossini, P. M., & Miniussi, C. (2003). The role of prefrontal cortex in verbal episodic memory: rTMS evidence. *Journal of Cognitive Neuroscience, 15*(6), 855–861.

Sandrini, M., Umiltà, C., & Rusconi, E. (2011). The use of transcranial magnetic stimulation in cognitive neuroscience: A new synthesis of methodological issues. *Neuroscience and Biobehavioral Reviews, 35*(3), 516–536.

Schacter, D. L., & Addis, D. R. (2007). Constructive memory: The ghosts of past and future. *Nature, 445*, 27.

Schambra, H. M., Abe, M., Luckenbaugh, D. A., Reis, J., Krakauer, J. W., & Cohen, L. G. (2011). Probing for hemispheric specialization for motor skill learning: A transcranial direct current stimulation study. *Journal of Neurophysiology, 106*(2), 652–661.

Schiller, D., & Phelps, E. A. (2011). Does reconsolidation occur in humans? *Frontiers in Behavioral Neuroscience, 5*, 24.

Scoville, W. B., & Milner, B. (1957). Loss of recent memory after bilateral hippocampal lesions. *Journal of Neurology, Neurosugery, and Psychiatry, 20*, 1151.

Seidler, R. D. (2010). Neural correlates of motor learning, transfer of learning, and learning to learn. *Exercise and Sport Sciences Reviews, 38*(1), 3–9.

Shea, J. B., & Morgan, R. L. (1979). Contextual interference effects on the acquisition, retention, and transfer of a motor skill. *Journal of Experimental Psychology: Human Learning and Memory, 5*, 179–187.

Simons, J. S., & Spiers, H. J. (2003). Prefrontal and medial temporal lobe interactions in long-term memory. *Nature Reviews. Neuroscience, 4*(8), 637–648.

Snyder, A. (2009). Explaining and inducing savant skills: Privileged access to lower level, less-processed information. *Philosophical Transactions of the Royal Society of London B: Biological Sciences, 364,* 1399–1405.

Song, S., Sharma, N., Buch, E. R., & Cohen, L. G. (2012). White matter microstructural correlates of superior long-term skill gained implicitly under randomized practice. *Cerebral Cortex, 22*(7), 1671–1677.

Sparing, R., Dafotakis, M., Meister, I. G., Thirugnanasambandam, N., & Fink, G. R. (2008). Enhancing language performance with non-invasive brain stimulation – A transcranial direct current stimulation study in healthy humans. *Neuropsychologia, 46*(1), 261–268.

Sparing, R., Mottaghy, F. M., Hungs, M., Brügmann, M., Foltys, H., Huber, W., et al. (2001). Repetitive transcranial magnetic stimulation effects on language function depend on the stimulation parameters. *Journal of Clinical Neurophysiology, 18*(4), 326–330.

Sporns, O. (2010). *Networks of the brain.* Cambridge, MA: MIT Press, p. 375.

Squire, L. R. (1992). Declarative and non-declarative memory: Multiple brain systems supporting learning and memory. *Journal of Cognitive Neuroscience, 4,* 232–243.

Squire, L. R., & Zola-Morgan, S. (1983). The neurology of memory: The case for correspondence between the findings for human and non-human primate. In J. A. Deutsch (Ed.), *The physiological basis of memory* (pp. 199–268). New York, NY: Academic.

Stagg, C. J., Jayaram, G., Pastor, D., Kincses, Z. T., Matthews, P. M., & Johansen-Berg, H. (2011). Polarity and timing-dependent effects of transcranial direct current stimulation in explicit motor learning. *Neuropsychologia, 49*(5), 800–804.

Steriade, M., & Timofeev, I. (2003). Neuronal plasticity in thalamocortical networks during sleep and waking oscillations. *Neuron, 37*(4), 563–576.

Tanaka, S., Honda, M., Hanakawa, T., & Cohen, L. G. (2010). Differential contribution of the supplementary motor area to stabilization of a procedural motor skill acquired through different practice schedules. *Cerebral Cortex, 20,* 2114–2121.

Taylor, J. A., & Ivry, R. B. (2012). The role of strategies in motor learning. *Annals of the New York Academy of Sciences, 1251,* 1–12.

Tecchio, F., Zappasodi, F., Assenza, G., Tombini, M., Vollaro, S., Barbati, G., et al. (2010). Anodal transcranial direct current stimulation enhances procedural consolidation. *Journal of Neurophysiology, 104*(2), 1134–1140.

Terney, D., Chaieb, L., Moliadze, V., Antal, A., & Paulus, W. (2008). Increasing human brain excitability by transcranial high-frequency random noise stimulation. *Journal of Neuroscience, 28*(52), 14147–14155.

Thompson-Schill, S. L., D'Esposito, M., Aguirre, G. K., & Farah, M. J. (1997). Role of left inferior prefrontal cortex in retrieval of semantic knowledge: A reevaluation. *Proceedings of the National Academy of Sciences of the United States of America, 94,* 14792–14797.

Thut, G., & Miniussi, C. (2009). New insights into rhythmic brain activity from TMS-EEG studies. *Trends in Cognitive Sciences, 13*(4), 182–189.

Tulving, E. (1983). *Elements of episodic memory.* London: Oxford University Press.

Tulving, E. (1985). How many memory systems are there? *American Psychologist, 40,* 385–398.

Tulving, E. (2002). Episodic memory: From mind to brain. *Annual Review in Psychology, 53,* 1–25.

Tulving, E., Kapur, S., Craik, F. I., Moscovitch, M., & Houle, S. (1994). Hemispheric encoding/retrieval asymmetry in episodic memory: Positron emission tomography findings. *Proceedings of the National Academy of Sciences of the United States of America, 91*(6), 2016–2020.

Venkatakrishnan, A., & Sandrini, M. (2012). Combining transcranial direct current stimulation and neuroimaging: Novel insights in understanding neuroplasticity. *Journal of Neurophysiology, 107*(1), 1–4.

Vidoni, E. D., & Boyd, L. A. (2007). Achieving enlightenment: What do we know about the implicit learning system and its interaction with explicit knowledge? *Journal of Neurological Physical Therapy, 31,* 145–154.

Vines, B. W., Cerruti, C., & Schlaug, G. (2008). Dual-hemisphere tDCS facilitates greater improvements for healthy subjects' non-dominant hand compared to uni-hemisphere stimulation. *BMC Neuroscience, 9*, 103.

Vines, B. W., Nair, D. G., & Schlaug, G. (2006). Contralateral and ipsilateral motor effects after transcranial direct current stimulation. *Neuroreport, 17*(6), 671–674.

Wagner, A. D., Shannon, B. J., Kahn, I., & Buckner, R. L. (2005). Parietal lobe contributions to episodic memory retrieval. *Trends in Cognitive Sciences, 9*, 445–453.

Walker, M. P., Brakefield, T., Morgan, A., Hobson, J. A., & Stickgold, R. (2002). Practice with sleep makes perfect: Sleep-dependent motor skill learning. *Neuron, 35*(1), 205–211.

Ward, N. S., & Cohen, L. G. (2004). Mechanisms underlying recovery of motor function after stroke. *Archives of Neurology, 61*(12), 1844–1848.

Willingham, D. B. (1997). Systems of memory in the human brain. *Neuron, 18*, 5–8.

Willingham, D. B. (1998). A neuropsychological theory of motor skill learning. *Psychological Review, 105*, 558–584.

Wirth, M., Rahman, R. A., Kuenecke, J., Koenig, T., Horn, H., Sommer, W., et al. (2011). Effects of transcranial direct current stimulation (tDCS) on behaviour and electrophysiology of language production. *Neuropsychologia, 49*(14), 3989–3998.

The Effects of Electrical Brain Stimulation Upon Visual Attention and Neglect

Maike D. Hesse and Gereon R. Fink

Cognitive Neuroscience, Institute of Neuroscience and Medicine (INM3), Research Center Juelich, Juelich, Germany; and Department of Neurology, University of Cologne, Germany

OUTLINE

The Stimulated Brain
http://dx.doi.org/10.1016/B978-0-12-404704-4.00010-7

INTRODUCTION

Deficits of attention are common in neurological diseases affecting the brain, irrespective of whether vascular, traumatic, or degenerative in origin. Attention deficits profoundly disable patients regarding active participation in daily life as well as during rehabilitation. To date, clinically relevant strategies to ameliorate deficits of attention remain scarce.

Transcranial electrical stimulation has been proven to be a promising tool for neurorehabilitation; it is easily applicable, non-invasive, and elicits prolonged effects exceeding the stimulation itself, which may even be potentiated by repetitive application (for reviews, see, for example, Edwards & Fregni, 2008; Harris-Love & Cohen, 2006; Hummel & Cohen, 2006). However, tDCS effects upon cognitive functions are more diverse than those observed in primary motor or sensory domains. In general, opposing effects of cathodal versus anodal stimulation of the primary motor (Nitsche & Paulus, 2000, 2001; Nitsche et al., 2005, 2008; Stagg et al., 2009), somatosensory (Antal et al., 2008; Dieckhöfer et al., 2006), and visual cortex (Accornero, Li Voti, La Riccia, & Gregori, 2007; Antal, Nitsche, & Paulus, 2001; Antal, Kincses, Nitsche, & Paulus, 2003a; 2003b; Antal, Kincses, Nitsche, Bartfai, & Paulus, 2004) have been described. While cathodal stimulation decreases cortical excitability, thus causing inhibition of function, anodal stimulation allows for facilitation by enhancing cortical excitability. This dichotomy is less clear in cognitive domains such as learning, working memory, language, or attention, where a greater variance of effects has been reported (see, for example, Berryhill, Wencil, Branch Coslett, & Olson, 2010; Flöel, Rösser, Michka, Knecht, & Breitenstein, 2008; Iyer et al., 2005; Jeon & Han, 2012; Kincses, Antal, Nitsche, Bártfai, & Paulus, 2004; Knoch et al., 2008; Loui, Hohmann, & Schlaug, 2010; Priori, Berardelli, Rona, Accornero, & Manfredi, 1998; Sparing & Mottaghy, 2008). At least in part, this greater variance may result from remote effects of network modulation.

Although TMS studies paved the way for the successive tDCS studies investigating not only the motor, but also sensory as well as cognitive functions, in this chapter, except for mentioning a few examples, we will refrain from compiling all related TMS studies.

The multifaceted presentation of attention and its deficits, and the tDCS effects in the cognitive context, certainly justify the multiple individual, specific, and circumscribed approaches taken in the past – but at the same time they call for a theoretical framework that may help to relate the individual and diverse findings to one another. We therefore sketch out such a framework in the hope of encouraging systematic, conscientious, and also basic, future studies to refer to it, thereby filling the current gaps.

THEORY OF ATTENTION

> Everyone knows what attention is. It is the taking of possession by the mind, in clear and vivid form, of one out of what seem several simultaneously possible objects or trains of thought. Focalisation, concentration, of consciousness are of its essence. It implies withdrawal from some things in order to deal efficiently with others, and it is a condition which has a real opposite in the confused, dazed and scatterbrained state. *(William James, 1890)*

In his often quoted statement, William James summarizes the key characteristics of attention: to optimize perception by selection of certain stimuli or events (and concurrent deselection of others) with the aim of allowing certain information to enter consciousness, guide thought and behavior, and support learning and memory. While indeed, in general, everyone seems to know what attention *is*, more and more sophisticated, differential, but also operationally more suitable views and concepts have evolved over time (Raz, 2006). Quite contrary to its initial comprehension as a unitary capacity, during recent decades the concept of attention has rather diversified into fragments supported by separable anatomical networks subserving specific differential aspects of attention. Within a clinical context, the three attentional networks model provided by Posner (Petersen & Posner, 2012; Posner, 1980), or variations thereof, have been proven valuable for patient studies not only of neglect (Corbetta, Kincade, Lewis, Snyder, & Sapir, 2005) but also of, for example, attention deficit hyperactivity disorder (Adólfsdóttir, Sørensen, & Lundervold, 2008; Booth, Carlson, & Tucker, 2007; Konrad et al., 2006; Tsal, Shalev, & Mevorach, 2005) or schizophrenia (Wang et al., 2005). With the application of tDCS for deficits of attention in mind, the three attentional networks model may provide a helpful theoretical framework to systematically evaluate the effects of neuromodulation. We will therefore discuss this model and its neuroanatomical basis in detail in order to refer to related tDCS studies.

ALERTING, ORIENTING, AND EXECUTIVE FUNCTIONS – THE THREE NETWORKS MODEL OF ATTENTION

According to Posner's concept, attention is based upon at least three separate networks, each subserving a distinct function. Michael Posner and colleagues explored and directly compared these differential aspects of attention by cueing paradigms, in which a cue, preceding the target to which subjects were to respond, indicated either the appearance (neutral cue) or the position (spatial cue) of the subsequent target (Fan, McCandliss, Fossella, Flombaum, & Posner, 2005; Posner, 1980; see also Fig. 10.1A). Valid cues, allowing for correct spatial orienting of attention, lead to measurable gains in reaction times compared to neutral (e.g., central) cues, which alert the subjects to the upcoming target but do not specify the target's position. Other studies addressed spatial reorienting by introducing invalid spatial cues, which incorrectly indicate the position of the following target. This causes an increase in reaction time, compared

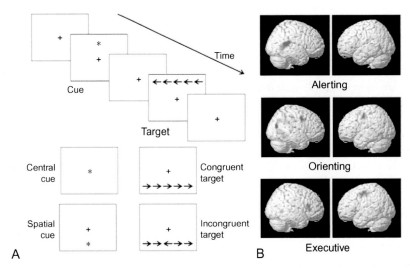

FIGURE 10.1   (A) Illustration of the attention network test. A central fixation cross is presented at the screen at all times. In all other but the "no cue" condition, a cue (central or spatial) appears for 200 ms at variable intervals (300 ms up to 11,800 ms) before the target, which is represented by the central arrow flanked by two (congruent or incongruent) arrows each to the left and right. After the participant's response by button press, the target and flankers disappear, until the next trial starts, again at variable delay (3000 and 15,000 ms). Effects of alerting, orienting, and executive attention are calculated by differences in reaction times (RT) between conditions (alerting = RT[no cue] – RT[central cue]; orienting = RT[central cue] – RT[spatial cue]; executive = RT[incongruent flanker] – RT[congruent flanker]). (B) fMRI results for the three attentional networks as projected to the cortical surface. *Figure adapted from Fan et al. (2005), with permission from Elsevier.*

to valid or neutral cues (see, for example, Corbetta & Shulman, 2002; Posner, Walker, Friedrich, & Rafal, 1984; Thiel, Zilles, & Fink, 2004). Executive or supervisory attention, such as is required to solve a response conflict, was concurrently assessed using a flanker task. In this task, the target stimulus is flanked on both the left and right sides by distractors which either afford the same response (congruent), thereby speeding up reactions, or the contrary response (incongruent), thus slowing down reactions, compared to a baseline condition in which neutral flankers, which do not indicate any response, are present. Intriguingly, alerting, orienting, and executive attention, when directly compared in a single paradigm, clearly showed their independence at the behavioral level, as there were no within subject correlations between the differential reaction time benefits. Whether spatial orienting may nevertheless be facilitated by an increase in alertness – i.e., whether the three networks interact – is still a matter of debate (see, for example, Raz, 2006, for review).

Using event-related fMRI and differential contrasts of a cued reaction time task with neutral and spatial cues, cortical structures specifically involved in alerting, orienting, and executive attention were differentiated (Fig. 10.1B). Neural correlates of the alerting effect were seen in extrastriatal cortex bilaterally (Thiel et al., 2004), as well as in the thalamus (Fan et al., 2005). Spatial orienting using central cues, requiring top-down orienting, involved the anterior cingulate cortex, while reorienting of attention following invalid cues recruited several brain regions, including the left and right intraparietal sulcus, right temporo-parietal junction, and middle frontal gyrus bilaterally (Corbetta & Shulman, 2002; Thiel et al., 2004). Peripheral spatial cues inducing bottom-up spatial orienting showed involvement of parietal areas and of the frontal eye fields (Fan et al., 2005). Finally, the network for executive control (assessed by the built-in flanker task) comprised the anterior cingulate cortex along with the thalamus, the left superior and right middle frontal gyrus, as well as, bilaterally, the inferior frontal gyrus and fusiform gyrus (Fan et al., 2005). Overall, the separable, hardly overlapping patterns of task-related neural activity changes confirmed the hypothesis of independent networks recruiting distinct cortical and subcortical anatomical structures for alerting, orienting, and supervisory executive functions of attention. Within these networks, cortical structures preferably located at the surface of the brain provide prime targets for intervention with tDCS.

In the following sections we will discuss the tDCS studies currently available in relation to the three attention networks. Where appropriate, we will also hint at the lessons to be learned from these studies with respect to the design and conduct of future studies applying tDCS in the field of attention. Using the three attentional networks model as a structure, but facing a great variety of tasks used to capture effects of tDCS, we ask readers to bear with us, even if the arrangement may not fully match the classification. We do so because it is our wish to encourage, for future tDCS studies, more systematic approaches to aspects of attention based on theoretical models, going beyond the mere comparison of individual attentional aspects.

Alertness (Phasic or Sustained) and Vigilance

The alertness or vigilance system aims at achieving and maintaining a state of high sensitivity to incoming stimuli, particularly when facing prolonged, dull tasks (Moruzzi & Magoun, 1949; Sturm & Willmes, 2001). While phasic alertness induced by neutral warning cues preceding a target reflects the capability to transiently increase response readiness by external cueing, sustained (also known as intrinsic or tonic) alertness denotes the ability to maintain attention to a task for a longer period of time in order to detect and respond to infrequent critical events (Parasuraman & Davies, 1976; Parasuraman, Nestor, & Greenwood, 1989; Warm, Parasuraman, & Matthews, 2008). Typically, in vigilance tasks, a decline in target detection rate or speed of response over time on task is observed: this effect is often referred to as vigilance decrement (Mackworth, 1964). Both sustained and phasic alerting systems have been attributed to a right-hemispheric network connecting frontal, parietal, and extrastriatal cortex, thalamus, and brainstem (Sturm & Willmes, 2001; Thiel et al., 2004; Fan et al., 2005). Norepinephrine (or noradrenaline) is considered to be the prevailing transmitter (Aston-Jones & Cohen, 2005). While some studies showed additional left hemispheric recruitment during phasic alertness, this was interpreted as basal aspects of attention selectivity rather than additional features of alerting (Coull et al., 2000; Fan et al., 2005; Sturm & Willmes, 2001).

Studying the effect of tDCS on sustained or intrinsic alertness, Nelson, McKinley, Golob, Warm, and Parasuraman (2012) showed that tDCS (1 mA for 10 minutes, pair of 3×5 cm^2 electrodes) applied bilaterally over the dorsolateral prefrontal cortex ("anodal": anode over left DLPFC (F3) and cathode over right DLPFC (F4); *vice versa* for "cathodal" stimulation) enhanced alertness. In a simulation of an air traffic control system, subjects watched a computer screen for 40 minutes with static symbols representing four airplanes in four quadrants of a circle, either facing clockwise or counterclockwise, in random order. Displays were presented once every second. Periodically (only 30 times per 10 minutes) there was a "critical event," with one airplane facing in the opposite direction than the others, thereby denoting the danger of a crash, which had to be indicated by button press. Hit rates during early online left anodal stimulation (from minutes 10 to 20 of the 40-minute task) were significantly higher than for both cathodal and sham stimulation (note that both electrodes should be regarded as active in this bilateral stimulation set-up; effects may thus not be differentially attributed to either one of them – see Chapter X). While hit rates largely remained at the initial level for the rest of the task for both early anodal and cathodal stimulation, they declined significantly under sham stimulation. Reaction times increased over time for all conditions, with no significant differential effects of stimulation on RTs. With slightly increasing false alarms, signal detection analysis further indicated that sensitivity and discriminability decreased significantly over time, independent of stimulation type, while, in particular, early anodal stimulation caused changes in response bias.

Unfortunately, as also alluded to by Nelson and his co-authors, baseline results prior to stimulation as well as during sham stimulation were not well replicated. This indicates increased unexplained variance between subjects and conditions over the 40 minutes of the vigilance task, which renders the interpretation of these data difficult and thus prohibits reliable conclusions regarding whether the same effects could be achieved by a late stimulation applied during the final 10 minutes of the task. Thus, further studies need to clarify and confirm these findings. Nevertheless, the data suggest that the choice of the time period of tDCS application is crucial for it becoming effective. In summary, the use of tDCS in a vigilance task on healthy subjects provides intriguing data in favor of the application of tDCS to enhance alertness. This offers potential for applications during neurorehabilitation: decline in attention, and particularly of alertness, is commonly observed following stroke, traumatic brain injury, or other brain lesions, and interferes with the process of rehabilitation (Robertson & Murre, 1999). Until alertness is increased, many severely affected brain injury patients may not be capable of participating successfully in rehabilitative treatment.

With this objective in mind, Kang and colleagues tested the effects of anodal tDCS applied over left DLPFC in 10 patients with post-stroke cognitive decline in a double-blind, sham-controlled, cross-over study (Kang, Baek, Kim, & Paik, 2009). While the 10 age-matched healthy controls did not show any improvement in either accuracy or reaction times in a computerized go/no-go task, discriminating between "1" (go) and "2" (no-go), response accuracy of the 10 stroke patients improved significantly after anodal tDCS (2 mA for 20 minutes, pair of $5 \times 5 \, cm^2$ electrodes) applied over the left DLPFC for at least 3 hours, compared to sham tDCS; reaction times improved independent of stimulation. These results suggest that non-invasive cortical modulation via tDCS could potentially be used during rehabilitative training to improve attention, which is often hampered following stroke. Unfortunately, the study does not further specify whether response accuracy rather reflected detection rate or response inhibition. It is thus difficult to judge whether this study serves as an example of tDCS improving alertness or rather of executive

. Furthermore, the study may indicate ceiling effects, which ask stimulation effects in healthy subjects. Therefore, stimulation based on basic behavioral paradigms lacking significant effects should not preclude successive studies on patients.

In a subsequent study, Kang, Kim, and Paik (2012) looked for comparable effects on nine patients following traumatic brain injury with intracranial hemorrhage and attention decline. In a non-spatial choice reaction time task (discriminating between the numbers "1" and "2" presented in random order at the center of the screen by pressing one of two different keys), reaction times immediately following 20 minutes of tDCS (2 mA, pair of 5×5 cm^2 electrodes) applied over the left DLPFC were slightly shortened relative to baseline prior to stimulation ($86.3\% \pm 7.8\%$; $P = 0.056$). No effect was observed 3 or 24 hours after stimulation or after sham stimulation. Moreover, the accuracy rate did not improve at any time after stimulation.

In direct comparison, the study of stroke patients showed specific effects upon response accuracy outlasting 3 hours, while the study of patients with traumatic brain injury found significant effects upon reaction times only. Whether these differences may be attributed to the two different tasks used (go/no-go vs choice reaction task), or to the fact that axonal damage following traumatic brain injury may be more diffuse, remains obscure. Certainly, more work on this topic is needed.

Orienting Attention

Orienting of attention may either be driven by sudden external events, such as a flashing light, or purposefully directed according to our internal interests, such as when looking left and right before crossing the street. Bottom-up orienting towards attention capturing changes in the environment – particularly towards those that are unexpected – is supported by a ventral attentional network that includes the inferior parietal lobe (IPL), temporo-parietal junction (TPJ), and ventral prefrontal cortex (vPFC) (Behrmann, Geng, & Shomstein, 2004; Corbetta & Shulman, 2002; Corbetta, Patel, & Shulman, 2008). In contrast, the dorsal attentional network, including the superior parietal cortex and the frontal eye fields bilaterally, is considered to mediate top-down modulation of attention when selecting spatial, temporal, or object-related features (Corbetta & Shulman, 2002; Corbetta et al., 2008).

Addressing bottom-up orienting of attention, in a visuospatial detection task with single and bilateral targets presented in the right and/or left visual hemifield at the detection threshold, Sparing et al. (2009) investigated the effects of tDCS on perception and extinction in 20 healthy subjects. Extinction denotes the phenomenon whereby a stimulus is detected when presented on its own but is missed when presented simultaneously with another stimulus. tDCS (1 mA for 10 minutes; 5×5 cm^2 stimulation electrode versus 5×7 cm^2 reference electrode) over the posterior parietal cortex (P3/P4 versus Cz) modulated visuospatial task performance bidirectionally depending on both the side of stimulation and the current polarity: anodal tDCS biased visuospatial attention towards the contralateral hemispace, thereby increasing the detection rate contralaterally. Following cathodal tDCS, however, contralateral attention deteriorated. Along with this deterioration, detection of bilateral visual stimuli was worse after cathodal stimulation, with mainly the contralateral stimulus being missed, consistent with contralateral extinction.

Crucially, as will be exposed below (see p. 288), this study serves as an example for a successful translational approach, in which insights into tDCS effects gained from healthy subjects were directly transferred into a proof-of-principle study in a patient population to pave the way for the potential use of tDCS in rehabilitation.

At variance with the lack of hemispheric asymmetries observed in the study of Sparing et al. (2009), Bolognini, Fregni, Casati, Olgiati, and Vallar (2010) trained subjects in a bimodal, visual, and auditory orienting task and found that modulation of right posterior parietal cortex (PPC; P4 vs left deltoid muscle, pair of 5×7 cm^2 electrodes) by anodal tDCS (2 mA for 30 minutes) improved visuo-spatial orienting, in both visual half-fields and for both valid and invalid spatial cueing. In contrast, left PPC anodal tDCS (P3 vs right deltoid muscle) had no significant effect. Furthermore, effects of right parietal tDCS were specific for orienting attention – i.e., no tDCS effect was observed for alertness or working memory. This observed hemispheric asymmetry re-emphasizes the role of right PPC in orienting, disengaging, and engaging – i.e., all major components of visuo-spatial orienting (Corbetta & Shulman, 2002; Posner et al., 1984).

In a sophisticated design, using a redundant signal effect (RSE) task, Bolognini and co-workers further investigated whether anodal tDCS applied over PPC (compared to sham stimulation as well as anodal stimulation over right occipital cortex) enhanced attentional orienting within and across the visual and auditory domain (Bolognini, Olgiati, Rossetti, & Maravita, 2010). Anodal tDCS over the right PPC (P4 vs left deltoid muscle; 2 mA for 15 minutes, pair of 5×7 cm^2 electrodes) significantly speeded up responses to contralateral targets, regardless of stimulus modality. Hence, up-regulating the level of excitability of right PPC by tDCS successfully enhanced spatial orienting independent of sensory modality (to unisensory as well as crossmodal stimuli). Furthermore, the effect of tDCS depended upon the nature of the audiovisual enhancement, being stronger when blue, rather than red, visual stimuli were presented together with the auditory stimuli. While multisensory *integration* of red visual with auditory stimuli, indicated by a neural coactivation mechanism, is known to be largely mediated at the subcortical level (Maravita, Bolognini, Bricolo, Marzi, & Savazzi, 2008), blue colored visual stimuli, mainly detected by S-cones, bypass the superior colliculus (de Monasterio, 1978; Leh, Ptito, Schönwiesner, Chakravarty, & Mullen, 2010; Marrocco & Li, 1977) to enter the PPC, where audiovisual *interactions* seem to rely on probabilistic mechanisms matching a race model (Bolognini, Miniussi, Savazzi, Bricolo, & Maravita, 2009). Therefore, the data demonstrate that anodal tDCS applied over PPC selectively enhanced audiovisual interactions occurring at a cortical level, while processes of multisensory integration at the subcortical level appeared less susceptible to polarization of the cortex.

With their study, Bolognini, Olgiati, Rossetti, & Maravita (2010) demonstrated how tDCS could fill an important gap in the investigation of multisensory processes by selectively facilitating and thereby allowing dissociating specific abilities in the multisensory domain. Crucially, their study benefitted from the careful choice of the paradigm and stimuli, and a profound knowledge of underlying neuroanatomy and mechanisms of stimulus processing, and thus serves as a good example of a theory-driven approach.

Attention may, however, not only be directed towards external events but also towards items encoded in visual working memory. Tanoue, Jones, Peterson, and Berryhill (2013) showed, in a change detection task, that "retro-cueing" by cues appearing after a display and to be memorized, and pre-cueing by cues indicating the to-be-probed item prior to the display, induce similar behavioral accuracy benefits, but are differentially disrupted by cathodal tDCS of the frontal and parietal cortices [which were shown to be differentially involved in pre- and retro-cueing; Lepsien & Nobre, 2006]). Cathodal tDCS (1.5 mA for 10 minutes, pair of 5×7 cm^2 electrodes) at right frontal (F4 vs left cheek) as well as parietal cortex (P4 vs left cheek) hindered performance, of both retro- and pre-cueing, but frontal tDCS had a greater negative impact on the retro-cued trials. The authors concluded that their findings indicate greater frontal involvement during shifts of internal attention.

Executive Attention

Executive attention constitutes the third attentional system in the Posner model. Apart from the anterior cingulate cortex, which, in the depth between the two hemispheres, is currently difficult to target by tDCS, the left superior and right middle frontal gyrus as well as (bilaterally) the inferior frontal gyrus have been suggested to support executive attention (Fan et al., 2005) and thus form appropriate targets for the modulation of executive attention by tDCS. In this paradigm, executive attention was assessed using a flanker task, in which flankers induce competing response tendencies, but executive aspects of attention are also captured in tasks of response inhibition and task switching.

In an attentional load paradigm in which irrelevant stimuli were processed only under low but not under high attentional load, Weiss and Lavidor (2012) showed that cathodal stimulation over the right PPC (P4 vs left supraorbital forehead; stimulating electrode 4×4 cm^2, reference electrode 5×7 cm^2; 1.5 mA for 15 minutes) enhanced cognitive performance by acting like a noise filter and increasing attentional resources. Cathodal, but not anodal, PPC tDCS enabled flanker processing even in high-loaded settings. In order to exclude that enhanced performance was related to altered attention allocation between center and surround, rather than increased attentional resources, a second experiment (in which the flankers were presented centrally) replicated these findings of improved flanker processing.

Given the current lack of more tDCS studies using the flanker task to represent the original definition of this aspect of attention, we discuss here a few aspects related to executive attention by looking at related studies of the executive domain.

While go/no-go tasks are often considered to tap aspects of alertness, one might also consider the inhibitory control required by this task to be related to executive aspects of attention. Consistent with this notion, brain regions underlying inhibitory control comprise frontal eye fields (FEFs, Curtis, Cole, Rao, & D'Esposito, 2005; Muggleton, Chen, Tzeng, Hung, & Juan, 2010), pre-supplementary motor cortex (pre-SMA, Isoda & Hikosaka, 2007), and supplementary eye fields (SEFs, Stuphorn & Schall, 2006; Stuphorn, Taylor, & Schall, 2000), while performance is monitored by the anterior cingulate cortex (ACC, Chevrier, Noseworthy, & Schachar, 2007; Ito, Stuphorn, Brown, & Schall, 2003). Hsu et al. (2011) found, in a go/no-go task, that anodal tDCS applied over the pre-SMA (Fz vs left cheek; 1.5 mA for 10 min, pair of 4×4 cm^2 electrodes) improved efficiency of inhibitory control, while cathodal tDCS showed a tendency towards impaired inhibitory control.

Transcranial direct current stimulation may not only facilitate inhibition, but also support training of an inhibition task. In the context of a learning paradigm, Ditye, Jacobson, Walsh, and Lavidor (2012) applied tDCS over right inferior frontal gyrus (rIFG; crossing point between T4–Fz and F8–Cz versus left orbitofrontal cortex above left eyebrow, pair of 5×7 cm^2 electrodes) repetitively over 4 consecutive days of training of a stop signal task (SST). Ten participants who received anodal tDCS (1.5 mA for 15 min) performed significantly better than 12 participants who received training without active stimulation. These findings indicate that tDCS combined with cognitive training not only improves the ability to inhibit responses, but also potentiates training effects. The effect, however, did not persist once the training was completed (i.e., at the fifth day after the 4-day training). The underlying mechanisms, as well as how persistence may be induced, need further exploration.

Finally, within the executive domain, task switching, thought to recruit prefrontal and parietal cortex, was shown to be selectively modulated by tDCS. In a task-switching paradigm, subjects are asked to switch at selected time points as indicated between two different tasks, generally performed on the same stimulus material. Task switching was modulated in a task- and hemisphere-specific way using a letter/digit naming task as well as a vowel–consonant/parity task by cross-hemispheric tDCS over PFC. In the letter/digit naming task, anodal stimulation of the left PFC (F3) and cathodal right PFC (F4) stimulation (2 mA for a maximum of 30 min, pair of 5×7 cm^2 electrodes) improved switching performance, while left cathodal vs right anodal stimulation increased response accuracy (Leite, Carvalho, Fregni, Boggio, & Gonçalves, 2013). However, in the vowel–consonant/parity task, left anodal vs right cathodal stimulation improved accuracy but decreased switching performance. The results suggest that the mechanisms underlying task switching are not a uniform entity but task dependent, and may be differentially lateralized to the left and right hemispheres.

As an interesting add-on, Plewnia et al. (2013) not only investigated effects of tDCS on executive attention by a parametric go/no-go task with different levels of task difficulty, but also searched for further explanations for interindividual variations in effectiveness of stimulation. They investigated whether differences of the Val158Met polymorphism of the catechol-O-methyltransferase (COMT) gene may affect tDCS interventions of executive attention. The COMT gene determines the prefrontal dopamine level, which plays an important role in executive functions, with COMT Met allele homozygosity associated with higher levels of prefrontal dopamine. In homozygous carriers only did 20 minutes of anodal tDCS applied over the left dorsolateral prefrontal cortex cause a deterioration of set-shifting ability as assessed by the most challenging level of a parametric go/no-go test. In contrast, sustained attention and response inhibition were unaffected by left DLPFC stimulation. Genetic screening may thus be used to interpret individual responsiveness to tDCS in executive tasks.

A more detailed discussion of tDCS effects on executive tasks goes beyond the scope of this chapter, and will be addressed in Chapter 11.

VISUAL SEARCH AND THE THEORY OF VISUAL ATTENTION BY BUNDESEN

Although the model of alerting, orienting, and executive attention provides a valuable framework, other theories of attention exist, based on different kinds of tasks, and these also merit discussion. In general, being surrounded by multiple objects and features, we need to search for the item of interest in our visual field among lots of distracting items. Bundesen (1990) developed a theory of visual attention (TVA) for such conditions. In contrast to the Posner model, which works more on the basis of a spatial "spotlight" of attention, shifting the respective spatial focus of attention, TVA is based on a race model of both selection and recognition of competing elements. These elements are encoded into the visual short-term memory based on their sensory load, and given subjective value (Bundesen, 1990; Kyllingsbaek, 2006). Importantly, the model provides a computational framework in which subcomponents of top-down control, attentional weighting, capacity of visual short-term memory, and processing speed may be calculated on the basis of differential reaction times.

Based on this computational model, Moos, Vossel, Weidner, Sparing, and Fink (2012) studied effects of tDCS (1 mA or 2 mA for 20 min) applied over right parietal cortex. In contrast to the other studies cited here, Moos et al. defined the position of their stimulation electrode over the right PPC using stereotactical neuronavigation based on high-resolution T1 MR images. The stimulation electrode $(5 \times 7 \, cm^2)$ was centered over the horizontal part of the right intraparietal sulcus, aligned in parallel to the mid-sagittal plane, while the reference electrode $(8 \times 12 \, cm^2)$ was placed contralaterally above the left orbit. Subjects verbally reported target letters presented visually on the screen, while ignoring potential letter distractors. Target letters were defined as targets by their color (e.g., red), with distractors being presented in a different color (e.g., green; color assignment was counterbalanced across subjects). Different displays of a target stimulus alone, or in combination with a second target stimulus or a distractor, within the same or the other hemifield, were presented. All letter displays were followed by a mask composed of superimposed red and green digits. Prior to the experiment, exposure duration of the letters was adapted individually to obtain a detection performance of 70% for the target-alone situation. Comparison of the different stimulus presentation conditions allowed for calculation of parameters reflecting attentional weights, top-down control as the ratio of distractor and target weights, and velocity of attentional processing (for details, see Bundesen, 1990; Dyrholm, Kyllingsbaek, Espeseth, & Bundesen, 2011; Kyllingsbaek, 2006).

Cathodal stimulation applied over the right PPC in the 2-mA condition only significantly enhanced top-down control of attention, reflected by a reduction of the alpha parameter of TVA, independent of the visual hemifield. (With attentional weights constituting the sensory evidence of relevance of each element displayed, the alpha parameter is defined as the ratio of attentional weights allocated to the distractors compared to attentional weights of the target, characterizing the spatial distribution of attention; values close to zero indicate perfect target selection, while values close to one indicate no selection between target and distractors.) With regard to performance scores, however, cathodal stimulation at 2 mA led to a decrease in performance in the target–target condition ($P = 0.031$), thus indicating overall increased distractibility by additional target letters, while there was hardly a trend for an increase in performance in presence of a distractor ($P = 0.158$). None of the other variables, referring to attentional weighting, capacity of visual short-term memory, and processing speed, was affected, nor did anodal or cathodal stimulation applied over the right PPC at 1 mA render significant effects. The data suggest that right parietal cortex may be involved in endogenous attentional control, without necessarily changing spatial attention. Moreover, the results suggest that a differentiation between relevant and irrelevant display elements can occur regardless of their spatial position. Top-down control is thus not bound to a spatial focus of attention.

This work also exemplifies the importance of stimulation strength (note that stimulation at 1 mA did not have a significant effect on any of the parameters) as well as that modulation of higher cognitive functions may not follow the simple dichotomy of cathodal-inhibitory/anodal-facilitatory effects (see also Jacobson, Koslowsky, & Lavidor, 2012, for a comprehensive review).

Signal detection theory was also applied by Clark, Coffmann, and colleagues (Clark et al., 2012; Coffman, Trumbo, Flores et al., 2012). In a different visual search task, placed in a more naturalistic (although still artificial) scenery, they trained participants for 1 hour to detect target objects concealed in a complex virtual environment, while applying anodal tDCS over right inferior frontal cortex (IFC, F10) or right parietal cortex (P4). Using fMRI prior to tDCS, these regions had been identified to be crucially involved in this visual search training (Clark et al., 2012). Right IFC tDCS during the training increased overall performance in a dose-dependent manner. In particular, performance improved for repeated stimuli with present targets, immediately after the training, and persisted for at least 1 hour after the training. Similar benefits were seen for stimulation of right parietal cortex.

Moreover, in a follow-up of their studies, Coffman, Trumbo, and Clark (2012) tested, by means of the attention network test (ANT; Fan et al., 2005), whether the positive tDCS effects exerted upon visual search training relate to enhanced alerting, orienting, and executive attention. Participants of the high-stimulation group receiving anodal stimulation of 2 mA for 30 minutes (right IFC [F10] vs left upper arm; pair of 11 cm^2 electrodes) along with the training had significantly higher alertness scores than the low-stimulation group at 0.1 mA. In contrast, scores of orienting or executive attention did not differ significantly between the two groups.

Unfortunately, as discussed by the authors, scores for all three networks were only obtained 1.5 hours after stimulation and training. With no baseline measures at hand to exclude group differences prior to stimulation, they could, however, show that for the 2-mA tDCS group only, post-stimulation alertness scores correlated with the percentage of hits in the visual search task after stimulation but not prior to stimulation. For the low-stimulation control group, post-stimulation alertness correlated neither with the hits before nor the hits after stimulation. Short-term effects of stimulation on either orienting or executive attention networks may not outlast the stimulation for 1.5 hours, and therefore not been captured at this delay. The results indicate that the increased search-task performance may relate to an increase of alertness by right frontal tDCS.

OBJECT-BASED FEATURES: GLOBAL VERSUS LOCAL ASPECTS, HIGH VERSUS LOW SALIENCY, ALLOCENTRIC VERSUS EGOCENTRIC REFERENCE FRAME

Further aspects, not touched by the models of attention discussed above, concern more object-based features of attention, namely saliency as well as global versus local aspects of hierarchical stimuli (Navon, 1977). While hierarchical letters as presented in the corresponding experiments may seem quite artificial, hierarchical arrangements of objects and their parts are regularly encountered in daily life: one may, for example, attend to a house across the street, its front door, or even the lock of the front door, etc.

In general, a global advantage is found, with global object aspects being perceived more quickly than local. Stimulus manipulations, such as number of local elements, shape, retinal projection, and saliency (Hughes, Fendrich, & Reuter-Lorenz, 1990; Lamb & Robertson, 1988; Mevorach, Hodsoll, Allen, Shalev, & Humphreys, 2010) may then be used to induce a bias towards processing of the local features (local advantage).

Hemispheric asymmetries for the processing of global versus local aspects have been suggested based upon neuropsychological studies of healthy subjects (Kimchi & Merhav, 1991; Martin, 1979) and patients (Delis, Robertson, & Efron, 1986; Lamb, Robertson, & Knight, 1990; Robertson, Lamb, & Knight, 1988), as well as neuroimaging (Fink et al., 1996, 1997) and ERP studies (Evans, Shedden, Hevenor, & Hahn, 2000; Han, Liu, Yund, & Woods, 2000, Han et al., 2002), with the left hemisphere preferring local and the right hemisphere preferring global aspects (see, however, Fink et al., 1997).

Stone and Tesche (2009) did not find any effect of left parietal tDCS (P3 versus outer arm below the right elbow; 2 mA for 20 min; either pair of 5×5 cm^2 electrodes or reference electrode 17.5×9 cm^2) on global versus local processing, but on switches between attention levels (global vs local). Furthermore, they reported disruptive effects of both anodal and cathodal stimulation: impaired performance was reported *during* cathodal tDCS for both switch types and *after* anodal tDCS (immediately after as well as 20 min later) for switches from local to global targets. In contrast, the main effects for time, stimulation, and their interactions were not significant. Based on the finding that baseline trials prior to each stimulation condition showed no significant main effect or interaction, baseline performance was subtracted from performance during and immediately after stimulation, and after a further delay of 20 minutes. Individual comparisons were made for anodal versus sham and cathodal versus sham conditions following Dunnett's procedure for comparing multiple groups with a control (Maxwell & Delaney, 2004). This analysis uncovered the differential effects of left parietal cathodal and anodal effects during and after stimulation. Critically, multiple comparisons between conditions only revealed marginal differences. This study may therefore also serve as an example for the difficulty encountered by a number of tDCS studies of higher cognitive functions in dealing with multiple conditions and relatively subtle behavioral effects induced by tDCS to be captured.

While initial tDCS studies mainly used supposedly inert areas to place the reference electrode, which was in addition larger than the active electrode for more diffuse distribution of the current below, some following studies aimed to potentiate effects by choosing a bilateral stimulation approach using both anodal and cathodal effects over two selected target areas at the same time. In such a bilateral stimulation procedure (see also Chapter 11), Bardi, Kanai, Mapelli, and Walsh (2013) found that anodal right PPC vs cathodal stimulation of the left PPC (thereby potentially facilitating right PPC while inhibiting left PPC) increased performance during a local task when the task was fixed in a block of trials, while an inverse stimulation protocol (anodal left PPC/cathodal right PPC) increased performance when selection at the global or local level was manipulated on a trial-by-trial basis. While congruent with a right/sustained and left/switch hypothesis of lateralization, the effect of the global/local task with right anodal stimulation facilitating the local task under sustained attention (i.e., when tasks were performed blockwise) was rather contrary to the prediction of left PPC preference for local aspects. Similarly, Antal, Nitsche et al. (2004) found that cathodal stimulation (V5 vs Cz, 1 mA for 7 min, pair of 5×7 cm electrodes), while deteriorating performance of simple detection of coherent motion as expected, paradoxically improved motion detection in a task with the target embedded in noise. Taken together, these studies demonstrate how subtle differences in experimental conditions may elicit inverse effects of tDCS stimulation.

The main aim of the study by Bardi et al. (2013) was, however, to assess whether hemispheric asymmetry in local versus global selection may alternatively be explained by salience-based selection of hierarchical stimuli (Fink, Marshall, Halligan, & Dolan, 1999). The dichotomy of global/right and local/left hemisphere preference has previously been challenged by arguments based on differential relative salience of the stimuli with respect to their global/local level. The left IPS has been suggested to prefer low-salient stimuli, as rTMS (70-mm figure-of-eight coil; 600×1-Hz pulses) of left IPS (P3) showed disruptive effects exerted upon the low-salient level with salient distractors at the irrelevant level, while right parietal TMS (over P4) conversely impaired performance on salient stimuli, indicative of the right hemispheric preference of high-salient stimuli (Mevorach, Humphreys, & Shalev, 2006).

Following the same paradigm, Bardi et al. (2013) manipulated saliency independent of global/local aspects during the same task using hierarchical stimuli. The results revealed a differential effect of stimulation with anodal tDCS (1.5 mA for 20 min, pair of 3×3 cm^2 electrodes) of the right PPC (P4) and concurrent cathodal tDCS of the left PPC (P3) increasing the participants' performance to select the letter presented at the more salient level and vice versa – as long as the global/local task was performed blockwise. In contrast, no asymmetries were found in the tDCS effects on salience-based selection when global/local attention was manipulated on a trial-by-trial basis. Altogether, the results demonstrate the preference of right vs left PPC for global vs local processing, sustained vs switching tasks, and high vs low saliency – processes that interact with each other, but do not fully explain each other.

Finally, somewhat related to global-local feature processing, although nevertheless distinct, the dichotomy of allocentric vs egocentric processing was addressed by Medina et al. (2013). Allocentric vs egocentric effects may present quite strikingly in patients with hemispatial neglect. In the experimental set-up by Medina and colleagues, healthy subjects had to indicate whether, within a display of four circles, there was an opening in one of them. Bilateral stimulation of the parietal cortex (CP4 versus CP3; 1.5 mA for 20 min, pair of 5×5 cm^2 electrodes) with right anodal and left cathodal orientation speeded up reaction times in general (potentially increasing attention over the entire visual field), but in particular for left-gapped compared to right-gapped targets, independent of their spatial location. This specific effect on allocentric processing was present during and up to 20 minutes after stimulation. Inverse stimulation did not show any effect upon reaction times compared to sham stimulation.

ATTENTION INVOLVED IN OTHER COGNITIVE DOMAINS

Encoding and memory require detection, selection, and perception – processes that are sensitive to attentional modulation. Performance in a visual short-term memory (VSTM) task may thus also depend upon attentional effects. If deficits in VSTM may result from a lack of visual attention, they might be overcome by enhancement of attention by using tDCS. Several studies on working memory suggest that modulation of attention may be a key factor leading to performance improvement (see, for example, Berryhill et al., 2010; Gladwin, den Uyl, Fregni, & Wiers, 2012). However, given that our focus here is on visual attention we will restrict the following discussion to one study, by Tseng et al. (2012), which addresses visual short-term memory. This study also allows us to indicate the risk of ceiling effects, which might lead to considerable interindividual differences in tDCS effects on healthy (compared to patient) subjects.

Preceding studies associated VSTM performance with right posterior parietal cortex (PPC): fMRI activity in right PPC (rPPC) was found to positively correlate with VSTM load (Todd & Marois, 2004, 2005; Xu & Chun, 2006). Likewise, sustained negativity from parietal cortex predicted VSTM performance in studies using event-related potentials (ERPs; Vogel & Machizawa, 2004; Vogel, Woodman, & Luck, 2005). Finally, patients with PPC damage may exhibit deficits in VSTM retrieval (Berryhill & Olson, 2008).

Based on these findings, Tseng et al. (2012) targeted the right PPC (P4 versus the left cheek, pair of $4 \times 4\,cm^2$ electrodes) by tDCS (1.5 mA for 15 min) to examine its effects upon a VSTM task. Subjects performed a well-established change detection task in which they memorized a display of 11 colored rectangles, presented for 200 ms, and compared it with a subsequent presentation 900 ms later to indicate a color change in any of the rectangles. Crucially, Tseng and colleagues detected differential effects in low and high performers of the VSTM task both with respect to (1) ERP findings, and (2) susceptibility to tDCS. Both, the N2pc as well as the sustained posterior contralateral negative ERP (SPCN), two negative deflections of the ERP at approximately 200 ms and 300–600 ms following stimulus onset, respectively, were smaller in low than in high performers. The N2pc at 200-ms peaks at posterior sites (PO7 and PO8) contralateral to the attended hemispace; its amplitude has been observed to be greater when people detect a change versus when a change is missed (Eimer & Mazza, 2005; Tseng et al., 2012) and has been closely related to the deployment of visual attention (Eimer, 1996; Jolicoeur, Brisson, & Robitaille, 2008; Luck & Hillyard, 1994; Woodman, 2010; Woodman, Arita, & Luck, 2009). The SPCN, following the N2pc at 300–600 ms (Jolicoeur et al., 2008), rather relates to the maintenance and access of visual short-term memory, as its amplitude varies according to memory load, persisting over the entire retention interval (Eimer & Kiss, 2010; Jolicoeur et al., 2008). Anodal tDCS increased both the N2pc as well as the SPCN. In low performers similar amplitudes were observed as in high performers, associated with improved performance – although not quite to the level of the high performers.

These findings of differential effects of tDCS based on prior performance as well as the initial electrophysiological trait as revealed by ERP are intriguing, since they suggest that future studies may benefit from characterizing individual performance prior to neuromodulation, as well as the collection of neurophysiological measures, in order to predict effectiveness of tDCS and to select suitable subjects. Also, they allude to the fact that negative findings, particularly with respect to enhancement of cognitive function, may be related to ceiling effects in high-performing subjects. Furthermore, studies on healthy subjects need to be complemented by studies on patients, who may respond quite differently. In the following we will thus present a brief description of neglect as a relevant deficit of spatial attention, along with two studies of tDCS applied in neglect patients, and then discuss a few aspects to be addressed in future studies of neglect using tDCS (see also Chapter 12).

SPATIAL NEGLECT – A MULTIFACETED SYNDROME

Spatial (hemi-)neglect or (hemi-)inattention are clinical terms used to describe several symptoms which share the feature that the patient fails to attend to, respond adequately to, or orient voluntarily to people or objects located at the side of space contralateral to the lesion (Bisiach & Vallar, 2000; Heilman, Watson, & Valenstein, 2003; Husain, 2008; Mesulam, 1981). Importantly, this syndrome is not a deficit of primary vision but of attention. Thus, the patient fails to attend to a certain part of the surrounding space (egocentric, extra- or peripersonal neglect), a part of an object (allocentric, object-based neglect), or part of the subject's own body (personal neglect). Of particular interest is the phenomenon of extinction observed in many patients with neglect, when objects or targets are omitted in the presence of stimuli presented in ipsilesional space, which "magnetically" attract attention. Although a widely distributed network of areas within the parietal and frontal cortices of both hemispheres mediates visuospatial attention, lesions within the right hemisphere, and in particular affecting the posterior parietal cortex (PPC) and the temporoparietal junction (TPJ), most frequently cause chronic visuospatial neglect (Corbetta, Kincade, Ollinger, McAvoy, & Shulman, 2000; Halligan, Fink, Marshall, & Vallar, 2003; Husain & Nachev, 2007; Mort et al., 2003; Vallar & Perani, 1986). While damage to cortical regions (if restricted) may provoke modular deficits, subcortical lesions disrupting fronto-parietal connections may affect several cortical modules within a disturbed network and thus aggravate the clinical presentation (Bartolomeo, Thiebaut de Schotten, & Doricchi, 2007; Doricchi & Tomaiuolo, 2003; Verdon, Schwartz, Lovblad, Hauert, & Vuilleumier, 2010).

Assessment of neglect comprises various neuropsychological tests, including the line bisection task, in which lines are typically bisected towards the ipsilesional side; the length judgement task of pre-bisected lines (also known as the Landmark task); and various letter- or object-cancellation tasks, scene copying, clock drawing, or text reading, in which contralesional targets, object parts, or words are omitted. Several dissociations of performance have been described for these tasks (see, for example, Binder, Marshall, Lazar, Benjamin, & Mohr, 1992; Halligan & Marshall, 1992; Vallar, 1998) indicating that the differentially addressed aspects of attention may have distinct cerebral representations. Likewise, spatial attention to personal or extrapersonal space may be differentially affected (Committeri et al., 2007; Halligan & Marshall, 1995; Weiss et al., 2000).

The Concept of Interhemispheric Rivalry

In addition to focusing on local disturbances of specialized brain functions, the impact of a lesion on the neural networks subserving the various aspects of attention also needs to be considered. Kinsbourne proposed the concept of interhemispheric rivalry and suggested reciprocal interhemispheric inhibition of both parietal cortices under physiological conditions (Kinsbourne, 1977, 1994). Disinhibition by damage to the right parietal cortex may then cause pathological overactivation of the left hemisphere, thereby aggravating the bias to attend to the right and hence to neglect the left side.

Support for the basic concept of interhemispheric rivalry stems from the clinical observation of a patient who suffered from sequential strokes in both hemispheres with a severe unilateral spatial neglect after a first right-sided parietal infarct (involving the caudalmost right angular gyrus) and abrupt disappearance of the neglect after a second left-sided frontal infarct involving the left frontal eye field (Vuilleumier, Hester, Assal, & Regli, 1996), as well as from fMRI studies showing hyperactivity of the undamaged left dorsal parietal cortex in neglect patients (Corbetta et al., 2005; see also Fig. 10.2). The concept of interhemispheric rivalry particularly provides an explanation for the phenomenon of extinction, with simultaneous presentation of a competing stimulus activating the intact parietal cortex, thereby leading to a further suppression of the corresponding lesioned contralateral cortex, which reduces the "perceptual weight" of the contralesional stimulus. It also provides the basis for the main strategy of therapeutic non-invasive brain stimulation attempting to countervail this interhemispheric imbalance by inhibiting the overactive contralesional hemisphere or by activating the lesioned hemisphere, as we will discuss later (see Chapter 12).

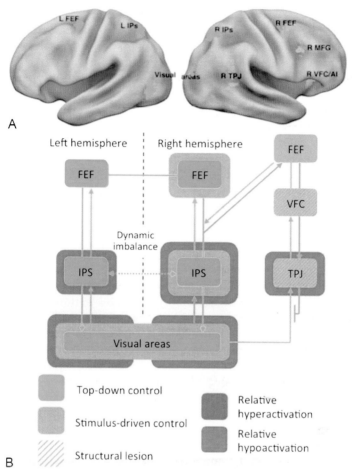

FIGURE 10.2 (A) Schematic capture of the bilateral dorsal fronto-parietal network for top-down orienting of attention (green) and the right lateralized ventral attention network for bottom-up detection of unexpected stimuli outside the attentional focus (orange). (B) In neglect patients suffering from a structural lesion within the right ventral network (shaded in gray), hypoactivation of the right parietal cortex and hyperactivity of the left parietal cortex cause a dynamic disequilibrium of the dorsal attention network and visual cortex (functional damage). FEF, frontal eye fields; MFG, middle frontal gyrus; VFC, ventral frontal cortex; IPS, intraparietal cortex; TPJ, temporoparietal junction. *Figure adapted from Corbetta et al. (2005, 2008), and Vossel and Kukolja (2009), with permission from Elsevier and Thieme Verlag, respectively.*

Brain stimulation studies using TMS allow testing the model of interhemispheric rivalry. Enhanced sensitivity and lowered detection thresholds within the hemispace ipsilateral to the stimulation have been interpreted as disinhibition of the contralateral hemisphere (Babiloni et al., 2007; Hilgetag, Théoret, & Pascual-Leone, 2001; Seyal,

Ro, & Rafal, 1995). Pathological hyperexcitability of the left hemisphere has recently been shown by a twin-coil approach, using a conditioning pulse over the left PPC prior to the stimulation of the left motor cortex, showing increased left PPC motor-cortex circuit excitability of neglect patients compared with right hemispheric stroke patients without neglect (Koch et al., 2008).

Most importantly, however, restorative features could be demonstrated in healthy subjects using bilateral stimulation. Extinction-like phenomena induced by unilateral TMS applied to right parietal cortex in a cued-target detection (Dambeck et al., 2006) or a line-bisection task (Fierro, Brighina, & Bisiach, 2006) were prevented by paired bilateral TMS, most likely by "rebalancing" the system.

"Virtual Lesion Models" to Subserve Treatment Development?

In a similar vein, "virtual lesion" models may be developed to test treatment strategies on a larger group of (more readily available) healthy subjects, with neglect symptoms transiently induced by stimulation (see, for example, Bien, Goebel, & Sack, 2012). So far, similar to Dambeck et al. (2006), the set-up by Bien et al. (2012) has served rather to clarify the underlying neuronal mechanisms quite specifically than to fully model treatment or disease yet. They investigated whether covert spatial attention (induced by cueing) affected lateralized visual extinction induced by TMS. While TMS showed clear effects of contralateral extinction, the respective ANOVA, unfortunately, did not show a significant interaction between the stimulated hemisphere and the type of cueing (but between absence or presence of TMS and cueing). The authors stressed that their *post hoc* analysis indicated hemispheric lateralization, in which only after right parietal stimulation did ipsilateral cueing significantly aggravate left hemifield extinction, while right hemifield extinction following left stimulation was hardly affected by ipsilateral cueing.

The point to make here with respect to future studies is, however, that Bien and colleagues used online triple-pulse TMS after target presentation to induce extinction. In neglect patients, processing of cues presented in the neglected hemifield might already be hampered. In addition, cueing only provides short-term effects on the subsequent individual event. Therefore, this set-up hardly meets the condition of a multifaceted, persisting syndrome as observed in neglect patients, or, as yet, addresses its treatment strategies. In the future, models for therapeutic strategies should take these aspects into account and strive for effects, that outlast the treatment session. With respect to tDCS, "virtual lesion" models might not only benefit from longer-lasting effects (which might also be elicited by repetitive TMS or TBS), but also from the more spatially distributed stimulation and thus more widespread interference inherent to this method. Similarly, treatment strategies should recognize the necessity for generalization and lasting effects.

Within this context, Giglia et al. (2011) investigated in healthy subjects whether tDCS may induce neglect-like symptoms outlasting stimulation. Neglect-like symptoms were assessed in 11 subjects when performing judgements on prebisected lines (i.e., the Landmark task). Furthermore, Giglia et al. (2011) investigated whether bilateral stimulation (at 1 mA for 15 min, pair of approx.. $4 \times 4\ cm^2$ electrodes) of right (P6) versus left parietal cortices (P5) compared with unilateral right cathodal stimulation (with the reference electrode at the left orbita) caused greater or longer-lasting effects. Both stimulation conditions, dual/bilateral as well as unilateral right PPC cathodal stimulation, induced a rightward bias in symmetry judgements compared with baseline and sham stimulation. Indeed, this bilateral approach more recently adopted by several studies should particularly suit application on interconnected areas facing inter-hemispheric rivalry. While the stimulation effect appeared earlier (after 10 vs 15 minutes of stimulation) and was significantly stronger in the bilateral than in the unilateral stimulation condition, effects had disappeared 5 minutes after stimulation in both conditions. In contrast, Loftus and Nicholls (2012) showed that right parietal tDCS – cathodal or anodal – did not affect pseudoneglect (i.e., the mild asymmetry in spatial attention often observed in healthy subjects who show leftward errors in line bisection, judgements of size or brightness) in a grayscale task (in which subjects had to judge which of two grayscale bars presented simultaneously was darker overall, with one gray scale going from white to black from left to right, the other in the opposite direction). Left parietal anodal stimulation, however, alleviated pseudoneglect in this task.

Taken together, further studies are required to establish adequate models of neglect that might serve to study treatment effects on a larger scale in healthy subjects. However, before following this appealing approach of establishing transient neglect models in healthy subjects, ethical aspects of inducing deficits in healthy subjects, even if transient and serving the development of new treatment strategies, also need to be thoroughly considered.

Neurorehabilitative Approaches in Neglect Patients by Means of tDCS

Based on the model of interhemispheric rivalry and the availability of facilitatory and inhibitory protocols, two complementary approaches using non-invasive brain stimulation in neglect patients are conceivable: inhibiting the contralesional hemisphere and enhancing the lesioned hemisphere. Though, for obvious reasons, full restoration of the functions of the lesioned site seems out of reach, facilitating protocols targeting the lesioned hemisphere may still contribute to the amelioration of neglect. Whether this effect is achieved by direct enhancement of attention-mediating right hemispheric structures and/or by interhemispheric inhibition of the contralesional intact cortex remains to be established.

To date, two studies investigated the effects of single tDCS sessions on neglect patients showing improved figure cancellation and/or line bisection immediately after ipsilesional anodal and/or contralesional cathodal tDCS (Ko, Han, Park, Seo, & Kim, 2008; Sparing et al., 2009).

Ko et al. (2008) demonstrated an enhancement of performance resulting from a facilitatory anodal stimulation of the lesioned right parietal cortex in 15 subacute stroke patients with spatial neglect. Severity of neglect, as identified by figure cancellation and line bisection, improved significantly immediately after 20 minutes of anodal tDCS at 2 mA over P4 (versus left supraorbital area; pair of 5×5 cm^2 electrodes) compared to sham stimulation in a double-blind protocol. A third letter-cancellation test showed comparable improvements after both interventions.

Similarly, Sparing et al. (2009) observed an amelioration of neglect symptoms with both contralesional inhibition as well as ipsilesional facilitation in 10 chronic stroke patients with neglect. The four stimulation conditions included facilitating anodal stimulation of the ipsilesional right PPC (P4 vs Cz) as well as inhibitory cathodal stimulation of the contralesional left PPC (P3 vs Cz), while ipsilesional sham stimulation and contralesional anodal stimulation served as controls. Despite a tendency towards faster responses and a slight increase in the number of stimuli detected in the "neglect" subtest of the TAP (Zimmermann & Fimm, 1995), none of the stimulation conditions improved the number of stimuli detected within the left hemifield and neither reaction times nor error rates showed significant effects. In the line-bisection task, however, both anodal tDCS of the lesioned hemisphere as well as cathodal tDCS of the non-lesioned hemisphere significantly reduced the pre-stimulation rightward deviations reflecting left visuospatial neglect, even leading to a small leftward bias after stimulation under both conditions. No significant effect on deviation was observed following the two control conditions – contralesional anodal as well as sham tDCS. Moreover, lesion size correlated negatively with the magnitude of improvement following cathodal tDCS of the unlesioned hemisphere.

Disturbed Networks of Attention

The model of interhemispheric rivalry may be extended by incorporating the two complementary networks mediating top-down and bottom-up regulation of attention, suggested by Corbetta et al. (2008) and

presented above. A bihemispheric dorsal frontoparietal netw
ing IPS, SPL, and FEF) was suggested to mediate top-down
voluntary attentional orientation to the contralateral hemisp
right-biased ventral frontoparietal network (including the
MFG, and IFG) is supposed to respond when behaviorally rel___ ___ _____
or targets are detected (Fig. 10.2; see also Corbetta & Shulman, 2002;
Corbetta et al., 2008; Hopfinger, Buonocore, & Mangun, 2000). Based on
this model, neglect and its predominant occurrence following right hemispheric lesions may be explained by two complementary pathomechan-
isms (Corbetta et al., 2005): diminished voluntary orienting towards the
contralesional left hemispace may arise from a disequilibrium between
an inhibited right and disinhibited (thus enhanced) left parietal cortex,
in addition to a general lack of stimulus-driven attentional orientation
by a right temporoparietal lesion. Left hemispheric lesions, in contrast,
preserve stimulus-driven orienting of attention, which may thus compensate for a diminished voluntary exploration of right hemispace. Further
differential effects may be envisioned by this model for lesions affecting
the right PPC versus the right TPJ. This much more complex model
may inform future treatment approaches addressing not only contralateral PPC but offering further frontal and TPJ targets to be addressed by
tDCS. These should be examined systematically in a standardized way.

DIVERSITY OF STIMULATION PROTOCOLS, BEHAVIORAL PARADIGMS, AND PATHOLOGY

Currently, a number of tDCS protocols exist. It is thus not surprising
that the studies summarized in this chapter show a variety of stimulation
sites, choice of location for reference electrode, current density, and stimulation duration applied. While optimal stimulation parameters are likely
to depend on the specific function targeted, on stimulation site, lesion
location, pathology, etc., only standardized stimulation protocols will
allow us to compare the individual studies and to draw conclusions that
can be generalized regarding the effects achieved. This is particularly relevant with respect to the limited availability of patients on the one hand,
and the large variance observed in patients calling for large sample sizes
on the other.

While tDCS may be quite effective in modulating a specific cognitive
function, its translational use in neurorehabilitation will depend on
whether or not tDCS shows a reliable and clinically relevant functional
impact across different types of lesion location and size in patients. Thus,
beyond the current pioneering state, standardization of protocols and systematic testing constitute the primary goal at present. Facing this dilemma
between the wish for individualized selection of parameters seeking

optimal treatment for an individual patient, and the need for standardized application to allow for direct comparability, we must become neither too "individual" nor too rigid with protocols in order to meet these diverse needs. (For a more detailed discussion of methodological aspects to be covered, see, for example, Hesse, Sparing, & Fink, 2011).

CONCLUSION

Studies on tDCS effects upon attention, both elementary and diverse, would benefit from a more systematic and standardized approach in order to allow for comparison and consolidation of the currently diverse stimulation studies on various aspects of attention. As described, the three networks model of attention proposed by Posner and colleagues provides a basic framework; however, this needs to be extended to include aspects of visual search as well as feature-based aspects of attention.

Although currently only a few proof-of-principle studies of non-invasive brain stimulation for the treatment of attention deficits such as neglect following brain injury are available, they provide promising results for applying neuromodulatory approaches in the neurorehabilitation of attention deficits. Nevertheless, before any widespread application in clinical routine may be pursued, large double-blind, placebo-controlled trials are needed that systematically study optimal, possibly individualized, stimulation protocols for site, intensity, frequency and duration of stimulation, onset of treatment, co-therapy, and prognostic criteria.

Acknowledgments

M. D. Hesse was supported by a grant of the Medical Faculty of the University of Cologne (Fortune No. 64/2010). Additional support to G. R. Fink from the Marga and Walter Boll Stiftung is gratefully acknowledged.

ABBREVIATIONS

ANG	angular gyrus
DLPFC	dorsolateral prefrontal cortex
DTI	diffusion tensor imaging
FEF	frontal eye field
fMRI	functional magnetic resonance imaging
IFG	inferior frontal gyrus
IPS	intraparietal sulcus
MFG	midfrontal gyrus
PFC	prefrontal cortex

PPC	posterior parietal cortex
rTMS	repetitive transcranial magnetic stimulation
SMG	supramarginal gyrus
SPL	superior parietal lobule
STG	superior temporal gyrus
TBS	theta burst stimulation
tDCS	transcranial direct current stimulation
TMS	transcranial magnetic stimulation
TPJ	temporoparietal junction

References

Accornero, N., Li Voti, P., La Riccia, M., & Gregori, B. (2007). Visual evoked potentials modulation during direct current cortical polarization. *Experimental Brain Research, 178,* 261–266.

Adólfsdóttir, S., Sørensen, L., & Lundervold, A. J. (2008). The attention network test: A characteristic pattern of deficits in children with ADHD. *Behavioral and Brain Functions, 4,* 9.

Antal, A., Brepohl, N., Poreisz, C., Boros, K., Csifcsak, G., & Paulus, W. (2008). Transcranial direct current stimulation over somatosensory cortex decreases experimentally induced acute pain perception. *The Clinical Journal of Pain, 24,* 56–63.

Antal, A., Kincses, T. Z., Nitsche, M. A., Bartfai, O., & Paulus, W. (2004). Excitability changes induced in the human primary visual cortex by transcranial direct current stimulation: Direct electrophysiological evidence. *Investigative Ophthalmology & Visual Science, 45,* 702–707.

Antal, A., Kincses, T. Z., Nitsche, M. A., & Paulus, W. (2003a). Manipulation of phosphene thresholds by transcranial direct current stimulation in man. *Experimental Brain Research, 150,* 375–378.

Antal, A., Kincses, T. Z., Nitsche, M. A., & Paulus, W. (2003b). Modulation of moving phosphene thresholds by transcranial direct current stimulation of V1 in human. *Neuropsychologia, 41,* 1802–1807.

Antal, A., Nitsche, M. A., Kruse, W., Kincses, T. Z., Hoffmann, K. P., & Paulus, W. (2004). Direct current stimulation over V5 enhances visuomotor coordination by improving motion perception in humans. *Journal of Cognitive Neuroscience, 16*(4), 521–527.

Antal, A., Nitsche, M. A., & Paulus, W. (2001). External modulation of visual perception in humans. *Neuroreport, 12,* 3553–3555.

Aston-Jones, G., & Cohen, J. D. (2005). An integrative theory of locus coeruleus–Norepinephrine function: Adaptive gain and optimal performance. *Annual Review of Neuroscience, 28,* 403–450.

Babiloni, C., Vecchio, F., Rossi, S., De Capua, A., Bartalini, S., Ulivelli, M., et al. (2007). Human ventral parietal cortex plays a functional role on visuospatial attention and primary consciousness. A repetitive transcranial magnetic stimulation study. *Cerebral Cortex, 17,* 1486–1492.

Bardi, L., Kanai, R., Mapelli, D., & Walsh, V. (2013). Direct current stimulation (tDCS) reveals parietal asymmetry in local/global and salience-based selection. *Cortex, 49*(3), 850–860.

Bartolomeo, P., Thiebaut de Schotten, M., & Doricchi, F. (2007). Left unilateral neglect as a disconnection syndrome. *Cerebral Cortex, 17,* 2479–2490.

Behrmann, M., Geng, J. J., & Shomstein, S. (2004). Parietal cortex and attention. *Current Opinion in Neurobiology, 14*(2), 212–217.

Berryhill, M. E., & Olson, I. R. (2008). Is the posterior parietal lobe involved in working memory retrieval? Evidence from patients with bilateral parietal lobe damage. *Neuropsychologia, 46*(7), 1775–1786.

Berryhill, M. E., Wencil, E. B., Branch Coslett, H., & Olson, I. R. (2010). A selective working memory impairment after transcranial direct current stimulation to the right parietal lobe. *Neuroscience Letters, 479*(3), 312–316.

Bien, N., Goebel, R., & Sack, A. T. (2012). Extinguishing extinction: Hemispheric differences in the modulation of TMS-induced visual extinction by directing covert spatial attention. *Journal of Cognitive Neuroscience, 24*(4), 809–818.

Binder, J., Marshall, R., Lazar, R., Benjamin, J., & Mohr, J. P. (1992). Distinct syndromes of hemineglect. *Archives of Neurology, 49*, 1187–1194.

Bisiach, E., & Vallar, G. (2000). Unilateral neglect in humans. In F. Boller, J. Grafman, & G. Rizzolatti (Eds.), *Handbook of neuropsychology: Vol. 1.* (pp. 459–502) (2nd ed.). Amsterdam, The Netherlands: Elsevier Science, B.V.

Bolognini, N., Fregni, F., Casati, C., Olgiati, E., & Vallar, G. (2010). Brain polarization of parietal cortex augments training-induced improvement of visual exploratory and attentional skills. *Brain Research, 1349*, 76–89.

Bolognini, N., Miniussi, C., Savazzi, S., Bricolo, E., & Maravita, A. (2009). TMS modulation of visual and auditory processing in the posterior parietal cortex. *Experimental Brain Research, 195*(4), 509–517.

Bolognini, N., Olgiati, E., Rossetti, A., & Maravita, A. (2010). Enhancing multisensory spatial orienting by brain polarization of the parietal cortex. *The European Journal of Neuroscience, 31*(10), 1800–1806.

Booth, J. E., Carlson, C. L., & Tucker, D. M. (2007). Performance on a neurocognitive measure of alerting differentiates ADHD combined and inattentive subtypes: A preliminary report. *Archives of Clinical Neuropsychology, 22*(4), 423–432.

Bundesen, C. (1990). A theory of visual attention. *Psychological Review, 97*(4), 523–547.

Chevrier, A. D., Noseworthy, M. D., & Schachar, R. (2007). Dissociation of response inhibition and performance monitoring in the stop signal task using event-related fMRI. *Human Brain Mapping, 28*(12), 1347–1358.

Clark, V. P., Coffman, B. A., Mayer, A. R., Weisend, M. P., Lane, T. D., Calhoun, V. D., et al. (2012). TDCS guided using fMRI significantly accelerates learning to identify concealed objects. *NeuroImage, 59*(1), 117–128.

Coffman, B. A., Trumbo, M. C., & Clark, V. P. (2012). Enhancement of object detection with transcranial direct current stimulation is associated with increased attention. *BMC Neuroscience, 13*, 108.

Coffman, B. A., Trumbo, M. C., Flores, R. A., Garcia, C. M., van der Merwe, A. J., Wassermann, E. M., et al. (2012). Impact of tDCS on performance and learning of target detection: Interaction with stimulus characteristics and experimental design. *Neuropsychologia, 50*(7), 1594–1602.

Committeri, G., Pitzalis, S., Galati, G., Patria, F., Pelle, G., Sabatini, U., et al. (2007). Neural bases of personal and extrapersonal neglect in humans. *Brain, 130*, 431–441.

Corbetta, M., Kincade, M. J., Lewis, C., Snyder, A. Z., & Sapir, A. (2005). Neural basis and recovery of spatial attention deficits in spatial neglect. *Nature Neuroscience, 8*, 1603–1610.

Corbetta, M., Kincade, J. M., Ollinger, J. M., McAvoy, M. P., & Shulman, G. L. (2000). Voluntary orienting is dissociated from target detection in human posterior parietal cortex. *Nature Neuroscience, 3*, 292–297.

Corbetta, M., Patel, G., & Shulman, G. L. (2008). The reorienting system of the human brain: From environment to theory of mind. *Neuron, 58*(3), 306–324.

Corbetta, M., & Shulman, G. L. (2002). Control of goal-directed and stimulus-driven attention in the brain. *Nature Reviews. Neuroscience, 3*, 201–215.

Coull, J. T., Frith, C. D., Büchel, C., & Nobre, A. C. (2000). Orienting attention in time: Behavioural and neuroanatomical distinction between exogenous and endogenous shifts. *Neuropsychologia, 38*(6), 808–819.

Curtis, C. E., Cole, M. W., Rao, V. Y., & D'Esposito, M. (2005). Canceling planned action: An FMRI study of countermanding saccades. *Cerebral Cortex, 15*(9), 1281–1289.

Dambeck, N., Sparing, R., Meister, I. G., Wienemann, M., Weidemann, J., Topper, R., et al. (2006). Interhemispheric imbalance during visuospatial attention investigated by unilateral and bilateral TMS over human parietal cortices. *Brain Research, 1072*, 194–199.

de Monasterio, F. M. (1978). Properties of ganglion cells with atypical receptive-field organization in retina of macaques. *Journal of Neurophysiology, 41*(6), 1435–1449.

Delis, D. C., Robertson, L. C., & Efron, R. (1986). Hemispheric specialization of memory for visual hierarchical stimuli. *Neuropsychologia, 24*(2), 205–214.

Dieckhöfer, A., Waberski, T. D., Nitsche, M., Paulus, W., Buchner, H., & Gobbelé, R. (2006). Transcranial direct current stimulation applied over the somatosensory cortex - differential effect on low and high frequency SEPs. *Clinical Neurophysiology, 117*(10), 2221–2227.

Ditye, T., Jacobson, L., Walsh, V., & Lavidor, M. (2012). Modulating behavioral inhibition by tDCS combined with cognitive training. *Experimental Brain Research, 219*(3), 363–368.

Doricchi, F., & Tomaiuolo, F. (2003). The anatomy of neglect without hemianopia: A key role for parietal-frontal disconnection? *NeuroReport, 14*, 2239–2243.

Dyrholm, M., Kyllingsbaek, S., Espeseth, T., & Bundesen, C. (2011). Generalizing parametric models by introducing trial-by-trial parameter variability: The case of TVA. *Journal of Mathematical Psychology, 55*, 416–429.

Edwards, D., & Fregni, F. (2008). Modulating the healthy and affected motor cortex with repetitive transcranial magnetic stimulation in stroke: Development of new strategies for neurorehabilitation. *Neuro Rehabilitation, 23*, 3–14.

Eimer, M. (1996). The N2pc component as an indicator of attentional selectivity. *Electroencephalography and Clinical Neurophysiology, 99*, 225–234.

Eimer, M., & Kiss, M. (2010). An electrophysiological measure of access to representations in visual working memory. *Psychophysiology, 47*, 197–200.

Eimer, M., & Mazza, V. (2005). Electrophysiological correlates of change detection. *Psychophysiology, 42*, 328–342.

Evans, M. A., Shedden, J. M., Hevenor, S. J., & Hahn, M. C. (2000). The effect of variability of unattended information on global and local processing: Evidence for lateralization at early stages of processing. *Neuropsychologia, 38*(3), 225–239.

Fan, J., McCandliss, B. D., Fossella, J., Flombaum, J. I., & Posner, M. I. (2005). The activation of attentional networks. *NeuroImage, 26*(2), 471–479.

Fierro, B., Brighina, F., & Bisiach (2006). Improving neglect bei TMS. *Behavioural Neurology, 17*, 169–176.

Fink, G. R., Halligan, P. W., Marshall, J. C., Frith, C. D., Frackowiak, R. S., & Dolan, R. J. (1996). Where in the brain does visual attention select the forest and the trees? *Nature, 382*(6592), 626–628.

Fink, G. R., Marshall, J. C., Halligan, P. W., & Dolan, R. J. (1999). Hemispheric asymmetries in global/local processing are modulated by perceptual salience. *Neuropsychologia, 37*(1), 31–40.

Fink, G. R., Marshall, J. C., Halligan, P. W., Frith, C. D., Frackowiak, R. S., & Dolan, R. J. (1997). Hemispheric specialization for global and local processing: The effect of stimulus category. *Proceedings of the Biological Sciences, 264*(1381), 487–494.

Flöel, A., Rösser, N., Michka, O., Knecht, S., & Breitenstein, C. (2008). Noninvasive brain stimulation improves language learning. *Journal of Cognitive Neuroscience, 20*(8), 1415–1422.

Giglia, G., Mattaliano, P., Puma, A., Rizzo, S., Fierro, B., & Brighina, F. (2011). Neglect-like effects induced by tDCS modulation of posterior parietal cortices in healthy subjects. *Brain Stimulation, 4*(4), 294–299.

Gladwin, T. E., den Uyl, T. E., Fregni, F. F., & Wiers, R. W. (2012). Enhancement of selective attention by tDCS: Interaction with interference in a Sternberg task. *Neuroscience Letters, 512*(1), 33–37.

Halligan, P. W., Fink, G. R., Marshall, J. C., & Vallar, G. (2003). Spatial cognition: Evidence from visual neglect. *Trends in Cognitive Sciences, 7*, 125–133.

Halligan, P. W., & Marshall, J. C. (1992). Left visuo-spatial neglect: A meaningless entity? *Cortex, 28*, 525–535.

Halligan, P. W., & Marshall, J. C. (1995). Lateral and radial neglect as a function of spatial position: A case study. *Neuropsychologia, 33*, 1697–1702.

Han, S., Liu, W., Yund, E. W., & Woods, D. L. (2000). Interactions between spatial attention and global/local feature selection: An ERP study. *Neuroreport, 11*(12), 2753–2758.

Han, S., Weaver, J. A., Murray, S. O., Kang, X., Yund, E. W., & Woods, D. L. (2002). Hemispheric asymmetry in global/local processing: Effects of stimulus position and spatial frequency. *NeuroImage, 17*(3), 1290–1299.

Harris-Love, M. L., & Cohen, L. G. (2006). Noninvasive cortical stimulation in neurorehabilitation: A review. *Archives of Physical Medicine and Rehabilitation, 87*, 84–93.

Heilman, K. M., Watson, R. T., & Valenstein, E. (2003). Neglect and related disorders. In K. M. Heilman & E. Valenstein (Eds.), *Clinical neuropsychology* (pp. 296–346). (4th ed.). New York, NY: Oxford University Press.

Hesse, M. D., Sparing, R., & Fink, G. R. (2011). Ameliorating spatial neglect with non-invasive brain stimulation: From pathophysiological concepts to novel treatment strategies. *Neuropsychological Rehabilitation, 21*(5), 676–702.

Hilgetag, C. C., Théoret, H., & Pascual-Leone, A. (2001). Enhanced visual spatial attention ipsilateral to rTMS-induced 'virtual lesions' of human parietal cortex. *Nature Neuroscience, 4*, 953–957.

Hopfinger, J. B., Buonocore, M. H., & Mangun, G. R. (2000). The neural mechanisms of top-down attentional control. *Nature Neuroscience, 3*, 284–291.

Hsu, T. Y., Tseng, L. Y., Yu, J. X., Kuo, W. J., Hung, D. L., Tzeng, O. J., et al. (2011). Modulating inhibitory control with direct current stimulation of the superior medial frontal cortex. *NeuroImage, 56*(4), 2249–2257.

Hughes, H. C., Fendrich, R., & Reuter-Lorenz, P. A. (1990). Global versus local processing in the absence of low spatial frequencies. *Journal of Cognitive Neuroscience, 2*(3), 272–282.

Hummel, F. C., & Cohen, L. G. (2006). Non-invasive brain stimulation: A new strategy to improve neurorehabilitation after stroke? *Lancet Neurology, 5*, 708–712.

Husain, M. (2008). Hemispatial neglect. In G. Goldenberg & B. L. Miller (Eds.), *Handbook of clinical neurology: Vol. 88.* (pp. 359–372). Amsterdam, The Netherlands: Elsevier, B. V.

Husain, M., & Nachev, P. (2007). Space and the parietal cortex. *Trends in Cognitive Sciences, 11*, 30–36.

Isoda, M., & Hikosaka, O. (2007). Switching from automatic to controlled action by monkey medial frontal cortex. *Nature Neuroscience, 10*(2), 240–248.

Ito, S., Stuphorn, V., Brown, J. W., & Schall, J. D. (2003). Performance monitoring by the anterior cingulate cortex during saccade countermanding. *Science, 302*(5642), 120–122.

Iyer, M. B., Mattu, U., Grafman, J., Lomarev, M., Sato, S., & Wassermann, E. M. (2005). Safety and cognitive effect of frontal DC brain polarization in healthy individuals. *Neurology, 64*(5), 872–875.

Jacobson, L., Koslowsky, M., & Lavidor, M. (2012). tDCS polarity effects in motor and cognitive domains: A meta-analytical review. *Experimental Brain Research, 216*(1), 1–10.

James, W. (1890). *The principles of psychology.* New York, NY: Holt.

Jeon, S. Y., & Han, S. J. (2012). Improvement of the working memory and naming by transcranial direct current stimulation. *Annals of Rehabilitation Medicine, 36*(5), 585–595.

Jolicoeur, P., Brisson, B., & Robitaille, N. (2008). Dissociation of the N2pc and sustained posterior contralateral negativity in a choice response task. *Brain Research, 1215,* 160–172.

Kang, E. K., Baek, M. J., Kim, S., & Paik, N. J. (2009). Non-invasive cortical stimulation improves post-stroke attention decline. *Restorative Neurology and Neuroscience, 27*(6), 645–650.

Kang, E. K., Kim, D. Y., & Paik, N. J. (2012). Transcranial direct current stimulation of the left prefrontal cortex improves attention in patients with traumatic brain injury: A pilot study. *Journal of Rehabilitation Medicine, 44*(4), 346–350.

Kimchi, R., & Merhav, I. (1991). Hemispheric processing of global form, local form, and texture. *Acta Psychologica, 76*(2), 133–147.

Kincses, T. Z., Antal, A., Nitsche, M. A., Bártfai, O., & Paulus, W. (2004). Facilitation of probabilistic classification learning by transcranial direct current stimulation of the prefrontal cortex in the human. *Neuropsychologia, 42*(1), 113–117.

Kinsbourne, M. (1977). Hemi-neglect and hemisphere rivalry. *Advances in Neurology, 18,* 41–49.

Kinsbourne, M. (1994). Mechanisms of neglect: Implications for rehabilitation. *Neuropsychological Rehabilitation, 4,* 151–153.

Knoch, D., Nitsche, M. A., Fischbacher, U., Eisenegger, C., Pascual-Leone, A., & Fehr, E. (2008). Studying the neurobiology of social interaction with transcranial direct current stimulation – The example of punishing unfairness. *Cerebral Cortex, 18*(9), 1987–1990.

Ko, M. H., Han, S. H., Park, S. H., Seo, J. H., & Kim, Y. H. (2008). Improvement of visual scanning after DC brain polarization of parietal cortex in stroke patients with spatial neglect. *Neuroscience Letters, 448,* 171–174.

Koch, G., Oliveri, M., Cheeran, B., Ruge, D., Lo Gerfo, E., Salerno, S., et al. (2008). Hyperexcitability of parietal–Motor functional connections in the intact left-hemisphere of patients with neglect. *Brain, 131,* 3147–3155.

Konrad, K., Neufang, S., Hanisch, C., Fink, G. R., & Herpertz-Dahlmann, B. (2006). Dysfunctional attentional networks in children with attention deficit/hyperactivity disorder: Evidence from an event-related functional magnetic resonance imaging study. *Biological Psychiatry, 59*(7), 643–651.

Kyllingsbaek, S. (2006). Modeling visual attention. *Behavior Research Methods, 38*(1), 123–133.

Lamb, M. R., & Robertson, L. C. (1988). The processing of hierarchical stimuli: Effects of retinal locus, locational uncertainty, and stimulus identity. *Perception & Psychophysics, 44*(2), 172–181.

Lamb, M. R., Robertson, L. C., & Knight, R. T. (1990). Component mechanisms underlying the processing of hierarchically organized patterns: Inferences from patients with unilateral cortical lesions. *Journal of Experimental Psychology. Learning, Memory, and Cognition, 16*(3), 471–483.

Leh, S. E., Ptito, A., Schönwiesner, M., Chakravarty, M. M., & Mullen, K. T. (2010). Blindsight mediated by an S-cone-independent collicular pathway: An fMRI study in hemispherectomized subjects. *Journal of Cognitive Neuroscience, 22*(4), 670–682.

Leite, J., Carvalho, S., Fregni, F., Boggio, P. S., & Gonçalves, O. F. (2013). The effects of cross-hemispheric dorsolateral prefrontal cortex transcranial direct current stimulation (tDCS) on task switching. *Brain Stimulation, 6*(4), 660–667.

Lepsien, J., & Nobre, A. C. (2006). Cognitive control of attention in the human brain: Insights from orienting attention to mental representations. *Brain Research, 1105*(1), 20–31.

Loftus, A. M., & Nicholls, M. E. (2012). Testing the activation-orientation account of spatial attentional asymmetries using transcranial direct current stimulation. *Neuropsychologia, 50*(11), 2573–2576.

Loui, P., Hohmann, A., & Schlaug, G. (2010). Inducing disorders in pitch perception and production: A reverse-engineering approach. *Proceedings of Meetings on Acoustics, 9*(1), 50002.

Luck, S. J., & Hillyard, S. A. (1994). Spatial filtering during visual search: Evidence from human electrophysiology. *Journal of Experimental Psychology. Human Perception and Performance, 20*(5), 1000–1014.

Mackworth, J. F. (1964). Performance decrement in vigilance, threshold, and high-speed perceptual motor tasks. *Canadian Journal of Psychology, 18*, 209–223.

Maravita, A., Bolognini, N., Bricolo, E., Marzi, C. A., & Savazzi, S. (2008). Is audiovisual integration subserved by the superior colliculus in humans? *Neuroreport, 19*(3), 271–275.

Marrocco, R. T., & Li, R. H. (1977). Monkey superior colliculus: Properties of single cells and their afferent inputs. *Journal of Neurophysiology, 40*(4), 844–860.

Martin, M. (1979). Hemispheric specialization for local and global processing. *Neuropsychologia, 17*(1), 33–40.

Maxwell, S. E., & Delaney, H. D. (2004). *Designing experiments and analyzing data: A model comparison perspective* (2nd ed.). Mahwah, NJ: Lawrence Erlbaum Associates.

Medina, J., Beauvais, J., Datta, A., Bikson, M., Coslett, H. B., & Hamilton, R. H. (2013). Transcranial direct current stimulation accelerates allocentric target detection. *Brain Stimulation, 6*(3), 433–439.

Mesulam, M. M. (1981). A cortical network for directed attention and unilateral neglect. *Annals of Neurology, 10*, 309–325.

Mevorach, C., Hodsoll, J., Allen, H., Shalev, L., & Humphreys, G. (2010). Ignoring the elephant in the room: A neural circuit to downregulate salience. *Journal of Neuroscience: The Official Journal of the Society for Neuroscience, 30*(17), 6072–6079.

Mevorach, C., Humphreys, G. W., & Shalev, L. (2006). Opposite biases in salience-based selection for the left and right posterior parietal cortex. *Nature Neuroscience, 9*(6), 740–742.

Moos, K., Vossel, S., Weidner, R., Sparing, R., & Fink, G. R. (2012). Modulation of top-down control of visual attention by cathodal tDCS over right IPS. *Journal of Neuroscience: The Official Journal of the Society for Neuroscience, 32*(46), 16360–16368.

Mort, D. J., Malhotra, P., Mannan, S. K., Rorden, C., Pambakian, A., Kennard, C., et al. (2003). The anatomy of visual neglect. *Brain, 126*, 1986–1997.

Moruzzi, G., & Magoun, H. W. (1949). Brain stem reticular formation and activation of the EEG. *Electroencephalography and Clinical Neurophysiology, 1*(4), 455–473.

Muggleton, N. G., Chen, C. Y., Tzeng, O. J., Hung, D. L., & Juan, C. H. (2010). Inhibitory control and the frontal eye fields. *Journal of Cognitive Neuroscience, 22*(12), 2804–2812.

Navon, D. (1977). Forest before trees: The precedence of global features in visual perception. *Cognitive Psychology, 9*, 353–383.

Nelson, J. T., McKinley, R. A., Golob, E. J., Warm, J. S., & Parasuraman, R. (2012). Enhancing vigilance in operators with prefrontal cortex transcranial direct current stimulation (tDCS). *NeuroImage*, (Epub ahead of print).

Nitsche, M. A., Cohen, L. G., Wassermann, E. M., Priori, A., Lang, N., Antal, A., et al. (2008). Transcranial direct current stimulation: State of the art 2008. *Brain Stimulation, 1*, 206–223.

Nitsche, M. A., & Paulus, W. (2000). Excitability changes induced in the human motor cortex by weak transcranial direct current stimulation. *The Journal of Physiology, 527*, 633–639.

Nitsche, M. A., & Paulus, W. (2001). Sustained excitability elevations induced by transcranial DC motor cortex stimulation in humans. *Neurology, 57*, 1899–1901.

Nitsche, M. A., Seeber, A., Frommann, K., Klein, C. C., Rochford, C., Nitsche, M. S., et al. (2005). Modulating parameters of excitability during and after transcranial direct current stimulation of the human motor cortex. *The Journal of Physiology, 568*, 291–303.

Parasuraman, R., & Davies, D. R. (1976). Decision theory analysis of response latencies in vigilance. *Journal of Experimental Psychology Human Perception and Performance, 2*(4), 578–590.

Parasuraman, R., Nestor, P., & Greenwood, P. (1989). Sustained-attention capacity in young and older adults. *Psychology and Aging, 4*(3), 339–345.

Petersen, S. E., & Posner, M. I. (2012). The attention system of the human brain: 20 years after. *Annual Review of Neuroscience, 35*, 73–89.

Plewnia, C., Zwissler, B., Längst, I., Maurer, B., Giel, K., & Krüger, R. (2013). Effects of transcranial direct current stimulation (tDCS) on executive functions: Influence of COMT Val/Met polymorphism. *Cortex, 49*(7), 1801–1807.

Posner, M. I. (1980). Orienting of attention. *The Quarterly Journal of Experimental Psychology, 32*, 3–25.

Posner, M. I., Walker, J. A., Friedrich, F. J., & Rafal, R. D. (1984). Effects of parietal injury on covert orienting of attention. *Journal of Neuroscience: The Official Journal of the Society for Neuroscience, 4*(7), 1863–1874.

Priori, A., Berardelli, A., Rona, S., Accornero, N., & Manfredi, M. (1998). Polarization of the human motor cortex through the scalp. *Neuroreport, 9*(10), 2257–2260.

Raz, A. (2006). Individual differences and attentional varieties. *Europa Medicophysica, 42*(1), 53–58.

Robertson, L. C., Lamb, M. R., & Knight, R. T. (1988). Effects of lesions of temporal-parietal junction on perceptual and attentional processing in humans. *Journal of Neuroscience: The Official Journal of the Society for Neuroscience, 8*(10), 3757–3769.

Robertson, I. H., & Murre, J. M. (1999). Rehabilitation of brain damage: Brain plasticity and principles of guided recovery. *Psychological Bulletin, 125*(5), 544–575.

Seyal, M., Ro, T., & Rafal, R. (1995). Increased sensitivity to ipsilateral cutaneous stimuli following transcranial magnetic stimulation of the parietal lobe. *Annals of Neurology, 38*, 264–267.

Sparing, R., & Mottaghy, F. M. (2008). Noninvasive brain stimulation with transcranial magnetic or direct current stimulation (TMS/tDCS) – From insights into human memory to therapy of its dysfunction. *Methods, 44*, 287–348.

Sparing, R., Thimm, M., Hesse, M. D., Küst, J., Karbe, H., & Fink, G. R. (2009). Bidirectional alterations of interhemispheric parietal balance by non-invasive cortical stimulation. *Brain, 132*, 3011–3020.

Stagg, C. J., O'Shea, J., Kincses, Z. T., Woolrich, M., Matthews, P. M., & Johansen-Berg, H. (2009). Modulation of movement-associated cortical activation by transcranial direct current stimulation. *The European Journal of Neuroscience, 30*(7), 1412–1423.

Stone, D. B., & Tesche, C. D. (2009). Transcranial direct current stimulation modulates shifts in global/local attention. *Neuroreport, 20*(12), 1115–1119.

Stuphorn, V., & Schall, J. D. (2006). Executive control of countermanding saccades by the supplementary eye field. *Nature Neuroscience, 9*(7), 925–931.

Stuphorn, V., Taylor, T. L., & Schall, J. D. (2000). Performance monitoring by the supplementary eye field. *Nature, 408*(6814), 857–860.

Sturm, W., & Willmes, K. (2001). On the functional neuroanatomy of intrinsic and phasic alertness. *NeuroImage, 14*(1 Pt 2), S76–S84.

Tanoue, R. T., Jones, K. T., Peterson, D. J., & Berryhill, M. E. (2013). Differential frontal involvement in shifts of internal and perceptual attention. *Brain Stimulation, 6*(4), 675–682.

Thiel, C. M., Zilles, K., & Fink, G. R. (2004). Cerebral correlates of alerting, orienting and reorienting of visuospatial attention: An event-related fMRI study. *NeuroImage, 21*(1), 318–328.

Todd, J. J., & Marois, R. (2004). Capacity limit of visual short-term memory in human posterior parietal cortex. *Nature, 428*(6984), 751–754.

Todd, J. J., & Marois, R. (2005). Posterior parietal cortex activity predicts individual differences in visual short-term memory capacity. *Cognitive, Affective, & Behavioral Neuroscience, 5*(2), 144–155.

Tsal, Y., Shalev, L., & Mevorach, C. (2005). The diversity of attention deficits in ADHD: The prevalence of four cognitive factors in ADHD versus controls. *Journal of Learning Disabilities, 38*(2), 142–157.

Tseng, P., Hsu, T. Y., Chang, C. F., Tzeng, O. J., Hung, D. L., Muggleton, N. G., et al. (2012). Unleashing potential: Transcranial direct current stimulation over the right posterior parietal cortex improves change detection in low-performing individuals. *Journal of Neuroscience: The Official Journal of the Society for Neuroscience, 32*(31), 10554–10561.

Vallar, G. (1998). Spatial hemineglect in humans. *Trends Cognitive Sciences, 2,* 87–97.

Vallar, G., & Perani, D. (1986). The anatomy of unilateral neglect after right-hemisphere stroke lesions. A clinical/CT-scan correlation study in man. *Neuropsychologia, 24,* 609–622.

Verdon, V., Schwartz, S., Lovblad, K. O., Hauert, C. A., & Vuilleumier, P. (2010). Neuroanatomy of hemispatial neglect and its functional components: A study using voxel-based lesion-symptom mapping. *Brain, 133,* 880–894.

Vogel, E. K., & Machizawa, M. G. (2004). Neural activity predicts individual differences in visual working memory capacity. *Nature, 428*(6984), 748–751.

Vogel, E. K., Woodman, G. F., & Luck, S. J. (2005). Pushing around the locus of selection: Evidence for the flexible-selection hypothesis. *Journal of Cognitive Neuroscience, 17*(12), 1907–1922.

Vossel, S., & Kukolja, J. (2009). Neglect. *Klinische Neurophysiologie, 40,* 255–262.

Vuilleumier, P., Hester, D., Assal, G., & Regli, F. (1996). Unilateral spatial neglect recovery after sequential strokes. *Neurology, 46,* 184–189.

Wang, K., Fan, J., Dong, Y., Wang, C. Q., Lee, T. M., & Posner, M. I. (2005). Selective impairment of attentional networks of orienting and executive control in schizophrenia. *Schizophrenia Research, 78*(2–3), 235–241.

Warm, J. S., Parasuraman, R., & Matthews, G. (2008). Vigilance requires hard mental work an is stressful. *Human Factors, 50*(3), 433–441.

Weiss, M., & Lavidor, M. (2012). When less is more: Evidence for a facilitative cathodal tDCS effect in attentional abilities. *Journal of Cognitive Neuroscience, 24*(9), 1826–1833.

Weiss, P. H., Marshall, J. C., Wunderlich, G., Tellmann, L., Halligan, P. W., Freund, H. J., et al. (2000). Neural consequences of acting in near versus far space: A physiological basis for clinical dissociations. *Brain, 123*(Pt 12), 2531–2541.

Woodman, G. F. (2010). A brief introduction to the use of event-related potentials in studies of perception and attention. *Attention, Perception, & Psychophysics, 72*(8), 2031–2046.

Woodman, G. F., Arita, J. T., & Luck, S. J. (2009). A cuing study of the N2pc component: An index of attentional deployment to objects rather than spatial locations. *Brain Research, 1297,* 101–111.

Xu, Y., & Chun, M. M. (2006). Dissociable neural mechanisms supporting visual short-term memory for objects. *Nature, 440*(7080), 91–95.

Zimmermann, P., & Fimm, B. (1995). *Test battery for attention performance (TAP).* Wuerselen, Germany: Psytest.

CHAPTER

11

High-Level Cognitive Functions in Healthy Subjects

Tal Sela and Michal Lavidor

Department of Psychology, and The Gonda Multidisciplinary Brain Research
Center, Bar Ilan University, Ramat Gan, Israel

OUTLINE

The Stimulated Brain
http://dx.doi.org/10.1016/B978-0-12-404704-4.00011-9

INTRODUCTION

Cognitive enhancement is in widespread use today, but is not always recognized as such. The automated spelling software in word processors, smart phones, and tweets are all part of our cognitive and language enhancement infrastructure that help us produce, receive, retrieve, and transfer information. Transcranial electrical stimulation (tES) methods such as transcranial direct current stimulation (tDCS), transcranial alternating current stimulation (tACS), and transcranial random noise stimulation (tRNS) are used to enhance cognitive and language capabilities in the healthy brain; as such, these techniques have enormous potential for research and rehabilitation in the short term, and eventually may be used on a daily basis to enhance our cognitive functioning.

Cognitive enhancement is best defined as the amplification or extension of core capacities of the mind by improving or augmenting internal or external information processing systems (Farah et al., 2004; Sandberg & Bostrom, 2006). Cognition is defined as the processes an organism uses to organize information. This includes acquiring information (sensation and perception), selecting (attention), communicating (language, numbers), representing (understanding) and retaining (memory) information, and using it to guide behavior (reasoning and coordination of motor outputs).

Interventions to improve cognitive function may be directed at any one of these core faculties. An intervention aimed at correcting a specific pathology or defect of a cognitive subsystem may be characterized as therapeutic. An enhancement is an intervention that improves a subsystem in some way other than repairing something that was damaged or remedying a specific dysfunction. In practice, the distinction between therapy and enhancement is often difficult to discern, and it could be argued that it lacks practical significance (see Chapter 18).

This chapter presents contemporary cutting-edge brain stimulation techniques that have been successful in enhancing cognitive functions in healthy individuals. Their applications to higher cognitive functions are discussed, and focus primarily on language, but also examine various cognitive functions and learning.

THE tES FAMILY: tDCS, tACS, AND tRNS

Transcranial direct current stimulation (tDCS) induces stimulation polarity-dependent cortical activity and excitability enhancements or reductions that emerge during stimulation, but can persist for 1 hour after stimulation (Nitsche & Paulus, 2000, 2001; Nitsche et al., 2003, 2008), although some studies have reported effects lasting for 90 minutes post-stimulation, and longer (Batsikadze, Moliadze, Paulus, Kuo, & Nitsche, 2013). The primary mechanism of tDCS is thought to be a modulation of spontaneous cortical activity via the resting membrane potential, where anodal tDCS causes neural depolarization and thus enhances cortical excitability, and cathodal tDCS causes neural hyperpolarization and decreased cortical excitability (Nitsche & Paulus, 2000, 2001). tDCS to the motor cortex has proven to be a powerful method to modulate excitability and has been suggested to be related to long-term potentiation (LTP-like: anodal tDCS) and long-term depression (LTD-like: cathodal tDCS) (Liebetanz, 2002; Nitsche et al., 2003; see also Stagg & Nitsche, 2011, and Chapters 5–6, for a comprehensive review of the physiological bases of tDCS in animals and humans). In addition, this method makes it possible to test a highly reliable sham condition (Gandiga, Hummel, & Cohen, 2006), in which the stimulation is turned on and off over a relatively short period of time, where the participants are unable to distinguish this condition from the real stimulation.

Behaviorally, tDCS studies have examined cognitive performance across a number of task domains, including working memory (Fregni et al., 2005), visual recognition memory (Boggio et al., 2009), probabilistic classification (Kincses, Antal, Nitsche, Bartfai, & Paulus, 2004), and probabilistic guessing (Hecht, Walsh, & Lavidor, 2010). The idea that anodal tDCS may promote upregulation whereas cathodal stimulation may promote downregulation, as found and replicated in motor or visual domains, has been challenged with respect to cathodal tDCS effects on cognition, as shown by a recent meta-analysis (Jacobson, Koslowsky, & Lavidor, 2012). There is, of course, no necessary correspondence between excitation/inhibition and behavioral improvements/impairments (Hecht et al., 2010). Depending on task specifications, and the stimulated brain region(s), cathodal tDCS could be used to impair cognition in a lesion-type approach (e.g., Sparing, Dafotakis, Meister, Thirugnanasambandam, & Fink, 2008) or to improve a behavioral function (e.g., Pope & Miall, 2012; Weiss & Lavidor, 2012).

Other forms of transcranial electrical brain stimulation, such as transcranial alternating current stimulation (tACS) and transcranial random noise stimulation (tRNS), are assumed to modulate neuronal membrane potentials by oscillatory electrical stimulation with specific or random frequencies (Antal et al., 2008; Terney, Chaieb, Moliadze, Antal, & Paulus, 2008). These methods are thought to interact with ongoing rhythmic cortical activities during cognitive processes and hence could be useful tools to investigate the underlying mechanisms of human cognition (Kuo & Nitsche, 2012; see also Chapter 2). However, so far only a few studies have been conducted to determine how these techniques alter perception and cognition (Fertonani, Pirulli, & Miniussi, 2011; Snowball et al., 2013; Terney et al., 2008).

EFFECTS OF tDCS ON LANGUAGE

The modern-day endeavor to understand the neural substrates of language, which dates back to the seminal work of Broca (1865) and Wernicke (1874), may be one area that benefits from brain stimulation research, as it provides tools that enable strong causal inferences (see Silvanto & Pascual-Leone, 2012).

To date, several tDCS studies have explored naming, picture naming, and verbal fluency. Naming is a basic, fundamental capacity of the human brain that requires a number of cognitive processes involving perception of the visual stimuli, the semantic and lexical processing of its features, the selection and retrieval of relevant information, and finally the articulation of a target concept.

In the context of naming and verbal fluency, several studies have used tDCS to improve performance by utilizing the facilitatory mode of anodal tDCS. For example, in a large, single-blind design, Iyer and colleagues investigated the effects of tDCS on prefrontal cortex-related functions (Iyer et al., 2005). The target location for the anodal stimulation was the left DLPFC, with the reference electrode placed over the right supraorbital area. There were no significant effects on performance with 1 mA tDCS. However, at 2 mA, verbal fluency improved during anodal stimulation but there were no effects on a range of other tasks (e.g., attention, reaction time, memory, and psychomotor speed). However, cathodal polarization did not produce the expected decrement in performance and showed no difference from sham in any of the experiments. Although not explicitly detailed in Iyer's report (Iyer et al., 2005; see also Wassermann & Grafman, 2005), the effect size for the 2-mA anodal stimulation montage was medium (~0.5; Jacobson, Koslowsky, & Lavidor, 2012). Iyer and colleagues' study provided the first direct evidence for cognitive enhancement in the context of language production by showing that it is possible to transiently change the human verbal fluency capacity through electrical stimulation, and showed that this effect depended on intensity (Iyer et al., 2005).

In another study, Sparing and colleagues explored whether tDCS could enhance visual picture naming (Sparing et al., 2008). Fifteen healthy participants performed the task before, during, and after tDCS was applied over the posterior perisylvian region (PPR). This position corresponds to the location of Wernicke's area, including the posterior part of the left superior temporal gyrus (STG), and has been used in a number of transcranial magnetic stimulation (TMS) studies (e.g., Mottaghy et al., 1999). Using a double-blind, within-subject design, participants underwent four different 2-mA stimulation sessions: anodal and cathodal stimulation of left PPR as the main target stimulation, and anodal stimulation of the homologous region of the right hemisphere and sham stimulation as control conditions. The results showed that participants responded significantly faster following anodal tDCS to the left PPR, with an effect size indicating an improvement of about 6% in naming latencies (effect size estimated as medium-high ∼ 0.6; Jacobson, Koslowsky, & Lavidor, 2012). This significant decrease in naming latency was found at the end of anodal tDCS to the left PPR, and was not evident during stimulation, but the facilitation effect ceased 5 and 10 minutes' post-stimulation.

Similarly, Fertonani, Rosini, Cotelli, Rossini, and Miniussi (2010) explored tDCS effects on picture naming in young healthy participants by using the DLPFC as the target region of interest, given the importance of this region in action naming (Cappa, Sandrini, Rossini, Sosta, & Miniussi, 2002). In a single-blind, within-subject design, anodal, cathodal, or sham tDCS (10-min stimulation; 2 mA) was applied to the left DLPFC, with the reference electrode located on the right shoulder. The results showed that anodal tDCS of the left DLPFC improved naming performance and facilitated verbal reaction times after the end of the stimulation, whereas cathodal stimulation had no effect. The authors suggested that the cerebral network dedicated to lexical retrieval processing was facilitated by anodal tDCS to left DLPFC.

Similar to Sparing et al. (2008), tDCS facilitation effects were the result of an anodal aftereffect that was manifested in faster response time, whereas accuracy scores remained intact. Furthermore, both studies failed to show any effect of cathodal stimulation on naming performance. Interestingly, though not explicitly reported by Fertonani et al. (2010), the mean effect was estimated as an improvement of about 6% in naming latencies. This means that, in essence, anodal tDCS produced small yet consistent and significant differences in the studies reviewed above. Interestingly, though different regions of interest were used in these studies (PPR and DLPFC), naming/verbal fluency performance improved, suggesting that tDCS can directly impact the neural mechanism that underlies the function (PPR for example) or a remote terminal that is a part of the network that underlies the function (e.g., DLPFC). This seems reasonable in that picture naming and word generation involve a massive activation of temporal and frontal regions (Indefrey & Levelt, 2004), and is consistent with the idea that multiple sites are effective by active stimulation, since the locus of tDCS effects occurs at the network level (e.g., Keeser et al., 2011).

Another major contribution to the study of naming via tDCS was made by Ross and colleagues, who investigated whether stimulation of the anterior temporal lobes (ATL) by means of tDCS was effective in modulating the memory of known people's proper names (Ross, McCoy, Wolk, Coslett, & Olson, 2010). The ATL is considered the anatomical site that mediates the semantic network which links person-specific information and includes proper names. Subjects were given left anodal, right anodal (1.5 mA, 15 min), or sham stimulation of the ATL, while naming pictures of famous individuals and landmarks. The reference electrode was placed over the contralateral cheekbone. The results showed that anodal stimulation to the right ATL significantly improved face-naming accuracy for people but not for landmarks. This effect was considerable (11%; effect size estimated as medium ~0.45; Jacobson, Koslowsky, & Lavidor, 2012) and highly consistent, as 13 out of the 15 participants showed an increase in naming performance after right anodal stimulation. The Ross et al. (2010) study is also worthy of note because it included a control condition (landmarks), a design that made it possible to assess a selective and specific effect which thus significantly enhanced the study's validity.

It has been argued that word retrieval during verbal fluency tasks involves both automatic processes that are associated with left posterior temporal-parietal regions, and controlled processes that are associated with the left prefrontal region (Hirshorn & Thompson-Schill, 2006). Vannorsdall et al. (2012) investigated whether tDCS can differentially modify controlled or automatic processes that support lexical retrieval on verbal fluency tasks, as assessed by clustering, which was taken to reflect relatively automatic processing, and switching, which is thought to require a more controlled type of processing. In a single-blind, sham-controlled experiment with a mixed-subject design, 24 participants were randomly assigned to receive 1 mA for 30 minutes of either anodal or cathodal tDCS over the left DLFPC cortex, or sham stimulation. The reference electrode was placed over the vertex. Results showed that anodal tDCS was associated with an increase in overall productivity during a category-guided verbal fluency task, and that anodal stimulation led to a relative increase in clustering, whereas cathodal stimulation had the opposite effect (a 6.6% increase in the percent of words in clusters for active anodal stimulation, whereas active cathodal stimulation produced a 2.2% reduction in the percent words in clusters). This study showed that tDCS could selectively alter automatic aspects of speeded lexical retrieval during a category-guided fluency task, and provided more modest evidence for a cathodal stimulation effect in the context of language research.

EFFECTS OF tDCS ON EXECUTIVE FUNCTIONS

Executive functions refer to a broad domain of functions that are involved in monitoring and regulating cognitive processes, and in goal-focused processes, inhibition, planning, working memory, performance monitoring, and problem solving (Alvarez & Emory, 2006). Executive functions play a major role in normal development, are critical for managing daily life, and are also related to occupational and social functioning. It has long been argued that the prefrontal cortex (PFC) subserves executive control, the ability to select actions on the basis of internal plans or goals

(Koechlin, Basso, Pietrini, Panzer, & Grafman, 1999; Koechlin, Ody, & Kouneiher, 2003; Miller & Cohen, 2001).

To date, several studies have attempted to target executive functions with tDCS. tDCS has already been shown to improve higher-order cognitive functions in decision-making (Hecht et al., 2010), risk taking (Fecteau, Knoch et al., 2007; Fecteau, Pascual-Leone et al., 2007; see also Chapter 14), and probabilistic classification (Kincses et al., 2004). It is postulated that even with respect to relatively complex functions that underlie different types of tasks, facilitation (or inhibition) by using basic designs of tDCS can modify performance. One mechanism that accounts for the overwhelming tDCS findings in the context of PFC stimulation may be related to the idea that tDCS effects are not local (see Holland et al., 2011) but rather distributed as suggested by Keeser et al. (2011), who showed that after anodal tDCS to the left DLPFC, a distributed network was activated rather than only the stimulated brain region.

In this manner, Sela and colleagues used tDCS to test the hypothesis that a prefrontal cognitive control network is involved in directing semantic decisions needed for the comprehension of idioms (Sela, Ivry, & Lavidor, 2012). A recent conceptualization argues in favor of a broad role of this brain region in figurative language comprehension (Lauro, Tettamanti, Cappa, & Papagno, 2008; Papagno, 2010; see also the meta-analysis by Rapp, Mutschler, & Erb, 2012), and claims that prefrontal regions are responsible for the suppression of alternative interpretations and response monitoring during idiom comprehension and for higher-order cognitive processes tapped for other types of figurative language (Lauro et al., 2008; Papagno, 2010).

Sela et al. (2012) used a double-blind, sham-controlled mixed design to explore this "PFC regulation hypothesis". Participants were randomly allocated to one of two stimulation groups (left DLPFC anodal/right DLPFC cathodal, or left DLPFC cathodal/right DLPFC anodal). The stimulation lasted 15 minutes, with an intensity of 1.5 mA. Over a 1-week interval, participants were tested twice, and were administered a semantic decision task and a control task (a spoonerism task, which assesses phonological awareness; Romani, Ward, & Olson, 1999) after receiving either active or sham stimulation. The semantic decision task required participants to judge the relatedness of an idiom and a target word, where the idiom was predictable or not. Targets were figuratively related, literally related, or unrelated to the idiom. The results showed that after tDCS stimulation, a general deceleration (around 10%) in reaction times to targets was found. In addition, the results indicated that the neural enhancement of a left lateralized prefrontal network (left DLPFC anodal/right DLPFC cathodal) improved performance when participants had to make decisions about the figurative targets of highly predictable idioms, whereas the neural enhancement of the opposite network (left DLPFC cathodal /right DLPFC anodal) improved performance for literal targets of unpredictable idioms (see Fig. 11.1). These effects were highly robust, and explained 28% and 23% of the variance, respectively. Finally, the results showed no difference with respect to performance in the control task.

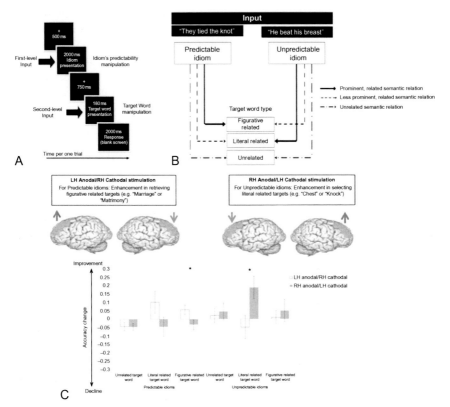

FIGURE 11.1   (A) Semantic decision task procedure: the trial began with the presentation of a fixation cross for 500 ms. The cross was replaced by an idiom which remained on the screen for 2000 ms. Participants were instructed to read the idioms silently. The fixation cross reappeared for 750 ms and was followed by the target word for 180 ms. Participants were instructed to indicate whether the idiomatic expression and the target word were related by pressing the right or left mouse keys. They were instructed to respond rapidly while maintaining a high level of accuracy. The next trial began after a 2000-ms interval. (B) Six experimental conditions: two experimental manipulations (2 × 3) were used – idiom predictability with two levels (predictable and unpredictable), and target word type with three levels (figurative related, literal related, and unrelated). The conditions were *a priori* defined as prominent, related semantic relations (continuous line); less prominent, related semantic relations (dashed line); or unrelated semantic relations (dashed–dot line). (C) Main finding reported in Sela et al. (2012) reflected in accuracy change scores (mean ± standard error of mean). The three-way interaction revealed that the tDCS effects were limited to specific idiom–target pairings. *$P < 0.05$. *Data from Sela et al. (2012), with permission from Elsevier.*

Additionally, tDCS effects were more pronounced in individuals who were rated as being most sensitive to reward likelihood. More specifically, a variation on a trait motivation propensity (BAS reward responsiveness; BAS–RR+, part of the BIS/BAS scale; Carver & White, 1994) moderated the effects of tDCS for the most canonical form of idioms (predictable idioms followed by their figurative meaning; see Fig. 11.2). This finding has important implications regarding the impact of trait motivation on cognitive control, and, in this context, on top-down regulation of language comprehension.

The Sela et al. (2012) findings corroborated the hypothesis put forward by Papagno and colleagues (Lauro et al., 2008; Papagno, 2010) that the PFC is implicated in selection processes. Sela et al. (2012) showed that the PFC regulates selection processes by using top-down bias based on stimulus characteristics (e.g., idiom predictability), and that individual differences in trait motivations are linked to the magnitude of the effect caused by tDCS.

It was also found that anodal tDCS over the left DLPFC enhances complex verbal insight problem-solving. A study by Cerruti and Schlaug (2009) tested whether prefrontal stimulation could enhance performance on the remote associates test (RAT). Typically, in RAT problems, subjects are presented with three words – e.g., AGE/MILE/SAND – and must find a common linguistic association in the form of a compound noun or a two-word phrase with each cue word – in this case, STONE (STONE-AGE, MILESTONE, and SANDSTONE). This task requires strong executive function capacities, since lateral associations and internal production of many words is needed until a key decision stage is reached in which the subject must select or generate a single answer.

In the Cerruti and Schlaug (2009) study, subjects read the problems and were asked to say the answer aloud while they were recorded. In the first experiment by Cerruti & Schlaug, 18 subjects underwent 3 stimulation conditions (anodal, cathodal, and sham) in one 3-h session, with the order of stimulation randomized across subjects. The washout period between stimulation sessions was 30 minutes. Stimulation duration was 20 minutes, and stimulation intensity was 1 mA. The target location was the left DLPFC, and the reference electrode was fixed over the right supraorbital region. Subjects performed the RAT task, which was administered immediately after the end of each stimulation session. The results showed a significant increase in performance after anodal stimulation. In their second experiment, Cerruti & Schlaug used an anodal stimulation to the left DLPFC or its homolog in the right hemisphere. The anodal effect for the left DLPFC was replicated, and the results showed that anodal stimulation of the right DLPFC had no effect on RAT performance. This experiment provided valuable information with respect to site specification, and the effect that was reported in Experiment 1 was quite robust ($\sim 20\%$; effect size estimated as ~ 0.5; Jacobson, Koslowsky, & Lavidor, 2012).

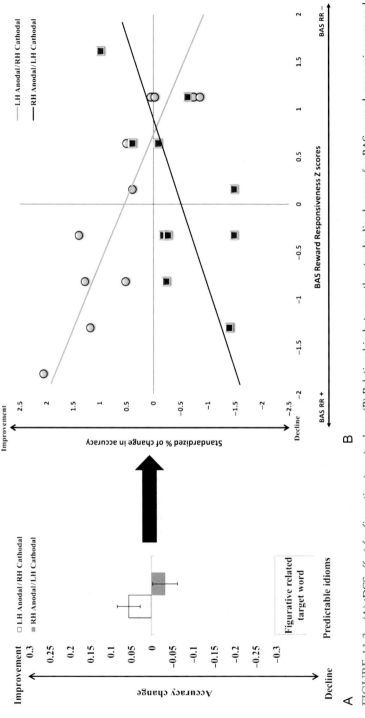

FIGURE 11.2   (A) tDCS effect for figurative targets alone. (B) Relationship between the standardized scores for BAS reward responsiveness and accuracy change differed following left and right DLPFC tDCS enhancement, with a pronounced effect for individuals with negative BAS reward responsiveness scores (BAS−RR+). *Data from Sela et al. (2012), with permission from Elsevier.*

To conclude, the Cerruti and Schlaug (2009) study provided evidence that anodal stimulation of the left DLPFC, a region associated with executive control and working memory functioning, can improve performance on a complex verbal problem-solving task which is believed to require significant executive function capacity.

The Cerruti and Schlaug (2009) findings indicated that stimulating the left DLPFC led to increased fluency when it came to the generation of solutions. Their findings raise interesting questions regarding the influence of tDCS on cognitive control processing, and the role of the left DLPFC in supporting the executive control processes needed to solve verbal insight problems. To describe the underlying neurocognitive processes that may modulate verbal problem solving, Metuki, Sela, and Lavidor (2012) created a stimulation study with a few methodological modifications compared with the procedure used by Cerruti & Schlaug (2009).

First, in order to probe solution recognition separately from solution generation, a different methodological variation of the task was used. Participants were presented with the problem words for a shorter duration of time, and then presented with a target word. Participants were requested to solve the problem while the prime words were presented, and indicate whether the target word was the correct solution or not. Teasing apart the processes enabled sensitive exploration of the specific processes that were modulated by anodal tDCS over the left DLPFC. Then, in order to better characterize the instances in which DLPFC supported cognitive control, items were *a priori* assigned to two groups on the basis of grouped difficulty. Using two problem difficulty levels allowed for a closer examination of the hypothesis that higher complexity or cognitive load calls for more executive control that is supported by the DLPFC.

The Metuki et al., study employed a sham-controlled within design. Twenty-one participants completed two identical experimental sessions administered 1 week apart. Subjects received 1 mA for 11 minutes, with the anodal electrode over the left DLPFC and the reference electrode over the right supraorbital region. The results indicated that for difficult problems alone the anodal tDCS over the left DLPFC enhanced solution recognition, but did not enhance solution generation (see Fig. 11.3). Metuki et al. argued that prefrontal LH cognitive control mechanisms modulate linguistic processing, and suggested the conditions where the facilitation effect was effective and substantial. Both the Cerruti & Schlaug (2009) and Metuki et al. (2012) studies show how the interpretation of facilitation effects is constrained by physiological and cognitive hypotheses as regards site specification (Cerruti & Schlaug, 2009) and experimental conditions (Metuki et al., 2012). Hence, the explanations for the improvement induced by tDCS stimulation draw on a combined cognitive and anatomical theoretical framework (Fecteau & Walsh, 2012) and thus enhance the validity of the results.

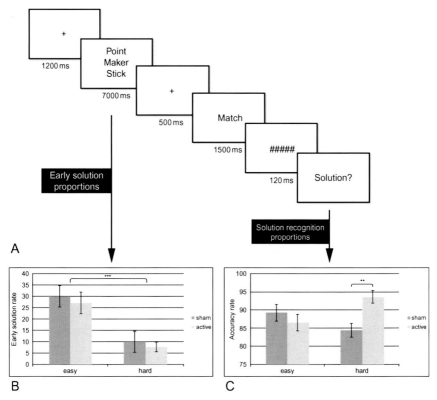

FIGURE 11.3 (A) Task procedure: Each trial began with a central fixation cross which was presented for 1200 milliseconds. The three prime words were then presented simultaneously, above, at, and below the center of the screen. The words remained on the screen for 7 seconds, during which the participants were asked to solve the problem. After a solution was indicated or the time limit was exceeded, a fixation cross reappeared for an additional 500 ms, followed by a presentation of the target word for 1500 ms. Then the word "Solution?" appeared on the screen, and the participants were instructed to indicate whether the target word was the correct solution to the problem or not. On half of the trials the target was the correct solution word, and on the other half it was an unrelated distractor. In this example, the correct solution followed the three problem words. (B) Solution generation: mean early solution rates and SE, by stimulation condition and item difficulty. ***$P < 0.001$. (C) Solution generation: mean early solution rates and SE, by stimulation condition and item difficulty. ***$P < 0.00$. *Data from Metuki et al., 2012, with permission from Elsevier.*

EFFECTS OF tDCS ON COGNITIVE CONTROL

A common feature of human existence is the ability to reverse decisions after they have been made but before they are implemented. This cognitive control process, termed response inhibition, allows individuals to recover from potentially harmful situations before it is too late – for example, avoiding touching a stove after realizing it is hot, or not commenting negatively about a co-worker who suddenly materializes. Cognitive control in general and response inhibition in particular are impaired in several neuropsychiatric disorders, such as attention deficit hyperactivity disorder (ADHD; Aron & Poldrack, 2005), and appear to be critically dependent upon intact function of the right inferior frontal gyrus (rIFG; Aron, Robbins, & Poldrack, 2004).

Response inhibition can be evaluated by the stop-signal task (SST; Logan & Cowan, 1984). In the SST there are two types of trials: *"go"* trials and *"stop"* trials. In the *"go"* trials, subjects are required to make a simple discrimination task within a pre-specified time window; the *"go"* trials are more frequent, thus setting up a pre-potent response tendency. The *"stop"* trials are less frequent, and require subjects to refrain from making the response when a stop signal is randomly presented following the *"go"* signal (Logan & Cowan, 1984).

Cognitive control processes, in general, are attributed mainly to the PFC. Response inhibition has been localized more specifically to the rIFG, based upon both functional brain-imaging and lesion-based approaches. For example, in an fMRI study, Li et al. (2008) showed that successful inhibition was associated with greater activation of multiple cortical areas, and in particular the right inferior and middle frontal gyri. Rubia et al. (2001) also reported common activation foci across different stop task versions in bilateral, but predominantly the right hemispheric inferior, prefrontal cortex. Studies employing temporary deactivation using TMS over the rIFG indeed found impaired inhibitory control (Chambers et al., 2006), supporting the potential role of the rIFG in response inhibition. However, although TMS was successful in establishing an interference stimulation protocol that impaired cognitive control (Figner et al., 2010; Muggleton, Chen, Tzeng, Hung, & Juan, 2010), there are conflicting results as well. For example, the same repetitive stimulation protocol resulted in facilitative effects in several reported studies (Bloch et al., 2010; Cho et al., 2010). The inconsistent effects and other practical limitations of TMS, such as mobility and subjects' comfort, make it less than optimal for developing enhancement stimulation protocols. To date, two teams have employed tDCS on SST tasks using different sites, as described below.

Jacobson, Javitt, and Lavidor (2011) demonstrated that anodal stimulation applied over the rIFG led to significant improvement in SST performance, but not for response time, in a control task that used SST stimuli but did not employ the response inhibition task. In addition, stimulation over the right angular gyrus, an area known to be unrelated to the SST (Chambers et al., 2006), did not affect response inhibition, demonstrating the regional selectivity of the effect. The Jacobson et al. (2011) results support theories of the brain mechanisms underlying response inhibition, and provide a potential method for behavioral modification.

A different research team targeted a different area, since other cortical areas are also involved in the cognitive control network. Li, Huang, Constable, and Sinha (2006) systematically investigated the neural correlates of motor inhibition with the stop-signal task, and found a linear correlation between the blood oxygen-level dependent (BOLD) activation of the pre-supplementary motor area (pre-SMA) and SST performance. More recently, Hsu et al. (2011) conducted a tDCS SST study to investigate the functional role of the pre-SMA in motor inhibition. Three tDCS conditions were employed: pre-SMA anodal/left cheek cathodal, left cheek anodal/ pre-SMA cathodal, and a control group with no tDCS stimulation. The current intensity was set at 1.5 mA for 10 minutes. Hsu et al. (2011) found that the effects of inhibitory (cathodal) tDCS replicated previous TMS findings by impairing performance on the task. The pattern was similar to TMS findings in the sense that there was marked failure to inhibit responses when a stop signal was presented (an elevated non-cancelled rate). Furthermore, facilitatory effects were observed after applying excitatory (anodal) tDCS over the pre-SMA. These decreased non-cancelled rates suggested an improvement in the inhibition of responses when a stop signal was presented. Such improvement or decrement in non-cancelled rates implies that neuronal excitability was modulated by tDCS, as many studies have suggested (Nitsche & Paulus, 2000). These findings also suggest a critical role for the pre-SMA in suppressing unwanted actions and facilitating desired ones, as seen in a microstimulaton study (Isoda & Hikosaka, 2007). Together, such effects on non-cancelled rates provide direct evidence that the region containing the pre-SMA is also important for inhibitory control.

Whether they involve the pre-SMA or the rIFG, SST studies clearly demonstrate a potential for clinical tDCS intervention in individuals experiencing difficulties with inhibitory control. However, further research is needed to more fully understand the nature of the neuronal changes following tDCS that enable modification of cognitive control (which here was measured by SST performance). Jacobson, Ezra, Berger, and Lavidor (2012) conducted an electroencephalography (EEG)-tDCS study that points to a possible neuronal mechanism for tDCS effects in the SST. They found that the rIFG stimulation protocol implemented in their behavioral SST study (Jacobson et al., 2011) generated a significant and selective diminution of the power of the theta band (4–7 Hz). The theta diminution was observed in the rIFG area (represented by the anode electrode), and was not found in the contralateral supraorbital region (represented by the cathode electrode). A significant effect was only observed in the theta but not in other bands. Since there is evidence that the electrophysiological activity associated with behavioral inhibition is theta band activity (Lansbergen, Schutter, & Kenemans, 2007; Wienbruch, Paul, Bauer, & Kivelitz, 2005), these results may help account for the improvement in behavioral inhibition following tDCS over the rIFG (see Fig. 11.4).

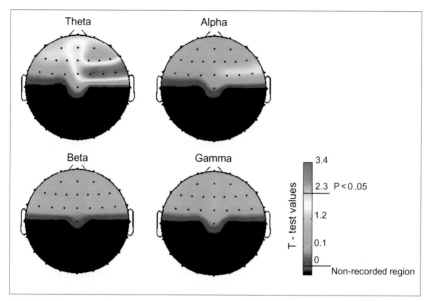

FIGURE 11.4   Electrophysiological changes following anodal stimulation of the rIFG. T-maps representing the difference in the power for each of the four analyzed bands (theta, alpha, beta, gamma) between anodal and sham stimulation conditions. Red indicates significant difference ($P < 0.05$); black represents non-recorded regions. *Data from Jacobson et al., 2012, with permission from MIT Press.*

EFFECTS OF tDCS ON LEARNING AND MEMORY

Flöel and colleagues examined tDCS effects on language learning and the acquisition of novel vocabulary (Flöel, Rösser, Michka, Knecht, & Breitenstein, 2008). In their experiment, tDCS stimulation was applied over the posterior part of the left perisylvian area in 19 young right-handed individuals, while participants had to acquire a miniature lexicon of 30 novel object names. This study employed a double-blind, sham-controlled within design. Each participant was given anodal, cathodal (each 20 min of 1 mA), and sham sessions in a randomized, counterbalanced manner. The results showed that with anodal stimulation, participants exhibited better associative learning in the fifth block as compared to sham and cathodal stimulation. Mood ratings, blood pressure, heart rate, discomfort, RTs, and response styles were similar across stimulation conditions. Importantly, transfer of the vocabulary into participants' native language was also significantly better after learning under anodal tDCS than under cathodal tDCS and sham. However, no significant difference between the conditions was found for the lexical knowledge test after 1 week. This study was the first to show that anodal tDCS, when applied on the left hemisphere, significantly improves the acquisition of a novel vocabulary (faster learning and higher overall success) in healthy subjects.

The De Vries et al. (2010) study was the first to demonstrate how tDCS facilitates the acquisition of grammatical knowledge. In this study, tDCS was used to investigate putative causal relationships between Broca's area and the learning of novel grammar. Artificial grammar learning constitutes a well-established model for the acquisition of grammatical knowledge in a natural setting. Thirty-eight healthy subjects participated in a between-subject, sham-controlled design. Stimulation included either anodal tDCS (20 min, 1 mA) over Broca's area during the acquisition of an artificial grammar or sham stimulation. The reference electrode was placed over the contralateral supraorbital region. The experiment consisted of an acquisition phase, which was presented as a working memory task (for 25 minutes) and a classification phase. Performance during the acquisition phase was comparable between groups. In the subsequent classification task, detecting syntactic violations improved significantly after anodal tDCS, resulting in overall better performance. Specifically, anodal tDCS over Broca's area during the acquisition process of an artificial grammar enhanced subsequent classification performance. Enhanced performance was manifested by better performance on syntactic violation detection and rule-based decisions. The authors argued that Broca's area is specifically involved in rule-based knowledge, and showed that it is possible to improve subjects' ability to detect syntactic violations.

Fiori and colleagues investigated potential tDCS enhancement of associative learning in healthy participants (Fiori et al., 2011: Experiment 1). Three experimental conditions were used in a randomized counterbalanced double-blind design over a 3-week period: anodal stimulation of the left Wernicke's area, and, as a control group, sham stimulation in the left Wernicke's area and anodal stimulation of the right occipitoparietal area. The experiment involved three phases: training, verification, and word retrieval. tDCS was only applied during the third phase. Ten healthy individuals were tested individually in a single daily session, and had to learn 20 new "words" (legal non-words which were arbitrarily assigned to 20 different pictures). Left anodal stimulation led to significant facilitation in picture naming with regard to vocal response times but not to naming accuracy. The authors highlighted the fact that their results showed that tDCS improves performance not only during the recognition of new words (Flöel et al., 2008) but also during word retrieval.

EFFECTS OF tDCS ON WORKING MEMORY

In "active maintenance" working memory (WM) tasks such as the n-back task, participants are required to continuously load and unload potential targets in WM, since the unexpected presentation of the probe demands that they match the current item to an item that appeared n items ago. In addition, on the n-back task, the neural substrates (e.g., DLPFC) involved constantly attempting to inhibit the activation of non-relevant items that appeared in previously encountered non-target displays. Therefore, this type of cognitive effort is likely to recruit executive control mechanisms (e.g., DLPFC), which are conceptualized to regulate goals so as to enable coherent and contextually appropriate behaviors in interference-rich conditions (Kane & Engle, 2002; Sandrini, Rossini, & Miniussi, 2008). Fregni et al. (2005) reported greater accuracy on a three-back WM task during anodal tDCS of the left PFC, whereas cathodal tDCS of the same area or anodal stimulation of the primary motor cortex (M1) had no effect. The authors concluded that left-PFC anodal stimulation leads to enhancement of WM performance. Their results were later confirmed by other investigators (Andrews, Hoy, Enticott, Daskalakis, & Fitzgerald, 2011; Ohn et al., 2008). In addition, the neurophysiological basis for modulation of WM by the left DLPFC was investigated by recording the underlying electroencephalographic activity (Zaehle, Sandmann, Thorne, Jäncke, & Herrmann, 2011). After anodal tDCS, oscillatory power in the theta and alpha bands was amplified and WM performance enhanced; on the other hand, cathodal tDCS decreased alpha and theta oscillatory activity and disrupted WM.

Although left PFC anodal stimulation increases accuracy without changing response times, bifrontal tDCS has been found to slow reaction times in a WM task (Marshall, Mölle, Siebner, & Born, 2005). The protocol in this experiment was rather unusual, and included 15 minutes of non-continuous stimulation (15 s on/15 s off), while subjects performed a modified Sternberg task. In contrast to these findings, in a more conventional protocol, Ferrucci et al. (2008) reported no increase in accuracy using bilateral prefrontal tDCS and faster reaction times after cathodal bilateral tDCS of the prefrontal cortices during a modified Sternberg task.

However, other brain regions have also been successfully stimulated to affect WM performance. A brief period of practice or even increased familiarity with a task can improve WM performance and lead to activation changes in the PPC in neuroimaging studies. Parietal tDCS was shown to be capable of hampering improvement in performance, thus lending further weight to the role of the PPC in this kind of task (Sandrini, Fertonani, Cohen, & Miniussi, 2012). Normal subjects underwent cathodal tDCS to the right inferior PPC, and then performed separate blocks of an object WM task probed by recall or recognition. WM was selectively impaired in recognition tasks, as is usually the case for patients with parietal lesions (Berryhill, Wencil, Coslett, & Olson, 2010). Thus, parietal involvement in WM performance may depend on both WM capacity and WM task demands (Jones & Berryhill, 2012).

The consensus is that anodal tDCS over the left DLPFC is most likely to affect WM when measured by the n-back task. The combination of anodal tDCS applied to the DLPFC with a WM task was shown to be superior to either tDCS or the cognitive task alone in improving the performance of a subsequent digit span forward task (Andrews et al., 2011). The effect of tRNS of the left DLPFC on a WM task was compared to the effects of tDCS applied to the same region (Mulquiney, Hoy, Daskalakis, & Fitzgerald, 2011). Whereas tDCS increased the speed of performance of the two-back WM task, tRNS had no effect.

EFFECTS OF tDCS ON NUMERICAL COGNITION

Numerical cognition is a fundamental ability that is essential for everyday life. Dyscalculia, a deficit in mastering the manipulation of abstract concepts and symbols such as numbers, can lead to serious personal, social, and economic difficulties (Lepage & Théoret, 2010). Neuroimaging studies focusing at the neural basis of numerical ability have repeatedly shown that the involvement of the posterior parietal cortex is crucial for this type of processing, and, more specifically, the intra-parietal sulcus (IPS; see Dehaene, Piazza, Pinel, & Cohen, 2003; Eger, Sterzer, Russ, Giraud, & Kleinschmidt, 2003). TMS studies reviewed by Sandrini and Rusconi (2009) confirmed the causal role of parietal cortex in numerical processing. Cohen Kadosh, Soskic, Iuculano, Kanai, and Walsh (2010) investigated whether tDCS to the parietal lobe during numerical learning can selectively improve numerical abilities.

In their experiment, subjects were trained over 6 days to assign a magnitude value to a series of abstract symbols, with each artificial digit represented by a number. Subjects were asked to repeatedly compare two symbols presented side by side, and to indicate which was of greater magnitude. Feedback was provided online to participants in order to generate learning. After each training session, numerical ability with the abstract symbols was evaluated using two standard tasks (numerical Stroop and number-to-space tests). At the beginning of each training day, when the learning phase started, a current of 1 mA was applied over the parietal cortex. Electrodes were positioned over the left and right parietal lobes. A total of 15 subjects were randomly assigned to one of three groups: right anodal/left cathodal, right cathodal/left anodal, and sham stimulation. The results showed that the polarity of the brain stimulation specifically enhanced or impaired the acquisition of automatic number processing and the mapping of numbers into space, which are both important indices of numerical proficiency. Right cathodal/left anodal stimulation led to impaired numerical ability on abstract symbols, whereas right anodal/left cathodal tDCS improved learning such that improvements in numerical ability occurred more rapidly and were of greater magnitude than in the sham stimulation. Furthermore, control tasks revealed that the effect of the stimulation was specific to the representation of the newly acquired artificial numerical symbols, although proficiency with everyday digits remained unchanged with stimulation.

Remarkably, the improvement was still present 6 months after the training. The authors argued that this long-lasting improvement in numerical abilities may be a first stage toward establishing a tool for intervention in cases of atypical numerical development or loss of numerical abilities as a result of stroke or degenerative illnesses.

Cohen Kadosh et al. (2010) suggested that tDCS could be used as a tool to improve cognitive functioning among healthy individuals, with long-lived beneficial aftereffects. However, more recently Iuculano and Cohen Kadosh (2013) noted a possible drawback in the form of a possible cognitive side-effect after repeated sessions of tDCS combined with training. Based on available reports from different tDCS studies (see Brunoni et al., 2011, for a systematic review of adverse effects; see also Chapter 3), the general impression is that tDCS is a safe technique with mild and transient adverse effects, including itching, tingling, headache, and discomfort. However, these reports mainly come from single-session studies in healthy volunteers, and not from studies in which subjects underwent multiple stimulation sessions. Furthermore, most studies did not focus on cognitive side effects.

In the Iuculano and Cohen Kadosh (2013) study, healthy subjects underwent cognitive training for 6 days on a new numerical set while receiving tDCS to the posterior parietal cortex or the DLPFC. Stimulation to the posterior parietal cortex facilitated numerical learning, whereas automaticity for the learned material was impaired. In contrast, stimulation to the DLPFC impaired the learning process, whereas automaticity for the learned material was enhanced. This finding may indicate that cognitive enhancement can occur at the expense of other cognitive functions.

Nonetheless, it is important to note that performance with everyday digits was not modulated by tDCS, which suggests that the cognitive cost was limited to the specific learned material, and did not interact with well-established fundamental numerical abilities. Moreover, since the Iuculano and Cohen Kadosh, (2013) study was the first to report a cognitive side-effect, much work still needs to be done to determine whether this "mental cost" is domain (or task) specific, or whether in general the enhancement of a specific cognitive ability might have adverse effects on another.

NEURAL UNDERPINNING OF tDCS EFFECTS ON COGNITION

Behavioral changes resulting from tDCS manipulation are the prime criteria for assessing whether a particular set of stimulation parameters (e.g., electrode positions and sizes, stimulation intensity and length) have transient or long-lasting effects. Neuroimaging and electroencephalography methods are employed to evaluate the nature of the changes that occur after anodal or cathodal stimulation.

Based on the finding that anodal tDCS over the left DLPFC results in better naming performance in healthy participants (Fertonani et al., 2010; Iyer et al., 2005), Wirth and others used EEG to investigate the putative neurophysiological mechanism underpinning language production (Wirth et al., 2011). Behavioral results showed a reduction in semantic interference after anodal stimulation, whereas no change in performance was found for the picture-naming task. The electrophysiological data showed that the behavioral reduction in semantic interference correlated with an enhancement over left temporal scalp-electrode sites compared to right temporal scalp-electrode sites. This modulation was suggested to reflect a tuning of neural responses within language-related generators. After anodal tDCS there was a reduction in delta activity during picture naming and the resting state, which was interpreted to indicate neural disinhibition. The authors suggested that anodal tDCS is capable of enhancing neural processes during and after application, and claimed that the null effects with respect to their offline naming task can be explained by a variety of methodological limitations, such as tDCS inter-electrode distance (cf. Moliadze, Antal, & Paulus, 2010), protocol characteristics, and the stimulation duration (cf. Fricke et al., 2011; Moliadze et al., 2010; Nitsche et al., 2008). However, it is important to note one shortcoming in the Wirth et al. (2011) study: it is highly possible that the null effect resulted from a basic problem with their experimental design. Crucially, the inclusion of an extensive activation of the language system (30 minutes of semantic blocking and tDCS stimulation during this period) may have confounded possible interpretations for the null effect. It is hard to determine whether the stimulation by itself did not produce an effect on the naming task, or whether the procedure caused the failure to replicate the effect.

Holland and colleagues tested whether tDCS over the left inferior frontal cortex (IFC) can be used to increase spoken picture-naming performance in neurologically unimpaired individuals (Holland et al., 2011). For all participants, the anode was placed over the left IFC with the cathode placed over the contralateral frontopolar cortex. The results showed a significant effect of left anodal tDCS on naming latency responses when compared to responses during sham stimulation. The fMRI measures showed that left anodal tDCS significantly reduced the BOLD signal in the left frontal cortex, including Broca's area, compared to sham responses. The imaging data also showed a regionally specific effect. Within the stimulated frontal cortex, not all regions were equally affected; Broca's area, but not other regions (e.g., precentral or anterior insular cortices), was modulated by anodal tDCS. Holland and colleagues suggested that the reduction of the BOLD signal in Broca's area might be analogous to the neural priming effects that are seen when utilizing behavioral priming paradigms.

More recently, Meinzer et al. (2012) used an fMRI design to assess the impact of anodal tDCS on semantic word-generation in 20 healthy young adults. In a cross-over sham-controlled study, fMRI was used to investigate neurofunctional correlations of improved language functions as induced by 1 mA anodal or sham tDCS over a core language area, the left IFG. The reference electrode was fixed over the contralateral supraorbital region. In general, the results showed that improved semantic word-generation during anodal tDCS compared with sham stimulation was associated with selectively reduced activity in the ventral portion of the IFG. Specifically, improved word-retrieval during anodal tDCS was paralleled by selectively reduced task-related activation in the left ventral IFG, an area which is specifically implicated in semantic retrieval processes. Moreover, under anodal tDCS, resting-state fMRI revealed increased connectivity of the left IFG and additional major hubs that overlap with the language network.

Keeser and colleagues investigated whether tDCS of the prefrontal cortex can modulate resting-state network connectivity as measured by fMRI (Keeser et al., 2011). In this study, 13 healthy subjects underwent real and sham tDCS in random order on separate days. tDCS was applied for 20 minutes at 2 mA with the anode positioned over the left DLPFC and the cathode over the right supraorbital region. Brain connectivity patterns of the resting-state network were assessed before and after tDCS or sham stimulation. The impact of active tDCS versus sham was examined based on observed activation changes in four resting-state networks, which included the default mode network, the left and right frontal-parietal networks, and the self-referential network. When the real tDCS was compared to the sham tDCS, the results showed that significant changes of regional brain connectivity were found for the default mode network and the frontal-parietal networks, both of which are close to the primary stimulation site and in connected brain regions. These findings suggest that prefrontal tDCS modulates resting-state functional connectivity in distinct functional networks of the human brain.

EFFECTS OF tDCS ON COGNITIVE FUNCTIONS: METHODOLOGICAL CONSIDERATIONS

A number of methodological considerations and caveats must be addressed in order to claim that a genuine effect has been found, and as such may be considered reliable and replicable. This section outlines some important steps for future experimental work in cognition using tDCS (see also Flöel 2012; Holland & Crinion, 2012).

Different stimulation montages are used to explore cognitive functions. In general, these can be divided into two types of montages. The first is the so-called unilateral stimulation method, in which the target location is excited or inhibited with the "active" electrode while the "reference" electrode is placed in an unrelated area (mostly contralateral frontopolar cortex; Sparing et al., 2008). The second, as in other studies of cognition (e.g., Hecht et al., 2010), involves bilateral placement (cf. Sela et al., 2012). The obvious advantage of the former is that it guarantees, to some extent, that the stimulation modifies a specific region of interest (but see modeling data reviewed in Chapter 4). The primary caveat of this method is that the use of the contralateral frontopolar cortex as the default region for the "reference" electrode may be reasonable when stimulating the motor cortex (Nitsche & Paulus, 2000), but not when the aim is to modify cognitive functions that may be related to the activation of this region or nearby regions. In any case, it is highly advisable to use a large reference electrode (e.g., 10×10 cm^2) when employing this type of montage, as reported for instance in the Meinzer et al. (2012) study, since the increased size of the reference electrode most likely renders the stimulation functionally inefficient without compromising tDCS effects under the active electrode (Stagg & Nitsche, 2011). The main advantage of the latter bilateral placement is based on the idea that if the two electrodes are both placed over cortical areas, tDCS can be used to simultaneously increase excitability in one region and decrease excitability in another region (cf. Sela et al., 2012) or affect interhemispheric connections between the stimulated regions (cf. Cohen Kadosh et al., 2010).

This method has advantages if the main hypothesis tackles issues of brain asymmetry and/or the combined involvement of the two cerebral hemispheres (or any other two regions) in a specific function (Hecht et al., 2010). Nevertheless, this method may suffer from potential confounding effects of two electrodes with opposite polarities over the brain, and may require further stimulation conditions in the form of unilateral stimulation. Alternatively, this shortcoming can be resolved by an experimental task design that includes two or more levels of the independent variable that are expected to be affected in inverse directions after bilateral stimulation. This way, one can argue that the effect is the result of a combined increased excitability in one region and decreased excitability in another region. For example, the design could employ stimulation type as one within-subject factor, with one sham condition and two bilateral active conditions (A & B, with inverse polarity), and one within-subject factor of the task with two or more levels (X_1, X_2). The idea is to be able to create an experiment that can test for a differential tDCS effect; for example, bilateral condition A will produce an effect on level X_1 but not on X_2, whereas the opposite bilateral condition (B) will exert its effect solely on level X_2 but not on level X_1. Moreover, a design in which one condition (A) shows enhancement of performance on one level and leads to a decline in performance on the other level, while the opposite bilateral condition (B) shows a reversed effect, would be even more persuasive.

Another option is to set up an experiment which explores double dissociations between tasks. For instance, a design could be used in which task (A, B) and location sites (frontal, occipital) serve as the within-subject factors. A valid result would be to show that performance for task A alone improved after frontal but not after occipital stimulation, with the complementary effect for task B.

Another possible electrode placement that is gaining in popularity is to use multiple small electrodes (i.e., around 1.2-cm diameter) to achieve effective targeted stimulation while ensuring the safety of the stimulation (see also Dmochowski, Datta, Bikson, Su, & Parra, 2011, and Chapter 4). As noted by Holland and Crinion (2012), the "best" approach is not always directly apparent. Deciding which of the above methods of placement to use involves consideration of other important parameters, such as stimuli duration, electrode size, and current intensity, in addition to more general considerations that include the nature of the function in question, the task at hand, and other design parameters.

Other key considerations that should be addressed include which would be the best design to use (within/between/mixed), when to start the stimulation (stimulation timing), how many control conditions should be included, optimal sample size, and so on. All these issues are inherent to the nature of the task and the task specifications. For example, including a control task may be important when the task by itself produces only one primary measure. In this case, it is recommended to include a control task to verify effect specificity. Including such a control has implications with respect to stimulation duration, the necessity of counterbalancing tasks presentation, and so on. Moreover, task properties should be examined carefully when deciding on the appropriate experimental design. For instance, tasks that are known to produce high inter-subject variability should naturally be tested with a within-subject design. However, what happens if the task involves learning, and the subject's performance is qualitatively changed after a single exposure? Another problem that arises frequently in cognitive research is that the number of stimuli is limited and there are many experimental conditions within the task, hence multiple sessions are not always an option. There are many ways to cope with these types of questions – a topic that goes beyond the scope of this chapter.

Nevertheless, the issue of controlling alternative explanations should be addressed thoroughly. It is obvious that a single study cannot cover all the bases, as doing so would result in endless control groups. However, it is highly advisable to deal with the most crucial alternative explanations for a given experiment, and at least use (1) a sham condition, (2) site control, (3) polarity control, and (4) a task or condition (within the main task) control. As in other domains of behavioral research, it is clear that any evidence for a "single dissociation" is good, but experimental designs should aim to produce evidence for a "double dissociation" (e.g., Iuculano & Cohen Kadosh, 2013). Finally, with respect to current intensity and the use of current density as a possible control (see Flöel, 2012; Nitsche et al., 2008), it is surprising that the Iyer et al. (2005) study is one of the few to examine how different levels of current intensity (1 mA and 2 mA) affect cognitive performance. It is clear that many other tDCS effects may be intensity-dependent; hence this parameter should be subjected to systematic manipulation in future studies.

DISCUSSION AND FUTURE DIRECTIONS

The utility of using tDCS to explore novel theoretical hypotheses and uncover the neural basis of the cognitive system is evident, though still in its early stages (see also Kuo & Nitsche, 2012). As shown in this chapter, studies have tackled intriguing questions such as the ability to improve WM (e.g., Andrews et al., 2011), the contribution of the PFC to language comprehension and production (e.g., Cerruti & Schlaug, 2009; Iyer et al., 2005), issues of connectivity (e.g., Meinzer et al., 2012), and other studies which may pave the way to improving cognitive control functioning among healthy subjects (e.g., Hsu et al., 2011) by using a simple, low-cost, and safe method.

Another tES method used to investigate and manipulate brain activity is tACS. tACS is thought to induce regional brain oscillations in a frequency-dependent manner, thereby interacting with specific functions of the stimulated region (Kanai, Chaieb, Antal, Walsh, & Paulus, 2008; Kanai, Paulus, & Walsh, 2010; Pogosyan, Gaynor, Eusebio, & Brown, 2009; Thut & Miniussi 2009; Zaehle, Rach, & Herrmann, 2010). Oscillatory activity is suggested to play an important role in linking crosstalk between brain areas (Thut & Miniussi, 2009), and it has been argued that oscillations are particularly instrumental in top-down processing (Engel, Fries, & Singer, 2001) or in the large-scale integration of bottom-up and top-down processes (Varela, Lachaux, Rodriguez, & Martinerie, 2001). Although this technique is still largely unexplored and volume conduction effects are not wholly understood (Feurra et al., 2011; Kanai et al., 2010; Schutter & Hortensius, 2011; Zaghi, Acar, Hultgren, Boggio, & Fregni, 2010), recent studies have demonstrated tACS efficiency in different domains. For instance, Kanai et al. (2010) showed that cortical excitability of the visual cortex as measured by the thresholds for TMS evoked phosphenes exhibits frequency dependency, where 20-Hz tACS over the visual cortex enhanced the sensitivity of the visual cortex. A recent study demonstrated that stimulation in the alpha and gamma bands over the associative sensory cortex induced positive sensory sensations (Feurra et al., 2011; for further examples and discussion see Chapter 7). It has also been demonstrated that tACS at prefrontal sites during sleep improved procedural memory consolidation (Marshall, Helgadóttir, Mölle, & Born, 2006), and Sela et al. (2012) showed that theta stimulation over the left DLPFC can alter decision-making strategies in a risk-taking game.

Given the enormous potential of tACS (Kuo & Nitsche, 2012), in the near future this method is likely to serve to explore basic questions in cognition by analyzing the huge amount of electrophysiological data gathered so far. For example, it has been proposed that an increase in theta activity (4–7 Hz) might mediate language and memory functions (Klimesch, 1999; Klimesch et al., 2001; Röhm, Klimesch, Haider, & Doppelmayr, 2001).

Another tES method, which although still in its infancy is beginning to receive a great deal of attention because some research (e.g., Fertonani et al., 2011) points to its superiority over tDCS, is tRNS. So far, only a few studies have used tRNS to explore and modify brain activity related to cognitive functions, but the findings are very promising. For example, Snowball et al. (2013) used 5 consecutive days of tRNS over the DLPFC interlaced with cognitive training to improve mathematical abilities. During tRNS or sham stimulation, subjects were engaged in a calculation task and a drill learning task. The results showed that the tRNS group was significantly better than the sham, showing an improvement in both calculation and drill learning. These behavioral improvements were accompanied by defined hemodynamic responses, as measured by near-infrared spectroscopy (NIRS), which is consistent with the claim that a more efficient neurovascular coupling within the left DLPFC may subserve mental arithmetic abilities. Six months later, about half of the subjects returned to the laboratory (12 subjects, 6 subjects from tRNS group) and were asked to answer similar mathematical problems. The results showed the tRNS groups showed behavioral improvement of extreme longevity relative to sham controls for trained and non-trained calculation material, whereas no differences were found with respect to drill learning. These results demonstrate that, depending on the learning domain, tRNS can induce long-term enhancement of neurocognitive functions.

CONCLUSION

The role of tDCS in boosting cognitive functions clearly makes it a major player in the contemporary effort to establish cognitive enhancement protocols. For example, behavioral experiments in the context of language production have provided crucial findings (e.g., Iyer et al., 2005) and have further documented the neural substructure of tDCS effects on the healthy brain (e.g., Holland et al., 2011; Wirth et al., 2011). These studies promote better understanding of the complex relationship between brain and behavior in the context of language production, and lay the groundwork for rehabilitation efforts (for a comprehensive review, see Flöel, 2012; Holland & Crinion, 2012; and Chapters 12–14). Future work within the realm of tDCS and cognitive functions will doubtless further refine the type of theoretical questions that are raised (e.g., Meinzer et al., 2012) and draw on the "proof of principle" established by current research to explore new areas of cognition.

Acknowledgments

This chapter presents studies that were supported by the Israel Academy of Sciences, grant no. 100/10; the Israeli Center of Research Excellence (I-CORE) in Cognition (I-CORE Program 51/11); and an ERC starting grant which was awarded to ML (Inspire 200512).

References

Alvarez, J. A., & Emory, E. (2006). Executive function and the frontal lobes: A meta-analytic review. *Neuropsychology Review, 16*(1), 17–42.

Andrews, S. C., Hoy, K. E., Enticott, P. G., Daskalakis, Z. J., & Fitzgerald, P. B. (2011). Improving working memory: The effect of combining cognitive activity and anodal transcranial direct current stimulation to the left dorsolateral prefrontal cortex. *Brain Stimulation, 4*, 84–89.

Antal, A., Boros, K., Poreisz, C., Chaieb, L., Terney, D., & Paulus, W. (2008). Comparatively weak after-effects of transcranial alternating current stimulation (tACS) on cortical excitability in humans. *Brain Stimulation, 1*(2), 97–105.

Aron, A. R., & Poldrack, R. A. (2005). The cognitive neuroscience of response inhibition: Relevance for genetic research in attention-deficit/hyperactivity disorder. *Biological Psychiatry, 57*, 1285–1292.

Aron, A. R., Robbins, T., & Poldrack, R. A. (2004). Inhibition and the right inferior frontal cortex. *Trends in Cognitive Sciences, 8*, 170–177.

Batsikadze, G., Moliadze, V., Paulus, W., Kuo, M. -F., & Nitsche, M. A. (2013). Partially non-linear stimulation intensity-dependent effects of direct current stimulation on motor cortex excitability in humans. *Journal of Physiology, 591*, 1987–2000.

Berryhill, M. E., Wencil, E. B., Coslett, H. B., & Olson, I. R. (2010). A selective working memory impairment after transcranial direct current stimulation to the right parietal lobe. *Neuroscience Letters, 479*, 312–316.

Bloch, Y., Harel, E. V., Aviram, S., Govezensky, J., Ratzoni, G., & Levkovitz, Y. (2010). Positive effects of repetitive transcranial magnetic stimulation on attention in ADHD Subjects: A randomized controlled pilot study. *World Journal of Biological Psychiatry, 11*, 755–758.

Boggio, P. S., Khoury, L. P., Martins, D. C. S., Martins, O. E. M. S., Macedo, E. C. D., & Fregni, F. (2009). Temporal cortex direct current stimulation enhances performance on a visual recognition memory task in Alzheimer disease. *Journal of Neurology, 80*(4), 444–447.

Broca, P. (1865). Sur le siège de la faculté du langage articulé. *Bulletins de la Société d'Anthropologie de Paris, 6*(1), 377–393.

Brunoni, A. R., Amadera, J., Berbel, B., Volz, M. S., Rizzerio, B. G., & Fregni, F. (2011). A systematic review on reporting and assessment of adverse effects associated with transcranial direct current stimulation. *International Journal of Neuropsychopharmacology, 14*(8), 1133–1145.

Cappa, S. F., Sandrini, M., Rossini, P. M., Sosta, K., & Miniussi, C. (2002). The role of the left frontal lobe in action naming: rTMS evidence. *Neurology, 59*(5), 720–723.

Carver, C. S., & White, T. L. (1994). Behavioral inhibition, behavioral activation, and affective responses to impending reward and punishment: The BIS/BAS scales *Journal of Personality and Social Psychology, 67*, 319.

Cerruti, C., & Schlaug, G. (2009). Anodal transcranial direct current stimulation of the prefrontal cortex enhances complex verbal associative thought. *Journal of Cognitive Neuroscience, 21*(10), 1980–1987.

Chambers, C. D., Bellgrove, M. A., Stokes, M. G., Henderson, T. R., Garavan, H., Robertson, I. H., et al. (2006). Executive "Brake Failure" following deactivation of human frontal lobe. *Journal of Cognitive Neuroscience, 18*, 444–455.

Cho, S. S., Ko, J. H., Pellecchia, G., Eimeren, T. V., Cilia, R., & Strafella, A. P. (2010). Continuous theta burst stimulation of right dorsolateral prefrontal cortex induces changes in impulsivity level. *Brain Stimulation, 3*, 170–176.

Cohen Kadosh, R., Soskic, S., Iuculano, T., Kanai, R., & Walsh, V. (2010). Modulating neuronal activity produces specific and long-lasting changes in numerical competence. *Current Biology, 20*(22), 2016–2020.

De Vries, M. H., Barth, A. C. R., Maiworm, S., Knecht, S., Zwitserlood, P., & Flöel, A. (2010). Electrical stimulation of Broca's area enhances implicit learning of an artificial grammar. *Journal of Cognitive Neuroscience, 22*(11), 2427–2436.

Dehaene, S., Piazza, M., Pinel, P., & Cohen, L. (2003). Three parietal circuits for number processing. *Cognitive Neuropsychology, 20*(3–6), 487–506.

Dmochowski, J. P., Datta, A., Bikson, M., Su, Y., & Parra, L. C. (2011). Optimized multi-electrode stimulation increases focality and intensity at target. *Journal of Neural Engineering, 8*(4), 046011.

Eger, E., Sterzer, P., Russ, M. O., Giraud, A. L., & Kleinschmidt, A. (2003). A supramodal number representation in human intraparietal cortex. *Neuron, 37*(4), 719–726.

Engel, A. K., Fries, P., & Singer, W. (2001). Dynamic predictions: Oscillations and synchrony in top-down processing. *Nature Reviews. Neuroscience, 2*(10), 704–716.

Farah, M. J., Illes, J., Cook-Deegan, R., Gardner, H., Kandel, E., King, P., et al. (2004). Neurocognitive enhancement: What can we do and what should we do? *Nature Reviews. Neuroscience, 5*(5), 421–425.

Fecteau, S., Knoch, D., Fregni, F., Sultani, N., Boggio, P., & Pascual-Leone, A. (2007). Diminishing risk-taking behavior by modulating activity in the prefrontal cortex: A direct current stimulation study. *Journal of Neuroscience, 27*(46), 12500–12505.

Fecteau, S., Pascual-Leone, A., Zald, D. H., Liguori, P., Theoret, H., Boggio, P. S., et al. (2007). Activation of prefrontal cortex by transcranial direct current stimulation reduces appetite for risk during ambiguous decision making. *Journal of Neuroscience, 27*(23), 6212–6218.

Fecteau, S., & Walsh, V. (2012). Introduction: Brain stimulation in cognitive neuroscience. *Brain Stimulation, 5*(2), 61–62.

Ferrucci, R., Marceglia, S., Vergari, M., Cogiamanian, F., Mrakic-Sposta, S., Mameli, F., et al. (2008). Cerebellar transcranial direct current stimulation impairs the practice-dependent proficiency increase in working memory. *Journal of Cognitive Neuroscience, 20*, 1687–1697.

Fertonani, A., Pirulli, C., & Miniussi, C. (2011). Random noise stimulation improves neuroplasticity in perceptual learning. *Journal of Neuroscience, 31*(43), 15416–15423.

Fertonani, A., Rosini, S., Cotelli, M., Rossini, P. M., & Miniussi, C. (2010). Naming facilitation induced by transcranial direct current stimulation. *Behavioural Brain Research, 208*(2), 311–318.

Feurra, M., Bianco, G., Santarnecchi, E., Del Testa, M., Rossi, A., & Rossi, S. (2011). Frequency-dependent tuning of the human motor system induced by transcranial oscillatory potentials. *Journal of Neuroscience, 31*(34), 12165–12170.

Figner, B., Knoch, D., Johnson, E. J., Krosch, A. R., Lisanby, S. H., Fehr, E., et al. (2010). Lateral prefrontal cortex and self-control in intertemporal choice. *Nature Neuroscience, 13*, 538–539.

Fiori, V., Coccia, M., Marinelli, C. V., Vecchi, V., Bonifazi, S., Ceravolo, M. G., et al. (2011). Transcranial direct current stimulation improves word retrieval in healthy and nonfluent aphasic subjects. *Journal of Cognitive Neuroscience, 23*(9), 2309–2323.

Flöel, A. (2012). Non-invasive brain stimulation and language processing in the healthy brain. *Aphasiology, 26*(9), 1082–1102.

Flöel, A., Rösser, N., Michka, O., Knecht, S., & Breitenstein, C. (2008). Noninvasive brain stimulation improves language learning. *Journal of Cognitive Neuroscience, 20*(8), 1415–1422.

Fregni, F., Boggio, P. S., Nitsche, M., Bermpohl, F., Antal, A., Feredoes, E., et al. (2005). Anodal transcranial direct current stimulation of prefrontal cortex enhances working memory. *Experimental Brain Research, 166*(1), 23–30.

Fricke, K., Seeber, A. A., Thirugnanasambandam, N., Paulus, W., Nitsche, M. A., & Rothwell, J. C. (2011). Time course of the induction of homeostatic plasticity generated by repeated transcranial direct current stimulation of the human motor cortex. *Journal of Neurophysiology, 105*(3), 1141–1149.

Gandiga, P. C., Hummel, F. C., & Cohen, L. G. (2006). Transcranial DC stimulation (tDCS): A tool for double-blind sham-controlled clinical studies in brain stimulation. *Clinical Neurophysiology, 117*(4), 845–850.

Hecht, D., Walsh, V., & Lavidor, M. (2010). Transcranial direct current stimulation facilitates decision making in a probabilistic guessing task. *The Journal of Neuroscience, 30*(12), 4241–4245.

Hirshorn, E. A., & Thompson-Schill, S. L. (2006). Role of the left inferior frontal gyrus in covert word retrieval: Neural correlates of switching during verbal fluency. *Neuropsychologia, 44* (12), 2547–2557.

Holland, R., & Crinion, J. (2012). Can tDCS enhance treatment of aphasia after stroke? *Aphasiology, 26*(9), 1169–1191.

Holland, R., Leff, A. P., Josephs, O., Galea, J. M., Desikan, M., Price, C. J., et al. (2011). Speech facilitation by left inferior frontal cortex stimulation. *Current Biology, 21*(16), 403–1407.

Hsu, T. U., Tseng, L. Y., Yu, J. X., Kuo, W. J., Hung, D. L., Tzeng, J. L., et al. (2011). Modulating inhibitory control with direct current stimulation of the superior medial frontal cortex. *NeuroImage, 56*(4), 2249–2257.

Indefrey, P., & Levelt, W. J. M. (2004). The spatial and temporal signatures of word production components. *Cognition, 92*(1–2), 101–144.

Isoda, M., & Hikosaka, O. (2007). Switching from automatic to controlled action by monkey medial frontal cortex. *Nature Neuroscience, 10*(2), 240–248.

Iuculano, T., & Cohen Kadosh (2013). The mental cost of cognitive enhancement. *Journal of Neuroscience, 33*(10), 4482–4486.

Iyer, M. B., Mattu, U., Grafman, J., Lomarev, M., Sato, S., & Wassermann, E. M. (2005). Safety and cognitive effect of frontal DC brain polarization in healthy individuals. *Neurology, 64*(5), 872.

Jacobson, L., Ezra, A., Berger, U., & Lavidor, M. (2012). Modulating oscillatory brain activity correlates of behavioral inhibition using transcranial direct current stimulation. *Clinical Neurophysiology, 123*(5), 979–984.

Jacobson, L., Javitt, D. C., & Lavidor, M. (2011). Activation of inhibition: Diminishing impulsive behavior by direct current stimulation ove rthe Inferior Frontal Gyrus. *Journal of Cognitive Neuroscience, 23*(11), 3380–3387.

Jacobson, L., Koslowsky, M., & Lavidor, M. (2012). tDCS polarity effects in motor and cognitive domains: A meta-analytical review. *Experimental Brain Research, 216*, 1–10.

Jones, K. T., & Berryhill, M. E. (2012). Parietal contributions to visual working memory depend on task difficulty. *Frontiers in Psychiatry, 3*, 81.

Kanai, R., Chaieb, L., Antal, A., Walsh, V., & Paulus, W. (2008). Frequency-dependent electrical stimulation of the visual cortex. *Current Biology, 18*(23), 1839–1843.

Kanai, R., Paulus, W., & Walsh, V. (2010). Transcranial alternating current stimulation (tACS) modulates cortical excitability as assessed by TMS-induced phosphene thresholds. *Clinical Neurophysiology, 121*(9), 1551–1554.

Kane, M. J., & Engle, R. W. (2002). The role of prefrontal cortex in working-memory capacity, executive attention, and general fluid intelligence: An individual-differences perspective. *Psychonomic Bulletin & Review, 9*(4), 637–671.

Keeser, D., Meindl, T., Bor, J., Palm, U., Pogarell, O., Mulert, C., et al. (2011). Prefrontal transcranial direct current stimulation changes connectivity of resting-state networks during fMRI. *Journal of Neuroscience, 31*(43), 15284–15293.

Kincses, T. Z., Antal, A., Nitsche, M. A., Bartfai, O., & Paulus, W. (2004). Facilitation of probabilistic classification learning by transcranial direct current stimulation of the prefrontal cortex in the human. *Neuropsychologia, 42*(1), 113–117.

Klimesch, W. (1999). EEG alpha and theta oscillations reflect cognitive and memory performance: A review and analysis. *Brain Research Reviews, 29*(2–3), 169–195.

Klimesch, W., Doppelmayr, M., Stadler, W., Pöllhuber, D., Sauseng, P., & Röhm, D. (2001). Episodic retrieval is reflected by a process specific increase in human electroencephalographic theta activity. *Neuroscience Letters, 302*(1), 49–52.

Koechlin, E., Basso, G., Pietrini, P., Panzer, S., & Grafman, J. (1999). The role of the anterior prefrontal cortex in human cognition. *Nature, 399*(6732), 148–151.

Koechlin, E., Ody, C., & Kouneiher, F. (2003). The architecture of cognitive control in the human prefrontal cortex. *Science, 302*(5648), 1181–1185.

Kuo, M. F., & Nitsche, M. A. (2012). Effects of transcranial electrical stimulation on cognition. *Clinical EEG and Neuroscience, 43*(3), 192–199.

Lansbergen, M. M., Schutter, D. J. L. G., & Kenemans, J. L. (2007). Subjective impulsivity and baseline EEG in relation to stopping performance. *Brain Research, 1148*, 161–169.

Lauro, L. J. R., Tettamanti, M., Cappa, S. F., & Papagno, C. (2008). Idiom comprehension: A prefrontal task? *Cerebral Cortex, 18*(1), 162–170.

Lepage, J. F., & Théoret, H. (2010). Numerical processing: Stimulating numbers. *Current Biology, 20*(22), R975–R977.

Li, C. S. R., Huang, R. T., Constable, R. T., & Sinha, R. (2006). Imaging response inhibition in a stop-signal task: Neural correlates independent of signal monitoring and post-response processing. *Journal of Neuroscience, 26*(1), 186–192.

Li, C. S. R., Huang, C., Yan, P., Paliwal, P., Constable, R. T., & Sinha, R. (2008). Neural correlates of post-error slowing during a stop signal task: A functional magnetic resonance imaging study. *Journal of Cognitive Neuroscience, 20*, 1021–1029.

Liebetanz, D. (2002). Pharmacological approach to the mechanisms of transcranial DC-stimulation-induced after-effects of human motor cortex excitability. *Brain, 125*(10), 2238–2247.

Logan, G. D., & Cowan, W. B. (1984). On the ability to inhibit thought and action: A theory of an act of control. *Psychological Review, 91*, 295–327.

Marshall, L., Helgadóttir, H., Mölle, M., & Born, J. (2006). Boosting slow oscillations during sleep potentiates memory. *Nature, 444*(7119), 610–613.

Marshall, L., Mölle, M., Siebner, H. R., & Born, J. (2005). Bifrontal transcranial direct current stimulation slows reaction time in a working memory task. *BMC Neuroscience, 6*, 23.

Meinzer, M., Antonenko, D., Lindenberg, R., Hetzer, S., Ulm, L., Avirame, K., et al. (2012). Electrical brain stimulation improves cognitive performance by modulating functional connectivity and task-specific activation. *The Journal of Neuroscience, 32*(5), 1859–1866.

Metuki, N., Sela, T., & Lavidor, M. (2012). Enhancing cognitive control components of insight problems solving by anodal tDCS of the left dorsolateral prefrontal cortex. *Brain Stimulation, 5*(2), 110–115.

Miller, E. K., & Cohen, J. D. (2001). An integrative theory of prefrontal cortex function. *Annual Review of Neuroscience, 24*(1), 167–202.

Moliadze, V., Antal, A., & Paulus, W. (2010). Electrode-distance dependent after-effects of transcranial direct and random noise stimulation with extracephalic reference electrodes. *Clinical Neurophysiology, 121*(12), 2165–2171.

Mottaghy, F. M., Hungs, M., Brügmann, M., Sparing, R., Boroojerdi, B., Foltys, H., et al. (1999). Facilitation of picture naming after repetitive transcranial magnetic stimulation. *Neurology, 53*(8), 1806–1812.

Muggleton, N. G., Chen, C. Y., Tzeng, O. J., Hung, D. L., & Juan, C. H. (2010). Inhibitory control and the frontal eye fields. *Journal of Cognitive Neuroscience, 22*(12), 2804–2812.

Mulquiney, P. G., Hoy, K. E., Daskalakis, Z. J., & Fitzgerald, P. B. (2011). Improving working memory: Exploring the effect of transcranial random noise stimulation and transcranial direct current stimulation on the dorsolateral prefrontal cortex. *Clinical Neurophysiology, 122*(12), 2384–2389.

Nitsche, M. A., Cohen, L. G., Wassermann, E. M., Priori, A., Lang, N., Antal, A., et al. (2008). Transcranial direct current stimulation: State of the art 2008. *Brain Stimulation, 1*(3), 206–223.

Nitsche, M. A., & Paulus, W. (2000). Excitability changes induced in the human motor cortex by weak transcranial direct current stimulation. *The Journal of Physiology, 527*(3), 633–639.

Nitsche, M. A., & Paulus, W. (2001). Sustained excitability elevations induced by transcranial DC motor cortex stimulation in humans. *Neurology, 57*(10), 1899.

Nitsche, M. A., Schauenburg, A., Lang, N., Liebetanz, D., Exner, C., Paulus, W., et al. (2003). Facilitation of implicit motor learning by weak transcranial direct current stimulation of the primary motor cortex in the human. *Journal of Cognitive Neuroscience, 15* (4), 619–626.

Ohn, S. H., Park, C. -I., Yoo, W. -K., Ko, M. -H., Choi, K. P., Kim, G. -M., et al. (2008). Time-dependent effect of transcranial direct current stimulation on the enhancement of working memory. *Neuroreport, 19*, 43–47.

Papagno, C. (2010). Idiomatic language comprehension: Neuropsychological evidence. In *Neuropsychology of communication* (pp. 111–129). Milan, Italy: Springer.

Pogosyan, A., Gaynor, L. D., Eusebio, A., & Brown, P. (2009). Boosting cortical activity at beta-band frequencies slows movement in humans. *Current Biology, 19*(19), 1637–1641.

Pope, P. A., & Miall, R. C. (2012). Task-specific facilitation of cognition by cathodal transcranial direct current stimulation of the cerebellum. *Brain Stimulation, 5*(2), 84–94.

Rapp, A. M., Mutschler, D. E., & Erb, M. (2012). Where in the brain is nonliteral language? A coordinate-based meta-analysis of functional magnetic resonance imaging studies. *NeuroImage, 63*(1), 600–610.

Röhm, D., Klimesch, W., Haider, H., & Doppelmayr, M. (2001). The role of theta and alpha oscillations for language comprehension in the human electroencephalogram. *Neuroscience Letters, 310*(2–3), 137–140.

Romani, C., Ward, J., & Olson, A. (1999). Developmental surface dysgraphia: What is the underlying cognitive impairment? *The Quarterly Journal of Experimental Psychology, 52* (1), 97–128.

Ross, L. A., McCoy, D., Wolk, D. A., Coslett, H. B., & Olson, I. R. (2010). Improved proper name recall by electrical stimulation of the anterior temporal lobes. *Neuropsychologia, 48* (12), 3671–3674.

Rubia, K., Russell, T., Overmeyer, S., Brammer, M. J., Bullmore, E. T., Sharma, T., et al. (2001). Mapping motor inhibition: Conjunctive brain activations across different versions of go/no-go and stop tasks. *NeuroImage, 13*(2), 250–261.

Sandberg, A., & Bostrom, N. (2006). Converging cognitive enhancements. *Annals of the New York Academy of Sciences, 1093*(1), 201–227.

Sandrini, M., Fertonani, A., Cohen, L. G., & Miniussi, C. (2012). Double dissociation of working memory load effects induced by bilateral parietal modulation. *Neuropsychologia, 50*, 396–402.

Sandrini, M., Rossini, P. M., & Miniussi, C. (2008). Lateralized contribution of prefrontal cortex in controlling task-irrelevant information during verbal and spatial working memory tasks: rTMS evidence. *Neuropsychologia, 46*, 2056–2063.

Sandrini, M., & Rusconi, E. (2009). A brain for numbers. *Cortex, 45*(7), 796–803.

Schutter, D. J. L. G., & Hortensius, R. (2011). Brain oscillations and frequency-dependent modulation of cortical excitability. *Brain Stimulation, 4*(2), 97–103.

Sela, T., Ivry, R. B., & Lavidor, M. (2012). Prefrontal control during a semantic decision task that involves idiom comprehension: A transcranial direct current stimulation study. *Neuropsychologia, 50*(9), 2271–2280.

Silvanto, J., & Pascual-Leone, A. (2012). Why the assessment of causality in brain-behavior relations requires brain stimulation. *Journal of Cognitive Neuroscience, 24*(4), 775–777.

Snowball, A., Tachtsidis, I., Popescu, T., Thompson, J., Delazer, M., Zamarian, L., et al. (2013). Long-term enhancement of brain function and cognition using cognitive training and brain stimulation. *Current Biology, 23*, 987–992.

Sparing, R., Dafotakis, M., Meister, I. G., Thirugnanasambandam, N., & Fink, G. R. (2008). Enhancing language performance with non-invasive brain stimulation – A transcranial direct current stimulation study in healthy humans. *Neuropsychologia, 46*(1), 261–268.

Stagg, C. J., & Nitsche, M. A. (2011). Physiological basis of transcranial direct current stimulation. *The Neuroscientist, 17*(1), 37–53.

Terney, D., Chaieb, L., Moliadze, V., Antal, A., & Paulus, W. (2008). Increasing human brain excitability by transcranial high-frequency random noise stimulation. *Journal of Neuroscience, 28*(52), 14147–14155.

Thut, G., & Miniussi, C. (2009). New insights into rhythmic brain activity from TMS-EEG studies. *Trends in Cognitive Sciences, 13*(4), 182–189.

Vannorsdall, T. D., Schretlen, D. J., Andrejczuk, M., Ledoux, K., Bosley, L. V., Weaver, J. R., et al. (2012). Altering automatic verbal processes with transcranial direct current stimulation. *Frontiers in Psychiatry, 3*, 73.

Varela, F., Lachaux, J. P., Rodriguez, E., & Martinerie, J. (2001). The brainweb: Phase synchronization and large-scale integration. *Nature Reviews. Neuroscience, 2*(4), 229–239.

Wassermann, E. M., & Grafman, J. (2005). Recharging cognition with DC brain polarization. *Trends in Cognitive Sciences, 9*(11), 503–505.

Weiss, M., & Lavidor, M. (2012). When less is more: Evidence for a facilitative cathodal tDCS effect in attentional abilities. *Journal of Cognitive Neuroscience, 24*(9), 1826–1833.

Wernicke, C. (1874). *Der aphasischeSymptomencomplex: EinepsychologischeStudie auf anatomischer Basis.* Cohn & Weigert.

Wienbruch, C., Paul, I., Bauer, S., & Kivelitz, H. (2005). The influence of methylphenidate on the power spectrum of ADHD children – An MEG study. *BMC Psychiatry, 5*(1), 29.

Wirth, M., Rahman, R. A., Kuenecke, J., Koenig, T., Horn, H., Sommer, W., et al. (2011). Effects of transcranial direct current stimulation (tDCS) on behaviour and electrophysiology of language production. *Neuropsychologia, 49*(14), 3989–3998.

Zaehle, T., Rach, S., & Herrmann, C. S. (2010). Transcranial alternating current stimulation enhances individual alpha activity in human EEG. *PLoS ONE, 5*(11), e13766.

Zaehle, T., Sandmann, P., Thorne, J. D., Jäncke, L., & Herrmann, C. S. (2011). Transcranial direct current stimulation of the prefrontal cortex modulates working memory performance: Combined behavioural and electrophysiological evidence. *BMC Neuroscience, 12*(1), 2.

Zaghi, S., Acar, M., Hultgren, B., Boggio, P. S., & Fregni, F. (2010). Noninvasive brain stimulation with low-intensity electrical currents: Putative mechanisms of action for direct and alternating current stimulation. *The Neuroscientist, 16*(3), 285–307.

IMPROVING FUNCTIONS IN THE ATYPICAL BRAIN

12

Brain Stimulation and its Role in Neurological Diseases

Maximo Zimerman[1,2] and Friedhelm C. Hummel[1,3]

[1]Brain Imaging and Neuro-Stimulation (BINS) Laboratory, Department
of Neurology, University Medical Center, Hamburg, Germany
[2]Institute of Cognitive Neurology (INECO), Buenos Aires, Argentina
[3]Medical School, Favoloro University, Buenos Aires, Argentina

The Stimulated Brain
http://dx.doi.org/10.1016/B978-0-12-404704-4.00012-0

INTRODUCTION

Since the pioneering study by Merton and Morton in 1980 demonstrating that transcranial electrical stimulation (tES) applied non-invasively through the scalp and skull can stimulate the corticospinal tract, generating motor evoked potentials (MEP), and the subsequent work by Barker, Jalinous, and Freeston (1985) showing similar results with magnetic pulses (for further details, see Barker et al., 1985; Merton & Morton, 1980), non-invasive brain stimulation techniques have been widely explored and have proven their unique potential to non-invasively modulate brain functions in healthy subjects and neurological patients.

It is well recognized that neurological disorders represent the consequences of dynamic plastic interactions in distributed neural networks (Dubovik et al., 2013; Grefkes & Fink, 2011; Ko et al., 2013). These plastic modifications include compensatory changes that prove to be adaptive for the patients, as well as changes that contribute to functional disability and are then consequently defined as maladaptive. The recent increase of interest in transcranial stimulation as a potential tool in neurological disorders was driven not only by the investigation of these methods for studying the abnormalities in the interactions of neural networks but also by the promising treatment potential in a variety of medical conditions. Both transcranial magnetic stimulation and transcranial direct current stimulation can induce lasting modulation of brain activity in the targeted brain region and across different brain networks even in aged and diseased subjects.

This chapter will start with a short overview of the plastic phenomena observed at the cortical level, as well as the main characteristics of non-invasive brain stimulation techniques; it will then review the scientific evidence achieved with these techniques to enhance our understanding of the neurobiological mechanisms of a variety of neurological disorders, including stroke, Alzheimer's, and Parkinson's disease; interventional treatment strategies for these diseases will be discussed and the chapter will be finished with a critical appraisal of this field as well as an outlook towards the next steps.

PLASTICITY IN THE CENTRAL NERVOUS SYSTEM: ANIMAL STUDIES

Neuronal plasticity is generally defined as the ability of the brain to change its structure and/or function in response to internal and external constraints or goals (Pascual-Leone, Amedi, Fregni, & Merabet, 2005). This process can occur at various levels of brain organization, from ultrastructural to synaptic, involving changes in the efficiency of transmission at existing synapses between two sites and/or changes in the number of connections between them. Originally demonstrated in hippocampal slices, long-term potentiation (LTP) and long-term depression (LTD) are the most studied forms of synaptic plasticity (Bliss & Collingridge, 1993). LTP can be induced experimentally by the application of stimuli at high frequency (e.g., at a theta burst pattern of 3–5 pulses applied at 100 Hz) increasing synaptic strength, whereas low-frequency stimulation (e.g., 1 Hz) leads to the opposite result (LTD, Malenka & Nicoll, 1999). In the motor domain at the cortical level, the best evidence for an involvement of synaptic plasticity in normal learning processes came from animal experiments. Rats had been first trained in a reaching task using one forelimb (Rioult-Pedotti, Friedman, & Donoghue, 2000). After training, motor cortical slices of each hemisphere (trained versus untrained) were examined to test whether training influenced synaptic plasticity. Interestingly, previous training made it more difficult to induce LTP in the contralateral hemisphere compared to the untrained hemisphere. This suggests that learning had induced LTP in the trained hemisphere, raising the threshold to further induce LTP by electrical stimulation. Testing LTD with the same experimental paradigm led to opposite results, with facilitated induction of LTD in the trained hemisphere compared with the untrained hemisphere.

Modification of synaptic plasticity may also occur after brain injury, and might play a crucial role in the process of recovery of function after central nervous system (CNS) damage. This notion was supported by the fact that a focal lesion of the hand area of the motor cortex in a monkey was accompanied by a shift in the representation of the hand into adjacent, perilesional areas of the cortex (Nudo, 2003). However, these findings were only observed if the animals received movement therapy for the affected extremity. Thus, functional recovery might significantly depend on cortical remodeling processes. At a synaptic level, the reorganization involves changing the strength of existing synaptic connections, as well as sprouting and formation of new connections in the area surrounding the lesion (Brown, Boyd, & Murphy, 2010). Strikingly, further interventional studies have shown that animals regain better hand motor function when an invasive, continuous, subthreshold electrical stimulation of the lesioned motor cortex is applied together with a rehabilitative training for several weeks, compared to rehabilitative training alone (Teskey, Flynn, Goertzen, Monfils, & Young, 2003).

METHODS OF NON-INVASIVE BRAIN STIMULATION (NIBS)

The introduction of techniques to non-invasively stimulate cortical areas of the brain has opened the way to influence behavior transiently in humans by altering spontaneous neural activity, resulting in facilitatory or inhibitory effects (Dayan, Censor, Buch, Sandrini, & Cohen, 2013; Hallett, 2007). Remarkably, the effects of NIBS have been shown to outlast the stimulation period, which is particularly important for rehabilitation purposes (Rothwell, 2010; Zimerman, Heise, Hoppe et al., 2012), sharing significant analogies to synaptic phenomena of LTP and LTD. Two methods are now in common use: transcranial magnetic stimulation (TMS), and transcranial direct current stimulation (tDCS). Although TMS has recently been approved in some countries for the treatment of depression, and growing numbers of other disorders are under treatment studies, both techniques can, to date, only be used with local ethical review board approvals (Rossi, Hallett, Rossini, & Pascual-Leone, 2009). In the following two sections we will introduce the abovementioned techniques only briefly, as a detailed description of these techniques is provided in Chapter 2.

Transcranial direct current stimulation

Non-invasive brain stimulation through tDCS is an effective and relatively simple method of polarizing cortical brain regions. Unlike other brain stimulation techniques (i.e., TMS and tES) it does not induce depolarization, which produces action potentials in neural membranes. In this way, tDCS provides a subthreshold stimulation that modulates spontaneous neuronal excitability by increasing or decreasing the respective transmembrane potentials. Based on this, tDCS has been considered a neuromodulatory intervention (Nitsche et al., 2008). Direct current has generally been delivered over the scalp, using electrodes that are enclosed in perforated sponge pockets (sized 25–35 cm^2 in most published studies) soaked with a saline solution or a conductive gel. Wires attach the sponge pockets to a constant current stimulator, which provides a small and steady flow of direct current while constantly monitoring the resistance in the system. The success of tDCS in inducing modifications of membrane polarity depends on current density, which determines the induced electrical field strength according to the quotient between the current strength and electrode size (Nitsche et al., 2007, 2008). The duration of the current determines the occurrence and length of the aftereffects (e.g., 10–20 minutes). The direction of the current flow determines the effects on the underlying cortical target area, which is defined generally by the electrodes' positions and polarity (anodal vs cathodal). Most frequently, one electrode is placed over a specific site while a reference electrode is placed over another location to complete the circuit of current flow. The anode is defined as the positively charged electrode, whereas the cathode is the negatively charged one. For instance, with an active electrode over the representation of the motor cortex and a reference electrode over a reference region (e.g., the contralateral supra-orbital region), the excitability of the

brain tissue under the anodal electrode is increased; when th'
is reversed, the excitability of the brain tissue under th'
decreased (i.e., the electrode that was previously the anode .
the cathode). Therefore, tDCS parameters such as: (1) current s.
(2) position, size, and shape of the electrodes, and (3) stimulation duratio..
should be stated in every protocol, for comparability between studies
(Gandiga, Hummel, & Cohen, 2006; Hummel & Cohen, 2006; Nitsche
et al., 2008).

Although tDCS is a painless method, at the beginning of the stimulation
it can induce short-lasting tingling or burning sensations which fade after
30–60 s, thereby making it ideal for blinding subjects (reliable sham/
placebo condition) by turning it off after the initial sensory experience
(Gandiga et al., 2006). Thus, with this procedure, naïve subjects cannot distinguish between real and sham tDCS, giving the opportunity to blind
both investigator and participants. None of the studies performed so far
has reported any serious adverse events, such as seizures, due to the intervention (in contrast to TMS). Nevertheless, well-documented side effects
include the sensation of itching or burning under the electrodes (rather
frequently) and headache (less frequently). Recently, uncommon side
effects such as eyelid myokymia and skin burning have been reported
in single-case studies (Brunoni et al., 2011; Wessel, Zimerman,
Timmermann, & Hummel, 2013).

Transcranial Magnetic Stimulation

TMS is a versatile technique that offers the opportunity to assess cortical excitability and effective connectivity of the human cortex, to induce
"virtual lesions" in order to test the functional relevance of the stimulated
neuronal network, or to induce long-lasting changes in excitability and
connectivity in certain cortical networks – which is especially important
for therapeutic purposes (Dayan et al., 2013; Hallett, 2007). TMS operates
by the principle of electromagnetic induction, in which an electrical capacitor is attached to a coil of loops of copper wire. When the circuit is made,
the capacitor discharges brief pulses of current through the wire, causing a
fluctuating magnetic field perpendicular to the plane of the coil that subsequently induces an orthogonal electric field into the brain capable of
depolarizing cortical neurons (right-hand rule). The induced current pulse
lasts about 200 µs and is similar in amplitude to that produced by conventional tES applied directly to the surface of the brain. Until now, most
studies have focused on the motor cortex, where an electromyographic
response to single-pulse TMS can be measured (MEP), providing
the opportunity to read out changes in cortical activation (for details,
see Hallett, 2007; Hummel et al., 2005). In addition, the application
of paired-pulse paradigms (paired-pulse TMS) allows exploration of

changes in cortical excitability by means of short-interval intracortical inhibition (SICI), long-interval intracortical inhibition (LICI), and intracortical facilitation (ICF) that may provide key information regarding GABA-A, GABA-B and glutamatergic neurotransmitters, respectively (Hummel et al., 2009; Kujirai et al., 1993).

Repetitive TMS (rTMS) refers to application of trains of repeated magnetic pulses capable of modulating brain activity beyond the stimulation period. Depending on the frequency, duration, and strength of the magnetic field, and the shape of the coil, rTMS can enhance or suppress activity in underlying cortical regions (Hallett, 2007). In general, "high-frequency stimulation" refers to frequencies above 5 Hz and is considered to produce an excitatory effect, whereas "low-frequency stimulation" (1 Hz or less) leads to reduction of excitability in the targeted cortical region. When applied to the motor cortex, low-frequency rTMS is able to reduce MEP size, while the reverse is true for high-frequency rTMS (Rossini & Rossi, 2007). Besides the classical rTMS procedures, other rTMS paradigms have recently been proposed; one of them, so-called "theta burst stimulation," can condition the human cortex for up to 90 minutes using short (less than 1 minute) asynchronous high-frequency rTMS trains (theta-frequency about 5 Hz). Applying theta bursts continuously induces an inhibitory effect, while applying theta bursts intermittently gives an excitatory effect (Huang, Edwards, Rounis, Bhatia, & Rothwell, 2005) (for a detailed description of the different rTMS protocols, see Dayan et al., 2013; Rossini & Rossi, 2007). Although, rTMS is a safe procedure, it has the potential to cause seizures even in healthy individuals. Recent guidelines recommend careful consideration of patient characteristics that may influence the seizure threshold (Rossi et al., 2009). Most frequent side effects include mild headaches responsive to common analgesics, local pain or paresthesias in the stimulated region, neck pain, tooth pain, and transient changes in audition (Machii, Cohen, Ramos-Estebanez, & Pascual-Leone, 2006; Rossi et al., 2009).

Besides their clear differences, both TMS and tDCS can induce long-term aftereffects on cortical excitability that may impact behavior. These long-term aftereffects are believed to engage mechanisms of neural plasticity, making these techniques ideally suited to promote functional recovery, particularly when combined with adequate behavioral interventions (e.g., in stroke patients; Zimerman, Heise, Hoppe et al., 2012). The intrinsic mechanisms underlying the NIBS-related effects are not completely understood; however, modulation of neurotransmitter levels appears to be a contributing factor (Ridding & Ziemann, 2010). Transcranial stimulation may result in changes in excitatory/inhibitory neurotransmitter systems (e.g., GABA and glutamate), which play an important role in the regulation of the neuronal activity in the cerebral cortex. To illustrate, rTMS effects do not occur if the subjects receive an oral dose of a drug that

interferes with NMDA receptors (Reis et al., 2006). Similarly, [
effects could be blocked by an NMDA antagonist, whereas
NMDA-agonist (d-cycloserine) selectively potentiated the du
motor cortical excitability by anodal tDCS (Nitsche et al., 2004).
MR spectroscopy study performed by Stagg and colleagues revealed new
insights into the role of neurotransmission under tDCS. Anodal tDCS
leads to a significant decrease in GABA concentration while cathodal
tDCS shows similar effects on glutamate over the motor cortex (Stagg
et al., 2009).

Another concept proposed that gene induction might be a potential
mechanism by which NIBS may exert longer-lasting plastic changes
(Fritsch et al., 2010). Using rTMS protocols, a significant enhancement of
brain-derived neurotrophic factor (BDNF) mRNA in the hippocampus,
parietal, and piriform cortices was described (Muller, Toschi, Kresse,
Post, & Keck, 2000). Interestingly, Fritsch et al. (2010) demonstrated that
BDNF might be a critical mediator of the tDCS-related effects by showing
that adult mice with deletion of the BDNF gene failed to exhibit the LTP-like
effect after tDCS exposure (Fritsch et al., 2010). As previously suggested,
BDNF is a member of the neurotrophin family and plays an important role
in synaptogenesis and synaptic mechanisms, related to learning and memory processes in healthy subjects as well as in neurological patients. Finally,
it is important to keep in mind that the effects of rTMS and tDCS are not
only restricted to the stimulation site but also, depending on the specific
parameters of stimulation, stimulation-induced changes can be observed
at distant points by proving an effective modulation of remote and interconnected networks (Plewnia, Lotze, & Gerloff, 2003; Zimerman, Heise, Hoppe
et al., 2012). This particular property of NIBS techniques has been recently
used in a number of "proof-of-principle" studies in neurorehabilitation,
with the purpose of enhancing and decreasing excitability of critical brain
regions involved in the recovery process after stroke (for further details, see
Hummel & Cohen, 2006; Nowak, Bosl, Podubecka, & Carey, 2010; Schulz,
Gerloff, & Hummel, 2013).

Recently, the repertoire of NIBS techniques has been enlarged by transcranial alternating current stimulation (tACS), transcranial random noise
stimulation (tRNS), and more complex rTMS protocols (quadri- and octa-
pulse rTMS). For example, tACS allows a frequency-specific modulation
of ongoing oscillatory activity. Recent studies performed by Wach et al.
(2013) revealed that 10-Hz and 20-Hz tACS over the motor cortex elicit different effects on motor behavior (Wach et al., 2013). The effects of these
novel approaches on behavioral and neurophysiological measures are
currently being tested with healthy subjects (Antal et al., 2008). However,
only few studies to date have applied these non-invasive procedures in
patients with neurological diseases (Angelakis et al., 2013; Chan
et al., 2012).

NIBS IN STROKE RECOVERY

In high-income countries, stroke is the most common cause of permanent disability among adults. The prevalence of stroke survivors with incomplete recovery has been estimated at 200–460/100,000 of the population (Kolominsky-Rabas, Weber, Gefeller, Neundoerfer, & Heuschmann, 2001). Two-thirds of the patients require assistance in activities of daily living (ADL), resulting in severe psychological, physical, and financial consequences for the individual and the community (Jorgensen et al., 1995; Taylor et al., 1996). Among the spectrum of persistent neurological impairments, hand function and aphasia are considered two major predictors for patients returning to their normal professional and private lives (Lai, Studenski, Duncan, & Perera, 2002; Patel, Duncan, Lai, & Studenski, 2000). To date, there is a general consensus that following the acute phase of a stroke, patients should be treated within multidisciplinary neurorehabilitative programs including intensive physical training in order to substantially promote recovery. However, despite recent technological and methodological developments in the field (e.g., constraint-induced therapy, robotic-aided, bilateral arm training, and virtual reality), recovery of motor function is still incomplete and not satisfactory. After 3 months 55–75% of the patients suffer from significant upper limb impairment, affecting functional independence and the normal integration into social and professional activities (Patel et al., 2000).

Changes in Cortical Networks and Stroke Recovery

Recent longitudinal and cross-sectional studies have started to describe the neural reorganization after stroke, using structural and functional neuroimaging (fMRI and PET) and TMS (Gerloff et al., 2006; Grefkes, Nowak et al., 2008; Johansen-Berg et al., 2002; Lotze et al., 2006; Ward, Brown, Thompson, & Frackowiak, 2003). Most of these studies revealed abnormal patterns of activation/excitability immediately after stroke and during the recovery process. As a matter of principle, focal subcortical lesions may not only directly affect the descending motor fibers, but also alter the functional network architecture of cortical areas in both hemispheres distant from the lesion.

In the motor domain, a typical pattern observed in the majority of neuroimaging studies investigating the changes in task-related neural activation demonstrated that movements of the paretic hand elicit a bilateral neural recruitment within motor areas in patients with a subcortical lesion –a pattern significantly different from healthy subjects or when patients move their unaffected hand (Ward et al., 2003). In this regard, patients with good functional outcome demonstrated a more lateralized (normal) neural activation pattern towards the ipsilesional (affected) hemisphere for movements of the paretic hand, while those patients whose motor deficit remained more severe recruited bilateral motor areas. The functional meaning of the bilateral activation, especially the contralesional activation, is under debate. Possible explanations vary from beneficial plastic changes of activation to a maladaptive phenomenon that interferes with the recovery process by abnormal interhemispheric interactions (Hummel et al., 2008; Lotze et al., 2006). Strikingly, recent studies revealed that in the first few weeks (subacute phase), increases of neural activity in the unaffected motor cortex are often associated with better recovery of the motor function during this period. However, if this pattern persists in the chronic phase after stroke (i.e., >6 months), it is rather associated with less favorable motor outcome (Rehme, Fink, von Cramon, & Grefkes, 2011).

Post-stroke patients exhibited changes in motor cortical excitability and abnormal levels of interhemispheric inhibition from the unaffected to the affected motor cortex. Using double-pulse TMS protocol, these interhemispheric interactions (IHIs) have been directly studied while individuals performed a unimanual task (Duque et al., 2007; Murase, Duque, Mazzocchio, & Cohen, 2004). Indeed, Murase et al. (2004) showed that chronic stroke patients had abnormally increased IHI from the healthy hemisphere onto the affected side relative to healthy subjects. This pathological IHI was significantly correlated with greater severity of hand motor impairment; patients with more motor impairment had larger abnormal inhibition targeting the lesioned hemisphere (Murase et al., 2004). Further support for these findings comes from neuroimaging studies, using fMRI to investigate effective connectivity by estimating the causal influence one area exerts over the activity of another, demonstrating that movements of the paretic hand were associated with inhibitory influences toward the affected M1 originating from the unaffected M1 (Grefkes, Eickhoff, Nowak, Dafotakis, & Fink, 2008). The current studies support the hypothesis that activation of the contralesional hemisphere may have a maladaptive negative modulatory effect on the ipsilesional side, resulting in impaired function of the affected side, at least in part of the patients (see Fig. 12.1). Therefore, strategies to enhance motor recovery may attempt to re-establish a normalized interhemispheric balance between the lesioned and the healthy hemisphere. This general model of interhemispheric rivalry has served as the foundation for a number of neurorehabilitation interventions not only for motor impairment but also for attention (Corbetta, Kincade, Lewis, Snyder, & Sapir, 2005) and language impairment after stroke (Chrysikou & Hamilton, 2011). Although an attractive model, supported by several studies, this idea cannot be generalized towards all stroke patients. The problem of studies in the field is that mainly relatively small and homogeneous groups of

Healthy controls

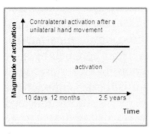 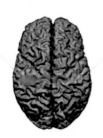 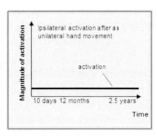

A

Subcortical stroke, good recovery

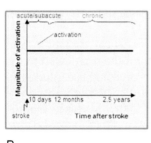 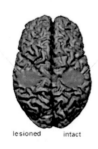 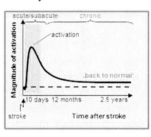

B

Cortical stroke, limited recovery

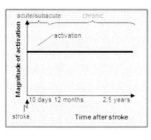 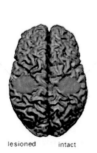 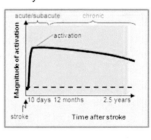

C

FIGURE 12.1   **Schematic of the development of bilateral motorcortical recruitment during an unimanual movement in healthy subjects and patients after stroke.** (A) Activation pattern in healthy subjects with normal contralateral dominant activation pattern. (B) Activation pattern during a unimanual movement of the paretic hand in patients with subcortical stroke. Note the changes of activation, especially in the intact hemisphere, over time with a pattern back to normal in the recovered stage. (C) In contrast, in not well-recovered patients with cortical stroke the additional activation in the intact hemisphere remains to support impaired upper extremity function (as a "second best solution"). In summary, there are clearly different patterns of functional reorganization after a stroke depending on different patient individual factors, such as lesion size, which might lead to an individualized application of NIBS in the future. *Figure adapted from Hummel and Gerloff (2012).*

patients have been studied cross-sectionally. Information from larger samples of heterogeneous patient groups evaluated in a longitudinal fashion is lacking. There is some evidence that the concept of maladaptive interhemispheric interactions does not hold true for all patients, especially for the more impaired with rather larger lesions. These patients might rely on the involvement and activity of the intact hemisphere to support the function of the paretic (ipsilateral) limb (Johansen-Berg et al., 2002; Lotze et al., 2006; Ward et al., 2003). Thus, the provided model is an interesting working model but has to be refined in more detail by upcoming studies.

How Can NIBS Promote Recovery After Stroke?

Two main strategies have been tested so far following the concept of interhemispheric competition between both motor cortices, which may be considered only a rough approximation to the complex network pathology to be observed after stroke: (1) inhibiting the motor cortex of the unaffected (contralesional – cM1) hemisphere to reduce the abnormal inhibitory drive towards the lesioned hemisphere, or (2) facilitating the motor cortex of the affected (ipsilesional – iM1) hemisphere. Both modalities have been suggested to normalize the balance of transcallosal inhibition between both hemispheres resulting in improved function of the affected side (Grefkes & Fink 2012; Hummel & Cohen, 2006). Enhancement of excitability can be achieved with either high-frequency rTMS or anodal tDCS, whereas inhibition of excitability can be accomplished with either low-frequency rTMS or cathodal tDCS.

Modulation of Impaired Motor Functions by NIBS

Over the past few years numerous studies have reported the beneficial effects of cortical stimulation techniques in improving motor recovery of the affected limb in patients after stroke. In the first double-blind sham-controlled study in the field, Hummel et al. (2005) demonstrated a transient improvement in performance of the Jebsen-Taylor hand function test (JTT), a set of tasks that mimic activities of daily living (ADL), after one single session of anodal tDCS stimulation targeting the affected hemisphere. This effect was not apparent with sham treatment. This transient improvement was evident in all patients studied and persisted for more than 30 minutes following the stimulation period. Interestingly, the beneficial behavioral effect was associated with increased motor cortical excitability and reduced SICI in the iM1 (Hummel et al., 2005). Using a single session of rTMS at inhibitory frequency, Mansur and colleagues reported an improvement in reaction times and motor performance measured by the Purdue pegboard test in eight patients with mild to moderate motor deficits (Mansur et al., 2005). Since these two pioneer "proof of principle" studies, the effects of NIBS methods have been frequently investigated in patients with chronic stroke (few clinical trials have been conducted in acute and subacute phases of the disease), most commonly in sham-controlled, double-blind experimental designs using a variety of motor tasks (Table 12.1 provides a summary of the studies). Independent of the stimulation technique (tDCS or rTMS), the targeted hemisphere (affected or unaffected hemisphere), and the heterogeneity of the study population (cortical or subcortical, acute or chronic), the effect size on hand motor function is usually in the range of 10% to 50% (depending on the outcome and experimental set-up) and often limited to the stimulation period (Nowak et al., 2010).

One important question is, how can these effects be augmented? Based on animal and healthy human studies (Fritsch et al., 2010; Reis et al., 2009; Zimerman et al., 2013), investigations explored whether additive or even supra-additive longer-lasting effects can be anticipated when NIBS is paired with motor training (see also Chapter 8). The possibility emerged that synchronous application of brain stimulation and motor learning might share synergistic impacts on synaptic plasticity and network reorganization, resulting in longer-lasting behavioral effects (Bolognini, Pascual-Leone, & Fregni, 2009). For instance, in a sample of chronic stroke patients with subcortical lesion, the application of cathodal tDCS to inhibit the cM1 concurrent with training enhanced the acquisition of a motor task. Importantly, these improvements in motor learning remained significant for up to 24 h by $\sim$20% of improvement compared with sham stimulation (Zimerman, Heise, Hoppe et al., 2012). In a long-term follow-up study performed in subacute stroke patients (between the fifth and tenth days post-stroke), Khedr et al. (2005) applied 10 consecutive days of rTMS to the iM1 as an add-on intervention to normal physical therapy. They found an enhancement on the NIH stroke scale (NIHSS) and Barthel Index scale with rTMS compared to sham stimulation, and these benefits lasted for at least 10 days after the intervention (Khedr et al., 2005). Notably, several studies that used NIBS alone without coupling it with any training or learning task did not find behavioral improvements (Liepert et al., 2007; Takeuchi et al., 2005; Talelli, Greenwood, & Rothwell, 2007).

Another strategy that has been explored to enhance the effects of brain stimulation is based on repetitive stimulation sessions. This methodology may provide additional benefits over a single session through cumulative effects, resulting in increased facilitation to subsequent stimulations (Baumer et al., 2003). For example, Avenanti et al. (2012) administered 1-Hz rTMS over cM1 for 10 days in a group of chronic stroke patients. The authors found that, compared with a sham stimulation group, suppressing excitability of cM1 prior to training was associated with a significant decrease of inhibition exerted on iM1 (reflected by a decreased ipsilateral silent period) and, more importantly, with behavioral

TABLE 12.1 Summary of Sham-Controlled Studies Performed with rTMS and tDCS in Motor Recovery After Stroke

	Number of Patients	Cortical/ subcortical	Ischemic/ hemorrhagic	Severity of Stroke	Stroke Duration	Motor Assessments and Outcomes	Concomitant Therapy	Study Design	NIBS Intervention	Number of Sessions	Follow-ups
Takeuchi, Chuma, Matsuo, Watanabe, and Ikoma (2005)	20	Subcortical	Ischemic	Mixed	26.95 months	FM, PA	NA	Randomized, parallel groups	1-Hz rTMS over cM1	1	NA
Hummel et al. (2005)	6	Subcortical 5, cortico-subcortical 1	Ischemic	Mild	44.4 months	MRC, FM, ASS, JTT	NA	Randomized, double-blinded, cross-over.	atDCS over iM1	1	10 days
Mansur et al. (2005)	10 stroke, 6 healthy	Cortico-subcortical	Ischemic	Mixed	<12 months	sRT, cRT, PP, FT	NA	Randomized, cross-over	1-Hz rTMS over cM1and cPM	1	NA
Khedr, Ahmed, Fathy, and Rothwell (2005)	52	Cortico-subcortical	Ischemic	Moderate to severe	5–10 days	SSS, NIHSS, BI	Standard physical therapy	Randomized, parallel groups	3-Hz rTMS; iM1	10 days	10 days
Fregni et al. (2005)	6	Cortico-subcortical	NM	Mild to moderate	27.1 months	MRC, ASS, JTT	NA	Randomized, double-blinded, cross-over.	ctDCS over cM1 and atDCS over iM1	1	NA

Continued

TABLE 12.1 Summary of Sham-Controlled Studies Performed with rTMS and tDCS in Motor Recovery After Stroke—cont'd

	Number of Patients	Cortical/ subcortical	Ischemic/ hemorrhagic	Severity of Stroke	Stroke Duration	Motor Assessments and Outcomes	Concomitant Therapy	Study Design	NIBS Intervention	Number of Sessions	Follow-ups
Fregni et al. (2006)	15	Cortical 1, subcortical 13, cortico-subcortical 1	Ischemic	Mild to moderate	44.05 months	MRC, ASS, JTT, sRT, cRT, PPT	NA	Randomized, parallel groups	1-Hz rTMS over cM1	5 days	2 weeks
Hummel and Cohen (2006)	11	subcortical	Ischemic	Mild to moderate	41.8 months	MRC, FM, ASS, sRT, PF	NA	Randomized, double-blinded, cross-over.	atDCS over iM1	1	NA
Liepert, Zittel, and Weiller (2007)	12	subcortical (2 pons)	NM	Mild	7.3 days	MRC, GF, NHPT	NA	Randomized, double-blinded, cross-over.	1-Hz rTMS over cM1	1	NA
Malcolm et al. (2007)	20	Cortico-subcortical	1 hemorrhagic	Mixed	45.6 months	WMFT, BBT, MAL	CIT	Randomized, parallel groups	20-Hz rTMS; iM1	10 days	6 months
Boggio et al. (2007)	9	Subcortical	NA	Mild to moderate	40.9 months	MRC, JTT, ASS	NA	Randomized, double-blinded, cross-over.	ctDCS over cM1 and atDCS over iM1	5 days	2 weeks

Study	N	Location	Type	Severity	Time since stroke	Outcome measures	Intervention	Design	rTMS protocol	Sessions	Follow-up
Nowak et al. (2008)	15	Subcortical	Ischemic	Mild	1.93 months	ARAT, MRC (4–5), finger tapping, reach to grasp	NA	Randomized, cross-over	1-Hz rTMS, cM1	1	NA
Takeuchi et al. (2008)	20	Subcortical	Ischemic	Mixed	29.9 months	FM, acceleration and PF	PF training	Randomized, parallel groups	1-Hz rTMS over cM1	1	1 week
Dafotakis et al. (2008)	12	Subcortical	Ischemic	Mild	1.88 months	MRC (4–5), NIHSS, ARAT, grip–lift task	Grasping and lifting	Randomized, cross-over	1-Hz rTMS over cM1	1	NA
Mally and Dinya (2008)	64	Cortical – large	Ischemic and hemorrhagic (18)	Severe	129.6 months	Spasticity score	NA	Randomized, parallel groups	1-Hz rTMS over cM1 and iM1	7 days	3 months
Ameli et al. (2009)	29	Cortical (13) and subcortical (16)	Ischemic	Mild to moderate	5.5 months	MRC, ARAT, MRS, NIHSS, index and FT	NA	Randomized, cross-over	10-Hz rTMS over iM1	1	NA
Khedr, Abdel-Fadeil, Farghali, and Qaid (2009)	36	Cortical (19) and subcortical (17)	Ischemic	Mild to moderate	0.57 months	MRC, NIHSS, BI, tapping, Purdue pegboard (PP)	NA	Randomized, parallel groups	1-Hz rTMS over cM1, 3 Hz over iM1	5	3 months

Continued

TABLE 12.1 Summary of Sham-Controlled Studies Performed with rTMS and tDCS in Motor Recovery After Stroke—cont'd

	Number of Patients	Cortical/subcortical	Ischemic/hemorrhagic	Severity of Stroke	Stroke Duration	Motor Assessments and Outcomes	Concomitant Therapy	Study Design	NIBS Intervention	Number of Sessions	Follow-ups
Takeuchi, Tada, Toshima, Matsuo, and Ikoma (2009)	30	Subcortical	Ischemic	Mixed	28.8 months	FM, acceleration and PF	Motor training (pinching task)	Randomized, parallel groups	1-Hz rTMS over cM1, 10 Hz over iM1, bilateral rTMS	1	1 week
Kim et al. (2010)	18	Cortical 5, subcortical 9, cortico-subcortical 4	Ischemic	Mixed	0.85	MRC (2–5) and FM (16–60), FM, BI	Occupational therapy	Randomized, parallel groups	ctDCS over cM1, atDCS over iM1	10	6 months
Lindenberg, Renga, Zhu, Nair, and Schlaug (2010)	20	Cortico-subcortical	Ischemic	Severe	35.4	FM(20–56), WMF	Occupational therapy		Bilateral tDCS	5	1 week
Grefkes et al. (2010)	11	Subcortical	Ischemic	Mild	1.91 months	MRC (4-5), ARAT, NIHSS, whole hand fist task	NA	Randomized, cross-over	1-Hz rTMS, cM1	1	NA

Study	N	Lesion location	Etiology	Severity	Time since stroke	Outcome measures	Intervention	Design	Stimulation	Sessions	Follow-up
Madhavan, Weber, and Stinear (2011)	9	Cortico-subcortical	NA	Lower extremity	130.8 months	FM-LE, dorsiflexion and plantar flexion movements	Tracking dorsiflexion and plantar flexion task	Randomized, cross-over	atDCS over iM1, atDCS over cM1	1	NA
Tanaka et al. (2011)	8	Subcortical	NA	Mixed, lower extremity	21.1 months	SIAS, knee extension, GF	Force knee extension	Randomized, cross-over	atDCS over iM1	1	NA
Nair, Renga, Lindenberg, Zhu, and Schlaug (2011)	14	Cortical 9, subcortical 5	NA	Moderate to severe	31 months	FM (30.1)	Occupational therapy	Randomized, parallel groups	ctDCS over cM1	15	1 week
Hesse et al. (2011)	96	Mixed cortico-subcortical	Ischemic	Severe	0.93 months	BI, FM (<18), BB, MAS, MRC	Robot-assisted arm training	Randomized, parallel groups, multileft	ctDCS over cM1 and atDCS over iM1	30 (6 weeks)	3 months
Bolognini et al. (2011)	14	Cortical 9, cortico-subcortical 5	Ischemic 12, hemorrhagic 2	Moderate to severe	35.21 months	FM, BI, JTT, HG, MAL	CIT	Randomized, parallel groups	Bilateral tDCS	10	4 weeks
Sasaki et al. (2013)	29	Subcortical	Ischemic 13, hemorrhagic 16	Mild to moderate	0.58 months	NIHSS, GF, FT	Standard physical therapy	Randomized, parallel groups	10-Hz rTMS over iM1, 1 Hz rTMS over cM1	5	NA

Continued

TABLE 12.1 Summary of Sham-Controlled Studies Performed with rTMS and tDCS in Motor Recovery After Stroke—cont'd

	Number of Patients	Cortical/ subcortical	Ischemic/ hemorrhagic	Severity of Stroke	Stroke Duration	Motor Assessments and Outcomes	Concomitant Therapy	Study Design	NIBS Intervention	Number of Sessions	Follow-ups
Stagg et al. (2012)	17	Cortical and subcortical	Ischemic 16, hemorrhagic 1	Mixed	37.9 months	FM, GF, response time task	NA	Randomized, double-blinded, cross-over	ctDCS over cM1 and atDCS over iM1	1	NA
Avenanti, Coccia, Ladavas, Provinciali, and Ceravolo (2012)	30	Cortical 3, cortico-subcortical 1, subcortical 26	Ischemic 20, hemorrhagic 10	Mild	31.47 months	JTT, NHPT, BB, PF	Standard physical therapy	Randomized, parallel groups	1-Hz rTMS, cM1	10	3 months
Conforto et al. (2012)	30	Subcortical 16, cortical 14	Ischemic	Mild to severe	0.92 months	MRC, NIHSS, JTT, PF	Standard physical therapy	Randomized, parallel groups	1-Hz rTMS, cM1	10	1 month
Zimerman, Heise, Gerloff, Cohen, and Hummel (2012)	12	Subcortical	Ischemic	Mild	30 months	MRC, FM, ASS, FT	FT, learning task	Randomized, double-blinded, cross-over.	ctDCS over cM1	10	3 months

cM1, contralesional motor cortex; iM1, ipsilesional motor cortex; cPM, contralesional pre motor cortex; PA, pinch acceleration; NA, not applicable; NM, not mentioned; MRC, Medical Research Council; PP, Purdue Pegboard Test; sRT, simple reaction time task; cRT, choice reaction time task; FT, finger tapping task; SSS, Scandinavian Stroke Scale; NIHSS, NIH Stroke Scale; BI, Barthel Index; JTT, Jebsen-Taylor Hand Function Test; GF, grip force; FM, Fugl-Meyer scale; PF, pinch force; CIT, constraint-induced therapy; WMFT, Wolf Motor Function Test; MAL, Motor Activity Log; BB, Box and Block test; ASS, Ashworth Spasticity Scale; MAS, Modified Ashworth Spasticity Scale.

improvements as indicated by enhanced grip force and dexterity persistent for up to 3 months post-intervention (Avenanti et al. 2012). Based on the successful results of either inhibiting the cM1 or enhancing the iM1, recent studies tried to apply these two concepts together to achieve additive functional effects. Using dual-mode tDCS for bihemispheric brain stimulation, Lindenberg et al. (2010) investigated whether modulation of bilateral motor cortices in combination with physical and occupational therapy improves motor outcome after stroke (Lindenberg et al., 2010). Although an additive effect in motor function scores has been proposed, it remains unclear whether the bilateral approach is superior to a unilateral one, due to lack of sufficient control conditions.

It should be noted that individual responses to NIBS are highly variable, and depend on a number of biological and technical factors (see Chapter 4). Whether the severity and localization of the stroke provides better or worse potential for NIBS-related improvement is an open question. Though to date there is not enough evidence to determine the aforementioned controversy, previous studies were able to demonstrate that even in highly impaired stroke patients NIBS contributed to enhance motor function (Boggio, Alonso-Alonso et al., 2006). Considering that the neuroplastic mechanisms involved in the process of stroke recovery and motor network reorganization are fundamentally distributed at the cortical level, one possible conjecture is that the magnitude of improvement is much more pronounced when stimulation is applied to subcortical versus cortical or cortico-subcortical strokes. Supporting this assumption, Ameli and colleagues described greater improvement of hand motor function after 10-Hz rTMS over iM1 in patients with subcortical stroke compared to ones with cortical lesions (Ameli et al., 2009). Factors such as stroke localization, functional impairment, time after stroke, and others might in future be used as means of patient stratification and as surrogate variables for the best individualized interventional strategy (Hummel et al., 2008; Schulz et al., 2012). Finally, parameters of functional or structural prerequisites, such as TMS excitability measurements (e.g., MEP, SICI, IHI, ICF, and silent period) combined with structural and functional MRI markers, might help to further predict which pattern of recovery an individual patient will follow and whether the patient will or will not benefit from specific neuromodulatory treatment protocols. Although this notion is still speculative in nature, current cross-sectional and longitudinal studies in stroke patients have started to yield valuable information (Schulz et al., 2012; Stinear & Ward, 2013). Taking together, the abovementioned questions, considerations, and controversies make it evident that longitudinal studies and more in-depth assessment of stroke characteristics are necessary for developing future stimulation protocols and tailoring them to the stroke patient's requirements for specific motor impairments.

We believe that with such an approach the effect size of NIBS on functional recovery after stroke can be significantly further increased.

NIBS to Enhance Language Recovery

Aphasia is a common consequence of dominant hemisphere strokes, occurring in 21–38% of acute-stroke patients (Pedersen, Jorgensen, Nakayama, Raaschou, & Olsen, 1995; Wade, Hewer, David, & Enderby, 1986). Individuals with aphasia are reported to have a lower quality of life and social participation. Despite the evidence that intensive speech and language therapy improves the functional communication abilities in these patients, 12% of stroke survivors persist with a relevant degree of chronic language deficits (Wade et al., 1986). Recently, a growing number of studies attempted to explore the application of NIBS as an adjuvant treatment for facilitating language recovery in post-stroke aphasia. Support for this intervention came from functional reorganizational studies of language networks following stroke demonstrating different mechanisms involved in recovery, including intrahemispheric cortical recruitment of adjacent areas in the left hemisphere and changes in trans-callosal interhemispheric interactions between homologous languages regions.

Evidence suggests that significant reacquisition of language ability after stroke is associated with reorganization of the injured dominant hemisphere by increased recruitment of residual perilesional regions. Functional studies revealed that non-fluent aphasic patients who demonstrated better language improvement showed larger activation of ipsilesional adjacent regions (Fridriksson 2010; Heiss & Thiel, 2006). By using NIBS techniques to facilitate cortical activity in the left hemisphere, Szaflarski et al. (2011) applied excitatory (intermittent) theta burst stimulation (TBS) to eight patients with moderate to severe chronic aphasia. Stimulation was applied to Broca's area, identified previously by fMRI activity during a semantic decision and tone decision task. Six of the eight patients demonstrated significant improvements in semantic fluency, and subsequent fMRI data demonstrated a leftward shift in language activation (Szaflarski et al., 2011). Improved language performance has been also observed after anodal tDCS to the left hemisphere. For example, Baker, Rorden, and Fridriksson (2010) described improved naming performance in 10 aphasic patients with left-hemisphere stroke after 5 consecutive days of anodal tDCS to the left frontal lobe (Baker et al., 2010). In another cross-over design study, the same investigators examined the effect of anodal tDCS on reaction times while fluent aphasic patients were receiving a computerized anomia treatment. Compared to a sham treatment, pairing tDCS with specific training significantly reduced naming reaction time immediately after treatment, and the improvement lasted for at least 3 weeks (Fridriksson, Richardson, Baker, & Rorden, 2011).

To date, the role of right non-dominant hemisphere in language functions and in the recovery process from aphasia remains more controversial. Different lines of evidence provide support for diverse hypotheses, suggesting right hemisphere to be deleterious, beneficial, or either one or the other depending on different factors such as time from aphasia onset, age, severity of the symptoms, and demands of the task, among others (for review, see Chrysikou & Hamilton, 2011). After left-hemisphere stroke, functional neuroimaging studies have revealed that there is an unusually robust activation in right homologous cortical regions (Martin et al., 2005; Naeser et al., 2004). Based on these findings, and supporting the concept of imbalanced interhemispheric interactions between both hemispheres after stroke, a number of studies have therefore employed inhibitory rTMS or cathodal tDCS to the right hemisphere with the goal of diminishing abnormal contralesional cortical activity. In six chronic non-fluent aphasic patients, Naeser et al. (2005) demonstrated that 1-Hz rTMS for 10 minutes to the anterior portion of the right Broca's area (pars triangularis) resulted in significant improvement in naming, while similar stimulation to the posterior portion (pars opercularis) transiently worsened performance (Naeser et al., 2005). In a second study from the same group, the right pars triangularis was targeted with 2 weeks of consecutive sessions of inhibitory rTMS (five sessions per week). A significant improvement on three naming tests was found even after 2 months of the rTMS intervention (Naeser et al., 2005).

According to recent findings, however, the previous approach has limited effects in patients with extensive left-hemispheric lesions. In these cases, contralesional language areas were suggested to play a crucial role in the recovery process, and should not be downregulated via NIBS techniques. Hence, anodal (excitatory) tDCS applied to the unaffected hemisphere led to variable language improvement, persisting for up to 2 weeks after stimulation (Flöel et al., 2011). One plausible explanation for the beneficial effect is the proposed hierarchical scheme of language recovery mechanisms (Heiss & Thiel, 2006). According to this model, the reacquisition of language functions in patients with small lesions in the left hemisphere tends to be mediated by recruitment of left perilesional areas with variable involvement of right-hemispheric structures (Heiss & Thiel, 2006; Hillis, 2007). These right-hemispheric regions are usually "mirror structures" of the lesioned left hemisphere, and they may become functionally relevant over time if they subserve language functions during recovery (i.e., homologous regions). In contrast, when left-hemispheric language networks are more severely impaired, as with relatively large lesions involving language-related structures of the fronto-temporal lobes, the only possible mechanism for recovery may be through the recruitment of homologous language and speech-motor regions in the right non-dominant hemisphere (Heiss & Thiel, 2006; Schlaug, Norton,

Marchina, Zipse, & Wan, 2010; Zipse, Norton, Marchina, & Schlaug, 2012). Although the mechanisms underlying the non-dominant engagement are not clear enough, some authors proposed that the right hemisphere assumes speech-motor output functions through a rudimentary arcuate fasciculus (for review, see Schlaug, Marchina, & Wan, 2011). In conclusion, future studies will need to take into account not only the stimulation parameters but also the location and extent of the lesion, timing of the intervention with regard to stroke onset, and patient information (e.g., severity of aphasia, age, medication, premorbid laterality for language, etc.), among other relevant factors.

Neglect

Unilateral neglect is a multimodal disorder, commonly defined as a failure to attend, respond adequately, or orient to stimuli located contralateral to the lesion (Heilman, Valenstein, & Watson, 2000). Stroke patients with neglect have longer rehabilitation hospital stays, are more prone to fall, and exhibit a diminished capacity to perform both basic self-care and more complex ADLs (Pedersen, Jorgensen, Nakayama, Raaschou, & Olsen, 1997).

Hemispatial neglect can be characterized as a dysfunction of the fronto-parietal network of attention. Within this network, spatial attention is controlled by both intra- and interhemispheric connections. Consistent with the model of interhemispheric interactions, concepts suggest that both parietal cortices exert reciprocal inhibition on one another (the left hemisphere directs the attention to the right side, while the right hemisphere accounts for both sides of the space). For instance, damage to right posterior parietal regions causes disinhibition and, thus, overactivation of the left hemisphere. This enhances the predisposition to attend to the right and, hence, to neglect the left hemi-space (Corbetta, Kincade, Lewis, Snyder and Sapir, 2005; Corbetta, Tansy et al., 2005). Further paired-pulse TMS studies provide evidence supporting a pathological hyperexcitability of the left hemisphere (Koch, Veniero, & Caltagirone, 2013). Thus, the applications of therapeutic NIBS attempt to countervail the present interhemispheric imbalance by reducing the overactivity of the contralesional hemisphere.

Until now, most of the studies performed have aimed to inhibit the contralesional parietal cortex. By using different rTMS and tDCS protocols, these studies demonstrated that downregulation of the healthy left (overactive) parietal cortex transiently improved contralateral visuospatial neglect and extinction (Fierro, Brighina, & Bisiach, 2006; Lim, Kang, & Paik, 2010). Indeed, low-frequency rTMS applied over left-sided posterior parietal cortex over 2 weeks improved visuospatial performance in three patients for up to 15 days after stimulation (Brighina et al., 2003). Similar benefits were demonstrated by an open-label study in seven neglect patients after 10 days of 1-Hz rTMS to the left parietal area immediately prior to occupational therapy, in comparison to seven control patients who received only occupational therapy (Lim et al., 2010). In an elegant cross-over, double-blind design, Sparing et al. (2009) applied three different stimulation sessions to 10 neglect patients, with (1) anodal tDCS to the ipsilesional parietal cortex, (2) cathodal tDCS to the left healthy parietal cortex, or (3) sham conditions. Interestingly, both interventional approaches reduced symptoms of visuospatial neglect as probed by reduction of the rightward bias in the line bisection task, suggesting that NIBS induced its beneficial effects by modulation of parietal interhemispheric imbalance in stroke patients with neglect (Sparing et al., 2009).

The presently available proof-of-principle studies of brain stimulation in the treatment of post-stroke neglect patients give rise to optimism regarding the application of neuromodulatory techniques in the clinical routine and combining them with current strategies such as prism adaptation or spatial training. However, larger double-blind, placebo-controlled trials that can potentially account for optimal stimulation protocols, and duration and site of stimulation, are needed.

NIBS IN ALZHEIMER'S DISEASE

Despite decades of intensive research in the field of Alzheimer's disease, a relevant pharmacological treatment remains out of reach. To date, most of these treatments attempt to slow down the progression of the disease by increasing cholinergic activity (Birks, Grimley Evans, Iakovidou, Tsolaki, & Holt, 2009; Feldman & Kertesz, 2001; Rosler et al., 1999). However, the benefit in terms of effect size is rather small. Therefore, alternative or complementary non-pharmacological adjuvant therapeutic strategies have gained increasing attention. In this regard, recent studies proposed neuromodulatory techniques as a possible treatment to enhance cognitive performance and learning in healthy elderly subjects (Zimerman & Hummel, 2010, Zimerman et al., 2013). Specifically, tDCS and rTMS demonstrated positive effects on different cognitive domains such as attention (Vanderhasselt et al., 2007), executive function as indexed by the Stroop task (Boggio et al., 2005), go/no-go tasks (Boggio et al., 2007), decision making (Fecteau et al., 2007), and a complex verbal problem-solving task (Cerruti & Schlaug, 2009). Based on these findings, recent work proposed NIBS as a suitable technique for patients affected by cognitive impairment (for review, see Nardone et al., 2012).

Preliminary studies have been carried out to assess the effects of rTMS on naming and language performance in patients with probable Alzheimer's disease (AD; see also Chapter 13). Two cross-over, sham-controlled studies performed by Cotelli and colleagues explored the application of a single-session facilitatory 20-Hz rTMS protocol over the dorsolateral prefrontal cortex (DLPFC) during the execution of a naming task (Cotelli et al., 2006, Cotelli, Manenti, Cappa, Zanetti, & Miniussi, 2008). First, Cotelli et al. (2006) investigated the effects of rTMS on 15 mild to moderate AD patients all receiving cholinesterase inhibitor treatment. They found a significant improvement in an action-naming task following both left and right DLPFC stimulation as compared with sham (Cotelli et al., 2006). In the second study, using the same paradigm, Cotelli et al. (2008) investigated the effects of rTMS on 24 AD patients with different degrees of cognitive decline, ranging from mild and moderate to severe AD. As previously described, rTMS of both DLPFC resulted in improved action-naming in the mild AD group (MMSE $\geq 17/30$). Strikingly, in patients with moderate to severe AD (MMSE $< 17/30$), both action- and object-naming were facilitated after both left and right DLPFC intervention (Cotelli et al., 2008). The present finding could potentially be explained by a "ceiling effect" for object-naming in mildly impaired AD patients, given that patients with moderate to severe AD have more room to improve. It is of interest that the bilateral facilitation effect observed after both left and right DLPFC intervention could potentially be attributed to compensatory mechanisms present in the aging brain, as previously found for the cognitive and even in the motor system using a variety of cognitive as well as motor tasks (Cabeza, 2002; Zimerman, Heise, Gerloff, Cohen, & Hummel, 2012).

Although the motor system is not primarily affected in the course of AD, further support for the use of NIBS in AD patients comes from alterations observed in intra- and intercortical excitability in mild to moderate AD patients in comparison with healthy subjects (Di Lazzaro et al., 2004, 2006). For instance, paired-pulse TMS protocols demonstrated reduced intracortical inhibition (evaluated with SICI) and significantly prolonged ipsilateral silent period latencies (a measure that likely reflects transcallosal inhibition) in AD patients (Hoeppner et al., 2011). In addition to these findings, it is of interest that reduction of GABA-mediated inhibition (probed by SICI at rest and during movement preparation) diminished as a function of increasing age, as recently demonstrated in a sample of 64 healthy participants between 20 and 88 years of age (Heise et al., 2013). Whether the changes in cortical excitability are specific phenomena related to AD or whether it is a general condition related to aging processes is a question that needs to be clarified in upcoming studies.

Since cognitive training may improve cognitive functions in AD, recent studies aimed to obtain a synergistic effect by combining rTMS with training in a group of eight patients with mild to moderate AD. Broca and Wernicke (language functions), right and left DLPFC (judgment, executive functions, and long-term memory), and right and left parietal association cortex (spatial and topographical orientation and praxias) were stimulated for 6 weeks, followed by maintenance sessions for an additional 3 months (Bentwich et al., 2011). Although an improvement in the Alzheimer's Disease Assessment Scale – Cognitive (ADAS-cog) and the Clinical Global Impression of Changes (CGIC) was reported, one important limitation of the study was the absence of adequate control conditions (e.g., cognitive training plus sham stimulation). By using tDCS, Boggio et al. (2009) investigated the effects of NIBS on a recognition memory test. Ten AD patients received tDCS in three different sessions: anodal tDCS over the left DLPFC, anodal tDCS over the left temporal cortex, and sham tDCS. Neuropsychological assessments included three cognitive domains: selective attention, working memory, and visual recognition memory. All tasks were performed during tDCS. The authors found an improvement in the visual recognition memory task during temporal and prefrontal cortex stimulation, which was not attributable to a non-specific attentional process, as assessed by the Stroop task. On the contrary, no effects were obtained on working memory (Boggio et al., 2009). Since a bipolar montage was used, it cannot be completely ruled out whether the present effects may be the result of the stimulation from the reference electrode (cathode). Moreover, the study did not measure whether the effects were longer lasting or only short and transient, and the authors did not perform any other behavioral assessments to assess whether the effects were clinically relevant.

Although promising, results from NIBS trials to enhance cognitive functions in AD have, to date, to be considered extremely preliminary. There are few articles on rTMS and even less on tDCS that investigate the effects of these tools as cognitive enhancers in AD. As recently demonstrated in healthy elderly subjects, one possible mechanism that can account for the effects of NIBS on cognitive performance represents the potential of these techniques to improve the ability to learn or to acquire new skills/strategies for carrying out behavioral tasks (Reis et al., 2009; Zimerman et al., 2013). On this basis, further studies should explore novel experimental paradigms and different stimulation targets in combination with reliable clinical, cognitive, and behavioral assessment tools.

NIBS IN THE TREATMENT OF PARKINSON'S DISEASE

Parkinson's disease (PD) is a progressive movement disorder caused by loss of dopaminergic neurons in the substantia nigra. In spite of recent advances, limitations in current therapies in PD remain. Dopaminergic medications are an effective therapy of current management, particularly for motor symptoms. However, dopamine-resistant symptoms, such as depression, cognitive deficits, freezing of gait, dementia, and hallucinations, also significantly contribute to morbidity (Poewe, 2008;

Storch et al., 2013). In addition, long-term treatment with L-Dopa may result in problematic motor fluctuations and dyskinesia (Nutt, 2001). While deep brain stimulation (DBS) demonstrated a beneficial option for medication-induced motor fluctuation, effects are still limited to a well-defined patient population and carry the risk of serious surgical complications and significant neuropsychiatric side effects (Skidmore et al., 2006).

The application of NIBS as an adjunctive treatment have been started to be investigated in PD (see also Chapter 13). One main obstacle for the use of NIBS techniques is that penetrance into the cortex is limited, and deeper structures, such as basal ganglia, cannot be directly targeted by these methods. However, altered network loops between the basal ganglia and cortical regions, as one major pathophysiological substrate for the motor symptoms, could be potentially targeted by non-invasive interventional techniques (Wu, Fregni, Simon, Deblieck, & Pascual-Leone, 2008). Ideally, NIBS would not only normalize the pathological subcortical–cortical circuitries but also the activation patterns and excitability levels of the cortical motor areas. For instance, changes of the cortical states in the course of PD were suggested to be related to motor symptom impairment such as early bradykinesia and later medication-induced dyskinesia (Haslinger et al., 2001). Accordingly, in early stages of PD mesial motor areas such as the supplementary motor area (SMA) regularly show decreased activity, whereas hyperactivity is found in more lateral regions, such as the primary motor cortex, in more advanced stages of the disease (Haslinger et al., 2001; Sabatini et al., 2000). While the hypoactive brain areas are usually interpreted as a "primary" dysfunction associated with parkinsonian symptoms, the hyperactivity has been interpreted as a neural correlate of adaptive plasticity within the motor system to compensate for the defective motor cortical–subcortical loop (Sabatini et al., 2000).

Based on the concept that striatal dopamine depletion results in an overinhibition of neuronal activity in the motor thalamus, and consequently in cortical motor regions, a series of controlled studies have investigated the potential of facilitatory NIBS applied to M1. rTMS in single- (Lefaucheur et al., 2004; Siebner, Rossmeier, Mentschel, Peinemann, & Conrad, 2000) and multisession studies (Khedr, Farweez, & Islam, 2003), as well as anodal tDCS (Fregni et al., 2006), demonstrated variable functional improvement. Interestingly, Lefaucheur et al. (2004) showed benefits of M1 rTMS with both low- and high-frequency rTMS. While 10-Hz rTMS reduced contralateral bradykinesia, 0.5-Hz rTMS reduced bilateral rigidity and improved gait speed. Thus, hypotheses of mechanisms for M1 stimulation might potentially account for modulation of both excitatory and inhibitory circuits (Lefaucheur et al., 2004).

The DLPFC is suggested to be an "entry port" to modulate prefrontal loops (Wu et al., 2008) which are suggested to be involved in non-motor symptoms in PD. On this basis, Fregni et al. (2004) demonstrated that 10 days of 15-Hz rTMS over left DLPFC (plus placebo medication) had an equivalent efficacy on depression rating scales as fluoxetine antidepressant (plus sham rTMS) which persisted for at least 8 weeks (Fregni et al., 2004). Except for some improvement in working memory (Boggio, Ferrucci et al., 2006), non-depressed PD patients do not seem to benefit in motor functions, either from activating rTMS (del Olmo, Bello, & Cudeiro, 2007) or tDCS applied to the DLPFC (Fregni et al., 2006).

Functional neuroimaging studies have supported the view that impaired activity of the SMA might play a crucial role in PD bradykinesia. Recent studies, however, were able to demonstrate overactivation of SMA in patients with drug-induced dyskinesia. Interestingly, the application of low-frequency rTMS to SMA (Brusa et al., 2006) transiently improved dyskinesia in these patients. Finally, as another potential target, Koch and colleagues provided evidence that 2-week sessions of bilateral cerebellar continuous TBS were capable of reducing peak-dose L-Dopa induced dyskinesia for up to 4 weeks (Koch et al., 2009).

In summary, although an increasing number of proof-of-principle studies yield some evidence of the beneficial effects of NIBS to treat motor and non-motor symptoms in PD patients, non-invasive techniques are still preliminary in nature and a long way from being therapeutically relevant, especially given the efficient current strategies based on pharmacological and DBS interventions. Moreover, there are several questions that need to be carefully answered in upcoming studies before an application in clinical practice can be envisaged.

REMARKS AND FUTURE DIRECTIONS

Overall, the available studies suggest that NIBS, by means of rTMS and tDCS, could serve as a potential complementary therapeutic tool in a variety of neurological conditions, such as stroke, Parkinson's and Alzheimer's disease, and a growing list of other neuropsychiatric disorders (e.g., depression, pain, epilepsy, and multiple sclerosis). Despite major advances over the past few decades, current neurological treatments, especially pharmacologic treatments, may be ineffective or cause treatment-interfering side effects. NIBS techniques, on the other hand, avoid systemic side effects and stimulate the brain with high temporal and spatial resolution that cannot currently be achieved pharmacologically or via other complementary therapies.

Although the outcomes of these initial "proof of principle" trials include some conflicting results, there is evidence that rTMS and tDCS may have a therapeutic value in different neurological conditions. Even in stroke, arguably the most suited to NIBS therapy, an increasing number of works are reported with no additional treatment benefit compared with physical therapy alone (Talelli et al., 2012). These negative findings could potentially be explained by interindividual differences in NIBS susceptibility, which seem to depend on a number of technical as well as biological factors. Brain damage can occur anywhere within the brain, including cerebral cortex, subcortical structures, white matter tracts and underlying white matter, brainstem, cerebellum, etc., and be of variable spatial extent and severity. Thus there is no such thing as "a" stroke, and NIBS approaches will need to accommodate this diversity. Furthermore, brain reorganization is a dynamic process, which differs considerably depending on time since stroke, and premorbid conditions such as age of the patient and even genetic profiles (Grefkes & Fink, 2012; Hummel et al., 2008; see also Fig. 12.1). All these different contributing factors make it unlikely that one stimulation protocol exists which is suitable for all patients and all diseases. It thus remains to be elucidated which patient should undergo which specific rTMS or tDCS protocol, and how these factors relate to stimulation location, and dose and frequency of the therapy. On this basis, the application of NIBS techniques will need to be refined to take into account the diversity of neurological symptoms, the fundamental differences between acute and rather stable (i.e., stroke) conditions, and chronic progressive disease processes (i.e., Parkinson's and Alzheimer's disease), and the differential part played by functional and dysfunctional plasticity in these diseases.

At present, the application of cortical stimulation is experimental and can only be recommended in the framework of controlled studies. Clinical trial evidence is still insufficient to allow endorsement of widespread use of the present NIBS techniques, despite the great margin of safety when appropriate guidelines and precautions are followed (Rossi et al., 2009). Further and larger studies on cortical stimulation are justified on the basis of multiple studies on laboratory animals, a large body of neurostimulation and neuroimaging data in young and aged healthy human volunteers, and "proof of principle" studies on rTMS and tDCS in different neurological diseases. Recently, the first multicenter longitudinal trial was set up to investigate the role of anodal tDCS applied in the subacute state after stroke combined with standardized physical training for motor recovery (Neuroregeneration Enhanced by Transcranial Direct Current Stimulation in Stroke [NETS, http://clinicaltrials.gov/ct2/show/NCT00909714]). Besides the evaluation of the functional effects of NIBS, this trial will hopefully contribute to the understanding of the temporal development of motor plasticity and regeneration. Thereby it could elucidate different recovery patterns, which might help to predict the effectiveness of brain stimulation using a multimodal approach.

References

Ameli, M., Grefkes, C., Kemper, F., Riegg, F. P., Rehme, A. K., Karbe, H., et al. (2009). Differential effects of high-frequency repetitive transcranial magnetic stimulation over ipsilesional primary motor cortex in cortical and subcortical middle cerebral artery stroke. *Annals of Neurology, 66*, 298–309.

Angelakis, E., Liouta, E., Andreadis, N., Leonardos, A., Ktonas, P., Stavrinou, L. C., et al. (2013). Transcranial alternating current stimulation reduces symptoms in intractable idiopathic cervical dystonia: A case study. *Neuroscience Letters, 533*, 39–43.

Antal, A., Boros, K., Poreisz, C., Chaieb, L., Terney, D., & Paulus, W. (2008). Comparatively weak after-effects of transcranial alternating current stimulation (tACS) on cortical excitability in humans. *Brain Stimulation, 1*, 97–105.

Avenanti, A., Coccia, M., Ladavas, E., Provinciali, L., & Ceravolo, M. G. (2012). Low-frequency rTMS promotes use-dependent motor plasticity in chronic stroke: A randomized trial. *Neurology, 78*, 256–264.

Baker, J. M., Rorden, C., & Fridriksson, J. (2010). Using transcranial direct-current stimulation to treat stroke patients with aphasia. *Stroke, 41*, 1229–1236.

Barker, A. T., Jalinous, R., & Freeston, I. L. (1985). Non-invasive magnetic stimulation of human motor cortex. *Lancet, 1*, 1106–1107.

Baumer, T., Lange, R., Liepert, J., Weiller, C., Siebner, H. R., Rothwell, J. C., et al. (2003). Repeated premotor rTMS leads to cumulative plastic changes of motor cortex excitability in humans. *NeuroImage, 20*, 550–560.

Bentwich, J., Dobronevsky, E., Aichenbaum, S., Shorer, R., Peretz, R., Khaigrekht, M., et al. (2011). Beneficial effect of repetitive transcranial magnetic stimulation combined with cognitive training for the treatment of Alzheimer's disease: A proof of concept study. *Journal of Neural Transmission, 118*, 463–471.

Birks, J., Grimley Evans, J., Iakovidou, V., Tsolaki, M., & Holt, F. E. (2009). Rivastigmine for Alzheimer's disease. *Cochrane Database of Systematic Reviews*, CD001191.

Bliss, T. V., & Collingridge, G. L. (1993). A synaptic model of memory: Long-term potentiation in the hippocampus. *Nature, 361*, 31–39.

Boggio, P. S., Alonso-Alonso, M., Mansur, C. G., Rigonatti, S. P., Schlaug, G., Pascual-Leone, A., et al. (2006). Hand function improvement with low-frequency repetitive transcranial magnetic stimulation of the unaffected hemisphere in a severe case of stroke. *American Journal of Physical Medicine and Rehabilitation, 85*, 927–930.

Boggio, P. S., Bermpohl, F., Vergara, A. O., Muniz, A. L., Nahas, F. H., Leme, P. B., et al. (2007). Go/no-go task performance improvement after anodal transcranial DC stimulation of the left dorsolateral prefrontal cortex in major depression. *Journal of Affective Disorders, 101*, 91–98.

Boggio, P. S., Ferrucci, R., Rigonatti, S. P., Covre, P., Nitsche, M., Pascual-Leone, A., et al. (2006). Effects of transcranial direct current stimulation on working memory in patients with Parkinson's disease. *Journal of the Neurological Sciences, 249*, 31–38.

Boggio, P. S., Fregni, F., Bermpohl, F., Mansur, C. G., Rosa, M., Rumi, D. O., et al. (2005). Effect of repetitive TMS and fluoxetine on cognitive function in patients with Parkinson's disease and concurrent depression. *Movement Disorders, 20*, 1178–1184.

Boggio, P. S., Khoury, L. P., Martins, D. C., Martins, O. E., de Macedo, E. C., & Fregni, F. (2009). Temporal cortex direct current stimulation enhances performance on a visual recognition memory task in Alzheimer disease. *Journal of Neurology, Neurosurgery, and Psychiatry, 80*, 444–447.

Bolognini, N., Pascual-Leone, A., & Fregni, F. (2009). Using non-invasive brain stimulation to augment motor training-induced plasticity. *Journal of Neuroengineering and Rehabilitation, 6*, 8.

Bolognini, N., Vallar, G., Casati, C., Latif, L. A., El-Nazer, R., Williams, J., et al. (2011). Neurophysiological and behavioral effects of tDCS combined with constraint-induced movement therapy in poststroke patients. *Neurorehabilitation and Neural Repair, 25*, 819–829.

Brighina, F., Bisiach, E., Oliveri, M., Piazza, A., La Bua, V., Daniele, O., et al. (2003). 1 Hz repetitive transcranial magnetic stimulation of the unaffected hemisphere ameliorates contralesional visuospatial neglect in humans. *Neuroscience Letters, 336*, 131–133.

Brown, C. E., Boyd, J. D., & Murphy, T. H. (2010). Longitudinal in vivo imaging reveals balanced and branch-specific remodeling of mature cortical pyramidal dendritic arbors after stroke. *Journal of Cerebral Blood Flow and Metabolism, 30*, 783–791.

Brunoni, A. R., Amadera, J., Berbel, B., Volz, M. S., Rizzerio, B. G., & Fregni, F. (2011). A systematic review on reporting and assessment of adverse effects associated with transcranial direct current stimulation. *The International Journal of Neuropsychopharmacology/ Official Scientific Journal of the Collegium Internationale Neuropsychopharmacologicum, 14*, 1133–1145.

Brusa, L., Versace, V., Koch, G., Iani, C., Stanzione, P., Bernardi, G., et al. (2006). Low frequency rTMS of the SMA transiently ameliorates peak-dose LID in Parkinson's disease. *Clinical Neurophysiology, 117*, 1917–1921.

Cabeza, R. (2002). Hemispheric asymmetry reduction in older adults: The HAROLD model. *Psychology and Aging, 17*, 85–100.

Cerruti, C., & Schlaug, G. (2009). Anodal transcranial direct current stimulation of the prefrontal cortex enhances complex verbal associative thought. *Journal of Cognitive Neuroscience, 21*, 1980–1987.

Chan, H. N., Alonzo, A., Martin, D. M., Player, M., Mitchell, P. B., Sachdev, P., et al. (2012). Treatment of major depressive disorder by transcranial random noise stimulation: Case report of a novel treatment. *Biological Psychiatry, 72*, e9–e10.

Chrysikou, E. G., & Hamilton, R. H. (2011). Noninvasive brain stimulation in the treatment of aphasia: Exploring interhemispheric relationships and their implications for neurorehabilitation. *Restorative Neurology and Neuroscience, 29*, 375–394.

Conforto, A. B., Anjos, S. M., Saposnik, G., Mello, E. A., Nagaya, E. M., Santos, W.Jr., et al. (2012). Transcranial magnetic stimulation in mild to severe hemiparesis early after stroke: A proof of principle and novel approach to improve motor function. *Journal of Neurology, 259*, 1399–1405.

Corbetta, M., Kincade, M. J., Lewis, C., Snyder, A. Z., & Sapir, A. (2005). Neural basis and recovery of spatial attention deficits in spatial neglect. *Nature Neuroscience, 8*, 1603–1610.

Corbetta, M., Tansy, A. P., Stanley, C. M., Astafiev, S. V., Snyder, A. Z., & Shulman, G. L. (2005). A functional MRI study of preparatory signals for spatial location and objects. *Neuropsychologia, 43*, 2041–2056.

Cotelli, M., Manenti, R., Cappa, S. F., Geroldi, C., Zanetti, O., Rossini, P. M., et al. (2006). Effect of transcranial magnetic stimulation on action naming in patients with Alzheimer disease. *Archives of Neurology, 63*, 1602–1604.

Cotelli, M., Manenti, R., Cappa, S. F., Zanetti, O., & Miniussi, C. (2008). Transcranial magnetic stimulation improves naming in Alzheimer disease patients at different stages of cognitive decline. *European Journal of Neurology, 15*, 1286–1292.

Dafotakis, M., Grefkes, C., Eickhoff, S. B., Karbe, H., Fink, G. R., & Nowak, D. A. (2008). Effects of rTMS on grip force control following subcortical stroke. *Experimental Neurology, 211*, 407–412.

Dayan, E., Censor, N., Buch, E. R., Sandrini, M., & Cohen, L. G. (2013). Noninvasive brain stimulation: From physiology to network dynamics and back. *Nature Neuroscience, 16*, 838–844.

del Olmo, M. F., Bello, O., & Cudeiro, J. (2007). Transcranial magnetic stimulation over dorsolateral prefrontal cortex in Parkinson's disease. *Clinical Neurophysiology, 118*, 131–139.

Di Lazzaro, V., Oliviero, A., Pilato, F., Saturno, E., Dileone, M., Marra, C., et al. (2004). Motor cortex hyperexcitability to transcranial magnetic stimulation in Alzheimer's disease. *Journal of Neurology, Neurosurgery, and Psychiatry, 75*, 555–559.

Di Lazzaro, V., Pilato, F., Dileone, M., Saturno, E., Oliviero, A., Marra, C., et al. (2006). *In vivo* cholinergic circuit evaluation in frontotemporal and Alzheimer dementias. *Neurology, 66*, 1111–1113.

Dubovik, S., Bouzerda-Wahlen, A., Nahum, L., Gold, G., Schnider, A., & Guggisberg, A. G. (2013). Adaptive reorganization of cortical networks in Alzheimer's disease. *Clinical Neurophysiology, 124*, 35–43.

Duque, J., Murase, N., Celnik, P., Hummel, F., Harris-Love, M., Mazzocchio, R., et al. (2007). Intermanual Differences in movement-related interhemispheric inhibition. *Journal of Cognitive Neuroscience, 19*, 204–213.

Fecteau, S., Knoch, D., Fregni, F., Sultani, N., Boggio, P., & Pascual-Leone, A. (2007). Diminishing risk-taking behavior by modulating activity in the prefrontal cortex: A direct current stimulation study. *Journal of Neuroscience: The Official Journal of the Society for Neuroscience, 27*, 12500–12505.

Feldman, H., & Kertesz, A. (2001). Diagnosis, classification and natural history of degenerative dementias. *The Canadian Journal of Neurological Sciences, 28*(Suppl. 1), S17–S27.

Fierro, B., Brighina, F., & Bisiach, E. (2006). Improving neglect by TMS. *Behavioural Neurology, 17*, 169–176.

Flöel, A., Meinzer, M., Kirstein, R., Nijhof, S., Deppe, M., Knecht, S., et al. (2011). Short-term anomia training and electrical brain stimulation. *Stroke, 42*, 2065–2067.

Fregni, F., Boggio, P. S., Mansur, C. G., Wagner, T., Ferreira, M. J., Lima, M. C., et al. (2005). Transcranial direct current stimulation of the unaffected hemisphere in stroke patients. *Neuroreport, 16*, 1551–1555.

Fregni, F., Boggio, P. S., Santos, M. C., Lima, M., Vieira, A. L., Rigonatti, S. P., et al. (2006). Noninvasive cortical stimulation with transcranial direct current stimulation in Parkinson's disease. *Movement Disorders, 21*, 1693–1702.

Fregni, F., Santos, C. M., Myczkowski, M. L., Rigolino, R., Gallucci-Neto, J., Barbosa, E. R., et al. (2004). Repetitive transcranial magnetic stimulation is as effective as fluoxetine in the treatment of depression in patients with Parkinson's disease. *Journal of Neurology, Neurosurgery, and Psychiatry, 75*, 1171–1174.

Fridriksson, J. (2010). Preservation and modulation of specific left hemisphere regions is vital for treated recovery from anomia in stroke. *Journal of Neuroscience: The Official Journal of the Society for Neuroscience, 30*, 11558–11564.

Fridriksson, J., Richardson, J. D., Baker, J. M., & Rorden, C. (2011). Transcranial direct current stimulation improves naming reaction time in fluent aphasia: A double-blind, sham-controlled study. *Stroke, 42*, 819–821.

Fritsch, B., Reis, J., Martinowich, K., Schambra, H. M., Ji, Y., Cohen, L. G., et al. (2010). Direct current stimulation promotes BDNF-dependent synaptic plasticity: Potential implications for motor learning. *Neuron, 66*, 198–204.

Gandiga, P. C., Hummel, F. C., & Cohen, L. G. (2006). Transcranial DC stimulation (tDCS): A tool for double-blind sham-controlled clinical studies in brain stimulation. *Clinical Neurophysiology, 117*, 845–850.

Gerloff, C., Bushara, K., Sailer, A., Wassermann, E. M., Chen, R., Matsuoka, T., et al. (2006). Multimodal imaging of brain reorganization in motor areas of the contralesional hemisphere of well recovered patients after capsular stroke. *Brain: A Journal of Neurology, 129*, 791–808.

Grefkes, C., Eickhoff, S. B., Nowak, D. A., Dafotakis, M., & Fink, G. R. (2008). Dynamic intra- and interhemispheric interactions during unilateral and bilateral hand movements assessed with fMRI and DCM. *NeuroImage, 41*, 1382–1394.

Grefkes, C., & Fink, G. R. (2011). Reorganization of cerebral networks after stroke: New insights from neuroimaging with connectivity approaches. *Brain: A Journal of Neurology, 134*, 1264–1276.

Grefkes, C., & Fink, G. R. (2012). Disruption of motor network connectivity post-stroke and its noninvasive neuromodulation. *Current Opinion in Neurology, 25*, 670–675.

Grefkes, C., Nowak, D. A., Eickhoff, S. B., Dafotakis, M., Kust, J., Karbe, H., et al. (2008). Cortical connectivity after subcortical stroke assessed with functional magnetic resonance imaging. *Annals of Neurology, 63*, 236–246.

Grefkes, C., Nowak, D. A., Wang, L. E., Dafotakis, M., Eickhoff, S. B., & Fink, G. R. (2010). Modulating cortical connectivity in stroke patients by rTMS assessed with fMRI and dynamic causal modeling. *NeuroImage, 50*, 233–242.

Hallett, M. (2007). Transcranial magnetic stimulation: A primer. *Neuron, 55*, 187–199.

Haslinger, B., Erhard, P., Kampfe, N., Boecker, H., Rummeny, E., Schwaiger, M., et al. (2001). Event-related functional magnetic resonance imaging in Parkinson's disease before and after levodopa. *Brain: A Journal of Neurology, 124*, 558–570.

Heilman, K. M., Valenstein, E., & Watson, R. T. (2000). Neglect and related disorders. *Seminars in Neurology, 20*, 463–470.

Heise, K. F., Zimerman, M., Hoppe, J., Gerloff, C., Wegscheider, K., & Hummel, F. C. (2013). The aging motor system as a model for plastic changes of GABA-mediated intracortical inhibition and their behavioral relevance. *Journal of Neuroscience: The Official Journal of the Society for Neuroscience, 33*, 9039–9049.

Heiss, W. D., & Thiel, A. (2006). A proposed regional hierarchy in recovery of post-stroke aphasia. *Brain and Language, 98*, 118–123.

Hesse, S., Waldner, A., Mehrholz, J., Tomelleri, C., Pohl, M., & Werner, C. (2011). Combined transcranial direct current stimulation and robot-assisted arm training in subacute stroke patients: An exploratory, randomized multicenter trial. *Neurorehabilitation and Neural Repair, 25*, 838–846.

Hillis, A. E. (2007). Magnetic resonance perfusion imaging in the study of language. *Brain and Language, 102*, 165–175.

Hoeppner, J., Wegrzyn, M., Thome, J., Bauer, A., Oltmann, I., Buchmann, J., et al. (2011). Intra- and inter-cortical motor excitability in Alzheimer's disease. *Journal of Neural Transmission, 119*, 605–612.

Huang, Y. Z., Edwards, M. J., Rounis, E., Bhatia, K. P., & Rothwell, J. C. (2005). Theta burst stimulation of the human motor cortex. *Neuron, 45*, 201–206.

Hummel, F., Celnik, P., Giraux, P., Flöel, A., Wu, W. H., Gerloff, C., et al. (2005). Effects of non-invasive cortical stimulation on skilled motor function in chronic stroke. *Brain: A Journal of Neurology, 128*, 490–499.

Hummel, F. C., Celnik, P., Pascual-Leone, A., Fregni, F., Byblow, W. D., Buetefisch, C. M., et al. (2008). Controversy: Noninvasive and invasive cortical stimulation show efficacy in treating stroke patients. *Brain Stimulation, 1*, 370–382.

Hummel, F. C., & Cohen, L. G. (2006). Non-invasive brain stimulation: A new strategy to improve neurorehabilitation after stroke? *Lancet Neurology, 5*, 708–712.

Hummel, F. C., & Gerloff, C. (2012). Transcranial brain stimulation after stroke. *Nervenarzt, 83*, 957–965.

Hummel, F. C., Steven, B., Hoppe, J., Heise, K., Thomalla, G., Cohen, L. G., et al. (2009). Deficient intracortical inhibition (SICI) during movement preparation after chronic stroke. *Neurology, 72*, 1766–1772.

Johansen-Berg, H., Dawes, H., Guy, C., Smith, S. M., Wade, D. T., & Matthews, P. M. (2002). Correlation between motor improvements and altered fMRI activity after rehabilitative therapy. *Brain: A Journal of Neurology, 125*, 2731–2742.

Jorgensen, H. S., Nakayama, H., Raaschou, H. O., Vive-Larsen, J., Stoier, M., & Olsen, T. S. (1995). Outcome and time course of recovery in stroke. Part I: Outcome. The Copenhagen Stroke Study. *Archives of Physical Medicine and Rehabilitation, 76*, 399–405.

Khedr, E. M., Abdel-Fadeil, M. R., Farghali, A., & Qaid, M. (2009). Role of 1 and 3 Hz repetitive transcranial magnetic stimulation on motor function recovery after acute ischaemic stroke. *European Journal of Neurology, 16*, 1323–1330.

Khedr, E. M., Ahmed, M. A., Fathy, N., & Rothwell, J. C. (2005). Therapeutic trial of repetitive transcranial magnetic stimulation after acute ischemic stroke. *Neurology, 65*, 466–468.

Khedr, E. M., Farweez, H. M., & Islam, H. (2003). Therapeutic effect of repetitive transcranial magnetic stimulation on motor function in Parkinson's disease patients. *European Journal of Neurology, 10*, 567–572.

Kim, D. Y., Lim, J. Y., Kang, E. K., You, D. S., Oh, M. K., Oh, B. M., et al. (2010). Effect of transcranial direct current stimulation on motor recovery in patients with subacute stroke. *American Journal of Physical Medicine and Rehabilitation, 89*, 879–886.

Ko, J. H., Mure, H., Tang, C. C., Ma, Y., Dhawan, V., Spetsieris, P., et al. (2013). Parkinson's disease: Increased motor network activity in the absence of movement. *Journal of Neuroscience: The Official Journal of the Society for Neuroscience, 33*, 4540–4549.

Koch, G., Brusa, L., Carrillo, F., Lo Gerfo, E., Torriero, S., Oliveri, M., et al. (2009). Cerebellar magnetic stimulation decreases levodopa-induced dyskinesias in Parkinson disease. *Neurology, 73*, 113–119.

Koch, G., Veniero, D., & Caltagirone, C. (2013). To the Other Side of the Neglected Brain: The Hyperexcitability of the Left Intact Hemisphere. *The Neuroscientist, 19*, 208–217.

Kolominsky-Rabas, P. L., Weber, M., Gefeller, O., Neundoerfer, B., & Heuschmann, P. U. (2001). Epidemiology of ischemic stroke subtypes according to TOAST criteria: incidence, recurrence, and long-term survival in ischemic stroke subtypes: A population-based study. *Stroke, 32*, 2735–2740.

Kujirai, T., Caramia, M. D., Rothwell, J. C., Day, B. L., Thompson, P. D., Ferbert, A., et al. (1993). Corticocortical inhibition in human motor cortex. *The Journal of Physiology, 471*, 501–519.

Lai, S. M., Studenski, S., Duncan, P. W., & Perera, S. (2002). Persisting consequences of stroke measured by the Stroke Impact Scale. *Stroke, 33*, 1840–1844.

Lefaucheur, J. P., Drouot, X., Von Raison, F., Menard-Lefaucheur, I., Cesaro, P., & Nguyen, J. P. (2004). Improvement of motor performance and modulation of cortical excitability by repetitive transcranial magnetic stimulation of the motor cortex in Parkinson's disease. *Clinical Neurophysiology, 115*, 2530–2541.

Liepert, J., Zittel, S., & Weiller, C. (2007). Improvement of dexterity by single session low-frequency repetitive transcranial magnetic stimulation over the contralesional motor cortex in acute stroke: A double-blind placebo-controlled crossover trial. *Restorative Neurology and Neuroscience, 25*, 461–465.

Lim, J. Y., Kang, E. K., & Paik, N. J. (2010). Repetitive transcranial magnetic stimulation to hemispatial neglect in patients after stroke: An open-label pilot study. *Journal of Rehabilitation Medicine, 42*, 447–452.

Lindenberg, R., Renga, V., Zhu, L. L., Nair, D., & Schlaug, G. (2010). Bihemispheric brain stimulation facilitates motor recovery in chronic stroke patients. *Neurology, 75*, 2176–2184.

Lotze, M., Markert, J., Sauseng, P., Hoppe, J., Plewnia, C., & Gerloff, C. (2006). The role of multiple contralesional motor areas for complex hand movements after internal capsular lesion. *Journal of Neuroscience: The Official Journal of the Society for Neuroscience, 26*, 6096–6102.

Machii, K., Cohen, D., Ramos-Estebanez, C., & Pascual-Leone, A. (2006). Safety of rTMS to non-motor cortical areas in healthy participants and patients. *Clinical Neurophysiology, 117*, 455–471.

Madhavan, S., Weber, K. A., 2nd., & Stinear, J. W. (2011). Non-invasive brain stimulation enhances fine motor control of the hemiparetic ankle: Implications for rehabilitation. *Experimental Brain Research, 209*, 9–17.

Malcolm, M. P., Triggs, W. J., Light, K. E., Gonzalez Rothi, L. J., Wu, S., Reid, K., et al. (2007). Repetitive transcranial magnetic stimulation as an adjunct to constraint-induced therapy: An exploratory randomized controlled trial. *American Journal of Physical Medicine and Rehabilitation, 86*, 707–715.

Malenka, R. C., & Nicoll, R. A. (1999). Long-term potentiation–A decade of progress? *Science, 285*, 1870–1874.

Mally, J., & Dinya, E. (2008). Recovery of motor disability and spasticity in post-stroke after repetitive transcranial magnetic stimulation (rTMS). *Brain Research Bulletin, 76*, 388–395.

Mansur, C. G., Fregni, F., Boggio, P. S., Riberto, M., Gallucci-Neto, J., Santos, C. M., et al. (2005). A sham stimulation-controlled trial of rTMS of the unaffected hemisphere in stroke patients. *Neurology, 64*, 1802–1804.

Martin, P. I., Naeser, M. A., Doron, K. W., Bogdan, A., Baker, E. H., Kurland, J., et al. (2005). Overt naming in aphasia studied with a functional MRI hemodynamic delay design. *NeuroImage, 28*, 194–204.

Merton, P. A., & Morton, H. B. (1980). Stimulation of the cerebral cortex in the intact human subject. *Nature, 285*.

Muller, M. B., Toschi, N., Kresse, A. E., Post, A., & Keck, M. E. (2000). Long-term repetitive transcranial magnetic stimulation increases the expression of brain-derived neurotrophic factor and cholecystokinin mRNA, but not neuropeptide tyrosine mRNA in specific areas of rat brain. *Neuropsychopharmacology, 23*, 205–215.

Murase, N., Duque, J., Mazzocchio, R., & Cohen, L. G. (2004). Influence of interhemispheric interactions on motor function in chronic stroke. *Annals of Neurology, 55*, 400–409.

Naeser, M. A., Martin, P. I., Baker, E. H., Hodge, S. M., Sczerzenie, S. E., Nicholas, M., et al. (2004). Overt propositional speech in chronic nonfluent aphasia studied with the dynamic susceptibility contrast fMRI method. *NeuroImage, 22*, 29–41.

Naeser, M. A., Martin, P. I., Nicholas, M., Baker, E. H., Seekins, H., Kobayashi, M., et al. (2005). Improved picture naming in chronic aphasia after TMS to part of right Broca's area: An open-protocol study. *Brain and Language, 93*, 95–105.

Nair, D. G., Renga, V., Lindenberg, R., Zhu, L., & Schlaug, G. (2011). Optimizing recovery potential through simultaneous occupational therapy and non-invasive brain-stimulation using tDCS. *Restorative Neurology and Neuroscience, 29*, 411–420.

Nardone, R., Bergmann, J., Christova, M., Caleri, F., Tezzon, F., Ladurner, G., et al. (2012). Effect of transcranial brain stimulation for the treatment of Alzheimer disease: A review. *International Journal of Alzheimer's Disease, 2012*, 687909.

Nitsche, M. A., Cohen, L., Wassermann, E., Priori, A., Lang, N., Antal, A., et al. (2008). Transcranial direct current stimulation: State of the art 2008. *Brain Stimulation, 1*, 206–223.

Nitsche, M. A., Doemkes, S., Karakose, T., Antal, A., Liebetanz, D., Lang, N., et al. (2007). Shaping the effects of transcranial direct current stimulation of the human motor cortex. *Journal of Neurophysiology, 97*, 3109–3117.

Nitsche, M. A., Jaussi, W., Liebetanz, D., Lang, N., Tergau, F., & Paulus, W. (2004). Consolidation of human motor cortical neuroplasticity by D-cycloserine. *Neuropsychopharmacology, 29*, 1573–1578.

Nowak, D. A., Bosl, K., Podubecka, J., & Carey, J. R. (2010). Noninvasive brain stimulation and motor recovery after stroke. *Restorative Neurology and Neuroscience, 28*, 531–544.

Nowak, D. A., Grefkes, C., Dafotakis, M., Eickhoff, S., Kust, J., Karbe, H., et al. (2008). Effects of low-frequency repetitive transcranial magnetic stimulation of the contralesional primary motor cortex on movement kinematics and neural activity in subcortical stroke. *Archives of Neurology, 65*, 741–747.

Nudo, R. J. (2003). Adaptive plasticity in motor cortex: Implications for rehabilitation after brain injury. *Journal of Rehabilitation Medicine*, 7–10.

Nutt, J. G. (2001). Motor fluctuations and dyskinesia in Parkinson's disease. *Parkinsonism & Related Disorders, 8*, 101–108.

Pascual-Leone, A., Amedi, A., Fregni, F., & Merabet, L. B. (2005). The plastic human brain cortex. *Annual Review of Neuroscience, 28*, 377–401.

Patel, A. T., Duncan, P. W., Lai, S. M., & Studenski, S. (2000). The relation between impairments and functional outcomes poststroke. *Archives of Physical Medicine and Rehabilitation, 81*, 1357–1363.

Pedersen, P. M., Jorgensen, H. S., Nakayama, H., Raaschou, H. O., & Olsen, T. S. (1995). Aphasia in acute stroke: Incidence, determinants, and recovery. *Annals of Neurology, 38*, 659–666.

Pedersen, P. M., Jorgensen, H. S., Nakayama, H., Raaschou, H. O., & Olsen, T. S. (1997). Hemineglect in acute stroke–Incidence and prognostic implications. The Copenhagen Stroke Study. *American Journal of Physical Medicine and Rehabilitation, 76*, 122–127.

Plewnia, C., Lotze, M., & Gerloff, C. (2003). Disinhibition of the contralateral motor cortex by low-frequency rTMS. *Neuroreport, 14*, 609–612.

Poewe, W. (2008). Non-motor symptoms in Parkinson's disease. *European Journal of Neurology, 15*(Suppl. 1), 14–20.

Rehme, A. K., Fink, G. R., von Cramon, D. Y., & Grefkes, C. (2011). The role of the contralesional motor cortex for motor recovery in the early days after stroke assessed with longitudinal FMRI. *Cerebral Cortex, 21*, 756–768.

Reis, J., John, D., Heimeroth, A., Mueller, H. H., Oertel, W. H., Arndt, T., et al. (2006). Modulation of human motor cortex excitability by single doses of amantadine. *Neuropsychopharmacology, 31*, 2758–2766.

Reis, J., Schambra, H. M., Cohen, L. G., Buch, E. R., Fritsch, B., Zarahn, E., et al. (2009). Non-invasive cortical stimulation enhances motor skill acquisition over multiple days through an effect on consolidation. *Proceedings of the National Academy of Sciences of the United States of America, 106*, 1590–1595.

Ridding, M. C., & Ziemann, U. (2010). Determinants of the induction of cortical plasticity by non-invasive brain stimulation in healthy subjects. *The Journal of Physiology, 588*, 2291–2304.

Rioult-Pedotti, M. S., Friedman, D., & Donoghue, J. P. (2000). Learning-induced LTP in neocortex. *Science, 290*, 533–536.

Rosler, M., Anand, R., Cicin-Sain, A., Gauthier, S., Agid, Y., Dal-Bianco, P., et al. (1999). Efficacy and safety of rivastigmine in patients with Alzheimer's disease: International randomised controlled trial. *BMJ, 318*, 633–638.

Rossi, S., Hallett, M., Rossini, P. M., & Pascual-Leone, A. (2009). Safety, ethical considerations, and application guidelines for the use of transcranial magnetic stimulation in clinical practice and research. *Clinical Neurophysiology, 120*, 2008–2039.

Rossini, P. M., & Rossi, S. (2007). Transcranial magnetic stimulation: Diagnostic, therapeutic, and research potential. *Neurology, 68*, 484–488.

Rothwell, J. C. (2010). Plasticity in the human motor system. *Folia Phoniatrica et Logopaedica: Official Organ of the International Association of Logopedics and Phoniatrics, 62*, 153–157.

Sabatini, U., Boulanouar, K., Fabre, N., Martin, F., Carel, C., Colonnese, C., et al. (2000). Cortical motor reorganization in akinetic patients with Parkinson's disease: A functional MRI study. *Brain: A Journal of Neurology, 123*(Pt 2), 394–403.

Sasaki, N., Mizutani, S., Kakuda, W., & Abo, M. (2013). Comparison of the effects of high- and low-frequency repetitive transcranial magnetic stimulation on upper limb hemiparesis in the early phase of stroke. *Journal of Stroke and Cerebrovascular Diseases, 22*, 413–418.

Schlaug, G., Marchina, S., & Wan, C. Y. (2011). The use of non-invasive brain stimulation techniques to facilitate recovery from post-stroke aphasia. *Neuropsychology Review, 21*, 288–301.

Schlaug, G., Norton, A., Marchina, S., Zipse, L., & Wan, C. Y. (2010). From singing to speaking: Facilitating recovery from nonfluent aphasia. *Future Neurology, 5*, 657–665.

Schulz, R., Gerloff, C., & Hummel, F. C. (2013). Non-invasive brain stimulation in neurological diseases. *Neuropharmacology, 64*, 579–587.

Schulz, R., Park, C. H., Boudrias, M. H., Gerloff, C., Hummel, F. C., & Ward, N. S. (2012). Assessing the integrity of corticospinal pathways from primary and secondary cortical motor areas after stroke. *Stroke, 43*, 2248–2251.

Siebner, H. R., Rossmeier, C., Mentschel, C., Peinemann, A., & Conrad, B. (2000). Short-term motor improvement after sub-threshold 5-Hz repetitive transcranial magnetic stimulation of the primary motor hand area in Parkinson's disease. *Journal of the Neurological Sciences, 178*, 91–94.

Skidmore, F. M., Rodriguez, R. L., Fernandez, H. H., Goodman, W. K., Foote, K. D., & Okun, M. S. (2006). Lessons learned in deep brain stimulation for movement and neuropsychiatric disorders. *CNS Spectrums, 11*, 521–536.

Sparing, R., Thimm, M., Hesse, M. D., Kust, J., Karbe, H., & Fink, G. R. (2009). Bidirectional alterations of interhemispheric parietal balance by non-invasive cortical stimulation. *Brain: A Journal of Neurology, 132,* 3011–3020.

Stagg, C. J., Bachtiar, V., O'Shea, J., Allman, C., Bosnell, R. A., Kischka, U., et al. (2012). Cortical activation changes underlying stimulation-induced behavioural gains in chronic stroke. *Brain, 135,* 276–284.

Stagg, C. J., Best, J. G., Stephenson, M. C., O'Shea, J., Wylezinska, M., Kincses, Z. T., et al. (2009). Polarity-sensitive modulation of cortical neurotransmitters by transcranial stimulation. *Journal of Neuroscience: The Official Journal of the Society for Neuroscience, 29,* 5202–5206.

Stinear, C. M., & Ward, N. S. (2013). How useful is imaging in predicting outcomes in stroke rehabilitation? *International Journal of Stroke, 8,* 33–37.

Storch, A., Schneider, C. B., Wolz, M., Sturwald, Y., Nebe, A., Odin, P., et al. (2013). Nonmotor fluctuations in Parkinson disease: Severity and correlation with motor complications. *Neurology, 80,* 800–809.

Szaflarski, J. P., Vannest, J., Wu, S. W., DiFrancesco, M. W., Banks, C., & Gilbert, D. L. (2011). Excitatory repetitive transcranial magnetic stimulation induces improvements in chronic post-stroke aphasia. *Medical Science Monitor, 17,* CR132–CR139.

Takeuchi, N., Chuma, T., Matsuo, Y., Watanabe, I., & Ikoma, K. (2005). Repetitive transcranial magnetic stimulation of contralesional primary motor cortex improves hand function after stroke. *Stroke, 36,* 2681–2686.

Takeuchi, N., Tada, T., Toshima, M., Chuma, T., Matsuo, Y., & Ikoma, K. (2008). Inhibition of the unaffected motor cortex by 1 Hz repetitive transcranical magnetic stimulation enhances motor performance and training effect of the paretic hand in patients with chronic stroke. *Journal of Rehabilitation Medicine, 40,* 298–303.

Takeuchi, N., Tada, T., Toshima, M., Matsuo, Y., & Ikoma, K. (2009). Repetitive transcranial magnetic stimulation over bilateral hemispheres enhances motor function and training effect of paretic hand in patients after stroke. *Journal of Rehabilitation Medicine, 41,* 1049–1054.

Talelli, P., Greenwood, R. J., & Rothwell, J. C. (2007). Exploring theta burst stimulation as an intervention to improve motor recovery in chronic stroke. *Clinical Neurophysiology, 118,* 333–342.

Talelli, P., Wallace, A., Dileone, M., Hoad, D., Cheeran, B., Oliver, R., et al. (2012). Theta burst stimulation in the rehabilitation of the upper limb: a semirandomized, placebo-controlled trial in chronic stroke patients. *Neurorehabilitation and Neural Repair, 26,* 976–987.

Tanaka, S., Takeda, K., Otaka, Y., Kita, K., Osu, R., Honda, M., et al. (2011). Single session of transcranial direct current stimulation transiently increases knee extensor force in patients with hemiparetic stroke. *Neurorehabilitation and Neural Repair, 25,* 565–569.

Taylor, T. N., Davis, P. H., Torner, J. C., Holmes, J., Meyer, J. W., & Jacobson, M. F. (1996). Lifetime cost of stroke in the United States. *Stroke, 27,* 1459–1466.

Teskey, G. C., Flynn, C., Goertzen, C. D., Monfils, M. H., & Young, N. A. (2003). Cortical stimulation improves skilled forelimb use following a focal ischemic infarct in the rat. *Neurological Research, 25,* 794–800.

Vanderhasselt, M. A., De Raedt, R., Baeken, C., Leyman, L., Clerinx, P., & D'Haenen, H. (2007). The influence of rTMS over the right dorsolateral prefrontal cortex on top-down attentional processes. *Brain Research, 1137,* 111–116.

Wach, C., Krause, V., Moliadze, V., Paulus, W., Schnitzler, A., & Pollok, B. (2013). Effects of 10 Hz and 20 Hz transcranial alternating current stimulation (tACS) on motor functions and motor cortical excitability. *Behavioural Brain Research, 241,* 1–6.

Wade, D. T., Hewer, R. L., David, R. M., & Enderby, P. M. (1986). Aphasia after stroke: Natural history and associated deficits. *Journal of Neurology, Neurosurgery, and Psychiatry, 49,* 11–16.

Ward, N. S., Brown, M. M., Thompson, A. J., & Frackowiak, R. S. (2003). Neural correlates of motor recovery after stroke: a longitudinal fMRI study. *Brain: A Journal of Neurology, 126,* 2476–2496.

Wessel, M., Zimerman, M., Timmermann, J. E., & Hummel, F. C. (2013). Eyelid myokymia in an older subject after repetitive sessions of anodal transcranial direct current stimulation. *Brain Stimulation, 6,* 463–465.

Wu, A. D., Fregni, F., Simon, D. K., Deblieck, C., & Pascual-Leone, A. (2008). Noninvasive brain stimulation for Parkinson's disease and dystonia. *Neurotherapeutics, 5,* 345–361.

Zimerman, M., Heise, K. F., Gerloff, C., Cohen, L. G., & Hummel, F. C. (2012). Disrupting the Ipsilateral motor cortex interferes with training of a complex motor task in older adults. *Cerebral Cortex.* http://dx.doi.org/10.1093/cercor/bhs38.

Zimerman, M., Heise, K. F., Hoppe, J., Cohen, L. G., Gerloff, C., & Hummel, F. C. (2012). Modulation of training by single-session transcranial direct current stimulation to the intact motor cortex enhances motor skill acquisition of the paretic hand. *Stroke, 43,* 2185–2191.

Zimerman, M., & Hummel, F. C. (2010). Non-invasive brain stimulation: Enhancing motor and cognitive functions in healthy old subjects. *Frontiers in Aging Neuroscience, 2,* 149.

Zimerman, M., Nitsch, M., Giraux, P., Gerloff, C., Cohen, L. G., & Hummel, F. C. (2013). Neuroenhancement of the aging brain: Restoring skill acquisition in old subjects. *Annals of Neurology, 73,* 10–15.

Zipse, L., Norton, A., Marchina, S., & Schlaug, G. (2012). When right is all that is left: Plasticity of right-hemisphere tracts in a young aphasic patient. *Annals of the New York Academy of Sciences, 1252,* 237–245.

13

Transcranial Direct Current Stimulation and Cognition in the Elderly

Francesca Mameli[1], Manuela Fumagalli[1], Roberta Ferrucci[1,2], and Alberto Priori[1,2]

[1]Centro Clinico per la Neurostimolazione, le Neurotecnologie ed i Disordini del Movimento, Fondazione IRCCS Ca' Granda, Ospedale Maggiore Policlinico, Milan, Italy

[2]Dipartimento di Fisiopatologia Medico-Chirurgica e dei Trapianti, Università degli Studi di Milano, Milan, Italy

OUTLINE

INTRODUCTION

Cognitive aging generally manifests with altered memory and executive functions. Healthy older people typically show declining processing speeds, working memory (WM), episodic memory and behavioral inflexibility (Hong & Rebec, 2012; Jagust, 2013). Region-specific changes in dendritic morphology, cellular connectivity, Ca^{2+} dysregulation, and gene expression can alter neuroplasticity and network dynamics in neural ensembles that support cognition, thus resulting in age-related behavioral impairment. The decline in episodic memory and executive functions reflects morphological alterations specifically in the temporal lobe memory system and the prefrontal cortex/striatal executive system (Hong & Rebec, 2012; Jagust, 2013; Zimerman & Hummel, 2010).

Transcranial direct current stimulation (tDCS) is a tool that can manipulate neuroplasticity and modulate cortical function with weak direct currents (Nitsche et al., 2008; Priori, 2003). It results in long-term potentiation (LTP)-like synaptic changes that accompany facilitatory effects on cortical excitability, neuroplasticity, and learning (Nitsche & Paulus, 2000; Nitsche et al., 2008). Previous studies showed that tDCS can enhance cognitive functions, such as memory, attention, learning, language, and motor functions, in young and in older healthy persons, and in the aged clinical population (Kuo & Nitsche, 2012; Monti et al., 2013; Nardone et al., 2012; Reis & Fritsch, 2011; Schulz, Gerloff, & Hummel, 2013).

This chapter reviews scientific data about the cognitive effects of tDCS in healthy older subjects and in neurodegenerative disorders typically manifesting in the elderly – Alzheimer's disease (AD), fronto-temporal dementia (FTD), and Parkinson's disease (PD) .

STUDIES IN HEALTHY OLDER SUBJECTS

Prompted by their previous results suggesting that non-invasive brain stimulation can improve decision-making in young participants (Fecteau et al., 2007), Boggio and colleagues (2010) applied tDCS in older subjects. In a double-blinded, randomized, and sham-controlled trial they investigated the effect of a single tDCS session on a decision-making task in 28 elderly subjects. Participants performed a gambling risk task, a test that measures decision-making under risk requiring minimum strategy and WM, while receiving anodal tDCS over the right and cathodal tDCS over the left dorsolateral prefrontal cortex (DLPFC), or anodal tDCS over the left with cathodal tDCS over the right DLPFC (2 mA, 15 minutes), or sham stimulation. tDCS started 5 minutes before the task and was delivered throughout the 10-minute task. During left anodal/right cathodal stimulation participants more often chose high-risk prospects than did participants receiving sham or those receiving right anodal/left cathodal stimulation (percentage choice of low-risk prospect: left anodal tDCS, about 53%; right anodal tDCS, about 78%; sham tDCS, about 73%). Because tDCS induced opposite behavioral effects in young and older subjects, Boggio and colleagues speculated that the observed effect in the elderly population reflects age-related changes in brain asymmetry, depending mainly on the reduced prefrontal right hemisphere activity – a change usually related to conservative behavior (Boggio et al., 2010). The non-specific tDCS-induced cognitive changes in the elderly (tDCS applied to either hemisphere tends to induce risk-taking behavior) is in line with the Hemispheric Asymmetry Reduction in Old Adults (HAROLD) model (Cabeza, Anderson, Locantore, & McIntosh, 2002) – the lower the functional asymmetry, the lower the probability of specific effects related to the stimulated hemisphere (Boggio et al., 2010).

To investigate the effects of anodal tDCS over the left inferior frontal cortex on spoken picture-naming performance in a healthy older sample, Holland and colleagues (2011) combined left frontal anodal tDCS (2 mA, 20 minutes) during an overt picture-naming task with functional magnetic resonance imaging (fMRI) (Holland et al., 2011). Half of the participants ($n=5$) received a sham stimulation run followed by an anodal tDCS run on their first fMRI scanning session. On their second session, the order of intervention was reversed. The results showed that anodal tDCS induced a significant improvement in naming response times (mean reaction times: tDCS, about 780 ms; sham, 800 ms). Anodal tDCS also reduced fMRI blood oxygen-level dependent signals in the left frontal cortex, including Broca's area. tDCS had significant behavioral and regionally specific blood oxygenation effects in the brain, supporting the importance of Broca's area in the naming network and pointing to this area as a candidate site for anodal tDCS in rehabilitation protocols aiming to improve anomia in patients whose brain damage spares this region.

In their study, Ross and colleagues (2011) extend previous results suggesting that anodal tDCS can enhance proper name recall for famous faces, in young participants (Ross, McCoy, Wolk, Coslett, & Olson, 2010; Ross et al., 2011) to the elderly population. In this study, 14 elderly subjects received left anodal, right anodal, or sham stimulation (15 mA, 15 minutes) applied to the anterior temporal lobes while naming pictures of famous individuals and landmarks. The results showed an improvement in face naming after left or right anterior temporal lobe stimulation, but a statistically significant effect was found only after left-lateralized tDCS (percentage of correct responses: left tDCS, 40; right tDCS, 34; sham, 29). The magnitude of the enhancing effect was similar in older and younger adults, but the lateralization of the effect differed depending on age.

In a double-blind, randomized, and sham-controlled study, Flöel and colleagues (2012) investigated the effect of tDCS on object-location learning and its retention (Flöel et al., 2012). Twenty healthy elderly subjects received tDCS (1 mA, 20 minutes) over the right temporo-parietal cortex, while they did an object-learning task requiring them to acquire the correct position for buildings on a street map. Each subject participated in two separate sessions, anodal tDCS and sham stimulation. tDCS and the task started simultaneously, but stimulation ended after 20 minutes and the task lasted for about 45 minutes. Outcome measures were learning success when each session ended, and immediate as well as delayed (1 week) free recall. Anodal tDCS enhanced free-recall performance by about 24% compared with sham (about 8%) rather than the learning curve itself or immediate free recall, and the cognitive effect became especially evident 1 week after the initial learning. tDCS could have benefited recall performance by directly modulating plasticity-enhancing processes within the right temporo-parietal region, or by acting indirectly on connected structures (Flöel et al., 2012). One such connected structure is the right hippocampus/parahippocampus, a brain area functionally involved in acquiring novel object-location knowledge (Rugg, Otten, & Henson 2002; Squire & Zola, 1996).

To investigate the WM function in a healthy older sample, in a randomized and sham-controlled study, Berryhill and Jones (2012) evaluated 25 healthy older participants performing verbal and visual two-back WM tasks at baseline and after three tDCS sessions: anodal tDCS to the left or to the right DLPFC (1.5 mA, 10 minutes), and sham. A distinctive finding was that WM performance improved in participants with higher education, whereas in the low education group tDCS left WM performance unchanged or even impaired (normalized difference indices [tDCS – sham]/[tDCS +sham]; mean low education right tDCS visual, −0.01, and verbal, 0.002; left tDCS visual, −0.06, and verbal, −0.01; high education right tDCS visual, 0.02, and verbal, 0.03; left tDCS visual, 0.03, and verbal, 0.03). To explain this result the authors suggested that, unlike the low education group, participants in the high education group might use a WM strategy that allows them to recruit the DLPFC during WM tasks (Berryhill & Jones, 2012).

In a cross-over within-subject, sham-controlled study, Meinzer and colleagues applied anodal tDCS to the left ventral frontal gyrus in older and younger subjects during overt semantic word generation, a task that is negatively affected by advanced age (Meinzer, Lindenberg, Antonenko, Flaisch, & Flöel, 2013). Twenty healthy elderly participants were assessed with fMRI and concurrent tDCS (1 mA, 20 minutes). In addition, resting state fMRI assessed changes induced by tDCS at network level independent of performance. Twenty matched younger subjects served as controls. The investigators found that anodal tDCS significantly improved word retrieval performance in older subjects up to the level of younger controls (older sham, 7 errors; older tDCS, about 6 errors; young controls, 5 errors). fMRI data demonstrated that tDCS-induced performance improvements resulted in reduced activity in bilateral prefrontal areas, and these areas were more active in older than in younger subjects. Additionally, fMRI analysis disclosed widespread connectivity changes in older than in younger participants, characterized by enhanced connectivity in sensory-motor and posterior regions. These data collectively demonstrated that a single stimulation session can temporarily reverse some age-associated changes in brain activity and connectivity (Meinzer et al., 2013).

These few studies collectively show that tDCS can improve cognitive processes, such as decision-making, visuo-spatial memory, language, and WM in healthy older people. Among factors influencing the results are education (Berryhill & Jones, 2012) and age (Boggio et al., 2010). Future tDCS studies on cognition in the elderly should take into account not only neurostimulation variables (brain area, duration, stimulation intensity), but also age-related changes in brain activity and participants' cultural and social features.

Age-related deficits in motor learning are well known and may at least partially reflect cognitive decline in control processes, poor memory consolidation, and reduced learning efficiency (Ren, Wu, Chan, & Yan, 2013). In a study seeking more information on these cognitive processes, Hummel and colleagues (2010) tested the hypothesis that anodal tDCS over left motor cortex (M1) could facilitate performance in right upper extremity tasks required for activities of daily living in older subjects in a double-blind, sham-controlled and cross-over study design. Ten aged healthy subjects participated in three experimental sessions: in the first session they familiarized themselves with the motor task, and in the other two sessions they received anodal tDCS (1 mA, 20 minutes) or sham in a pseudorandomized, counterbalanced order. The primary endpoint measure was the time required to complete the Jebsen-Taylor hand function test, a widely used well-validated test for functional motor assessment that reflects activities of daily living (Jebsen, Taylor, Trieschmann, Trotter, & Howard, 1969). Anodal tDCS applied over M1 in a single session led to significant improvement in performance of skilled motor tasks included in the Jebsen-Taylor hand function test (shorter total time by about 4 seconds to complete the Jebsen-Taylor hand function test compared with sham). These results are consistent with previous findings in younger individuals showing that this stimulation modality can facilitate motor function (Nitsche & Paulus, 2000; Nitsche, Liebetanz, et al., 2003; Nitsche, Schauenburg, et al., 2003; Vines, Nair, & Schlaug, 2006) and motor cortical excitability in the stimulated M1 (Nitsche et al., 2005). Because performance in skilled motor tasks requires accurate visuo-motor integration that relies on activity in primary motor and premotor cortical areas (Chouinard, Leonard, & Paus, 2006), given the tDCS technique's poor spatial resolution (Nitsche et al., 2007) and relatively large effect size reported in a previous study (Lang et al., 2005), stimulation applied over M1 could have spread to nearby premotor areas.

In a double-blind, sham-controlled, cross-over design study, Zimerman and colleagues (2014) compared the behavioral consequences induced by interfering with the ipsilateral motor cortex (iM1) during training for a complex motor skill in 13 healthy old and 10 young volunteers, who participated in a training session receiving cathodal tDCS (1 mA, 20 minutes) or sham to the iM1. Motor performance was evaluated before, during, 90 minutes, and 24 hours after training with a finger tapping task that consisted of sequentially pressing with the right hand five keys on a four-button electronic keyboard. Their results showed that cathodal tDCS to the iM1 impaired training and decreased correctly played sequences in old subjects (decrease by about 15 correct sequences compared with sham). The disruptive effect was more prominent the older the subject. Additionally, even after two consecutive retraining sessions without stimulation, the performance level achieved with sham remained unaccomplished with the cathodal tDCS condition (Zimerman et al., 2014). These findings strongly support the concept that the iM1 is involved in implementing and acquiring complex unimanual motor behavior in a healthy old population, but not in a young population, as previous neuroimaging studies suggest (Mattay et al., 2002; Naccarato et al., 2006).

In another double-blind, cross-over, sham-controlled study, Zimerman and colleagues (2013) tested whether tDCS can enhance complex motor skill acquisition in old and young participants. They enrolled 29 old and 24 young subjects who participated in a training session receiving anodal (1 mA, 20 minutes) or sham tDCS over the contralateral M1. The endpoint measure was the scoring obtained in the finger tapping task at 90 minutes and 24 hours after training (retention period). The main finding was that old participants experienced significant improvement (about 35% compared with sham) when training was applied concurrently with tDCS, and the benefits lasted for at least 24 hours (Fig. 13.1). This result could imply that tDCS modulates GABAergic neurotransmission, thus unmasking excitatory connections, as well as indirectly enhancing NMDA-dependent processes supporting LTP. The investigators speculated that anodal tDCS in old subjects influences the ability of the aged cortex to undergo plastic modification by preparing the cortical ground for successful plastic changes due to motor training (Zimerman et al., 2013).

In an old population, Lindenberg and colleagues studied the differential effect induced by unihemispheric and bihemispheric stimulation

Restoring skill acquisition

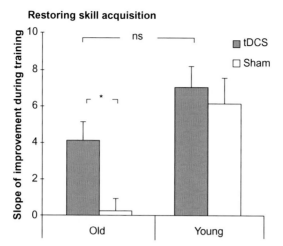

FIGURE 13.1 Effects of transcranial direct current stimulation (tDCS) over the right motor cortex on a finger tapping task in old and young healthy subjects. Anodal tDCS significantly improves motor learning. Error bars are standard error of the mean (SEM). *Figure reproduced from Zimerman et al. (2013), with permission.*

(Lindenberg, Nachtigall, Meinzer, Sieg, & Flöel, 2013). Bihemispheric (or "dual") tDCS using anodal stimulation is thought to upregulate M1 excitability whereas concurrent cathodal stimulation downregulates excitability in the contralateral M1. In this randomized, sham-controlled study, 20 older subjects underwent tDCS and simultaneous fMRI during a visually-cued choice reaction-time task and at rest. Additionally, in between resting-state and the visually-cued choice reaction-time task subjects performed an overt semantic word-retrieval task. Subjects participated in three sessions with concurrent dual, anodal (mA, 30 minutes), or sham tDCS. In the anodal condition the anode was applied over the left M1 and the reference electrode placed over the contralateral supraorbital region, whereas for dual stimulation the anode was placed over the left M1 and the cathode over the right M1. Results for the resting-state analysis showed that, compared with sham, both dual and anodal tDCS decreased connectivity in the right hippocampus and M1, but at the same time increased connectivity in the left prefrontal cortex. Notably, dual but not anodal tDCS enhanced connectivity in the left dorsal posterior cingulate cortex. Dual tDCS also yielded stronger bilateral M1 activations than anodal tDCS when participants used either their left or right hand during the motor task. The corresponding tDCS-induced changes in laterality of activations were related to the microstructural status of transcallosal motor fibers (Lindenberg et al., 2013). These results suggest that bihemispheric tDCS cannot be explained by mere add-on effects of anodal and concurrent cathodal stimulation, but rather by complex network modulations involving interhemispheric interactions and areas associated with motor control in the dorsal posterior cingulate cortex.

These studies collectively show that tDCS applied over M1 improves motor learning performance, and suggest that brain stimulation can enhance motor function in the aging brain. Hence tDCS can be successfully applied during motor training (online procedure) and before performance begins (offline procedure) (Hummel et al., 2010; Zimerman et al., 2013, 2014). Cathodal stimulation applied to the iM1 decreases performance, whereas anodal stimulation over contralateral M1 improves motor skills and the effect can persist for up to 24 hours after stimulation ends (Zimerman et al., 2013, 2014). In addition, a fMRI study on motor system activity and connectivity (Lindenberg et al., 2013) showed different effects of bihemispheric versus unihemispheric motor cortex stimulation in older adults (Table 13.1).

STUDIES IN NEURODEGENERATIVE DISEASES

Alzheimer's Disease

A clinical hallmark of AD is progressive episodic memory loss (Dickerson & Eichenbaum, 2010) associated with decline in other cognitive domains, including attention, perceptual–spatial abilities, language, and executive functions, as well as declining sensory and motor functions (Freitas, Mondragon-Llorca, & Pascual-Leone, 2011). To date no cure exists for AD, and interventions (including medications) can at best slow down disease progression by 6–12 months in half of the patients (Freitas et al., 2011). Current treatments still yield small effect sizes, and pharmacological treatments induce severe adverse effects (Shafqat, 2008). Given its increasing prevalence and debilitating impact, finding successful diagnostic and therapeutic interventions for AD is an immediate need.

Increasing evidence over recent years shows that memory test performance improves after patients with AD receive tDCS (Boggio et al., 2009, 2012; Ferrucci et al., 2008). Experiments conducted in our laboratory specifically sought to clarify memory changes in elderly patients with mild probable AD by applying tDCS over the temporo-parietal cortical areas bilaterally, and evaluating memory variables after anodal, cathodal, and sham stimulation. Before and 30 minutes after tDCS applied at 1.5 mA for 15 minutes, 10 patients were tested with a word recognition memory task and visual attention task. After anodal tDCS, accuracy in the word recognition task increased by about 17%. Conversely, after cathodal tDCS over the same areas memory performance worsened, showing that the improvement is polarity specific. tDCS failed to influence visual

TABLE 13.1 tDCS Studies on Cognitive Functions in Healthy Older Subjects.

Studies	Sample	Age (mean ± SD years)	Education (mean ± SD years)	Cognitive Function	Polarity	Stimulated Areas	Reference Electrode	Intensity/ Duration	Task	Online/ offline	Effects	Follow-up
Boggio et al., 2010	28 subjects (3 men)	50–85 (range years)	*(1)9.2 ± 5.2; (2)7.0 ± 5.2; (3)5.2 ± 4.5	Decision-making	A/C/S	Left or right DLPFC	Left or right DLPFC	2 mA 15 min/1 session	Gambling risk task	Online	Left anodal / right cathodal tDCS increases high-risk responses	No
Holland et al., 2011	10 subjects (3 men)	62–74 (range years)	DNR	Language	A/S	Left inferior frontal cortex	Contralateral frontopolar cortex	2 mA 20 min/2 sessions	Picture-naming task	Online	tDCS decreases naming response times and reduces fMRI blood oxygen-level dependent signals in the left frontal cortex	No
Ross et al., 2011	14 subjects (7 men)	55–69 (range years)	DNR	Language	A/S	Left/right anterior temporal lobes	Contralateral cheek	1.5 mA, 15 min/3 sessions	Picture-naming task	Online	Left tDCS improves naming performance	No
Flöel et al., 2012	20 subjects (10 men)	62.1 ± 9.2	13.2 ± 2.3	Learning	A/S	Right temporo-parietal cortex	Contralateral supraorbital area	1 mA, 20 min/2 sessions	Associative object-location learning task	Online and offline	tDCS improves performance only at 1 week after learning	1 week
Berryhill and Jones (2012)	25 subjects (gender DNR)	56–80 (range years)	High education: 16.9 ± DNR; Low education: 13.5 ± DNR.	Memory	A/S	Left or right DLPFC	Contralateral cheek	1.5 mA, 10 min/3 sessions	Verbal and visual two-back working memory tasks	Offline	tDCS selectively improves performance in participants with higher education	No

Continued

TABLE 13.1 tDCS Studies on Cognitive Functions in Healthy Older Subjects.—cont'd

Studies	Sample	Age (mean ± SD years)	Education (mean ± SD years)	Cognitive Function	Polarity	Stimulated Areas	Reference Electrode	Intensity/ Duration	Task	Online/ offline	Effects	Follow-up
Meinzer et al., 2013	20 old subjects (10 men), 20 young subjects (gender DNR)	Old subjects: 68.0 ± 5.7 Young subjects: 26.4 ± 3.4	DNR	Language	A/S	Left ventral frontal gyrus	Contralateral supraorbital area	1 mA, 20 min/2 sessions	Semantic word generation task	Online	tDCS improves word retrieval performance, reduces activity in bilateral prefrontal areas and change connectivity	No
Hummel et al., 2010	10 subjects (5 men)	69 ± 9.2	DNR	Motor learning	A/S	Left M1	Contralateral supraorbital area	1 mA, 20 min/3 sessions (the first session for training only)	Jebsen-Taylor hand function test	Online and offline	tDCS improves performance of skilled hand functions	No
Zimerman et al., 2014	13 old subjects (6 men), and 10 young subjects (4 men)	Old subjects: 58–85 Young subjects: 22–35 (range years)	DNR	Motor learning	C/S	Hand knob area of the right M1	Contralateral supraorbital area	1 mA, 20 min/2 sessions	Finger tapping task	Online and offline	tDCS impairs performance in old subjects	24 hours

Study	Sample	Age		Topic	Type	Target area	Reference electrode	Current/duration	Task	Online/offline	Results	Follow-up
Zimerman et al., 2013	29 old subjects (12 men), and 24 young subjects (10 men)	Old subjects: 55–88. Young subjects: 21–31 (range years)	DNR	Motor learning	A/S	Hand knob area of the left M1	Contralateral supraorbital area	1 mA, 20 min/2 sessions	Finger tapping task	Online and offline	In old participants tDCS improves performance during the training and at 24 hours post-stimulation	24 hours
Lindenberg et al., 2013	20 subjects (10 men)	68.2 ± 5.0	DNR	Motor learning and language	A/dual-A/S	Left M1	For A session: contralateral supraorbital area For dual-A: right M1	1 mA, 30 min/3 sessions	Visually cued choice reaction time task, semantic word-retrieval task	Online	In the resting state dual-A and anodal tDCS decreased connectivity of right hippocampus and M1 while increasing connectivity in the left prefrontal cortex Dual-A tDCS enhanced connectivity of the left dorsal posterior cingulate cortex During the motor task, dual-A tDCS increased activation in bilateral M1 compared with anodal tDCS	No

A, anodal tDCS; C, cathodal tDCS; S, sham tDCS; dual-A, dual anodal tDCS; mA, milliampere; offline, the subject receives stimulation before and after executing the task; online, the subject receives stimulation during the task; DLPFC, dorsolateral prefrontal cortex; M1, motor cortex; DNR, data not reported; *, three groups were studied separately.

attention (Ferrucci et al., 2008; see also Fig. 13.2). Because anodal tDCS increases cortical excitability, it presumably benefits patients' memory performance by focally improving function in temporo-parietal areas. The improvement could also arise from a tDCS-dependent functional improvement in cholinergic cortical circuits, as suggested by experiments with tDCS in healthy subjects (Scelzo et al., 2010). Conversely, cathodal tDCS presumably worsens memory performance by decreasing cortical excitability (Kuo & Nitsche, 2012; Pellicciari, Brignani, & Miniussi, 2013; Priori, 2003).

In a study designed to investigate how tDCS influences other cognitive functions, Boggio and colleagues (2009) investigated anodal tDCS-induced changes in visual recognition memory, WM, and selective attention in 10 elderly patients with mild-to-moderate AD (Boggio et al., 2009). Their tDCS protocol differed from that used by Ferrucci and colleagues (2008) because it had higher intensity (2 mA) and doubled the stimulation time (30 minutes). They applied anodal and sham tDCS over the left DLPFC and over the left temporal cortex. For both conditions, the reference cathode electrode was placed over the right supraorbital area. The main finding was that DLPFC tDCS enhanced performance in a visual recognition memory task by about 14% and left temporal cortex tDCS by about 18%, as compared with sham stimulation. These task-dependent changes may arise because the anodal tDCS electrode facilitates the stimulated brain areas and could therefore improve their functions. None of the other tests disclosed clinically important

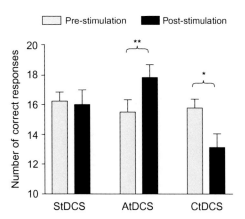

FIGURE 13.2   Effects of transcranial direct current stimulation (tDCS) over the bilateral temporo-parietal cortex on the word recognition task in patients with Alzheimer's disease. After anodal tDCS, word recognition task accuracy increased, whereas after cathodal tDCS it decreased. StDCS, sham tDCS; AtDCS, anodal tDCS; CtDCS, cathodal tDCS. Error bars are standard error of the mean (SEM). *Figure reproduced from Ferrucci et al. (2008), with permission.*

tDCS-induced changes. Although the tDCS-elicited cognitive enhancement observed by Ferrucci and colleagues (2008) is comparable to the improvement induced by Boggio and colleagues (2009), who used tDCS at a higher intensity and longer duration, both studies applied tDCS in a single session and neither study assessed possible long-lasting effects.

The aforementioned studies based upon a single tDCS session therefore prompted research to assess the effects induced by repeated tDCS sessions in patients with AD. Investigating long-term effects, Boggio and colleagues (2012) tested memory changes induced by anodal tDCS applied for 30 minutes, in five consecutive daily sessions, bilaterally over the temporal cortex (Boggio et al., 2012). They enrolled 15 elderly patients with mild-to-moderate AD in two independent clinical centers. Cognitive functions were assessed at four time points – before the first tDCS session for each condition (real and sham), at the end of treatment, 1 week later, and then 4 weeks later – using four different tasks: mini mental state examination, Alzheimer's disease assessment scale-cognitive subscale (ADAS-cog), visual recognition memory task, and visual attention task. They found that after patients received anodal tDCS their visual recognition memory improved by about 9% from baseline and the benefit persisted for at least 4 weeks after therapy, whereas after sham stimulation visual recognition memory decreased by 2.6%. These findings imply that the improvement is polarity specific and depends only on changes induced by temporal anodal tDCS (Fig. 13.3). tDCS failed to influence differentially general cognitive performance measures or a visual attention measure (Boggio et al., 2012; see also Table 13.2).

The long-lasting tDCS-induced changes could arise from its effect on long-term potentiation for memory (Kuo & Nitsche, 2012). In a recent review on the putative mechanisms that underlie tDCS-induced actions in AD, Hansen (2012) proposed that the technique could change membrane polarization and cerebral blood flow and induce synaptic and non-synaptic aftereffects with polarity-dependent changes in neurotransmitters – all mechanisms potentially altered in neurodegenerative diseases. A further intriguing hypothesis to test is whether tDCS modulates beta amyloid-induced neuronal damage (Hansen, 2012).

Although promising, the results from studies using tDCS to enhance cognitive functions in patients with AD remain preliminary. Apart from enrolling small sample sizes, none of these studies clarifies how the elicited memory changes will influence patients' daily life. To assess tDCS's clinical effectiveness in AD we also need more comprehensive outcome measures to evaluate behavioral and affective disorders such as agitation and depression. Equally important, we also need to evaluate patients in the different clinical disease stages (mild, moderate, or severe), because cognitive decline during disease progression depends on changes involving several neural networks. These data could further

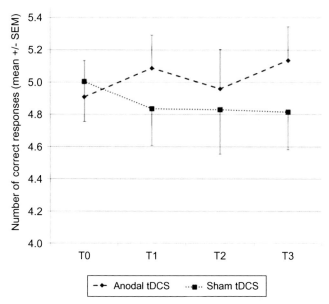

FIGURE 13.3   Effects of transcranial direct current stimulation (tDCS) over the temporo-parietal cortex on the visual recognition task in patients with Alzheimer's disease. Anodal tDCS improved mean accuracy. T0, baseline; T1, immediately after tDCS; T2, 1 week after tDCS; T3, 4 weeks after tDCS. Error bars are standard error of the mean (SEM). *Figure reproduced from Boggio et al. (2012), with permission.*

support applying tDCS to activate specific neural networks (Boggio et al., 2011). Finally, future studies should evaluate whether various procedures, including tDCS and behavioral interventions, might be combined (Boggio et al., 2011).

Fronto-Temporal Dementia

FTD results from degeneration in the frontal or anterior temporal lobes, or both, and manifests with behavioral and language disorders (Lund/Manchester, 1994) and with age at onset typically in the 50s and 60s. No effective treatment exists to stop or slow down neurodegeneration (Seltman & Matthews, 2012), and medical treatment aims only at the patient's key symptoms (Witt, Deuschl, & Bartsch, 2013). Seeking to fill this gap, Huey and colleagues (2007) studied language changes induced by tDCS in 10 patients with FTD and used the letter-cued verbal fluency test as the primary therapeutic outcome and the neuropsychiatric inventory as the secondary outcome (Huey et al., 2007). Patients received anodal and sham tDCS in separate sessions, with the anode electrode placed over the left DLPFC and the cathode over the right supraorbital

TABLE 13.2 tDCS Studies on Cognitive Functions in Patients with Neurodegenerative Diseases.

Studies	Sample	Age (mean ± SD years)	Education (mean ± SD years)	Cognitive Function	Polarity	Stimulated Areas	Reference Electrode	Intensity/ duration	Task	Online/ offline	Effects	Follow-up
STUDIES IN PATIENTS WITH ALZHEIMER'S DISEASE												
Ferrucci et al., 2008	10 patients (3 men)	65–84 (range years)	5–18 (range years)	Memory	A/C/S	Bilateral temporo-parietal cortex	Right deltoid muscle	1.5 mA, 15 min/3 sessions	Word recognition memory task	Offline	Anodal tDCS improves accuracy	No
Boggio et al., 2009	10 patients (4 men)	69–92 (range years)	4–16 (range years)	Memory	A/S	Left DLPFC, left temporal cortex	Contralateral supraorbital area	2 mA, 30 min /3 sessions	Visual recognition memory task	Online	Temporal and DLPFC tDCS increases accuracy	No
Boggio et al., 2012	15 patients (8 men)	65–93 (range years)	5–18 (range years)	Memory	A/S	Bilateral temporal cortex	Right deltoid muscle	2 mA, 30 min/ 5 days/2 sessions	Visual recognition memory task	Offline	tDCS improves performance	1 week, 4 weeks
STUDIES IN PATIENTS WITH FRONTO-TEMPORAL DEMENTIA												
Huey et al., 2007	10 patients (gender DNR)	46–80 (range years)	DNR	Verbal fluency	A/S	Left DLPFC	Contralateral supraorbital area	2 mA, 40 min/2 sessions	Phonemic verbal fluency task	Online	No significant effects	No

Continued

TABLE 13.2 tDCS Studies on Cognitive Functions in Patients with Neurodegenerative Diseases.—cont'd

Studies	Sample	Age (mean ± SD years)	Education (mean ± SD years)	Cognitive Function	Polarity	Stimulated Areas	Reference Electrode	Intensity/ duration	Task	Online/ offline	Effects	Follow-up
STUDIES IN PATIENTS WITH PARKINSON'S DISEASE												
Boggio et al., 2006	18 patients (12 men)	45–71 (range years)	*(1)4.7 ± 4.4; (2)5.3 ± 4.7	Memory	A/S	Left DLPFC, M1	Contralateral orbit area	1 mA and 2 mA, 20 min/3 sessions	Three-back working memory task	Online	tDCS of the left DLPFC/ 2 mA improves accuracy	No
Benninger et al., 2010	25 patients (16 men)	*(1) 64.26 ± 8.8; (2) 63.66 ± 9.0	DNR	Learning	A/S	Bilateral premotor/ motor cortex, prefrontal cortex	Mastoids	2 mA, 20 min/ 8 sessions	Serial reaction time task	Offline	No significant effects	24 h, 1 and 3 months
Pereira et al., 2012	16 patients (7 men)	61.5 ± 59.9	12. ± 36.1	Verbal fluency	A	Left DLPFC, left temporo-parietal cortex	Contralateral supraorbital area	2 mA, 20 min	Phonemic and semantic verbal fluency tasks	Offline	DLPFC tDCS increases performance on the phonemic fluency task	No

SD, standard deviation; A, anodal tDCS; C, cathodal tDCS; S, sham tDCS; mA, milliampere; offline, the subject receives stimulation before and after executing the task; online, the subject receives stimulation during the task; DLPFC, dorsolateral prefrontal cortex; M1, motor cortex; DNR, data not reported; *, two groups were studied separately.

area, in a randomized and counterbalanced order. The task was administered during the stimulation, current was delivered at 2 mA for 40 minutes, and started 20 minutes before the task began. Anodal tDCS left verbal fluency unchanged compared with sham, and treatment had no significant effect on the neuropsychiatric inventory scores (Huey et al., 2007; see also Table 13.2). tDCS failed to induce an improvement for several reasons: first, current could shunt through the increased space left by brain atrophy; second, neuronal depletion may leave the affected cortex unable to respond to polarization; and third, some patients with severe FTD find it difficult to cooperate during the experimental protocol. Another possible limitation is the study's sample characteristics, given that most patients had predominantly behavioral symptoms and only one patient had language symptoms – hence verbal fluency may not have been a reliable variable to assess. tDCS could also have left verbal fluency unchanged owing to several factors, including type of stimulation, outcome variables, and the lack of post-tDCS evaluation. Further investigations should therefore address the expected effects in experiments using an extra-cephalic reference montage, or offline procedures in which the subject receives stimulation before and after rather than during the task and different outcome measures to evaluate different executive functions. Although this study provides negative results, ample evidence from the literature supports tDCS's ability to enhance cortical function, thus encouraging further trials in cognitive and neurobehavioral disorders.

Parkinson's Disease

PD is a neurodegenerative disorder whose main pathological hallmark is dopamine cell loss within the substantia nigra and, more specifically, the ventral pars compacta, affecting up to 70% of the cells by the time death occurs (Davie, 2008). Clinical features include motor symptoms, such as tremor, postural instability, rigidity, and bradykinesia; cognitive disorders, including attention, memory, visuo-spatial, executive, and language functions and, in up to 80% of patients, dementia as a long-term outcome; and behavioral and psychiatric symptoms, such as impulsive control disorders, mood disturbances, apathy, and anxiety (Gallagher & Schrag, 2012; Pagonabarraga & Kulisevsky, 2012; Weintraub et al., 2011).

Available studies investigated tDCS-induced changes in cognitive functions, particularly WM, procedural learning, and language, in PD (Benninger et al., 2010; Boggio et al., 2006; Pereira et al., 2012).

The first study investigated whether anodal tDCS is associated with a change in a WM task performance in 18 patients with PD (Boggio et al., 2006). Patients did a three-back WM task during anodal tDCS applied to the left DLPFC, anodal tDCS to the M1, or sham tDCS. In all these tDCS montages, the cathode was placed over the contralateral right orbit. To test whether the effects depended on stimulation intensity, tDCS was delivered for 20 minutes at 1 mA or 2 mA. Antiparkinsonian medications were withheld for approximately 12 hours before the experiment. Whereas WM accuracy significantly increased from baseline by about 20% and error frequency decreased by about 35% after anodal tDCS to the left DLPFC at 2 mA, the other stimulation conditions (sham tDCS, anodal left DLPFC tDCS at 1 mA, and anodal M1 tDCS) elicited no significant changes in task performance (Fig. 13.4). Although the lack of follow-up precluded the investigators from assessing how long the effect lasted, these results suggest that tDCS applied at different intensities can induce differential changes in cognitive functions (Boggio et al., 2006).

In a double-blind, randomized, sham-controlled study, Benninger and colleagues (2010) investigated whether anodal tDCS applied to the motor and prefrontal cortices improves motor, cognitive, and psychological variables in 25 patients with PD, and whether these effects persist over time (Benninger et al., 2010). tDCS was applied in eight sessions over 2.5 weeks when patients were receiving dopaminergic medication. The motor area and the prefrontal area were alternately stimulated at 2 mA for 20 minutes. Patients attended for follow-up evaluations 24 hours, 1 month, and 3 months after the last tDCS intervention session. Evaluations include gait, bradykinesia, visuo-motor speed, and procedural learning (serial reaction

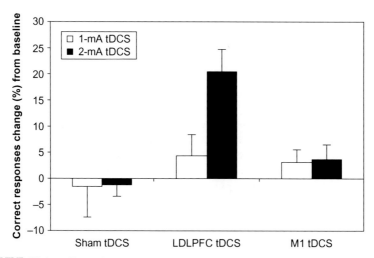

FIGURE 13.4 Effects of transcranial direct current stimulation (tDCS) over the left dorsolateral prefrontal cortex (LDLPFC) and motor cortex (M1) on the working memory task in patients with Parkinson's disease. After 2 mA anodal tDCS to the left DLPFC, word recognition task accuracy increased. Error bars are standard error of the mean (SEM). *Figure reproduced from Boggio et al. (2006), with permission.*

time task), mood, health, and wellbeing. The motor tests and the Unified Parkinson's Disease Rating Scale (UPDRS) scores were assessed while patients were on and off dopaminergic medication (overnight withdrawal for ≥ 12 h). Although gait improved significantly 24 h after tDCS – walking time decreased by about 22% and bradykinesia decreased by about 28% when patients were on medication, and by 36% when they were off medication, and this effect persists for longer than 3 months – no differences were found for changes in visuo-motor speed and procedural learning performance, mood, and wellbeing between tDCS and sham interventions. The investigators concluded that tDCS applied to the motor and prefrontal cortices may have a therapeutic potential in PD, but more powerful stimulation is needed (Benninger et al., 2010).

In a cross-over study using tDCS combined with fMRI, Pereira and colleagues (2012) aimed to assess the effects of tDCS over the left DLPFC or over the left temporo-parietal cortex on phonemic and semantic fluency functional networks in 16 patients with PD (Pereira et al., 2012). Patients did tasks inside the scanner immediately after tDCS delivered at 2-mA intensity for 20 minutes. Phonemic fluency performance, adjusted for baseline performance, time of the day for stimulation, and levodopa-equivalent doses, increased significantly more after DLPFC tDCS than after temporo-parietal stimulation (47 ± 11 words vs 44 ± 10 words). Although no significant main effects were found for semantic fluency, patients produced more words in response to a semantic category cue after DLPFC tDCS than after temporo-parietal stimulation. tDCS-induced changes in phonemic fluency were unrelated to clinical disease features, daily dopaminergic doses, or demographic variables. fMRI data showed that, in patients with PD, tDCS enhanced functional connectivity in verbal fluency and in deactivation task-related networks significantly more when applied over the DLPFC than when applied over the temporo-parietal cortex. During the verbal fluency tasks, DLPFC stimulation activated various brain areas, both near and contralateral to the stimulation site (Pereira et al., 2012). Because these brain regions are known to be involved in verbal abilities (Costafreda et al., 2006; Gurd et al., 2002; McCandliss, Cohen, & Dehaene, 2003), the study provides evidence that DLPFC tDCS specifically affects verbal fluency networks. Hence this technique might be useful to enhance phonemic fluency functions in patients with PD, although the study reports no data on how long the beneficial effect lasts. tDCS increases functional connectivity in various brain areas, and its effects spread trans-synaptically to distant cortical structures (Table 13.2).

In conclusion, because DLPFC is a key cortical station for the basal ganglia–thalamo-cortical associative circuit – a loop involved in cognitive processes, such as attention, WM, and mood regulation (Temel, Blokland, Steinbusch, & Visser-Vandewalle, 2005) – decreased activity in the DLPFC was interpreted as a "primary" dysfunction associated with PD (Fukuda, Edwards, & Eidelberg, 2001; Sabatini et al., 2000). Anodal tDCS specifically increases excitability and probably reverses decreased activity in the DLPFC, thus improving cognitive functions. Finally, tDCS interacts with the dopaminergic system in a complex way (Kuo, Paulus, & Nitsche, 2008; Nitsche et al., 2006) that could help to explain its cognitive (and motor) effects in PD.

AN OVERALL VIEW

tDCS holds considerable promise as a neurostimulation technique for improving cognitive function in healthy elderly persons, and for managing cognitive dysfunctions related to neurodegenerative disorders.

Normal aging and neurodegenerative diseases both induce changes in brain network functionality. To explain tDCS-induced cognitive changes in the healthy elderly, researchers have proposed a model for hemispheric asymmetry and aging. The HAROLD model (Cabeza et al., 2002) suggests that prefrontal activity during cognitive performance tends to be less lateralized in older adults than in younger people. This age-related asymmetry reduction acts as a compensatory mechanism that could help counteract age-related neurocognitive decline, or as a de-differentiation mechanism that reflects a difficulty in recruiting specialized neural mechanisms. Whether this model applies not only to the prefrontal cortex but also to other brain areas, thus reflecting a global reorganization in task-specific neurocognitive networks, needs confirmation (Dolcos, Rice, & Cabeza, 2002).

Only a few tDCS studies have directly compared young and old participants in experiments using the same methodology. In the decision-making study, the investigators found that tDCS applied to the same brain area has an opposite effect on risk behavior in young and in older subjects. These differences could depend on age-related changes in brain asymmetry, indicating reduced right hemisphere functioning (Boggio et al., 2010). In the language study, the investigators showed that tDCS induced its effects in the opposite hemisphere in older and younger subjects, whereas in the younger subjects face name recall improved after right tDCS while in the elderly it improved after left tDCS. These results are consistent with the HAROLD model showing compensatory recruitment in the homologous region contralateral to the area activated in younger subjects (Ross et al., 2010). In another study on semantic word generation, the different fMRI activation pattern found in the young and elderly is also coherent with the HAROLD model, and tDCS seems able to reverse age-related functional brain activity and behavioral performance (Meinzer et al., 2013). Two motor-learning studies showed tDCS-induced effects in elderly but not in young subjects by applying electrodes over both the left and right motor area (Zimerman et al., 2013, 2014). These findings are consistent with the HAROLD model, suggesting that not only contralateral, but also ipsilateral motor areas are functionally recruited in old adults as an adaptive response to aging (Zimerman et al., 2014). Finally, only one study compared elderly unihemispheric and bihemispheric tDCS-induced brain activation by fMRI, finding differential effects on motor areas and explaining these discrepancies with the age-dependent rebalancing effects of interhemispheric inhibition, according to the HAROLD model (Lindenberg et al., 2013). Differences in the experimental tasks, selection criteria for participants, and tDCS variables leave open to question whether tDCS has specific age-related effects, and, if so, the precise mechanisms involved.

The mechanisms underlying tDCS are probably highly complex. tDCS could act by increasing neuroplasticity, thereby improving function in the neural structures lying below the stimulating electrode or distant from it or at both sites. For example, in patients with PD and AD, tDCS might improve basal ganglia function throughout a distributed cortico-subcortical network (Benninger et al., 2010; Boggio et al., 2006, 2009, 2012; Ferrucci et al., 2008; Pereira et al., 2012).

tDCS is considered a safe procedure (Poreisz, Boros, Antal, & Paulus, 2007), no adverse effects were recorded in patients with AD even after five daily tDCS sessions (Boggio et al., 2012). Nonetheless, although tDCS appears safe in patients with AD, the long-term risks need further evaluation (Freitas et al., 2011; Nardone et al., 2012).

Finally, in interpreting the results reported in tDCS studies we also have to take into account other factors, such as education and the behavioral strategy used.

FUTURE DIRECTIONS

Although the clinical efficacy of tDCS awaits confirmation in large, clinical, randomized controlled studies, the results for managing cognitive dysfunctions in neurological disorders involving the elderly are encouraging and promising. Future research work should systematically assess the clinical features predicting an optimal response, tDCS interactions with other diseases and treatments, how long the beneficial effects last, and their real impact on the patient's life. Finally, tDCS's possible therapeutic effectiveness could also depend on several factors: for dementias, the severity of cognitive dysfunction and duration of disease; for PD, the motor symptoms. Other possible variables for assessing changes induced by tDCS are age, gender, genetic polymorphism (Plewnia et al., 2013), comorbidities, and drug-induced interactions.

The potential for therapeutically improving cognitive functions in the elderly with neurological diseases, and the possibility that this effect may be long lasting, could lead to the development of innovative therapeutic approaches. Owing to its simplicity, portability, safety, and low cost, tDCS holds great promise for clinical application in patients with various cognitive disorders.

References

Benninger, D. H., Lomarev, M., Lopez, G., Wassermann, E. M., Li, X., & Considine, E. (2010). Transcranial direct current stimulation for the treatment of Parkinson's disease. *Journal of Neurology, Neurosurgery, and Psychiatry, 81*(10), 1105–1111.

Berryhill, M. E., & Jones, K. T. (2012). tDCS selectively improves working memory in older adults with more education. *Neuroscience Letters, 521*(2), 148–151.

Boggio, P. S., Campanha, C., Valasek, C. A., Fecteau, S., Pascual-Leone, A., & Fregni, F. (2010). Modulation of decision-making in a gambling task in older adults with transcranial direct current stimulation. *The European Journal of Neuroscience, 31*(3), 593–597.

Boggio, P. S., Ferrucci, R., Mameli, F., Martins, D., Martins, O., & Vergari, M. (2012). Prolonged visual memory enhancement after direct current stimulation in Alzheimer's disease. *Brain Stimulation, 5*(3), 223–230.

Boggio, P. S., Ferrucci, R., Rigonatti, S. P., Covre, P., Nitsche, M., & Pascual-Leone, A. (2006). Effects of transcranial direct current stimulation on working memory in patients with Parkinson's disease. *Journal of the Neurological Sciences, 249*(1), 31–38.

Boggio, P. S., Khoury, L. P., Martins, D. C., Martins, O. E., de Macedo, E. C., & Fregni, F. (2009). Temporal cortex direct current stimulation enhances performance on a visual recognition memory task in Alzheimer disease. *Journal of Neurology, Neurosurgery, and Psychiatry, 80*(4), 444–447.

Boggio, P. S., Valasek, C. A., Campanha, C., Giglio, A. C., Baptista, N. I., & Lapenta, O. M. (2011). Non-invasive brain stimulation to assess and modulate neuroplasticity in Alzheimer's disease. *Neuropsychological Rehabilitation, 21*(5), 703–716.

Cabeza, R., Anderson, N. D., Locantore, J. K., & McIntosh, A. R. (2002). Aging gracefully: Compensatory brain activity in high-performing older adults. *NeuroImage, 17*(3), 1394–1402.

Chouinard, P. A., Leonard, G., & Paus, T. (2006). Changes in effective connectivity of the primary motor cortex in stroke patients after rehabilitative therapy. *Experimental Neurology, 201*(2), 375–387.

Costafreda, S. G., Fu, C. H., Lee, L., Everitt, B., Brammer, M. J., & David, A. S. (2006). A systematic review and quantitative appraisal of fMRI studies of verbal fluency: Role of the left inferior frontal gyrus. *Human Brain Mapping, 27*(10), 799–810.

Davie, C. A. (2008). A review of Parkinson's disease. *British Medical Bulletin, 86*, 109–127.

Dickerson, B. C., & Eichenbaum, H. (2010). The episodic memory system: Neurocircuitry and disorders. *Neuropsychopharmacology, 35*(1), 86–104.

Dolcos, F., Rice, H. J., & Cabeza, R. (2002). Hemispheric asymmetry and aging: Right hemisphere decline or asymmetry reduction. *Neuroscience and Biobehavioral Reviews, 26*(7), 819–825.

Fecteau, S., Knoch, D., Fregni, F., Sultani, N., Boggio, P., & Pascual-Leone, A. (2007). Diminishing risk-taking behavior by modulating activity in the prefrontal cortex: A direct current stimulation study. *Journal of Neuroscience: The Official Journal of the Society for Neuroscience, 27*(46), 12500–12505.

Ferrucci, R., Mameli, F., Guidi, I., Mrakic-Sposta, S., Vergari, M., & Marceglia, S. (2008). Transcranial direct current stimulation improves recognition memory in Alzheimer disease. *Neurology, 71*(7), 493–498.

Flöel, A., Suttorp, W., Kohl, O., Kurten, J., Lohmann, H., & Breitenstein, C. (2012). Noninvasive brain stimulation improves object-location learning in the elderly. *Neurobiology of Aging, 33*(8), 1682–1689.

Freitas, C., Mondragon-Llorca, H., & Pascual-Leone, A. (2011). Noninvasive brain stimulation in Alzheimer's disease: Systematic review and perspectives for the future. *Experimental Gerontology, 46*(8), 611–627.

Fukuda, M., Edwards, C., & Eidelberg, D. (2001). Functional brain networks in Parkinson's disease. *Parkinsonism & Related Disorders, 8*(2), 91–94.

Gallagher, D. A., & Schrag, A. (2012). Psychosis, apathy, depression and anxiety in Parkinson's disease. *Neurobiology of Disease, 46*(3), 581–589.

Gurd, J. M., Amunts, K., Weiss, P. H., Zafiris, O., Zilles, K., & Marshall, J. C. (2002). Posterior parietal cortex is implicated in continuous switching between verbal fluency tasks: An fMRI study with clinical implications. *Brain, 125*(Pt 5), 1024–1038.

Hansen, N. (2012). Action mechanisms of transcranial direct current stimulation in Alzheimer's disease and memory loss. *Front in Psychiatry, 3*, 48.

Holland, R., Leff, A. P., Josephs, O., Galea, J. M., Desikan, M., & Price, C. J. (2011). Speech facilitation by left inferior frontal cortex stimulation. *Current Biology, 21*(16), 1403–1407.

Hong, S. L., & Rebec, G. V. (2012). Biological sources of inflexibility in brain and behavior with aging and neurodegenerative diseases. *Frontiers in Systems Neuroscience, 6*, 77.

Huey, E. D., Probasco, J. C., Moll, J., Stocking, J., Ko, M. H., & Grafman, J. (2007). No effect of DC brain polarization on verbal fluency in patients with advanced frontotemporal dementia. *Clinical Neurophysiology, 118*(6), 1417–1418.

Hummel, F. C., Heise, K., Celnik, P., Flöel, A., Gerloff, C., & Cohen, L. G. (2010). Facilitating skilled right hand motor function in older subjects by anodal polarization over the left primary motor cortex. *Neurobiology of Aging, 31*(12), 2160–2168.

Jagust, W. (2013). Vulnerable neural systems and the borderland of brain aging and neurodegeneration. *Neuron, 77*(2), 219–234.

Jebsen, R. H., Taylor, N., Trieschmann, R. B., Trotter, M. J., & Howard, L. A. (1969). An objective and standardized test of hand function. *Archives of Physical Medicine and Rehabilitation, 50*(6), 311–319.

Kuo, M. F., & Nitsche, M. A. (2012). Effects of transcranial electrical stimulation on cognition. *Clinical EEG and Neuroscience, 43*(3), 192–199.

Kuo, M. F., Paulus, W., & Nitsche, M. A. (2008). Boosting focally-induced brain plasticity by dopamine. *Cerebral Cortex, 18*(3), 648–651.

Lang, N., Siebner, H. R., Ward, N. S., Lee, L., Nitsche, M. A., & Paulus, W. (2005). How does transcranial DC stimulation of the primary motor cortex alter regional neuronal activity in the human brain? *The European Journal of Neuroscience, 22*(2), 495–504.

Lindenberg, R., Nachtigall, L., Meinzer, M., Sieg, M. M., & Flöel, A. (2013). Differential effects of dual and unihemispheric motor cortex stimulation in older adults. *Journal of Neuroscience: The Official Journal of the Society for Neuroscience, 33*(21), 9176–9183.

Lund/Manchester. (1994). Clinical and neurophatological criteria for frontotemporal dementia. The Lund and Manchester Groups. *Journal of Neurology, Neurosurgery and Psychiatry, 57*, 416–418.

Mattay, V. S., Fera, F., Tessitore, A., Hariri, A. R., Das, S., & Callicott, J. H. (2002). Neurophysiological correlates of age-related changes in human motor function. *Neurology, 58*(4), 630–635.

McCandliss, B. D., Cohen, L., & Dehaene, S. (2003). The visual word form area: Expertise for reading in the fusiform gyrus. *Trends in Cognitive Sciences, 7*(7), 293–299.

III. IMPROVING FUNCTIONS IN THE ATYPICAL BRAIN

Meinzer, M., Lindenberg, R., Antonenko, D., Flaisch, T., & Flöel, A. (2013). Anodal transcranial direct current stimulation temporarily reverses age-associated cognitive decline and functional brain activity changes. *Journal of Neuroscience: The Official Journal of the Society for Neuroscience, 33*(30), 12470–12478.

Monti, A., Ferrucci, R., Fumagalli, M., Mameli, F., Cogiamanian, F., & Ardolino, G. (2013). Transcranial direct current stimulation (tDCS) and language. *Journal of Neurology, Neurosurgery, and Psychiatry.*

Naccarato, M., Calautti, C., Jones, P. S., Day, D. J., Carpenter, T. A., & Baron, J. C. (2006). Does healthy aging affect the hemispheric activation balance during paced index-to-thumb opposition task? An fMRI study. *NeuroImage, 32*(3), 1250–1256.

Nardone, R., Bergmann, J., Christova, M., Caleri, F., Tezzon, F., & Ladurner, G. (2012). Effect of transcranial brain stimulation for the treatment of Alzheimer disease: A review. *International Journal of Alzheimer's Disease, 2012,* 687909.

Nitsche, M. A., Cohen, L. G., Wassermann, E. M., Priori, A., Lang, N., & Antal, A. (2008). Transcranial direct current stimulation: State of the art 2008. *Brain Stimulation, 1*(3), 206–223.

Nitsche, M. A., Doemkes, S., Karakose, T., Antal, A., Liebetanz, D., & Lang, N. (2007). Shaping the effects of transcranial direct current stimulation of the human motor cortex. *Journal of Neurophysiology, 97*(4), 3109–3117.

Nitsche, M. A., Lampe, C., Antal, A., Liebetanz, D., Lang, N., & Tergau, F. (2006). Dopaminergic modulation of long-lasting direct current-induced cortical excitability changes in the human motor cortex. *The European Journal of Neuroscience, 23*(6), 1651–1657.

Nitsche, M. A., Liebetanz, D., Antal, A., Lang, N., Tergau, F., & Paulus, W. (2003). Modulation of cortical excitability by weak direct current stimulation – Technical, safety and functional aspects. *Supplements to Clinical Neurophysiology, 56,* 255–276.

Nitsche, M. A., & Paulus, W. (2000). Excitability changes induced in the human motor cortex by weak transcranial direct current stimulation. *The Journal of Physiology, 527*(Pt 3), 633–639.

Nitsche, M. A., Schauenburg, A., Lang, N., Liebetanz, D., Exner, C., & Paulus, W. (2003). Facilitation of implicit motor learning by weak transcranial direct current stimulation of the primary motor cortex in the human. *Journal of Cognitive Neuroscience, 15*(4), 619–626.

Nitsche, M. A., Seeber, A., Frommann, K., Klein, C. C., Rochford, C., & Nitsche, M. S. (2005). Modulating parameters of excitability during and after transcranial direct current stimulation of the human motor cortex. *The Journal of Physiology, 568*(Pt 1), 291–303.

Pagonabarraga, J., & Kulisevsky, J. (2012). Cognitive impairment and dementia in Parkinson's disease. *Neurobiology of Disease, 46*(3), 590–596.

Pellicciari, M. C., Brignani, D., & Miniussi, C. (2013). Excitability modulation of the motor system induced by transcranial direct current stimulation: A multimodal approach. *NeuroImage, 83,* 569–580.

Pereira, J. B., Junque, C., Bartres-Faz, D., Marti, M. J., Sala-Llonch, R., & Compta, Y. (2012). Modulation of verbal fluency networks by transcranial direct current stimulation (tDCS) in Parkinson's disease. *Brain Stimulation, 6,* 16–24.

Plewnia, C., Zwissler, B., Langst, I., Maurer, B., Giel, K., & Kruger, R. (2013). Effects of transcranial direct current stimulation (tDCS) on executive functions: Influence of COMT Val/Met polymorphism. *Cortex, 49*(7), 1801–1807.

Poreisz, C., Boros, K., Antal, A., & Paulus, W. (2007). Safety aspects of transcranial direct current stimulation concerning healthy subjects and patients. *Brain Research Bulletin, 72* (4–6), 208–214.

Priori, A. (2003). Brain polarization in humans: A reappraisal of an old tool for prolonged non-invasive modulation of brain excitability. *Clinical Neurophysiology, 114*(4), 589–595.

Reis, J., & Fritsch, B. (2011). Modulation of motor performance and motor learning by transcranial direct current stimulation. *Current Opinion in Neurology, 24*(6), 590–596.

Ren, J., Wu, Y. D., Chan, J. S., & Yan, J. H. (2013). Cognitive aging affects motor performance and learning. *Geriatrics & Gerontology International, 13*(1), 19–27.

Ross, L. A., McCoy, D., Coslett, H. B., Olson, I. R., & Wolk, D. A. (2011). Improved proper name recall in aging after electrical stimulation of the anterior temporal lobes. *Frontiers in Aging Neuroscience, 3,* 16.

Ross, L. A., McCoy, D., Wolk, D. A., Coslett, H. B., & Olson, I. R. (2010). Improved proper name recall by electrical stimulation of the anterior temporal lobes. *Neuropsychologia, 48*(12), 3671–3674.

Rugg, M. D., Otten, L. J., & Henson, R. N. (2002). The neural basis of episodic memory: Evidence from functional neuroimaging. *Philosophical Transactions of the Royal Society of London Series B: Biological Sciences, 357*(1424), 1097–1110.

Sabatini, U., Boulanouar, K., Fabre, N., Martin, F., Carel, C., & Colonnese, C. (2000). Cortical motor reorganization in akinetic patients with Parkinson's disease: A functional MRI study. *Brain, 123*(Pt 2), 394–403.

Scelzo, E., Giannicola, G., Rosa, M., Ciocca, M., Ardolino, G., & Cogiamanian, F. (2010). Increased short latency afferent inhibition after anodal transcranial direct current stimulation. *Neuroscience Letters, 498*(2), 167–170.

Schulz, R., Gerloff, C., & Hummel, F. C. (2013). Non-invasive brain stimulation in neurological diseases. *Neuropharmacology, 64,* 579–587.

Seltman, R. E., & Matthews, B. R. (2012). Frontotemporal lobar degeneration: Epidemiology, pathology, diagnosis and management. *CNS Drugs, 26*(10), 841–870.

Shafqat, S. (2008). Alzheimer disease therapeutics: Perspectives from the developing world. *Journal of Alzheimer's Disease, 15*(2), 285–287.

Squire, L. R., & Zola, S. M. (1996). Structure and function of declarative and nondeclarative memory systems. *Proceedings of the National Academy of Sciences of the United States of America, 93*(24), 13515–13522.

Temel, Y., Blokland, A., Steinbusch, H. W., & Visser-Vandewalle, V. (2005). The functional role of the subthalamic nucleus in cognitive and limbic circuits. *Progress in Neurobiology, 76*(6), 393–413.

Vines, B. W., Nair, D. G., & Schlaug, G. (2006). Contralateral and ipsilateral motor effects after transcranial direct current stimulation. *Neuroreport, 17*(6), 671–674.

Weintraub, D., Doshi, J., Koka, D., Davatzikos, C., Siderowf, A. D., & Duda, J. E. (2011). Neurodegeneration across stages of cognitive decline in Parkinson disease. *Archives of Neurology, 68*(12), 1562–1568.

Witt, K., Deuschl, G., & Bartsch, T. (2013). Frontotemporal dementias. *Nervenarzt, 84*(1), 20–32.

Zimerman, M., Heise, K. F., Gerloff, C., Cohen, L. G., & Hummel, F. C. (2014). Disrupting the ipsilateral motor cortex Interferes with training of a complex motor task in older adults. *Cerebral Cortex, 24*(4), 1030–1036.

Zimerman, M., & Hummel, F. C. (2010). Non-invasive brain stimulation: Enhancing motor and cognitive functions in healthy old subjects. *Frontiers in Aging Neuroscience, 2,* 149.

Zimerman, M., Nitsch, M., Giraux, P., Gerloff, C., Cohen, L. G., & Hummel, F. C. (2013). Neuroenhancement of the aging brain: Restoring skill acquisition in old subjects. *Annals of Neurology, 73*(1), 10–15.

14

Clinical use of Transcranial Direct Current Stimulation in Psychiatry

Andre Brunoni[1] and Paulo Boggio[2]

[1]Center for Clinical and Epidemiological Research & Interdisciplinary Center for Applied Neuromodulation, University Hospital, and University of São Paulo Medical School, University of São Paulo, São Paulo, Brazil
[2]Social and Cognitive Neuroscience Laboratory, Center for Health and Biological Sciences, Mackenzie Presbyterian University, São Paulo, Brazil

OUTLINE

HISTORICAL REMARKS: tDCS IN CLINICAL PSYCHIATRY

Although transcranial direct current stimulation (tDCS) is a technique referred to as "new" for the treatment of depression and other psychiatric disorders, there have been reports of its clinical use since the 1960s on mood and alertness in healthy volunteers. For example, in an article in 1964 ("Mental changes resulting from the passage of small direct current through the human brain"), Lippold and Redfearn (1964) wrote:

> We applied small voltages to the intact scalp of human volunteers, including ourselves. ... The effects perhaps could be summarized in the statement that scalp-negative stimulation often caused quietness and withdrawal, whereas scalp-positive stimulation tended to cause alertness or move involvement in the environment.

In the same year, Costain, Redfearn, and Lippold (1964) showed, in a double-blind, placebo-controlled experiment, that tDCS was effective in reducing depressive symptoms compared to sham stimulation. However, the authors did not use standardized psychiatric scales (which were not yet in widespread use at the time). Subsequently, other authors conducted open trials reporting a reduction in depressive symptoms after using tDCS with different protocols and parameters (Carney, Cashman, & Sheffield, 1970; Herjanic & Moss-Herjanic, 1967; Nias & Shapiro, 1974; Ramsay & Schlagenhauf, 1966). Finally, a second randomized, double-blind, placebo-controlled study conducted by another group (Arfai, Theano, Montagu, & Robin, 1970) was unable to demonstrate the antidepressant effects of brain stimulation.

tDCS was largely forgotten between 1970 and 2000, possibly due to the advancement of psychopharmacology and the social stigma of ECT that affected other forms of non-invasive brain stimulation such as tDCS (Nitsche, Boggio, Fregni, & Pascual-Leone, 2009). Note that tDCS parameters used at that time differ from those currently proposed, as will be shown below.

POTENTIAL ADVANTAGES OF USING tDCS IN CLINICAL PSYCHIATRY

Considering that tDCS could become an established, effective therapy for some psychiatric disorders, should it be used in clinical psychiatry? This question is of paramount importance since current evidence from clinical trials in depression, for instance, suggests that tDCS is an effective therapy – perhaps as effective as pharmacotherapy and repetitive transcranial magnetic stimulation (rTMS) (Brunoni, Ferrucci, Fregni, Boggio, & Priori, 2012; Kalu, Sexton, Loo, & Ebmeier, 2012; Schutter, 2009).

Vis-à-vis rTMS, tDCS is probably a more advantageous treatment (considering that both therapies have similar efficacy). tDCS is cheaper than rTMS, and easier to use (Priori, Hallett, & Rothwell, 2009). Also, rTMS is administered via a non-portable device that can be handled only by trained staff, meaning that patients must make daily visits to the clinic, whereas tDCS is delivered via a handheld device and patients could even be trained to use it at home (for instance, tailored head caps would assist the subject in placing the electrodes) (Brunoni, Ferrucci, Fregni, Boggio, & Priori, 2012).

Conversely, tDCS is less advantageous than pharmacotherapy. Actually, taking a pill is easier than using tDCS, even if a portable device were available. In selected groups, however, tDCS could be an interesting alternative. Examples include during pregnancy, depression associated with clinical comorbidities (where pharmacological interactions with antidepressants are an issue), and patients especially intolerant to the adverse effects of pharmacotherapy. Nevertheless, treatment with tDCS should be considered not only *instead of* but also *as well as* antidepressant drugs. Both treatments combined might theoretically induce increased and faster effects than each treatment alone (Brunoni, Ferrucci et al., 2013; Brunoni, Valiengo et al., 2013).

PSYCHIATRIC DISORDERS AND tDCS

Major Depressive Disorder

Major depressive disorder (MDD) is an incapacitating disorder associated with significant personal, social, and economic impairment. Patients with MDD present a "double burden," characterized by a lower quality of life associated with a higher prevalence of medical comorbidities (Wittchen, Knauper, & Kessler, 1994). The main symptoms of MDD include persistent low mood, anhedonia (i.e., diminished pleasure in previous significant activities), impairment in sleep, psychomotor retardation, weight changes, and negative thoughts that range from pessimism to guilt and suicidal ideation. Moreover, although only the most severe spectrum of depression is associated with suicide, its chronic, incapacitating symptoms make depression one of the most incapacitating conditions worldwide. Thus, MDD has been projected to be the second most disabling condition by 2020 (Murray & Lopez, 1997). MDD is known to be a recurrent and relapsing psychiatric condition, and approximately 50% of the patients who present with a depressive episode will undergo a new episode further in life (Eaton et al., 1997). Finally, nearly 30% of patients present in a refractory state – i.e., depressive symptoms are observed despite the appropriate psychological and pharmacological treatment (Rush et al., 2006). For these reasons, continuous research on MDD in terms of newer treatment techniques is imperative.

Pharmacotherapy

Antidepressant drugs are considered to be the cornerstone of treatment for depression. The pharmacological arsenal includes first-generation antidepressants (tricyclic antidepressants and monoamine oxidase inhibitors), SSRIs (serotonin selective reuptake inhibitors, such as sertraline and fluoxetine), SNRIs ("dual-inhibitors" such as venlafaxine and duloxetine), and others (e.g., bupropion and mirtazapine). A recent meta-analysis suggested that escitalopram and sertraline are the antidepressants that best combine effectiveness with tolerability, and therefore should be the first choice for treatment (Cipriani et al., 2010). Given the multiple pharmacological treatments available, the STAR*D (Sequenced Treatment Alternatives to Relieve Depression), a NIMH-sponsored trial, enrolled almost 3000 patients to evaluate the efficacy of several antidepressant treatments (Rush et al., 2006). STAR*D highlighted the importance of refractoriness in pharmacotherapy – i.e., remission rates decay as more antidepressant treatments fail, and in fact after four consecutive antidepressant interventions 30% of patients still show symptoms of depression. Also, drop-out rates are relatively high irrespective of the drug class assessed; the causes are multiple, and include side effects, the time gap between the initial treatment and consequent improvement of depressive symptoms, and the patient–physician relationship, all of which can affect relapse rates in the long-term (Warden et al., 2007). These issues reinforce the need for newer interventions in the treatment of MDD.

Transcranial Direct Current Stimulation

MECHANISMS OF ACTION

Four pathophysiological models are particularly compelling for understanding the antidepressant effects of tDCS: (1) the "bottom-up"/"top-down" dysfunction between subcortical and cortical structures (Koenigs & Grafman, 2009) observed in patients with MDD; (2) the prefrontal asymmetry hypothesis for affective processing, in which patients with MDD present relatively hypoactivity on the left DLPFC and overactivity of the right DLPFC (Vanderhasselt, De Raedt, Leyman, & Baeken, 2009); (3) the DMN/ACN (default-mode network/anticorrelated network) dysfunction, which is also observed in patients with MDD (Pizzagalli, 2011); and (4) the observation that MDD is associated with decreased neuroplasticity (Brunoni, Lopes, & Fregni, 2008), and tDCS might increase neuroplasticity (Fritsch et al., 2010). It should be emphasized that many of the findings from the studies described below were reproduced in healthy samples, and thereby should also apply as general models for understanding tDCS' mechanisms of action in the field of affective psychology, or even other psychiatric disorders that present affective impairment and/or deficits in DLPFC functioning.

Neuroimaging findings revealed that MDD is associated with both functional and structural alterations in the fronto-cingulo–striatal circuits. For instance, recent meta-analyses showed that patients with MDD, compared to healthy subjects, presented volumetric reductions in these circuits (Bora, Fornito, Pantelis, & Yucel, 2012), as well as decreased fractional anisotropy in these areas (Liao et al., 2013). In addition, antidepressant treatment with sertraline was able to increase gray matter volume over the left DLPFC (Smith, Chen, Baxter, Fort, & Lane, 2013), whereas a double-blind, randomized trial showed that antidepressant treatment with high-frequency rTMS increased fractional anisotropy in the left middle frontal gyrus (Peng et al., 2012). In fact, this imbalance between cortical and subcortical activity might also explain neurophysiological alterations observed in MDD, such as hypercortisolism and increased blood levels of inflammatory cytokines, triggered by an overactive hypothalamic–pituitary–adrenal (HPA) axis (Arnsten, 2009), and decreased heart rate variability, reflecting an overactive sympathetic–adrenal–medullary (SAM) system (Kemp et al., 2010). Theoretically, the focal effects of tDCS could increase cortical activity and consequently decrease subcortical activity, thus restoring the fronto-cingulo–striatal activity to physiological levels. In this context, Beeli, Casutt, Baumgartner, and Jancke (2008) were able to decrease skin conductance (a physiological marker of sympathetic activity) using cathodal stimulation over the right DLPFC in a stress-inducing, virtual reality test (a rollercoaster riding experience), suggesting top-down modulation of the brainstem. In addition, Brunoni, Vanderhasselt et al. (2013) found that anodal stimulation over the left DLPFC/cathodal stimulation over the right DLPFC decreased salivary cortisol levels and increased vagal activity in subjects viewing negative imagery. In fact, tDCS might primarily counterbalance stress activity than having a direct influence on brainstem activity, since other studies found that tDCS does not induce physiological changes during rest, at least in healthy subjects (Sampaio, Fraguas, Lotufo, Bensenor, & Brunoni, 2012).

MDD is also associated with dysfunctional processing in affective-related neural circuits (Clark, Chamberlain, & Sahakian 2009; Williams, Mathews, & MacLeod, 1996) – the "prefrontal asymmetry hypothesis" (Grimm et al., 2008; Koenigs & Grafman, 2009; Mayberg, 2003). Cognitive theories acknowledge that a biased, preferential processing of negative-valence information (also known as the "differential activation hypothesis") makes negative thinking patterns more easily available, which maintains the ruminative cognitive style of depression and might trigger and perpetuate depressive episodes (De Raedt & Koster, 2010). The anodal, excitability-enhancing effects and/or the cathodal, excitability-decreasing effects of tDCS could theoretically reverse such asymmetry. For instance, Boggio et al. (2007) found, in one single, double-blind tDCS session, that anodal DLPFC stimulation increased accuracy for positive imagery in a go/no-go task. Recently, Brunoni, Zanao et al. (2013) also reported that one single tDCS session induced an increase in positive affect processing, as compared to sham tDCS.

Recently, studies using resting-state MRI and multichannel EEG revealed that several mental disorders, notably MDD, are associated with DMN dysfunction (Andrade, 2013; Pizzagalli, 2011). Theoretically, patients with depression present decreased ACN and increased DMN activity, which could in turn be related to symptoms such as increased rumination and pessimistic thoughts (associated with the DMN) (Wang, Hermens, Hickie, & Lagopoulos, 2012) and psychomotor retardation and executive dysfunction (associated with the ACN) (Whitfield-Gabrieli & Ford, 2012). Recent studies showed, in healthy subjects, that tDCS modulates functional activity in large brain networks (Sehm et al., 2012), increasing synchrony in the ACN and reducing synchrony in the DMN (Pena-Gomez et al., 2011). Therefore, it is possible that the antidepressant effects of tDCS involve the dysregulation between DMN and ACN observed in depression.

Finally, MDD presents not only neuro-anatomic and functional alterations, but also dysfunction at a neurobiological level. In particular, BDNF (brain-derived neurotrophic factor), a neurotrophin critical to long-term synaptic potentiation (LTP), is decreased during the acute depressive episode, being partially restored to normal levels after depression is remitted (Brunoni et al., 2008; Sen, Duman, & Sanacora, 2008). Interestingly, an animal study using direct current stimulation showed that this technique induces BDNF-dependent synaptic plasticity (Fritsch et al., 2010), and studies exploring the electrophysiology of tDCS also demonstrate that tDCS induces neuroplasticity (Stagg & Nitsche, 2011). On the other hand, Brunoni, Kemp et al. (2013), using data from the SELECT-TDCS trial (described in the following section), found that the BDNF polymorphism Val66Met did not moderate tDCS antidepressant effects, and Palm, Fintescu et al. (2013) did not observe BDNF increasing after tDCS treatment in a depressed sample. Therefore, another putative mechanism of action that should be investigated for tDCS is its capacity to directly induce neuroplasticity, which is impaired in depression.

tDCS CLINICAL TRIALS FOR DEPRESSION IN THE 1960s AND 1970s

According to a review undertaken by Nitsche et al. (2009), eight clinical trials for MDD were performed between 1964 and 1974 using a technique named "brain polarization" which, although akin to tDCS, consisted of the application of *two* frontal anode electrodes and *one* extracephalic cathode (usually, but not only, in the knee). These early studies used low (<0.5 mA) direct currents for several (>6) hours once a day for 1 week. They presented mixed findings; however, such studies were methodologically weak (poor evaluation of depressive symptoms, insufficient description of the devices and montages used), hindering a proper evaluation of them (for earlier usage of electricity to treat mental illnesses, see Chapter 1).

"MODERN" tDCS TRIALS FOR MDD

From 2006 to late 2012, several clinical studies – including case reports, case series, open-label trials, and double-blind, randomized trials – evaluating tDCS as a treatment for MDD were performed (Table 14.1). Of note, the blinding of tDCS randomized clinical trials (RCTs) is considered effective since, for sham tDCS, the device is turned off after 30 seconds, mimicking the local effects that occur in the skin (e.g., redness, itching, tingling sensation) (Gandiga, Hummel, & Cohen, 2006). However, other adverse effects, such as skin reddening, might not be adequately mimicked by this method, since recent studies reported increased rates of this adverse effect in the active versus sham group (Brunoni, Valiengo et al., 2013; O'Connell et al., 2012; Palm, Reisinger et al., 2013). Nonetheless, although some studies have recently cast doubts regarding the blinding of investigators (at 1 mA) (Ambrus et al., 2012), and of both investigators and subjects (at 2 mA) (O'Connell et al., 2012), sham tDCS seems to be a more reliable method than, for instance, sham rTMS (Brunoni, Nitsche et al., 2012).

In a first RCT, Fregni, Boggio, Nitsche, Marcolin et al. (2006) enrolled 10 antidepressant-free patients with mild to moderate depression to receive either active or sham tDCS (anodal over the left DLPFC, cathode over the right supraorbital area; current intensity 1 mA, 20 minutes per day for 5 days), finding positive results with an improvement of 60% in the active versus only 12% in the sham group. In another RCT using the same tDCS set-up and stimulation parameters, Fregni, Boggio, Nitsche, Rigonatti and Pascual-Leone (2006) confirmed their previous findings, also finding significant improvement in the active versus sham group (58.5% vs 13.1%, respectively). Boggio et al. (2008) enrolled 40 patients with MDD, randomizing them to three groups: (1) active anodal tDCS over the DLPFC, (2) active anodal tDCS over the occipital cortex, and (3) sham tDCS (all participants received the cathode over the right supraorbital area). They used a current intensity of 2 mA, 20 minutes per day for 10 days, and found that the active DLPFC tDCS group presented a superior, significant improvement in Hamilton Depression Rating Scale (HDRS) scores compared with the other groups (improvement of 40% in active left PFC versus 20% in the occipital group and 10% in the sham group).

Subsequently, two other RCTs found that active tDCS was not superior to sham tDCS. Loo et al. (2010) enrolled 40 patients with severe MDD,

TABLE 14.1 Summary of Transcranial Direct Current Stimulation Clinical Studies for Major Depressive Disorder

Author	Sample Size	Depression Scale	Protocol Anode	Cathode	Current Density (A/m²)	Session Duration (min)	Number of Sessions	Frequency	Improvement (change in scores) Active tDCS	Sham tDCS	Endpoint (from 1st day of treatment)
RANDOMIZED, DOUBLE-BLIND, CONTROLLED TRIALS											
Fregni, Boggio, Nitsche, Marcolin et al. (2006)	10	HDRS	F3	R SO	0.28	20	5	Every other weekday	60%	12%	2 weeks
Fregni, Boggio, Nitsche, Rigonatti, and Pascual-Leone (2006)	18	HDRS	F3	R SO	0.28	20	5	Every other weekday	58.5%	13.1%	2 weeks
Boggio et al. (2008)	40	HDRS	F3	R SO	0.57	20	10	Consecutive weekdays	40.4%	10.4%	6 weeks
Loo et al. (2010)	40	MADRS	F3	R SO	0.28	20	5	Every other weekday	19.5%	19.2%	2 weeks
Palm et al. (2012)	22	HDRS	F3	R SO	0.28/0.57	20	10	Consecutive weekdays	14.6%/ 6.7%	9%	2 weeks
Loo et al. (2012)	64	MADRS	F3	R SO	0.57	20	15	Consecutive weekdays	28.4%	15.9%	2 weeks
Blumberger, Tran, Fitzgerald, Hoy, and Daskalakis (2012)	24	HDRS	F3	F4	0.57	20	15	Consecutive weekdays	21.3%	24.8%	3 weeks

Brunoni, Valiengo et al. (2013)	120	MADRS	F3	F4	0.8	30	10	Consecutive weekdays	47%	24%	6 weeks
OPEN-LABEL STUDIES										
Ferrucci, Bortolomasi, Vergari et al. (2009)	14	HDRS/BDI	F3	F4	0.57	20	10	2×/day (one weekday)	32.1%	–	5 weeks
Ferrucci, Bortolomasi, Brunoni et al. (2009)	32	HDRS/BDI	F3	F4	0.57	20	10	2×/day (one weekday)	27.7%	–	5 weeks
Brunoni, Ferrucci, Bortolomasi et al. (2011)	31	HDRS/BDI	F3	F4	0.57	20	10	2×/day (one weekday)	45.2%(*)	–	5 weeks
Dell'osso et al. (2012)	23	HDRS/MADRS	F3	F4	0.57	20	10	2×/day (one weekday)	31.3%	–	2 weeks
Martin et al. (2011)	11	MADRS	F3	R arm	0.57	20	20	Consecutive weekdays	43.8%	–	4 weeks
Brunoni, Ferrucci et al. (2013)	82	BDI	F3	F4	0.57	20	5	2×/day (one weekday)	29%	–	5 days

Continued

TABLE 14.1 Summary of Transcranial Direct Current Stimulation Clinical Studies for Major Depressive Disorder—cont'd

Author	Sample Size	Depression Scale	Protocol						Improvement (change in scores)		
			Anode	Cathode	Current Density (A/m²)	Session Duration (min)	Number of Sessions	Frequency	Active tDCS	Sham tDCS	Endpoint (from 1st day of treatment)
CASE REPORTS:									COMMENT:		
Palm et al. (2009)	1	HDRS/BDI	F3	R SO	0.28	20	16	Consecutive weekdays			Treatment-resistant depression modestly improved after tDCS
Arul-Anandam, Loo, and Mitchell (2010)	1	MADRS	F3	R SO	0.28	20	5	Consecutive weekdays			Transient hypomania episode that started after three sessions and resolved spontaneously
Baccaro, Brunoni, Bensenor, and Fregni (2010)	1	YMRS	F3	F4	0.8	30	10	Consecutive weekdays			Transient hypomania episode that started after six sessions and resolved spontaneously
Brunoni, Valiengo, Zanao et al. (2011)	1	YMRS	F3	F4	0.8	30	6	Consecutive weekdays			Full-blown manic episode after six sessions of tDCS+sertraline requiring pharmacological intervention
Bueno, Brunoni, Boggio, Bensenor, and Fregni (2011)	1	MADRS	F3	F4	0.8	30	10	Consecutive weekdays			Post-stroke depression that markedly improved after tDCS
Gálvez et al. (2011)	1	MADRS	F3	R arm	0.57	20	20	2×/day (one weekday)			Hypomanic episode in a bipolar depressed patient after fronto-extracephalic tDCS

III. IMPROVING FUNCTIONS IN THE ATYPICAL BRAIN

OTHERS

Study									
Rigonatti et al. (2008)	11	HDRS	F3	R SO	0.57	20	10	Consecutive weekdays	tDCS and fluoxetine had similar improvement rates at endpoint, tDCS was superior at 2 weeks
Kalu et al. (2012)	176	Hedges' g	F3	R SO	0.28/0.57	20	5/10/15	Daily/every other day	Hedges' g of 0.74 (95% CI 0.21–1.27) favoring active vs sham group although between-sample heterogeneity was important
Berlim, Van den Eynde, and Daskalakis (2013)	200	Odds Ratio	F3	R SO/ F4	0.28/0.57	20	5/10/15	Daily/every other day	No significant differences for clinical response and remission (ORs of 1.97, 95% CI 0.85–4.57 and 2.13, 95% CI 0.64–7.06)

HDRS, Hamilton Depression Rating Scale; MADRS, Montgomery-Asberg Depression Rating Scale; YMRS, Young Mania Rating Scale; BDI, Beck Depression Inventory; F3, left dorsolateral prefrontal cortex; F4, right dorsolateral prefrontal cortex; R SO, right supraorbital area; R arm, right arm; CI, confidence interval; OR, odds ratio.

finding similar improvements of approximately 19% in both groups; active tDCS to the DLPFC was only more effective during the open-label phase, in which patients received an additional five sessions. However, this study had some limitations: the dose applied was relatively low (1 mA) and there were only five stimulation sessions, which were alternated (i.e., performed every other day). Moreover, patients with personality disorders were not excluded – an issue that might have increased sample heterogeneity. In another RCT, Palm et al. (2012) randomized 22 patients to receive 1 mA or 2 mA for 20 minutes per day per 2 weeks, finding similar improvement in active versus sham tDCS groups. Possible reasons for this negative finding were the high degree of treatment resistance, and the concomitant use of antidepressant medications. In a large RCT, Loo et al. (2012), in contrast with their previous study, found positive results in 64 patients that were randomized to receive 3-week active or sham anodal tDCS to the left DLPFC (2 mA/20 min), showing an improvement of 28.4% in the active group versus 15.9% in the sham group. In this trial, the sample was composed of bipolar and unipolar depressed patients, mostly (67%) on antidepressant treatment and with chronic, treatment-resistant depression. Lastly, Blumberger et al. (2012) randomized 24 patients to receive active tDCS (anodal over the left and cathode over the right DLPFC) or sham tDCS at 2 mA (20 minutes per day, for 15 days) showing that the remission rates did not differ between both groups. The authors acknowledged that some methodological limitations might have hindered a positive outcome, such as the small sample size and that more subjects in the active tDCS group had failed an ECT course in the current depressive episode.

THE SELECT-TDCS STUDY

Recently, our group published a large trial named SELECT-TDCS (the Sertraline versus Electrical Current Therapy for Treating Depression Clinical Study) (Brunoni, Valiengo et al., 2013). In this RCT, we enrolled 120 antidepressant-free patients that were randomized to four groups, in a factorial design: sham tDCS/placebo pill; sham tDCS/sertraline; active tDCS/placebo; and active tDCS/sertraline. The sample size was powered to assess three main questions: (1) whether active tDCS is superior to sham tDCS; (2) whether active tDCS is as effective as sertraline 50 mg/day, and (3) whether the combined treatment (active tDCS/sertraline) is superior to each treatment alone (Brunoni, Valiengo, Baccaro et al., 2011). Of 850 volunteers, we included only those with moderate to severe depression, low suicidal ideation, absence of other psychiatric and medical comorbidities, and either not currently on antidepressants or using and agreeing to discontinue their use. We did not enrol patients on sertraline and that had ever used sertraline during the current major depressive episode. tDCS was applied at 2 mA/25 cm^2, with the anode and the cathode over the left and right DLPFC, respectively, for 30 minutes daily, for 10 weekdays. Thereafter, tDCS was applied every other week, until the endpoint at 6 weeks (i.e., two extra sessions). For sham tDCS, the device was turned off after 30 seconds of stimulation. We performed an intention-to-treat analysis in the 103 patients who finished the study. The Montgomery-Asberg depression rating scale (MADRS) was the primary outcome. The four groups were similar at baseline. At week 6, the combined treatment group was significantly more effective ($P \leq 0.01$ for all comparisons) than placebo (mean difference of 11.5 points, 95% Confidence Interval [CI] $=6$–17), sertraline (8.5 points, 95% CI $=2.9$–14), and tDCS (5.9 points, 95% CI $=0.36$–11.43). tDCS and sertraline presented similar efficacy (2.6 points, 95% CI $= -2.9$ to 8.1, $P = 0.35$). Other depression scales yielded similar results.

The SELECT-TDCS contributes to the literature of tDCS and MDD treatment, being the first phase II/III study to date. It also has important clinical repercussions, since the combined treatment group was also more effective than the other groups at week 2, and it presented greater efficacy than the other groups at week 6. tDCS could, therefore, be applied in inpatient settings, with the aim of hastening clinical response and decreasing hospitalization costs. Of note, we also showed that tDCS is as effective as sertraline 50 mg/day, a dosage commonly used for those with mild depression. tDCS might be an effective alternative in such cases, especially because in mild MDD the discontinuation rates due to adverse effects of the medications are higher.

OPEN-LABEL STUDIES AND CASE REPORTS

Several open-label studies have also investigated tDCS effects in MDD. Some open-label studies found positive results using the "bifrontal montage" – i.e., anode over F3 and cathode over F4. Ferrucci, Bortolomasi, Vergari et al. (2009) stimulated 14 patients with severe MDD using 2 mA for 20 minutes for 5 days twice a day (total 10 sessions), showing 32.1% depression improvement in 5 weeks. In another study with 32 patients, Ferrucci, Bortolomasi, Brunoni et al. (2009) used the same tDCS protocol and observed a similar (27.7%) improvement. In this study, the effects seemed to be more robust in more severe patients. Dell'osso et al. (2012), also using the same tDCS protocol, observed 31.3% improvement 5 weeks after treatment onset in 23 patients with refractory depression. Martin et al. (2011) also found clinical benefits in 11 patients with depression after tDCS; in this study, the cathode was positioned over the right deltoid muscle (extracephalic position). Finally, in a recent study, Brunoni, Ferrucci et al. (2013) investigated whether tDCS clinical effects could be modulated by the chronic use of antidepressant drugs and benzodiazepines. This is a key question in clinical scenarios, where the use of several medications is common. The authors found that the overall effects of anodal tDCS over the left DLPFC were positive, although the use of benzodiazepines was associated with a worse outcome, and the use of antidepressants was associated with increased antidepressant effects.

Two case reports described tDCS effects in special situations. Bueno et al. (2011) reported dramatic improvement of a woman with post-stroke depression after tDCS, whereas Palm et al. (2009) described moderate depression improvement and significant cognitive improvement in a patient with treatment-resistant depression. These case reports are useful because they highlight tDCS antidepressant effects in different populations, thus generating hypotheses for novel studies.

ADVERSE EFFECTS

Liebetanz et al. (2009) showed, in an animal study of safety, that brain lesions only occurred when rats received cathodal tDCS stimulation almost 100-fold higher than used in clinical studies (Liebetanz et al., 2009). In a recent systematic review of clinical studies using tDCS, Brunoni, Amadera, Berbel et al. (2011) observed the lack of serious adverse effects associated with tDCS, with the exception of one case of skin burn (Palm et al., 2008). In the SELECT-TDCS, the only adverse effect significantly more associated with the active tDCS was skin redness on the stimulated scalp region (Brunoni, Valiengo et al., 2013). Importantly, tDCS, used in the context of MDD treatment, is also not associated with adverse cognitive effects (Brunoni, Valiengo et al., 2013; Loo et al., 2012).

Nonetheless, most studies only applied single sessions of tDCS in healthy volunteers, whereas clinical use of tDCS involves repeated, daily tDCS sessions. In this context, treatment-emergent (hypo)mania associated with tDCS might be an issue for patients with MDD. Three case reports (Arul-Anandam et al., 2010; Baccaro et al., 2010; Gálvez et al., 2011) described hypomanic episodes that were generally benign and directly associated with the tDCS course. Brunoni, Valiengo, Zanao et al. (2011), however, described a severe manic, psychotic episode after 6 treatment days with concomitant use of tDCS and sertraline that required pharmacological intervention. In the SELECT-TDCS trial we described seven cases of treatment-emergent (hypo)mania; one in the sertraline-only group, one in the active tDCS-only group, and five in the combined treatment group. Future studies should be aware of this risk, especially when combining tDCS with antidepressant drugs.

FOLLOW-UP STUDIES

Recently, Martin et al. (2013) reported data regarding the antidepressant effects of tDCS following acute treatment – i.e., during the maintenance treatment phase of the depressive episode. They followed 26 participants for 6 months, performing tDCS on a weekly basis for 3 months and thereafter once per fortnight for the last 6 months. They found probabilities of surviving without relapse of 83.7% at 3 months and 51.1% at 6 months, with medication resistance being a predictor of relapse during continuation tDCS.

During the follow-up phase of the SELECT-TDCS, 42 remitted patients were followed for 6 months, performing tDCS every other week during the first 3 months and once a month in the 3 subsequent months. With similar results to Martin et al. (2011), a survival rate of 47% at 6 months was found. Treatment-resistant depression at baseline was a predictor of relapse, as patients with treatment-resistant depression presented a much lower 24-week survival rate as compared to non-refractory patients (10% vs 77%, odds ratio = 5.52, $P < 0.01$) (Valiengo et al., 2013).

Bipolar Disorder and tDCS

Bipolar disorder (BD) is a recurrent, chronic, and severe disease. It has a significant impact on quality of life and also causes considerable distress to the relatives of the patients and society in general. The prevalence of BD in the United States varies from around 0.4% to 3.7%. The functional incapacity of the disease is comparable to that of most chronic diseases, such as cardiac conditions, since its comorbidity, both physical and psychiatric, is due to low adherence to the prescribed treatment.

Currently, there are no trials that have investigated tDCS as a treatment for the manic episode. For the depressive episode, Brunoni, Ferrucci, Bortolomasi et al. (2011) used anodal tDCS over the left DLPFC in 31 patients (14 with BD, 17 with MDD). Depressive symptoms in both study groups improved immediately after the fifth session. The beneficial effect persisted after 1 week and 1 month. Nonetheless, this trial did not use a sham group, which further limits its generalizability.

Schizophrenia

Schizophrenia is a common psychiatric disorder with an overall prevalence of 1–1.5% and a chronic course through life. The disease onset is in early adulthood, although preclinical symptoms might be present in childhood and adolescence (McGlashan & Johannessen, 1996). Its symptoms can be grouped into three relatively distinct phenomenological presentations: (1) positive symptoms; (2) impairment or "negative" symptoms; and (3) cognitive dysfunction. Positive symptoms are characterized by hallucinations and delusions; negative symptoms by impairments in sociability, expression of affect, and motivation; and cognitive dysfunction by deficits in executive functioning (attention and/or memory) (APA, 2000).

Diagnostic criteria according to the *DSM-IV* are based on the presence of at least two of five symptoms (hallucinations, delirium, disorganized speech, disorganized or catatonic behavior, and negative symptoms) (APA, 2000). Traditionally, positive symptoms occur within the first 10–15 years of the disease, while negative and cognitive symptoms exhibit a more chronic, persistent, and sometimes progressive presentation (Weickert et al., 2000).

Patients with schizophrenia have, in general, low functionality in performing daily life activities, lower quality of life, and greater incidence of comorbidities such as depressive symptoms, substance related disorders, suicidal behavior, and cardiovascular risk (Bensenor et al., 2012; Conley, 2009).

Pharmacological Treatment

Several antipsychotics, both "typical" (first generation, developed between 1950 and 1970) and "atypical" (second generation, developed since the 1990s), are available for the pharmacological treatment of schizophrenia. However, recent clinical studies using some of these drugs have failed to show efficacy of any particular medication, with clozapine being the sole exception (Leucht et al., 2013). However, although effective, clozapine has its use limited by potentially severe collateral effects such as neutropenia and agranulocytosis (Chong & Remington, 2000). The treatment of schizophrenia usually starts with either a typical or atypical antipsychotic, with expected clinical response within 4 to 6 weeks, although approximately 25% of patients with schizophrenia do not respond to conventional drug treatment (Leucht et al., 2013). In these cases, several strategies are available, with discrete levels of evidence, such as electroconvulsive therapy (ECT), repetitive transcranial magnetic stimulation (rTMS), and the combination of antipsychotics with other drugs such as lamotrigine.

Transcranial Direct Current Stimulation

MECHANISMS OF ACTION

From a neurobiological perspective, schizophrenia is a disorder of dopaminergic dysfunction in which there is phasic hyperactivity in the mesolimbic pathway (a pathway from the ventral tegmental area to the ventral striatum) which is associated with positive symptoms; and a sustained hypoactivity of the mesocortical pathway (from the ventral tegmental area to the DLPFC) which is associated with negative symptoms (Stahl, 2008). This framework explains the inherent difficulties of antipsychotic agents, in which successful dopaminergic receptor blocking in the mesolimbic pathway controls positive symptoms but may paradoxically worsen negative/cognitive symptoms due to excessive blocking in the mesocortical pathway (Moritz, Andreou, Klingberg, Thoering, & Peters, 2013).

In this regard, non-pharmacological therapies might be particularly useful as they can target one pathway separately. In fact, low-frequency, inhibitory rTMS over the temporo-parietal cortex, an area directly involved with auditory hallucinations, is an effective treatment for such hallucinations, as demonstrated by recent several meta-analyses (Demeulemeester et al., 2012; Freitas, Fregni, & Pascual-Leone, 2009; Prikryl, 2011). On the other hand, studies using high-frequency rTMS over the DLPFC did not show improvement of cognitive and negative symptoms (see, for instance, Barr, Farzan, Tran, Fitzgerald, & Daskalakis, 2012), possibly due to the severity of the disorder and/or the need to further optimize stimulation parameters.

The same rationale used for rTMS is valid when designing tDCS trials for the treatment of schizophrenia (see following section). The inhibitory electrode (cathode) is placed over the dominant language area (left tempoparietal cortex), aiming to reduce auditory hallucinations. The same rationale applies for using the cathode over the occipital area to control visual hallucinations (Shiozawa, da Silva, Cordeiro, Fregni, & Brunoni, 2013a). In turn, the excitability-increasing electrode (anode) is placed over the left DLPFC so as to improve symptoms related to cognitive impairment, apathy, and emotional blunting.

CLINICAL TRIALS

Although clinical studies evaluating tDCS efficacy for schizophrenia are currently limited to a few case reports and one randomized sham-controlled trial, the results are encouraging. Homan and colleagues described a patient with refractory auditory verbal hallucinations who underwent tDCS treatment, with the cathode positioned over the "Wernicke area" (left temporoparietal cortex) and the anode over the right supraorbital cortex (Homan et al., 2011). After 10 consecutive daily sessions of 1 mA/20 min of stimulation, the patient improved not only in positive symptoms, but also in negative and global symptoms. Moreover, this was accompanied by a regional decrease of cerebral blood flow, indexed by arterial spin labeling. In another report, Rakesh and colleagues used tDCS in monotherapy to treat a full-blown paranoid schizophrenia on an outpatient basis. The cathode was positioned over the left temporo-parietal junction (T3P3) and the anode over the left DLPFC (midpoint between F3 and Fp1); tDCS was applied twice daily at 2 mA/20 min for 5 consecutive days (Rakesh et al., 2013). The authors reported full cessation of verbal hallucinations. Shiozawa and colleagues explored the use of tDCS in severe forms of schizophrenia (Shiozawa, da Silva, Cordeiro, Fregni, & Brunoni, 2013b). In one case, tDCS (anode over the left and cathode over the right DLPFC, 2 mA/20 min, 10 consecutive sessions) was used to treat a severe catatonic, schizophrenic patient refractory to clozapine and ECT. Improvement was remarkable, with virtually full remission of catatonia 30–60 days after tDCS onset. In another study (Shiozawa et al., 2013a), the authors used cathodal stimulation consecutively over the occipital cortex and the temporo-parietal cortex (anode over the left DLPFC) to treat visual and auditory hallucinations, with a partial response that nevertheless enhanced global functioning. Finally, Andrade explored the long-term use of tDCS (cathode over T3P3, anode over F3), with once- to twice-daily tDCS sessions for nearly 3 years, with sustained improvement, in a clozapine-refractory patient with schizophrenia (Andrade, 2013). Interestingly, when the sessions were performed on alternate days the benefits were attenuated or lost.

To date, only one randomized clinical trial has investigated tDCS for the treatment of auditory hallucinations (AH) in schizophrenia. Thirty patients with persistent AH were randomized to receive either active or sham tDCS. The cathode was placed on the left temporo-parietal region and the anode on the left DLPFC. The rationale was to simultaneously perform an inhibitory stimulation over the area related to positive symptoms (AH), and an excitatory stimulation over the area correlated with negative symptoms. tDCS was applied twice daily for 5 days. The authors showed an improvement of AH (primary endpoint) after the end of stimulation, with sustained clinical response after 1 and 3 months of treatment (Brunelin et al., 2012).

Finally, Mattai and colleagues investigated the safety and tolerability of tDCS in childhood-onset schizophrenia in 12 adolescent (10- to 17-year-old) patients (Mattai et al., 2011). Two double-blinded, randomized, sham-controlled trials were carried out with different tDCS set-ups (bilateral anodal prefrontal stimulation for cognitive improvement, and bilateral cathodal temporo-parietal stimulation for hallucinatory control, both with an extracephalic reference). The treatment was well tolerated, with mild adverse effects such as tingling, itching, and fatigue sensations that, although frequent (30–50%), presented similar rates in both active and sham groups.

Obsessive-Compulsive Disorder

Obsessive-compulsive disorder (OCD) has a prevalence of approximately 2–3% in the general population (APA, 2000). This makes OCD the fourth most prevalent psychiatric disorder. Among adults the prevalence is equivalent in men and women, differing only in adolescents and children, where there are higher rates for males. The mean age is 20 years. This syndrome is characterized by the presence of obsessions and compulsions sufficiently severe to cause disruption in the patient's life, resulting in considerable suffering. Common treatments include the antidepressant clomipramine, followed by selective serotonin reuptake inhibitors (SSRIs) such as paroxetine, sertraline, fluoxetine, citalopram, and fluvoxamine. The protocol used for medical intervention consists of starting with SSRIs, followed by the use of three different SSRIs and, after that, by a trial with clomipramine. The addition of an atypical antipsychotic such as risperidone is an option, although cognitive–behavioral therapy (CBT), such as exposure and response prevention, should be the first approach to treatment, along with family counseling for children and adolescents. For adults, CBT can initially be combined with pharmaco-therapy (Bandelow et al., 2012).

Transcranial Direct Current Stimulation

There is only one case report investigating tDCS efficacy for OCD. Volpato et al. (2012) studied one patient with severe OCD, performing rTMS and tDCS (cathode over the left DLPFC and anode over the posterior neck-base). Interestingly, neither rTMS nor tDCS improved obsessive-compulsive symptoms, although tDCS (but not rTMS) was able to improve symptoms of depression and anxiety. In fact, the optimal param-eters for OCD treatment are unknown even for rTMS. In a recent meta-analysis of 10 randomized clinical trials using rTMS for OCD, Berlim, Neufeld, and Van den Eynde (2013) observed that larger, significant effect sizes were found for inhibitory (low-frequency) and non-DLPFC stimula-tions such as the orbito-frontal cortex and the supplementary motor area. This is in agreement with the findings that OCD is associated with impaired cortico-subcortical circuits, especially the fronto-striatal and orbito-frontal loops (Saxena & Rauch, 2000). Gonçalves et al. (2011) hypothesized that OCD patients present an interhemispheric functional imbalance, possibly due to inadequate thalamic filtering, and that tDCS and rTMS could be used to restore this interhemispheric imbalance by simultaneously activating and deactivating several cortical areas related to these impaired circuits.

Attention Deficit Hyperactivity Disorder (ADHD)

ADHD is a syndrome defined by a persistent pattern of lack of attention and/or hyperactive behavior and impulsiveness, which tends to be more severe than would be expected in children of the same age and at the same level of cognitive development (APA, 2000). ADHD is one of the most fre-quent diagnoses made in neuropsychiatric childhood disorders. A core symptom is motor hyperactivity. It accounts for approximately 3–8% of the diagnoses made in childhood. Over the past decade, the use of medication for treating ADHD has increased considerably.

Pharmacotherapy

The treatment of ADHD involves a multidimensional approach combining psychosocial and psychopharmacological interventions. When considering the psychosocial treatment, efforts should be directed towards providing family members with information regarding the clinical aspects of the disorder. A special training program for parents in order to learn how to manage their children's symptoms can be endorsed. The school environment also has to be organized to accommodate the needs of these children, and teachers should have special training so that external stimuli can be minimized. Physical activities are an important therapeutic tool in terms of enhancing concentration in other school activities. Also, psychomotor re-education for motor control can be necessary in some cases. In terms of psychosocial interventions, clinical psychotherapy can be introduced to cope with comorbidities such as depressive and anxiety symptoms, self-esteem issues, lack of control of hyperactivity, and impulse symptoms (de Mathis et al., 2013).

Psychostimulants are the first line of pharmacological treatment for ADHD. Effectiveness is similar for adolescents and children. Methylphenidate is used at between 20 mg/d and 60 mg/d (0.3 mg/kg per day to 1 mg/kg per day); it acts through increasing dopaminergic and noradrenergic synaptic efflux throughout the brain, and presents a rapid onset of action (Ramos-Quiroga, Montoya, Kutzelnigg, Deberdt, & Sobanski, 2013).

Transcranial Direct Current Stimulation

Although there have been no tDCS trials for ADHD to date, evidence from neuroimaging (Makris, Biederman, Monuteaux, & Seidman, 2009) and rTMS studies suggests that the DLPFC might be the preferred target for DC stimulation. One pilot single-session, sham-controlled trial found that high-frequency rTMS over the right DLPFC improved attention difficulties in ADHD patients (Bloch et al., 2010), although another study applying 10 consecutive sessions of high-frequency rTMS over the right DLPFC did not show significant differences in attention compared to sham rTMS (Weaver et al., 2012). It should be emphasized that not only the DLPFC but also other brain areas, such as the anterior cingulate cortex and the basal ganglia, are involved (Frodl & Skokauskas, 2012); nevertheless, for non-invasive brain stimulation purposes the DLPFC might be the most accessible gateway to modulate the cortico-subcortical pathways involved in ADHD.

There have also been experiments with healthy volunteers on the effects of tDCS on attention and inhibitory control. Beeli et al. (2008) showed that tDCS over the right DLPFC modulates skin conductance response and impulsiveness responses. Hsu et al. (2011) also demonstrated the effect of tDCS on response inhibition. They showed that tDCS over the pre-supplementary motor area modulates the inhibitory control in a polarity-specific manner. Similarly, Jacobson, Javitt, and Lavidor (2011) showed that anodal tDCS of the right inferior frontal gyrus improved the performance of healthy volunteers on a response inhibition task. The same group extended these findings, showing that tDCS over this area reduces the power of the theta band (Jacobson, Ezra, Berger, & Lavidor, 2012). Considering the well-known changes on theta band observed in ADHD patients, these findings open an avenue of new studies regarding the potential use of tDCS as a non-invasive therapeutic tool to treat attentional deficits and behavioral inhibitory control. Interestingly, the use of tDCS in impulse control disorders such as drug addiction has shown positive results (see Chapter 15).

CONCLUSIONS

As seen in this chapter, tDCS is gaining a reputation as an important non-invasive tool for treatment in neuropsychiatry, particularly depression. As it is cheap, easy to apply, and has no significant adverse effects, its use will probably increase in future years, as more research is being developed for other psychiatric disorders than schizophrenia and major depression – such as bipolar disorder, ADHD, and OCD. In fact, tDCS is a versatile, relatively focal therapy that can be applied in a wide range of neuropsychiatric disorders. One current limitation of tDCS is the need for patients to return to the clinical center/hospital to have tDCS delivered, although the development of domestic tDCS devices (currently under research) might aid in overcoming this issue. In addition, other forms of transcranial electric stimulation, such as random noise stimulation (tRNS) and alternating current stimulation (tACS), are also showing preliminary encouraging results in the treatment of depression (Chan et al., 2012) and the modulation of cognitive processes (Herrmann, Rach, Neuling, & Struber, 2013), respectively. As tDCS moves from bench to bedside and is being increasingly investigated in neuropsychiatric disorders, another interesting aspect is its growing potential either as a substitute for or augmentation to pharmacotherapy – in the former, as an alternative for patients that cannot use medication for several reasons (e.g., intolerable side effects, other medical conditions, etc.); in the latter, as a potentiation therapy to boost efficacy without increasing the rate of side effects. For these reasons, it is expected that the role of tDCS in the arsenal of neuropsychiatric treatments will increase in importance in the years to come.

References

Ambrus, G. G., Al-Moyed, H., Chaieb, L., Sarp, L., Antal, A., & Paulus, W. (2012). The fade-in - Short stimulation - Fade out approach to sham tDCS – Reliable at 1 mA for naive and experienced subjects, but not investigators. *Brain Stimulation*, *5*(4), 499–504.

Andrade, C. (2013). Once- to twice-daily, 3-year domiciliary maintenance transcranial direct current stimulation for severe, disabling, clozapine-refractory continuous auditory hallucinations in schizophrenia. *The Journal of ECT*, *74*(11), e1054–e1058.

APA (American Psychiatric Association). (2000). *Diagnostic and statistic manual of mental disorders*. (IV-TR ed.). Arlington, VA: American Psychiatric Association.

Arfai, E., Theano, G., Montagu, J. D., & Robin, A. A. (1970). A controlled study of polarization in depression. *The British Journal of Psychiatry*, *116*(533), 433–434.

Arnsten, A. F. (2009). Stress signalling pathways that impair prefrontal cortex structure and function. *Nature Reviews. Neuroscience*, *10*(6), 410–422.

Arul-Anandam, A. P., Loo, C., & Mitchell, P. (2010). Induction of hypomanic episode with transcranial direct current stimulation. *The Journal of ECT*, *26*(1), 68–69.

Baccaro, A., Brunoni, A. R., Bensenor, I. M., & Fregni, F. (2010). Hypomanic episode in unipolar depression during transcranial direct current stimulation. *Acta Neuropsychiatrica*, *22*(6), 316–318.

Bandelow, B., Sher, L., Bunevicius, R., Hollander, E., Kasper, S., Zohar, J., et al. (2012). Guidelines for the pharmacological treatment of anxiety disorders, obsessive-compulsive disorder and posttraumatic stress disorder in primary care. *International Journal of Psychiatry in Clinical Practice*, *16*(2), 77–84.

Barr, M. S., Farzan, F., Tran, L. C., Fitzgerald, P. B., & Daskalakis, Z. J. (2012). A randomized controlled trial of sequentially bilateral prefrontal cortex repetitive transcranial magnetic stimulation in the treatment of negative symptoms in schizophrenia. *Brain Stimulation*, *5*(3), 337–346.

Beeli, G., Casutt, G., Baumgartner, T., & Jancke, L. (2008). Modulating presence and impulsiveness by external stimulation of the brain. *Behavioral and Brain Functions*, *4*, 33.

Bensenor, I. M., Brunoni, A. R., Pilan, L. A., Goulart, A. C., Busatto, G. F., Lotufo, P. A., et al. (2012). Cardiovascular risk factors in patients with first-episode psychosis in Sao Paulo, Brazil. *General Hospital Psychiatry*, *34*(3), 268–275.

Berlim, M. T., Neufeld, N. H., & Van den Eynde, F. (2013). Repetitive transcranial magnetic stimulation (rTMS) for obsessive-compulsive disorder (OCD): An exploratory meta-analysis of randomized and sham-controlled trials. *Journal of Psychiatric Research*, *47*(8), 999–1006.

Berlim, M. T., Van den Eynde, F., & Daskalakis, Z. J. (2013). Clinical utility of transcranial direct current stimulation (tDCS) for treating major depression: A systematic review and meta-analysis of randomized, double-blind and sham-controlled trials. *Journal of Psychiatric Research*, *47*(1), 1–7.

Bloch, Y., Harel, E. V., Aviram, S., Govezensky, J., Ratzoni, G., & Levkovitz, Y. (2010). Positive effects of repetitive transcranial magnetic stimulation on attention in ADHD Subjects: A randomized controlled pilot study. *The World Journal of Biological Psychiatry*, *11*(5), 755–758.

Blumberger, D. M., Tran, L. C., Fitzgerald, P. B., Hoy, K. E., & Daskalakis, Z. J. (2012). A randomized double-blind sham-controlled study of transcranial direct current stimulation for treatment-resistant major depression. *Frontiers in Psychiatry/Frontiers Research Foundation*, *3*, 74.

Boggio, P. S., Bermpohl, F., Vergara, A. O., Muniz, A. L., Nahas, F. H., Leme, P. B., et al. (2007). Go/no-go task performance improvement after anodal transcranial DC stimulation of the left dorsolateral prefrontal cortex in major depression. *Journal of Affective Disorders*, *101*(1–3), 91–98.

Boggio, P. S., Rigonatti, S. P., Ribeiro, R. B., Myczkowski, M. L., Nitsche, M. A., Pascual-Leone, A., et al. (2008). A randomized, double-blind clinical trial on the efficacy of cortical direct current stimulation for the treatment of major depression. *The International Journal of Neuropsychopharmacology*, *11*(2), 249–254.

Bora, E., Fornito, A., Pantelis, C., & Yucel, M. (2012). Gray matter abnormalities in major depressive disorder: A meta-analysis of voxel based morphometry studies. *Journal of Affective Disorders*, *138*(1–2), 9–18.

Brunelin, J., Mondino, M., Gassab, L., Haesebaert, F., Gaha, L., Suaud-Chagny, M. F., et al. (2012). Examining transcranial direct-current stimulation (tDCS) as a treatment for hallucinations in schizophrenia. *The American Journal of Psychiatry*, *169*(7), 719–724.

Brunoni, A. R., Amadera, J., Berbel, B., Volz, M. S., Rizzerio, B. G., & Fregni, F. (2011). A systematic review on reporting and assessment of adverse effects associated with transcranial direct current stimulation. *The International Journal of Neuropsychopharmacology*, *14*(8), 1133–1145.

Brunoni, A. R., Ferrucci, R., Bortolomasi, M., Scelzo, E., Boggio, P. S., Fregni, F., et al. (2013). Interactions between transcranial direct current stimulation (tDCS) and pharmacological interventions in the major depressive episode: Findings from a naturalistic study. *European Psychiatry*, *28*(6), 356–361.

Brunoni, A. R., Ferrucci, R., Bortolomasi, M., Vergari, M., Tadini, L., Boggio, P. S., et al. (2011). Transcranial direct current stimulation (tDCS) in unipolar vs bipolar depressive disorder. *Progress in Neuro-Psychopharmacology & Biological Psychiatry*, *35*(1), 96–101.

Brunoni, A. R., Ferrucci, R., Fregni, F., Boggio, P. S., & Priori, A. (2012). Transcranial direct current stimulation for the treatment of major depressive disorder: A summary of preclinical, clinical and translational findings. *Progress in Neuro-Psychopharmacology & Biological Psychiatry*, *39*(1), 9–16.

Brunoni, A. R., Kemp, A. H., Shiozawa, P., Cordeiro, Q., Valiengo, L. C., Goulart, A. C., et al. (2013). Impact of 5-HTTLPR and BDNF polymorphisms on response to sertraline versus transcranial direct current stimulation: Implications for the serotonergic system. *European Neuropsychopharmacology*, *23*(11), 1530–1540.

Brunoni, A. R., Lopes, M., & Fregni, F. (2008). A systematic review and meta-analysis of clinical studies on major depression and BDNF levels: Implications for the role of neuroplasticity in depression. *The International Journal of Neuropsychopharmacology*, *11*(8), 1169–1180.

Brunoni, A. R., Nitsche, M. A., Bolognini, N., Bikson, M., Wagner, T., Merabet, L., et al. (2012). Clinical research with transcranial direct current stimulation (tDCS): Challenges and future directions. *Brain Stimulation*, *5*(3), 175–195.

Brunoni, A. R., Valiengo, L., Baccaro, A., Zanao, T. A., de Oliveira, J. F., Vieira, G. P., et al. (2011). Sertraline vs electrical current therapy for treating depression clinical trial – SELECT-TDCS: Design, rationale and objectives. *Contemporary Clinical Trials*, *32*(1), 90–98.

Brunoni, A. R., Valiengo, L., Baccaro, A., Zanao, T. A., Oliveira, A. C., Goulart, A. C., et al. (2013). The sertraline versus electrical current therapy for treating depression clinical study: Results from a factorial, randomized, controlled trial. *JAMA Psychiatry*, *70*(4), 383–391.

Brunoni, A. R., Valiengo, L., Zanao, T., de Oliveira, J. F., Bensenor, I. M., & Fregni, F. (2011). Manic psychosis after sertraline and transcranial direct-current stimulation. *Journal of Neuropsychiatry and Clinical Neurosciences*, *23*(3), E4–E5.

Brunoni, A. R., Vanderhasselt, M. A., Boggio, P. S., Fregni, F., Dantas, E. M., Mill, J. G., et al. (2013). Polarity- and valence-dependent effects of prefrontal transcranial direct current stimulation on heart rate variability and salivary cortisol. *Psychoneuroendocrinology*, *38* (1), 58–66.

Brunoni, A. R., Zanao, T. A., Vanderhasselt, M. A., Valiengo, L., de Oliveira, J. F., Boggio, P. S., et al. (2013). Enhancement of affective processing induced by bifrontal transcranial direct current stimulation in patients with major depression. *Neuromodulation: Journal of the International Neuromodulation Society*, (Epub ahead of print).

Bueno, V. F., Brunoni, A. R., Boggio, P. S., Bensenor, I. M., & Fregni, F. (2011). Mood and cognitive effects of transcranial direct current stimulation in post-stroke depression. *Neurocase*, 17(4), 318–322.

Carney, M. W., Cashman, M. D., & Sheffield, B. F. (1970). Polarization in depression. *The British Journal of Psychiatry*, 117(539), 474–475.

Chan, H. N., Alonzo, A., Martin, D. M., Player, M., Mitchell, P. B., Sachdev, P., et al. (2012). Treatment of major depressive disorder by transcranial random noise stimulation: Case report of a novel treatment. *Biological Psychiatry*, 72(4), e9–e10.

Chong, S. A., & Remington, G. (2000). Clozapine augmentation: Safety and efficacy. *Schizophrenia Bulletin*, 26(2), 421–440.

Cipriani, A., La Ferla, T., Furukawa, T. A., Signoretti, A., Nakagawa, A., Churchill, R., et al. (2010). Sertraline versus other antidepressive agents for depression. *Cochrane Database of Systematic Reviews*, 4, CD006117.

Clark, L., Chamberlain, S. R., & Sahakian, B. J. (2009). Neurocognitive mechanisms in depression: Implications for treatment. *Annual Review of Neuroscience*, 32, 57–74.

Conley, R. R. (2009). The burden of depressive symptoms in people with schizophrenia. *The Psychiatric Clinics of North America*, 32(4), 853–861.

Costain, R., Redfearn, J. W., & Lippold, O. C. (1964). A controlled trial of the therapeutic effect of polarization of the brain in depressive illness. *The British Journal of Psychiatry*, 110, 786–799.

de Mathis, M. A., Diniz, J. B., Hounie, A. G., Shavitt, R. G., Fossaluza, V., Ferrao, Y., et al. (2013). Trajectory in obsessive-compulsive disorder comorbidities. *European Neuropsychopharmacology*, 23(7), 594–601.

De Raedt, R., & Koster, E. H. (2010). Understanding vulnerability for depression from a cognitive neuroscience perspective: A reappraisal of attentional factors and a new conceptual framework. *Cognitive, Affective, & Behavioral Neuroscience*, 10(1), 50–70.

Dell'osso, B., Zanoni, S., Ferrucci, R., Vergari, M., Castellano, F., D'Urso, N., et al. (2012). Transcranial direct current stimulation for the outpatient treatment of poor-responder depressed patients. *European Psychiatry*, 27(7), 513–517.

Demeulemeester, M., Amad, A., Bubrovszky, M., Pins, D., Thomas, P., & Jardri, R. (2012). What is the real effect of 1-Hz repetitive transcranial magnetic stimulation on hallucinations? Controlling for publication bias in neuromodulation trials. *Biological Psychiatry*, 71(6), e15–e16.

Eaton, W. W., Anthony, J. C., Gallo, J., Cai, G., Tien, A., Romanoski, A., et al. (1997). Natural history of Diagnostic Interview Schedule/DSM-IV major depression. The Baltimore Epidemiologic Catchment area follow-up. *Archives of General Psychiatry*, 54(11), 993–999.

Ferrucci, R., Bortolomasi, M., Brunoni, A. R., Vergares, M., Tadini, L., Giacopuzzi, M., et al. (2009). Comparative benefits of transcranial direct current stimulation (tDCS) treatment in patients with mild/moderate vs severe depression. *Clinical Neuropsychiatry*, 6, 246–251.

Ferrucci, R., Bortolomasi, M., Vergari, M., Tadini, L., Salvoro, B., Giacopuzzi, M., et al. (2009). Transcranial direct current stimulation in severe, drug-resistant major depression. *Journal of Affective Disorders*, 118(1–3), 215–219.

Fregni, F., Boggio, P. S., Nitsche, M. A., Marcolin, M. A., Rigonatti, S. P., & Pascual-Leone, A. (2006). Treatment of major depression with transcranial direct current stimulation. *Bipolar Disorders*, 8(2), 203–204.

Fregni, F., Boggio, P. S., Nitsche, M. A., Rigonatti, S. P., & Pascual-Leone, A. (2006). Cognitive effects of repeated sessions of transcranial direct current stimulation in patients with depression. *Depression and Anxiety*, 23(8), 482–484.

Freitas, C., Fregni, F., & Pascual-Leone, A. (2009). Meta-analysis of the effects of repetitive transcranial magnetic stimulation (rTMS) on negative and positive symptoms in schizophrenia. *Schizophrenia Research, 108*(1–3), 11–24.

Fritsch, B., Reis, J., Martinowich, K., Schambra, H. M., Ji, Y., Cohen, L. G., et al. (2010). Direct current stimulation promotes BDNF-dependent synaptic plasticity: Potential implications for motor learning. *Neuron, 66*(2), 198–204.

Frodl, T., & Skokauskas, N. (2012). Meta-analysis of structural MRI studies in children and adults with attention deficit hyperactivity disorder indicates treatment effects. *Acta Psychiatrica Scandinavica, 125*(2), 114–126.

Gálvez, V., Alonzo, A., Martin, D., Mitchell, P. B., Sachdev, P., & Loo, C. K. (2011). Hypomania induction in a patient with bipolar II disorder by transcranial direct current stimulation (tDCS). *The Journal of ECT, 27*(3), 256–258.

Gandiga, P. C., Hummel, F. C., & Cohen, L. G. (2006). Transcranial DC stimulation (tDCS): A tool for double-blind sham-controlled clinical studies in brain stimulation. *Clinical Neurophysiology, 117*(4), 845–850.

Gonçalves, O. F., Carvalho, S., Leite, J., Pocinho, F., Relvas, J., & Fregni, F. (2011). Obsessive Compulsive Disorder as a functional interhemispheric imbalance at the thalamic level. *Medical Hypotheses, 77*(3), 445–447.

Grimm, S., Beck, J., Schuepbach, D., Hell, D., Boesiger, P., Bermpohl, F., et al. (2008). Imbalance between left and right dorsolateral prefrontal cortex in major depression is linked to negative emotional judgment: An fMRI study in severe major depressive disorder. *Biological Psychiatry, 63*(4), 369–376.

Herjanic, M., & Moss-Herjanic, B. (1967). Clinical report on a new therapeutic technique: Polarization. *Canadian Psychiatric Association Journal, 12*(4), 423–424.

Herrmann, C. S., Rach, S., Neuling, T., & Struber, D. (2013). Transcranial alternating current stimulation: A review of the underlying mechanisms and modulation of cognitive processes. *Frontiers in Human Neuroscience, 7*, 279.

Homan, P., Kindler, J., Federspiel, A., Flury, R., Hubl, D., Hauf, M., et al. (2011). Muting the voice: A case of arterial spin labeling-monitored transcranial direct current stimulation treatment of auditory verbal hallucinations. *The American Journal of Psychiatry, 168*(8), 853–854.

Hsu, T. Y., Tseng, L. Y., Yu, J. X., Kuo, W. J., Hung, D. L., Tzeng, O. J., et al. (2011). Modulating inhibitory control with direct current stimulation of the superior medial frontal cortex. *NeuroImage, 56*(4), 2249–2257.

Jacobson, L., Ezra, A., Berger, U., & Lavidor, M. (2012). Modulating oscillatory brain activity correlates of behavioral inhibition using transcranial direct current stimulation. *Clinical Neurophysiology, 123*(5), 979–984.

Jacobson, L., Javitt, D. C., & Lavidor, M. (2011). Activation of inhibition: Diminishing impulsive behavior by direct current stimulation over the inferior frontal gyrus. *Journal of Cognitive Neuroscience, 23*(11), 3380–3387.

Kalu, U. G., Sexton, C. E., Loo, C. K., & Ebmeier, K. P. (2012). Transcranial direct current stimulation in the treatment of major depression: A meta-analysis. *Psychological Medicine, 42*(9), 1791–1800.

Kemp, A. H., Quintana, D. S., Gray, M. A., Felmingham, K. L., Brown, K., & Gatt, J. (2010). Impact of depression and antidepressant treatment on heart rate variability: A review and meta-analysis. *Biological Psychiatry, 67*(11), 1067–1074.

Koenigs, M., & Grafman, J. (2009). The functional neuroanatomy of depression: Distinct roles for ventromedial and dorsolateral prefrontal cortex. *Behavioural Brain Research, 201*(2), 239–243.

Leucht, S., Cipriani, A., Spineli, L., Mavridis, D., Orey, D., Richter, F., et al. (2013). Comparative efficacy and tolerability of 15 antipsychotic drugs in schizophrenia: A multiple-treatments meta-analysis. *Lancet, 382*(9896), 951–962.

Liao, Y., Huang, X., Wu, Q., Yang, C., Kuang, W., Du, M., et al. (2013). Is depression a disconnection syndrome? Meta-analysis of diffusion tensor imaging studies in patients with MDD. *Journal of Psychiatry & Neuroscience, 38*(1), 49–56.

Liebetanz, D., Koch, R., Mayenfels, S., Konig, F., Paulus, W., & Nitsche, M. A. (2009). Safety limits of cathodal transcranial direct current stimulation in rats. *Clinical Neurophysiology, 120*(6), 1161–1167.

Lippold, O. C., & Redfearn, J. W. (1964). Mental changes resulting from the passage of small direct currents through the human brain. *British Journal of Psychiatry, 110*, 768–772.

Loo, C. K., Alonzo, A., Martin, D., Mitchell, P. B., Gálvez, V., & Sachdev, P. (2012). Transcranial direct current stimulation for depression: 3-week, randomised, sham-controlled trial. *The British Journal of Psychiatry, 200*(1), 52–59.

Loo, C. K., Sachdev, P., Martin, D., Pigot, M., Alonzo, A., Malhi, G. S., et al. (2010). A double-blind, sham-controlled trial of transcranial direct current stimulation for the treatment of depression. *The International Journal of Neuropsychopharmacology, 13*(1), 61–69.

Makris, N., Biederman, J., Monuteaux, M. C., & Seidman, L. J. (2009). Towards conceptualizing a neural systems-based anatomy of attention-deficit/hyperactivity disorder. *Developmental Neuroscience, 31*(1–2), 36–49.

Martin, D. M., Alonzo, A., Ho, K. A., Player, M., Mitchell, P. B., Sachdev, P., et al. (2013). Continuation transcranial direct current stimulation for the prevention of relapse in major depression. *Journal of Affective Disorders, 144*(3), 274–278.

Martin, D. M., Alonzo, A., Mitchell, P. B., Sachdev, P., Gálvez, V., & Loo, C. K. (2011). Fronto-extracephalic transcranial direct current stimulation as a treatment for major depression: An open-label pilot study. *Journal of Affective Disorders, 134*(1–3), 459–463.

Mattai, A., Miller, R., Weisinger, B., Greenstein, D., Bakalar, J., Tossell, J., et al. (2011). Tolerability of transcranial direct current stimulation in childhood-onset schizophrenia. *Brain Stimulation, 4*(4), 275–280.

Mayberg, H. S. (2003). Positron emission tomography imaging in depression: A neural systems perspective. *Neuroimaging Clinics of North America, 13*(4), 805–815.

McGlashan, T. H., & Johannessen, J. O. (1996). Early detection and intervention with schizophrenia: Rationale. *Schizophrenia Bulletin, 22*(2), 201–222.

Moritz, S., Andreou, C., Klingberg, S., Thoering, T., & Peters, M. J. (2013). Assessment of subjective cognitive and emotional effects of antipsychotic drugs. Effect by defect? *Neuropharmacology, 72C*, 179–186.

Murray, C. J., & Lopez, A. D. (1997). Alternative projections of mortality and disability by cause 1990–2020: Global Burden of Disease Study. *Lancet, 349*(9064), 1498–1504.

Nias, D. K., & Shapiro, M. B. (1974). The effects of small electrical currents upon depressive symptoms. *The British Journal of Psychiatry, 125*, 414–415.

Nitsche, M. A., Boggio, P. S., Fregni, F., & Pascual-Leone, A. (2009). Treatment of depression with transcranial direct current stimulation (tDCS): A review. *Experimental Neurology, 219*(1), 14–19.

O'Connell, N. E., Cossar, J., Marston, L., Wand, B. M., Bunce, D., Moseley, G. L., et al. (2012). Rethinking clinical trials of transcranial direct current stimulation: Participant and assessor blinding is inadequate at intensities of 2 mA. *PLoS One, 7*(10), e47514.

Palm, U., Fintescu, Z., Obermeier, M., Schiller, C., Reisinger, E., Keeser, D., et al. (2013). Serum levels of brain-derived neurotrophic factor are unchanged after transcranial direct current stimulation in treatment-resistant depression. *Journal of Affective Disorders, 150*(2), 659–663.

Palm, U., Keeser, D., Schiller, C., Fintescu, Z., Reisinger, E., Baghai, T. C., et al. (2009). Transcranial direct current stimulation in a patient with therapy-resistant major depression. *The World Journal of Biological Psychiatry, 10*(4 Pt 2), 632–635.

Palm, U., Keeser, D., Schiller, C., Fintescu, Z., Reisinger, E., Nitsche, M., et al. (2008). Skin lesions after treatment with transcranial direct current stimulation (tDCS). *Brain Stimulation, 1*(4), 386–387.

Palm, U., Reisinger, E., Keeser, D., Kuo, M. F., Pogarell, O., Leicht, G., et al. (2013). Evaluation of sham transcranial direct current stimulation for randomized, placebo-controlled clinical trials. *Brain Stimulation, 6*(4), 690–695.

Palm, U., Schiller, C., Fintescu, Z., Obermeier, M., Keeser, D., Reisinger, E., et al. (2012). Transcranial direct current stimulation in treatment resistant depression: A randomized double-blind, placebo-controlled study. *Brain Stimulation, 5*(3), 242–251.

Pena-Gomez, C., Sala-Lonch, R., Junque, C., Clemente, I. C., Vidal, D., Bargallo, N., et al. (2011). Modulation of large-scale brain networks by transcranial direct current stimulation evidenced by resting-state functional MRI. *Brain Stimulation, 5*(3), 252–263.

Peng, H., Zheng, H., Li, L., Liu, J., Zhang, Y., Shan, B., et al. (2012). High-frequency rTMS treatment increases white matter FA in the left middle frontal gyrus in young patients with treatment-resistant depression. *Journal of Affective Disorders, 136*(3), 249–257.

Pizzagalli, D. A. (2011). Frontocingulate dysfunction in depression: Toward biomarkers of treatment response. *Neuropsychopharmacology, 36*(1), 183–206.

Prikryl, R. (2011). Repetitive transcranial magnetic stimulation and treatment of negative symptoms of schizophrenia. *Neuroendocrinology Letters, 32*(2), 121–126.

Priori, A., Hallett, M., & Rothwell, J. C. (2009). Repetitive transcranial magnetic stimulation or transcranial direct current stimulation? *Brain Stimulation, 2*(4), 241–245.

Rakesh, G., Shivakumar, V., Subramaniam, A., Nawani, H., Amaresha, A. C., Narayanaswamy, J. C., et al. (2013). Monotherapy with tDCS for Schizophrenia: A case report. *Brain Stimulation, 6*(4), 708–709.

Ramos-Quiroga, J. A., Montoya, A., Kutzelnigg, A., Deberdt, W., & Sobanski, E. (2013). Attention deficit hyperactivity disorder in the European adult population: Prevalence, disease awareness, and treatment guidelines. *Current Medical Research and Opinion,* (in press).

Ramsay, J. C., & Schlagenhauf, G. (1966). Treatment of depression with low voltage direct current. *Southern Medical Journal, 59*(8), 932–934.

Rigonatti, S. P., Boggio, P. S., Myczkowski, M. L., Otta, E., Fiquer, J. T., Ribeiro, R. B., et al. (2008). Transcranial direct stimulation and fluoxetine for the treatment of depression. *European Psychiatry, 23*(1), 74–76.

Rush, A. J., Trivedi, M. H., Wisniewski, S. R., Nierenberg, A. A., Stewart, J. W., Warden, D., et al. (2006). Acute and longer-term outcomes in depressed outpatients requiring one or several treatment steps: A STAR*D report. *The American Journal of Psychiatry, 163*(11), 1905–1917.

Sampaio, L. A., Fraguas, R., Lotufo, P. A., Bensenor, I. M., & Brunoni, A. R. (2012). A systematic review of non-invasive brain stimulation therapies and cardiovascular risk: Implications for the treatment of major depressive disorder. *Frontiers in Psychiatry/Frontiers Research Foundation, 3*, 87.

Saxena, S., & Rauch, S. L. (2000). Functional neuroimaging and the neuroanatomy of obsessive-compulsive disorder. *The Psychiatric Clinics of North America, 23*(3), 563–586.

Schutter, D. J. (2009). Antidepressant efficacy of high-frequency transcranial magnetic stimulation over the left dorsolateral prefrontal cortex in double-blind sham-controlled designs: A meta-analysis. *Psychological Medicine, 39*(1), 65–75.

Sehm, B., Schaefer, A., Kipping, J., Margulies, D., Conde, V., Taubert, M., et al. (2012). Dynamic modulation of intrinsic functional connectivity by transcranial direct current stimulation. *Journal of Neurophysiology, 108*(12), 3253–3263.

Sen, S., Duman, R., & Sanacora, G. (2008). Serum brain-derived neurotrophic factor, depression, and antidepressant medications: Meta-analyses and implications. *Biological Psychiatry, 64*(6), 527–532.

Shiozawa, P., da Silva, M. E., Cordeiro, Q., Fregni, F., & Brunoni, A. R. (2013a). Transcranial direct current stimulation (tDCS) for catatonic schizophrenia: A case study. *Schizophrenia Research, 146*(1–3), 374–375.

Shiozawa, P., da Silva, M. E., Cordeiro, Q., Fregni, F., & Brunoni, A. R. (2013b). Transcranial direct current stimulation (tDCS) for the treatment of persistent visual and auditory hallucinations in schizophrenia: A case study. *Brain Stimulation, 6*(5), 831–833.

Smith, R., Chen, K., Baxter, L., Fort, C., & Lane, R. D. (2013). Antidepressant effects of sertraline associated with volume increases in dorsolateral prefrontal cortex. *Journal of Affective Disorders, 146*(3), 414–419.

Stagg, C. J., & Nitsche, M. A. (2011). Physiological basis of transcranial direct current stimulation. *The Neuroscientist, 17*(1), 37–53.

Stahl, S. S. (2008). *Stahl's essential psychopharmacology: Neuroscientific basis and practical aplications.* Cambridge, UK: Cambridge Medicine.

Valiengo, L., Bensenor, I. M., Goulart, A. C., de Oliveira, J. F., Zanao, T. A., Boggio, P. S., et al. (2013). The sertraline versus electrical current therapy for treating depression clinical study (SELECT-tDCS): Results of the crossover and follow-up phases. *Depression and Anxiety, 30*(7), 646–653.

Vanderhasselt, M. A., De Raedt, R., Leyman, L., & Baeken, C. (2009). Acute effects of repetitive transcranial magnetic stimulation on attentional control are related to antidepressant outcomes. *Journal of Psychiatry & Neuroscience, 34*(2), 119–126.

Volpato, C., Piccione, F., Cavinato, M., Duzzi, D., Schiff, S., Foscolo, L., et al. (2012). Modulation of affective symptoms and resting state activity by brain stimulation in a treatment-resistant case of obsessive-compulsive disorder. *Neurocase, 19*(4), 360–370.

Wang, L., Hermens, D. F., Hickie, I. B., & Lagopoulos, J. (2012). A systematic review of resting-state functional-MRI studies in major depression. *Journal of Affective Disorders, 142*(1–3), 6–12.

Warden, D., Trivedi, M. H., Wisniewski, S. R., Davis, L., Nierenberg, A. A., Gaynes, B. N., et al. (2007). Predictors of attrition during initial (citalopram) treatment for depression: A STAR*D report. *The American Journal of Psychiatry, 164*(8), 1189–1197.

Weaver, L., Rostain, A. L., Mace, W., Akhtar, U., Moss, E., & O'Reardon, J. P. (2012). Transcranial magnetic stimulation (TMS) in the treatment of attention-deficit/hyperactivity disorder in adolescents and young adults: A pilot study. *The Journal of ECT, 28*(2), 98–103.

Weickert, T. W., Goldberg, T. E., Gold, J. M., Bigelow, L. B., Egan, M. F., & Weinberger, D. R. (2000). Cognitive impairments in patients with schizophrenia displaying preserved and compromised intellect. *Archives of General Psychiatry, 57*(9), 907–913.

Whitfield-Gabrieli, S., & Ford, J. M. (2012). Default mode network activity and connectivity in psychopathology. *Annual Review of Clinical Psychology, 8*, 49–76.

Williams, J. M., Mathews, A., & MacLeod, C. (1996). The emotional Stroop task and psychopathology. *Psychological Bulletin, 120*(1), 3–24.

Wittchen, H. U., Knauper, B., & Kessler, R. C. (1994). Lifetime risk of depression. *The British Journal of Psychiatry. Supplement,* (26), 16–22.

CHAPTER

15

The Use of Non-Invasive Brain Stimulation in Drug Addictions

Antoine Hone-Blanchet[1] and Shirley Fecteau[1,2]

[1]Centre Interdisciplinaire de Recherche en Réadaptation et Intégration Sociale, Centre de Recherche de l'Institut Universitaire en Santé Mentale de Québec, Medical School, Laval University, Québec, Canada
[2]Berenson-Allen Center for Noninvasive Brain Stimulation, Beth Israel Deaconess Medical Center, Harvard Medical School, Harvard University, Boston, MA

OUTLINE

INTRODUCTION

Drug addictions are having a growing impact on healthcare worldwide. They are chronically relapsing disorders, and current treatments, such as pharmacological and behavioral therapies, are not fully efficient on a long-term basis and rarely prevent relapses. Addiction has been extensively studied in animal and human models in recent decades, and growing evidence suggests that it consists of a neuroadaptative pathology. It is the result of the pharmacological usurpation of neural mechanisms of reward, motivated learning, and memory (Hyman, 2007; Kalivas & O'Brien, 2007; Koob & Volkow, 2009).

Non-invasive brain stimulation (NIBS) has been of increasing interest in the past few years as a novel means for modulating the brain's plastic potential. More than a simple tool to assess cortical excitability, its lasting physiological effects on cortical and subcortical structures have proven to efficiently modulate drug-seeking behavioral patterns and tone down cravings in addicted individuals. Although the method is still experimental, many convincing results mean that it is emerging as a potential clinical tool in the treatment of various addiction diseases (Feil & Zangen, 2010).

Hence, in this chapter we present the current understanding of addiction, and how NIBS has become an object of interest in this field. The first section describes the different phases of drug addiction. In subsequent sections, we present available results focusing on the neuroplasticity-inducing potential of NIBS in the context of addiction to diverse psychoactive substances. More specifically, we review findings on nicotine, alcohol, and cocaine, as well as food.

THE ADDICTION CYCLE AND NEUROCIRCUITRY

Chronic use and abuse of legal or illegal psychoactive drugs leads to substance dependence and drug addiction. Drug addiction is a chronically relapsing disorder characterized by the compulsive seeking and use of a substance despite its negative or adverse effects. It also implies a loss of direct control regarding substance intake, and results in negative affects when access to the substance is restrained (Koob, 2011).

The development and maintenance of addictive behavior have been described extensively in the past decade, and a general consensus has arisen regarding the three main different components of the addiction cycle (Koob & Volkow, 2009). The first phase is *intoxication*, in which an individual repeatedly abuses a psychoactive substance. This recurrent bingeing phase is followed by one of *withdrawal* from the substance, during which the individual experiences various symptoms of the withdrawal syndrome, including the emergence of a negative emotional state. The final phase of this spiraling cycle is one of *preoccupation* and craving, in which memories and sensory inputs act as conditioned cues leading to intoxication, and reinforce the addictive behavior (Koob & Volkow, 2009).

Neural changes related to these phases have also been studied. The meso-corticolimbic dopamine system comprises pathways from dopamine neurons in the ventral tegmental area (VTA) to the dopaminoceptive targets in the (ventral striatum) nucleus accumbens (NA), and mesolimbic and pre-frontal cortex (mesocortical) areas (for review, see Russo, Mazei-Robison, Ables, & Nestler 2009; Russo et al., 2010). Its activation, naturally or by phar-macological means, associates incentive salience to external stimuli, and ini-tiates goal-directed actions and motivational behavior (Koob, 2011). This system is therefore majorly responsible for the rewarding effects obtained during the intoxication/bingeing phase. Although the NA and VTA are immensely important in drug reward, results also point towards the involvement of the central nucleus of the amygdala (CeA) in the reinforcing actions of nicotine and alcohol, the ventral pallidum (VP) in the motivation of drug-seeking, and the dorsal striatum in the development of compulsive drug-seeking (Franken, Booij, & Vandenbrink, 2005; Koob & Volkow, 2009).

In the second phase of the addiction cycle, the lack of stimulation of the aforementioned pathways engages the individual in various withdrawal symptoms. The shift from acute drug reward to acute drug abstinence recruits, on a neurobiological level, the extended amygdala (including the CeA and the shell part of NA), a complex cluster of nuclei involved in mediating limbic and efferent motor influx, fear conditioning, and pain processing (Koob, 2011). The decrease in activity of reward-related struc-tures (VTA-NA) is thought to increase the brain reward threshold, which leads to biochemical changes defining the physiological symptoms of with-drawal and the vulnerability to relapse (Koob, 2011). Such biochemical changes are thought to impact on brain stress systems. Indeed, a common withdrawal feature of all types of drugs of abuse is the elevation in concen-tration of corticotropin-releasing factor (CRF) in the CeA. Corticotropin and corticosterone levels are also increased during acute withdrawal. Deregulation of the brain stress systems may also bear further negative consequences in the development of addiction, as they could possibly enhance the effect of stressors on the vulnerability to relapse. It is also a key player in the increase of anxiety during the abstinence period (Koob & Kreek, 2007). Development of addiction is fueled by negative reinforce-ment mechanisms, which are represented by the negative emotional state that results in withdrawing from the acute rewarding effect of drug intake. The additional activation of brain stress systems during withdrawal would then provide a supplemental force in the development of craving.

The last phase of the addiction cycle characterizes addiction as a persis-tent relapsing disorder, and its hallmark is the emergence of craving. Craving is defined as the desire for the previously experienced effects of a psychoactive drug; this desire is technically motivated by internal and external cues (Hyman, 2007). The reinstatement of drug-seeking behavior after a more or less prolonged period of abstinence is thought, in animal models, to be induced by stress or the presence of an envi-ronmental stimulus previously associated with the substance of abuse

(Koob, 2011). Drug-induced reinstatement is thought to be dependent on the activation of a glutamatergic pathway, from the medial prefrontal cortex (PFC) to the NA. The involvement of the basolateral amygdala and PFC in the attribution of cues and their emotional value is also likely to be decisive. Stress-induced reinstatement of drug-seeking behavior depends largely on the sustained action of CRF in the extended amygdala, as described previously. This final phase of the addiction cycle elicits the importance of the prefrontal systems in decision-making processes and cognitive control (Goldstein & Volkow, 2002). Ultimately, the orbitofrontal cortex (OFC), dorsolateral prefrontal cortex (DLPFC), and anterior cingulate cortex (ACC) take into account all cues coming from the basal ganglia, amygdala, and hippocampus to determine whether or not the individual will resist the craving. Cognitive impairments and deficits are frequent among drug-users and, unsurprisingly, are correlated with higher rates of relapse (Goldstein & Volkow, 2011). Although all drugs have their own pharmacological, neurotoxic, and cognitive effects, addiction as a global process is characterized by dysfunctional inhibitory control and decision-making capacities (see Fig. 15.1). In sum, addiction is a

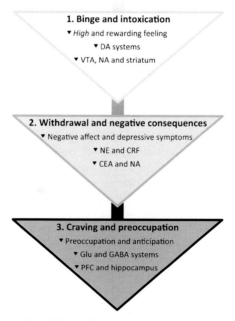

FIGURE 15.1   **Illustration of the Addiction Cycle and its Different Stages.** All stages are described from top to bottom with their main characteristics (behavioral correlate, main neurotransmitters associated, cerebral structures involved). DA, dopamine; VTA,: ventral tegmental area; NA, nucleus accumbens; NE, norepinephrine; CRF, corticotropin-releasing factor; CEA, central nucleus of the amygdala; Glu, glutamate; GABA, gamma-aminobutyric acid; PFC, prefrontal cortex.

complex medical condition, a pathology of neuroplasticity (Kauer & Malenka, 2007), which comprises the usurpation of normal reward systems, the rise of neurocognitive reinforcements and cues, the loss of control over compulsive behavior, and impulsive decision-making.

NON-INVASIVE BRAIN STIMULATION IN DRUG ADDICTIONS

Studies using NIBS to modulate addictive behaviors have mainly targeted the DLPFC, a major cortical player in drug addictions. This structure, encompassing Brodmann areas 9 and 46, part of the prefrontal cortex complex along with the ACC and the OFC, is associated with decision making, working memory, attention, and control of interference (Goldstein, Moeller, & Volkow, 2011). The role of the DLPFC has been extensively studied in decision-making tasks within neuroimaging and brain stimulation paradigms. Although its functions are not completely defined, it is essential in the valuation and computation of reward and the subsequent decision-making processes (Camus et al., 2009; Philiastides, Auksztulewicz, Heekeren, & Blankenburg, 2011). Moreover, a meta-analysis of neuroimaging studies in decision making has highlighted the importance of the DLPFC and OFC in taking decisions in tasks involving ambiguity and risk (Krain, Wilson, Arbuckle, Castellanos, & Milham, 2006). Inappropriate risk-taking and dysfunctional inhibitory control are believed to be critical in the occurrence of relapses and maintenance of addictive disorder (Bechara, 2005). Decision making in healthy individuals can be disrupted with NIBS, which resembles the risk-taking behavior characteristic of drug-addicted patients (Knoch et al., 2006). This risk-taking behavior can also be toned down in healthy or addicted participants in decision-making tasks involving taking risks (Fecteau et al., 2007, Fecteau, Fregni, Boggio, Camprodon, & Pascual-Leone, 2010). Several other neuroimaging results have also demonstrated that hypoactivation of the DLPFC and ACC in cognitive tasks is characteristic of addicted patients (Goldstein & Volkow, 2011; Goldstein et al., 2011). Hence, non-invasively targeting the DLPFC may potentially tone down maladaptive decision-making and promote healthy behaviors in addicts on a long-term basis (Fecteau et al., 2010). These hypotheses regarding the role of the DLPFC and prefrontal areas in addiction explain their ubiquity in the studies using NIBS reviewed in the following sections.

The mechanisms of action of NIBS in toning down addiction-prone behaviors are still vague and in need of characterization. Current explanations for the therapeutic effects of tDCS and rTMS are focused on their ability to modify cortical excitability over a long period (for reviews, see Fregni & Pascual-Leone, 2007; Wagner, Valero-Cabre, & Pascual-Leone, 2007).

These effects are largely based on early works on the use of rTMS in refractory major depression (George et al., 1997; Pascual-Leone, Rubio, Pallardò, & Català, 1996). In addictive disorders, beneficial effects have been found when targeting the right or the left DLPFC with rTMS, or both DLPFCs with tDCS. This is in line with imaging data, which also remain unclear regarding the hemispheric specificity in cravings. Cravings have been associated with prefrontal metabolic variations in both hemispheres (Brody et al., 2002; Volkow et al., 2010). Moreover, stimulating the DLPFC with rTMS on one side may result in modulating the contralateral DLPFC, due to a network effect, but evidence is still scarce (Nahas et al., 2001). Studies using tDCS in addictions have placed the two electrodes on both DLPFCs (anodal over the right DLPFC coupled with cathodal over the left DLPFC, or the opposite electrode montage), thus very likely modulating activity in both hemispheres without knowing whether the effect is of greater importance for one hemisphere or not (Stagg & Nitsche, 2011). Future work is warranted to elucidate the potential hemispheric specificity in addictions, and determine the optimal stimulation localizations. These will also be of significant interest in correlations with clinical effects of NIBS in neuropsychiatry.

Changes in neurotransmission are also ascribable to NIBS, as rTMS has been proven to enhance dopamine transmission in the mesolimbic pathway (Keck et al., 2002), striatum (Pogarell et al., 2007; Strafella, Paus, Barrett, & Dagher, 2001), and ACC and OFC (Ko & Strafella, 2011). tDCS can also affect dopamine transmission in a similar way, and induce prolonged alterations in cortical excitability (Nitsche, 2003; Nitsche et al., 2006, see also Chapters 5 and 6). NIBS has been used in the past to measure cortical excitability within addicted populations. However, with the emergence of several lines of study demonstrating the long-term neuromodulatory potential of repetitive NIBS in psychiatric and neurologic conditions, it has also been studied in the context of drug addictions. The following sections will review the current state of knowledge on addressing addictions with NIBS. We will review data on nicotine, alcohol, cocaine, and food cravings, as these substances comprise the most results in the literature, with respect to the research conducted on other substances. Table 15.1 provides a summary of the findings.

Nicotine

Cigarette smoking is a widely encountered habit, causing many diseases and premature deaths worldwide. Even though nicotine cannot be held directly accountable for the various smoking-induced illnesses, it is the primary addictive agent driving chronic cigarette smoking (Schwartz & Benowitz, 2010). Various pharmacotherapeutical options

TABLE 15.1 Description of Studies Reporting NIBS-Induced Modulation of Drug Consumption and Craving

Author, Year	Subjects (n)	Design	NIBS	NIBS Parameters	Targeted Regions	Main Results
NICOTINE						
Johann et al., 2003	Addicted to nicotine smoking (11)	Sham-controlled Crossover	rTMS	1 session 20 Hz 90% RMT 1000 pulses	L DLPFC	Decreased cigarette craving when comparing active to sham rTMS.
Eichhammer et al., 2003	Addicted to nicotine smoking (14)	Sham-controlled Crossover	rTMS	2 sessions 20 Hz 90% RMT 1000 pulses	L DLPFC	Reduced cigarette consumption when comparing active to sham rTMS. No change in cigarette craving when comparing active to sham rTMS.
Amiaz, Levy, Vainiger, Grunhaus, & Zangen, 2009	Treatment seeking, addicted to nicotine smoking (48)	Sham-controlled Parallel	rTMS	10 sessions 10 Hz 100% RMT 1000 pulses	L DLPFC	Decreased cigarette consumption and cue-induced cigarette craving when comparing active to sham rTMS. The reduction in cigarette consumption was not significant 6 months after the end of the rTMS sessions.
Rose et al., 2011	Addicted to nicotine smoking (15)	Sham-controlled Crossover	rTMS	1 Hz 90% RMT 450 pulses 10 Hz 90% RMT 4500 pulses	SFG	Following the presentation of smoking cues, increased cigarette craving when comparing 10-Hz rTMS over the SFG to 1-Hz rTMS over the SFG and to 1-Hz rTMS over M1. Following the presentation of neutral cues, decreased cigarette craving when comparing 10-Hz rTMS over the SFG, to 1-Hz rTMS over the SFG and to 1-Hz rTMS over M1.

Continued

TABLE 15.1 Description of Studies Reporting NIBS-Induced Modulation of Drug Consumption and Craving—cont'd

Author, Year	Subjects (n)	Design	NIBS	NIBS Parameters	Targeted Regions	Main Results
Fregni, Liguori, Fecteau, & Nitsche, 2008	Addicted to nicotine smoking (24)	Sham-controlled Crossover	tDCS	3 sessions 2 mA 20 min	Anodal LDLPFC coupled with cathodal R DLPFC; Anodal R DLPFC coupled with cathodal L DLPFC	Decreased cigarette craving when comparing active tDCS (both configurations: anodal tDCS over the R DLPFC with cathodal over the LDLPFC and anodal tDCS over the L DLPFC with cathodal over the R DLPFC) to sham tDCS.
Boggio, Liguori, Sultani, & Rezende, 2009	Addicted to nicotine smoking (27)	Sham-controlled Parallel	tDCS	5 sessions 2 mA 10 min	Anodal L DLPFC coupled with cathodal R DLPFC	Decreased consumption of cigarettes in a dose-dependant effect when comparing active to sham tDCS. Decreased cravings for cigarettes when comparing active to sham tDCS.
ALCOHOL						
Mishra, Nizamie, Das, & Praharaj, 2011	Addicted to alcohol (45)	Sham-controlled Parallel	rTMS	10 sessions 10 Hz 110% RMT 1000 pulses	R DLPFC	Reduced alcohol cravings when comparing active to sham rTMS immediately after the stimulation period and after 1 month.
Höppner et al., 2011	Addicted to alcohol (19)	Sham-controlled Parallel	rTMS	10 sessions 20 Hz 90% RMT 1000 pulses	L DLPFC	No difference between active and sham stimulation in alcohol cravings and no effects on mood enhancement.
De Ridder, Vanneste, Kovacs, Sunaert, & Dom, 2011	Detoxified, addicted to alcohol (1)	Case report	rTMS	15 sessions 1 Hz 600 pulses	dACC	Reduced alcohol cravings and consumption during the stimulation protocol. Reduction of withdrawal symptoms and sustained reduction of craving lasted for 3 months after termination of the stimulation protocol.

Study	Population (n)	Design	Technique	Parameters	Target	Findings
Herremans et al., 2012	Detoxified, addicted to alcohol (36)	Sham-controlled Parallel	rTMS	1 session 20 Hz 110% RMT 1560 pulses	R DLPFC	No difference between active and sham rTMS in alcohol craving.
Boggio, Sultani, Fecteau, & Merabet, 2008	Detoxified, addicted to alcohol (13)	Sham-controlled Crossover	tDCS	1 session 10 mA 20 min	Anodal L DLPFC coupled with cathodal R DLPFC; Anodal R DLPFC coupled with cathodal L DLPFC	Reduced cue-induced alcohol craving when comparing active (both configurations: anodal tDCS over the R DLPFC with cathodal over the L DLPFC and anodal tDCS over the L DLPFC with cathodal over the R DLPFC) to sham tDCS.

COCAINE

Study	Population (n)	Design	Technique	Parameters	Target	Findings
Camprodon, Martinez-Raga, Alonso-Alonso, Shih, & Pascual-Leone, 2007	Hospitalized, detoxified, addicted to cocaine (6)	Crossover	rTMS	1 session 10 Hz 90% RMT 2000 pulses	L DLPFC R DLPFC	Reduced cocaine craving when comparing ratings before and after rTMS to the R DLPFC. No effect on cocaine cravings when comparing ratings before and after rTMS to the L DLPFC.
Politi, Fauci, Santoro, & Smeraldi, 2008	Detoxified, addicted to cocaine (36)		rTMS	10 sessions 15 Hz 100% RMT 600 pulses	L DLPFC	Reduced cocaine craving gradually along the course of stimulation protocol.

FOOD

Study	Population (n)	Design	Technique	Parameters	Target	Findings
Uher, Yoganathan, Mogg, & Eranti, 2005	Healthy women with high levels of self-reported food cravings (28)	Sham-controlled Parallel	rTMS	1 session 15 Hz 110% RMT 1000 pulses	L DLPFC	Reduced cue-induced food craving when comparing active to sham rTMS. No effect on consumption of snack foods between active and sham rTMS.

Continued

III. IMPROVING FUNCTIONS IN THE ATYPICAL BRAIN

TABLE 15.1 Description of Studies Reporting NIBS-Induced Modulation of Drug Consumption and Craving—cont'd

Author, Year	Subjects (n)	Design	NIBS	NIBS Parameters	Targeted Regions	Main Results
Van den Eynde et al., 2010	Bulimic patients (38)	Sham-controlled Parallel	rTMS	1 session 15 Hz 110% RMT 1000 pulses	L DLPFC	Reduced food craving and binge eating 24 h after the stimulation period when comparing active to sham rTMS.
Fregni, Orsati et al., 2008	Healthy subjects reporting frequent food cravings (23)	Sham-controlled Crossover	tDCS	1 session 2 mA 20 min	Anodal L DLPFC coupled with cathodal R DLPFC; Anodal R DLPFC coupled with cathodal L DLPFC	Reduced cue-induced food craving when comparing active anodal tDCS over the RDLPFC with cathodal tDCS over the LDLPFC to sham tDCS. Lower caloric ingestion when comparing active (both configurations) to sham tDCS.
Goldman et al., 2011	Healthy subjects reporting frequent food cravings (19)	Sham-controlled Crossover	tDCS	1 session 2 mA 20 min	Anodal R-DLPFC	Reduced cravings in both sham and active tDCS conditions. Decreased ratings for specific food items when comparing active to sham tDCS.

N, sample size; NIBS, non-invasive brain stimulation; tDCS, transcranial direct current stimulation; rTMS, repetitive transcranial magnetic stimulation; RMT, resting motor threshold; L, left; R, right; DLPFC, dorsolateral prefrontal cortex; SFG, superior frontal gyrus; M1, primary motor cortex; dACC, dorsal anterior cingulate cortex.

are currently available to smokers, such as nicotine replacement therapies (patches, gums, inhalers, etc.), bupropion, and varenicline. However, absolute smoking cessation rates appear to not exceed 35% despite pharmacological treatment (Benowitz, 2009).

Following the inhalation of smoke, nicotine is quickly carried from the lungs to the brain, where it selectively binds to nicotinic cholinergic receptors (nAChRs). Stimulation of the receptors leads to the liberation of various neurotransmitters, including dopamine in the mesocortico-limbic pathways. Acute and chronic effects of nicotine intake result in the activation of the prefrontal cortex, visual areas, and thalamus, and an increase in dopamine concentration in the VTA, NA, and striatum. The release of dopamine in the aforementioned areas is responsible for nicotine's pleasurable, stimulating, and arousing effects. Nicotine intake also stimulates the liberation of GABA and glutamate, neurotransmitters that have inhibiting and facilitating effects, respectively, on dopamine transmission. Chronic use of nicotine tones down the inhibitory action of GABA release but maintains the release of glutamate, which facilitates the release of dopamine, enhancing the reinforcing effects of nicotine and stimulating neuromodulatory changes. Several lines of evidence also point to the reduction of the activity of monoamine oxidase A and B (MAO-A and MAO-B), both enzymes responsible for catalysis of catecholamines such as dopamine, in the development of nicotine addiction (Schwartz & Benowitz, 2010). It is worth noting that nicotine also stimulates the release of acetylcholine, serotonin, norepinephrine, and endorphins, triggering a whole-brain response. Moreover, chronic nicotine intake can induce alterations in neuronal activity and excitability (for review, see Markou, 2008). Single-pulse and paired-pulse paradigms used in the study by Lang, Hasan, Sueske, Paulus, and Nitsche (2007) have suggested that chronic nicotine intake may increase cortical inhibition. TMS measurements of cortical excitability in 22 heavy smokers and 22 controls have highlighted the different cortical responses in smokers, with smaller amplitude of motor evoked potentials and increased afferent inhibition (Lang et al., 2007).

A few studies have investigated the effects of tDCS and rTMS on the modulation of consumption and craving for cigarettes. Several studies are still required to determine the precise mechanisms of action of rTMS in the context of nicotine addiction. Nevertheless, its action on dopamine and GABA levels within cortical and subcortical structures provides an interesting insight into its plausibility and possible efficacy in diminishing addictive behavior regarding nicotine. Studies in healthy subjects have unveiled the potential of rTMS in increasing the release of dopamine in the mesocortico-limbic system (Strafella et al., 2003; Strafella et al., 2001) and cortex (Cho & Strafella, 2009), subsequently modulating cortical GABA transmission. Keck and colleagues have also demonstrated rTMS modulates levels of dopamine in the hippocampus and NA in rats (Keck et al., 2002). In nicotine smokers, most studies have investigated the effect of rTMS (intensity 1–20 Hz at 90–100% of resting motor threshold [RMT]) over the left DLPFC. Initial studies from Johann et al. (2003) and Eichhammer et al. (2003) were conducted in a similar fashion to evaluate the impact of rTMS (left DLPFC) on cigarette craving. Johann and colleagues found that nicotine-addicted individuals rated their own cravings for cigarettes as lower on a visual analog scale (VAS) after an active high-frequency TMS session (one active, one sham session; 20 Hz; 90% RMT), compared to a sham group (Johann et al., 2003). Similarly, Eichhammer and colleagues evaluated cravings with a similar scale, although the study was conducted as a double-blind cross-over trial (two active, two sham sessions; 20 Hz; 90% RMT). The results were more modest, as they found no difference in craving levels between the sham and active conditions. However, they also measured the number of smoked cigarettes before and after each session, and found that active TMS reduced cigarette consumption (Eichhammer et al., 2003). The authors concluded that the sample size was inadequate and the subjective evaluations of craving may not have been sensitive enough. However, those two pioneering studies provided an interesting insight regarding the possibility of interfering with craving and smoking habits by using rTMS. Amiaz et al. (2009) went further by assessing the impact of visual cues in the initiation of craving, and measuring biometrically the levels of consumed nicotine with urinary cotinine levels. In this trial, 48 treatment-seeking smokers were individually assigned to one of the following four categories: rTMS with smoking cues, rTMS with neutral cues, sham stimulation with smoking cues, and sham stimulation with neutral cues. Again, craving was assessed using the VAS (Amiaz et al., 2009). To induce long-lasting effects, rTMS and sham sessions were given 10 times daily (10 Hz; 100% RMT). Results demonstrated a significant decrease in cigarette consumption, craving intensity, and overall nicotine addiction in active rTMS groups. However, the effects did not last long, and the results were not significant after the follow-up period of 6 months post-experimentation (Amiaz et al., 2009). Recently, Rose et al. (2011) investigated the effects of low-frequency (1 Hz; 90% RMT) and high-frequency (10 Hz; 90% RMT) rTMS on the superior frontal gyrus (SFG) of nicotine-addicted individuals (all participants received both types of stimulation and a low-frequencystimulation of M1 as baseline). Participants were also presented with neutral and smoking cues and with cigarette smoke to induce nicotine craving. Interestingly, high-frequency rTMS to the SFG induced greater craving during smoking cue presentations than low-frequency rTMS (Rose et al., 2011). These results provide interesting insights regarding the role of the SFG in the magnitude of craving and the reactivity to craving intensity.

tDCS can also provide long-lasting cortical and subcortical changes and affect addictive behavior when targeting the DLPFC. In nicotine addiction, a pioneering study by Fregni, Liguori, Fecteau and Nitsche (2008) used a randomized, double-blind, sham-controlled cross-over paradigm to determine whether tDCS can modulate nicotine cravings within nicotine-addicted individuals. The craving levels were determined before and after the presentation of a smoking video cue with the VAS. Interestingly, anodal stimulation of both the right and left DLPFC decreased the craving levels when compared to sham stimulation (Fregni, Liguori, Fecteau, & Nitsche, 2008). A similar study by Boggio et al. (2009) followed up to determine whether repeated sessions of anodal tDCS on the left DLPFC could impact the consumption of cigarettes (Boggio et al., 2009). They found that active stimulation decreased the number of smoked cigarettes when compared to sham and the effect was dose-dependent, as the effect of tDCS seemed to gain magnitude according to the number of sessions. Overall, these results provide excellent introductive data on the potential for reducing nicotine cravings and cigarette consumption by tDCS. However, as also determined in rTMS studies, it is not yet possible to determine whether the addiction-relieving effects are long-lasting or definitive. The general consensus regarding the use of NIBS in nicotine addiction is that it represents a plausible treatment modality.

Alcohol

Alcohol use disorder (AUD) is the most frequent addictive disorder, with alcohol being the most widely used psychoactive substance. However, various mechanistic components of alcohol addiction are still elusive in the initiation, withdrawal, or preoccupation stages of the addiction cycle. This lack of certainty and the various concomitant psychiatric conditions encountered among alcoholic patients, such as major depressive disorders, contribute to make alcoholism a very complex disorder (Vengeliene, Bilbao, Molander, & Spanagel, 2009).

Alcohol, and its psychoactive ingredient ethanol, acts as a CNS depressant and sedative. It is a non-selective pharmacological agent, which easily penetrates the blood–brain barrier following consumption. It acts primarily by disrupting receptors and ion channels, mediating effects on a broad range of neurotransmitter systems, and hence it is extremely difficult to identify which effects are directly ascribable to a particular system or receptor interaction. During intoxication, alcohol has a direct action on ion channels, inhibiting L-type Ca^{2+} channels and opening G-protein activated K^+ channels. Thus it induces the inhibition of NMDA subtypes of glutamate receptor activation, thereby reducing excitation, and enhances the function of $GABA_A$ receptors, thereby enhancing inhibition. These primary actions on various ion channels, GABA receptors, and glutamate receptors are thought to be dependent on diverse variables, most importantly the concentration of ethanol in blood and the affinity of the subunit for the receptor or channel (for review, see Vengeliene et al., 2009). However, the modulation of intrinsic membrane properties leads to a broad range of molecular mechanisms implicating other neurotransmitters and second messengers. Serotoninergic ($5\text{-}HT_3$) receptors present on GABAergic or other interneurons are also potentiated by alcohol consumption and enhance the inhibitory action of GABA. Activation of $5\text{-}HT_3$ and nicotinic cholinergic receptors (nAChRs), also present on the same neurons, increases the release of dopamine and modulates the release of glutamate, GABA, acetylcholineb and norepinephrine (Vengeliene et al., 2009). The reinforcing effects of ethanol are thought to be caused primarily by the release of dopamine in the mesolimbic pathway, mediated by the disinhibition of dopamine neurons at GABA receptors and by the modulation of glutamatergic systems. It is also thought that ethanol may directly excite dopamine neurons in the VTA and stimulate the release of dopamine (Sulzer, 2011). An additional theory for the ethanol-initiated release of dopamine is the increase of dopamine neurons firing caused by the decrease in K^+ currents and activation of inward currents by acetaldehyde, a metabolite of ethanol (Sulzer, 2011). However, strong as dopamine may be as a mediator of ethanol-based reward, opiates and cannabinoids are also released and participate in the initiation and maintenance of ethanol addiction. Blocking CB1 receptors in animals suppresses chronic alcohol consumption and blocking opiate receptors with naltrexone, an opioid receptor antagonist with high affinity for κ- and μ-opioid receptors, reduces cravings for alcohol in alcohol-addicted animals (Herz, 1997; Hillemacher, Heberlein, Muschler, Bleich, & Frieling, 2011; Stahl, 2005; Trigo, Martin-García, Berrendero, Robledo, & Maldonado, 2010; Vengeliene et al., 2009). Available pharmacotherapies for AUD target the previously stated mechanisms, and are relatively effective. Disulfiram (an acetaldehyde dehydrogenase inhibitor), naltrexone (an opioid-receptor antagonist), and acamprosate (acts by normalizing NMDA hyperexcitability during withdrawal) are the currently used compounds (Lev-Ran, Balchand, Lefebvre, Araki, & Le Foll, 2012). However, concurrent psychiatric disorders are frequently encountered within alcoholic populations, and these have proved to be an obstruction to proper diagnosis and drug prescription.

Following alcohol's modulation of glutamate and GABA neurotransmission, a few studies have focused on its obvious effects on cortical excitability and physiology. Ziemann, Lönnecker, and Paulus (1995) pioneered this specific field by demonstrating that acute alcohol consumption induces cortical inhibition in the motor cortex, and that this effect is dose-dependent (Ziemann et al., 1995). It has also been found that acute consumption of alcohol reduces cortical excitability in the prefrontal cortex, which may explain the mood, attention, and judgment impairments associated with this substance (Kähkönen, Wilenius, Nikulin, Ollikainen and Ilmoniemi, 2003). Interestingly, it has been shown that young subjects at high risk of developing AUD (i.e., offspring of treatment-seeking AUD patients) exhibit relative impairments in cortico-cortical and transcallosal inhibitory mechanisms (Muralidharan, Venkatasubramanian, Pal, & Benegal, 2008). Conte et al. (2008) also addressed the question of cortical excitability and alcohol use by comparing acute alcohol intake in healthy subjects to chronic alcohol intake in patients with AUD. They found decreased cortical excitability as well as suppressed rTMS-induced motor evoked-potential facilitation in subjects with chronic AUD, compared to healthy subjects. They postulated that these results may be caused by long-lasting effects on glutamate transmission (Conte et al., 2008). These studies demonstrate how AUD can be investigated successfully using electrophysiological methods. Further results on functional connectivity, central motor conduction, and cortical plasticity are available in the literature (Nardone et al., 2012); however, these are beyond the scope of this chapter.

The previously described results indicate the past and present interest in studying AUD with EEG and NIBS. We will now focus on recent results on NIBS as a potential treatment for alcohol addiction. Mishra et al. (2011) designed a sham-controlled, single-blind study and used 10 sessions of 10-Hz rTMS on the right DLPFC in 45 patients (15 received sham stimulation) with AUD. They evaluated the severity of cravings for alcohol with a specific questionnaire following the rTMS sessions, and after a month-long follow-up period. The subjects had been abstinent for 10 consecutive days before the start of the experiment. The results indicated that active rTMS significantly reduced craving scores when compared to craving scores of sham-stimulated patients. The authors suggest that stimulation of the right DLPFC may modulate the activity of the mesolimbic dopamine pathway through mesofronto-limbic connections, as increased dopaminergic activity in this pathway is associated with alcohol cravings, and dopaminergic antagonists (clozapine and olanzapine) are known to tone down these cravings. They also point out the possible trans-synaptic suppression of the left DLPFC, resulting from the stimulation of the right DLPFC, which may have reduced cravings for alcohol (Mishra et al., 2011). Although this study was not double-blinded, it highlights the potential efficacy of high-frequency rTMS in diminishing craving intensity in AUD. Höppner, Broese, Wendler, Berger, & Thome (2011) have also investigated the effect of high-frequency rTMS in alcoholics, using 20-Hz rTMS, on 10 consecutive days, on the left DLPFC in 19 women struggling with AUD. They measured alcohol cravings with the Obsessive Compulsive Drinking Scale, and depressive symptoms with two depression measurements (the Hamilton Scale, and Beck's Inventory). Although they found some interesting results concerning the attentional blink in alcohol-addicted patients, they did not identify significant differences between sham- and active-stimulated groups in terms of mood enhancement or reduction of craving (Höppner et al., 2011). Herremans et al. (2012) investigated the effect of a single session of high-frequency rTMS (right DLPFC) on alcohol cravings in 36 detoxified patients with AUD. Again, the craving intensity was assessed with the Obsessive Compulsive Drinking Scale before and after the rTMS session. There were no significant differences in the magnitude of alcohol cravings when comparing active- to sham-stimulated patients. However, this study was the first to evaluate cravings in detoxified patients in their natural environment, and highlights the importance of the number of active stimulations needed to achieve a clinical effect. It is also worth noting that these patients had stopped taking benzodiazepine shortly before the rTMS experiment, which may also explain the craving measurements (Herremans et al., 2012). The final available published paper on TMS as a treatment option for AUD is a case report, from De Ridder et al. (2011), on a woman with severe alcoholism and a chronic history of drinking. They used rTMS to try to tone down her intractable alcohol cravings. The stimulation sessions were delivered each day for 3 weeks, at a frequency of 1 Hz, on the medial frontal cortex. There was a significant reduction in alcohol consumption for the duration of the treatment, and significantly reduced cravings and withdrawal symptoms for 3 months. After 3 months the patient relapsed and was treated again with a week of rTMS, with the same parameters. She relapsed again after a further 3 weeks and became completely unresponsive to the subsequent rTMS sessions (De Ridder et al., 2011). The studies by Mishra et al. and De Ridder et al. are the only two showing positive results among a total of four presently available studies evaluating rTMS in alcohol addiction. Of note, stimulation parameters and brain targets were different across studies and no control sites for stimulation were used (active parameters were compared to sham). Hence, it is difficult to come to a conclusion regarding the efficacy of rTMS on alcohol addiction.

Boggio and colleagues have provided the only published study on tDCS for alcohol cravings (Boggio et al., 2008). This randomized, sham-controlled study of 13 subjects with AUD sought to determine whether bilateral active tDCS could reduce the intensity of alcohol cravings. Subjects were presented with alcohol-depicting visual cues to increase their cravings. Both anodal left/cathodal right and cathodal left/anodal right electrode conformations in active tDCS significantly reduced cravings associated with alcohol stimuli, compared to sham stimulation. Interestingly, the reduced intensity of craving was sustained after the treatment among patients who received active tDCS. The authors propose that these effects may in part be mediated by the mesofronto-limbic connections of the DLPFC with the mesolimbic dopamine pathways. They also suggest that these effects may be mediated by the connections from the OFC to the striatum and amygdala, which regulate motivational behavior and reward. The aforementioned networks are known to undergo changes in activity following tDCS (Boggio et al., 2008).

To summarize, rTMS and tDCS are promising means of reducing cravings and withdrawal symptoms in alcoholism and AUD. However, tDCS data are limited to a single study with a positive outcome. Results are mitigated across four rTMS studies, as these have slightly different methodologies in assessing cravings and withdrawal, brain targets, and technical parameters. Again, it is hard to determine precisely how NIBS is effective in AUD, as alcohol affects a broad range of neurotransmitter systems in the human brain. Obviously, more studies are needed to determine the mechanisms of action of NIBS in general, but also on how it can modulate AUD-related behaviors.

Cocaine

Cocaine addiction is a very serious social issue, with 1.7 million people currently struggling with this condition in the US (NIDA, 2012). The available literature on cocaine addiction is immense – a revealing fact regarding this drug's history in medicine and neurosciences. Like amphetamines, cocaine is a psychostimulant of the CNS and acts directly on dopamine pathways, hence its notorious reinforcing effects and addictive properties. Indeed, cocaine addiction is strongly characterized by relapse and recidivism (Dackis & O'Brien, 2001; Stahl, 2005).

Other than its effects as a local anesthetic, acute cocaine administration induces intense euphoria and reduces fatigue; higher doses can also induce tremors, panic, paranoia, and stereotyped behaviors (Dackis & O'Brien, 2001). Cocaine is an indirect agonist at dopamine receptors and an inhibitor of monoamine transporters (such as DAT, the dopamine transporter); it thus blocks the reuptake mechanism of mesolimbic and mesocortical dopamine neurons (Stahl, 2005). This causes an accumulation of dopamine in the synaptic cleft, increasing its length of action and causing dopamine concentration to rise to a non-physiological level, thereby increasing neurotransmission. The behavioral effects on cocaine users are mainly mediated by this mechanism, although it also has similar but less important effects on norepinephrinergic and serotoninergic neurons. Chronic cocaine intake increases dopamine release in the mesocortical pathway, as with any other drug, and downregulates the concentration of D2 receptors in the prefrontal cortex, which leads to an increase in D1 signaling. This is thought to facilitate an increase in glutamate release in cortico-limbic projections and eventually to lead to changes in the postsynaptic density (PSD) of GABA medium spiny neurons of the nucleus accumbens, which will affect the metabotropic glutamate receptors (mGluRs) present in this very density. Such changes include the augmentation of dendritic spines, the insertion of AMPA receptors in the PSD, and an increase in receptor sensitivity (Kalivas 2007a; Kalivas, Volkow, & Seamans, 2005). Targeting mGluRs is in fact one of many pharmacological experimental avenues used to suppress cocaine addiction, as is the partial inhibition of glutamate release in the PFC. Indeed, studies have demonstrated that the blocking of AMPA receptors in the NA inhibits relapse in cocaine addiction (Cornish & Kalivas, 2000; Kalivas, 2007a). Augmentation of glutamate release near limbic structures is thought to influence GABA transmission and its GABAergic projections from the NA to the VP, among other structures. Targeting GABA transmission is another valuable therapeutic avenue, as GABA levels in the VP of cocaine addicts are lower than normal. Decrease in GABA concentrations in this structure is associated with cocaine-seeking behaviors and the development of cocaine sensitization (Kalivas, 2007b). Outputs from the NA to the VP are also peptidergic, and chronic psychostimulant intake can induce long-term changes in opioid peptide regulation and gene expression. Indeed, acute and chronic cocaine administration increases levels of β-endorphin in the NA and dynorphin in striato-nigral neurons. Chronic cocaine administration is also known to modulate opioid receptor gene expression in the basal ganglia and associated receptive structures, especially μ- and δ-opioid receptors. However, all opioid receptors are likely implicated in the rewarding effect of cocaine (Trigo et al., 2010).

Changes in diversely important neurotransmitter systems have important effects on cortical excitability. Two studies by Boutros and colleagues have investigated the impact of chronic cocaine consumption on the RMT. Using single-pulse TMS, they found that cocaine-dependent subjects had a significantly higher RMT when compared to controls (Boutros et al., 2001). Interestingly, this effect was also present in 3-weeks' post-abstinence ex-cocaine users (Boutros et al., 2005). Sundaresan, Ziemann, Stanley, and Boutros (2007) provided similar results (higher RMT) in abstinent cocaine-dependent individuals, using single-pulse and paired-pulse TMS. Hence, three studies have provided evidence linking chronic cocaine consumption with a long-lasting decrease in cortical excitability. This characteristic indicates that chronic cocaine abuse increases cortical inhibition, in spite of the reduction in prefrontal GABA concentrations. The authors suggest that this phenomenon may elicit a compensatory mechanism for the effects of repetitive cocaine intake (Boutros et al., 2001), or a protective effect against cocaine-induced seizures and other effects (Sundaresan et al., 2007; Feil & Zangen, 2010).

To date, only two studies have investigated the clinical potential of NIBS in cocaine addiction, and these only with rTMS. Camprodon et al. (2007) administered two sessions of rTMS (10 Hz) on the right and left DLPFC at intensity level of 90% of RMT. Each patient received the treatment on each hemisphere in a randomized fashion, and completed a craving VAS before the stimulation, directly afterwards, and 4 hours afterwards. One session of rTMS applied to the right but not left hemisphere significantly and transiently decreased the craving for cocaine. The authors, along with Strafella et al. (2001), propose that stimulation of the DLPFC can induce dopamine release in the dorsal striatum and this may, in part, explain the observed positive outcome. It is worth noting that the patients participating in this study were all trying to quit cocaine abuse (Camprodon et al., 2007). The second available study report focused on 36 patients post-detoxification (Politi et al., 2008), and used 10 sessions of 15-Hz rTMS to the left DLPFC at intensity level of 100% of RMT. Psychopathologic symptoms of cocaine craving were assessed on each day of experimentation. The intensity of craving diminished significantly, and gradually, following the duration of treatment. The authors reported that the most significant changes occurred at the seventh session. Although data are still scarce, it seems likely that rTMS may become a useful tool in treating cocaine addiction. As discussed in Fecteau et al. (2010), the shared and differential effects related to targeting the right or left DLPFC need to be further investigated. As studies combining NIBS with neuroimaging suggest, rTMS over the right or the left DLPFC modulates a complex network involving ipsilateral and contralateral sides of the targeted regions.

Food

So far, this chapter has focused on reviewing results and data on NIBS and substance addictions. Although substances such as alcohol, cocaine, and nicotine are widely used and are central to the addiction treatment issue, growing interest is emerging from the study of compulsive activities that are not yet characterized as substance-use disorders or addictions, such as gambling, internet use, and shopping (Davis & Carter, 2009). Furthermore, natural rewards such as food, sexual behavior, and social interactions, which are intrinsically essential for survival but also comprise hedonic characteristics, are proven to engage similar brain pathways as do drugs of abuse. Moreover, they can modulate and induce neuroplasticity in the reward pathways, similarly to traditional pharmacological agents used as drugs (Olsen, 2011; Pitchers, Balfour, & Lehman, 2010).

Food has both homeostatic and hedonic components, which makes it a potent natural reward and conditioning stimulus (Volkow, Wang,

& Baler, 2011). The relationship between overeating, compulsive behavior, and obesity has drawn attention to similarities with drug use in addiction. In fact, sources have proposed the idea of defining obesity as a brain disorder, a pathology of neuroadaptation (Kenny, 2011a, 2011b).

Food addiction is not yet recognized as a proper addictive disorder, for different reasons. First of all, it is not clear yet whether food addiction can specifically describe a human phenotype. Obesity, metabolic syndrome, binge-eating disorder, and bulimia are all medical and/or psychiatric conditions sharing characteristics with food addiction and compulsive overeating, but nevertheless are very distinct pathologies. It is also thought that alternative psychosocial explanations are still plausible in explaining the phenomenon and its relation to the development of obesity. Second, there is a lack of evidence regarding withdrawal and tolerance, which are critical in the definition of addiction. Finally, apart from the interaction with striatal dopamine and PFC activation in craving conditions, neurobiological mechanisms of food addiction are still elusive. It is also worth noting that although serious pieces of evidence are demonstrating food addiction in animals (in the form of sucrose-bingeing and sugar-addicted rat models; for review see Avena & Rada, 2008), the translation to humans is not scientifically obvious (Benton, 2010; Ziauddeen, Farooqi, & Fletcher, 2012). Unfortunately, clinical human data concerning withdrawal, sensitization, and tolerance in compulsive overeating are still largely anecdotal (Davis & Carter, 2009).

Several studies using human neuroimaging have, however, highlighted and identified compelling clues linking obesity to a modulation of reward mechanisms, advocating a food addiction model. Indeed, obese individuals show greater activation of the OFC, ACC, amygdala, and striatum in response to food cues and anticipated palatable food receipt than lean individuals (Stice, Spoor, Ng, & Zald 2009; Stoeckel et al., 2009). Moreover, individuals with a greater food addiction score (on the Yale Food Addiction Scale) show greater activation in the DLPFC and striatum in response to anticipated receipt of palatable food, but show less activation when actually receiving food (Gearhardt et al., 2011). These observations are striking in their resemblance to traditional drug use (Volkow & Wise, 2005; Volkow, Wang, Fowler, Tomasi, & Baler, 2011).

Other parameters are also intriguingly similar between drug- and food-craving individuals, such as reward hypersensitivity, impulsivity, and deficits in decision-making (Volkow, Wang, Fowler, Tomasi, & Baler, 2011). Finally, a valuable hypothesis in appreciating the complexity of compulsive overeating is that it represents a combination of two addictive components: (1) food, the substance, is a dopamine-activating substance which triggers the brain reward mechanisms; and (2) eating, the activity, is a rewarding and reinforcing behavior (Davis & Carter, 2009).

No matter how controversial this issue might be, understanding compulsive overeating may help in dealing with the severe obesity epidemic spreading worldwide. Indeed, several NIBS studies have investigated the possibility of reducing food cravings in healthy subjects. Uher and colleagues used a single session of rTMS (15 Hz; 110% RMT) in a double-blind, randomized parallel study (Uher et al., 2005). They stimulated the left DLPFC of 28 healthy women reported to experience frequent food cravings. The subjects were exposed to palatable food items before and after the stimulation, and rated their own desire for food, using the VAS. Subjects who received active rTMS lacked the increase in food cravings observed in subjects receiving sham stimulation. The authors concluded that prefrontal stimulation inhibits the development of craving, and therefore it may be considered as a therapeutic tool against binge eating (Uher et al., 2005). The only other study to date that has used rTMS to investigate food cravings was developed by Van den Eynde et al. (2010), and focused on the effect of rTMS in bulimic patients. This double-blinded study sought to determine whether a dysfunction of the DLPFC could cause the severe food cravings characteristic of bulimic eating disorder. Patients were shown real palatable food items following the presentation of video sequences showing people eating the same items, in order to stimulate craving, and were asked to rate their sensation of craving on the VAS and the Food Craving Questionnaire before and 24 h after the only rTMS session (frequency and RMT were not specified). They found a significant reduction in the urge to eat among the participants who received the real rTMS. Moreover, they observed a significant reduction in binge eating 24 h after the stimulation, which constitutes a proof-of-concept result in the development of a tool for the treatment of bulimia. However, they did not investigate the sustained effect of rTMS in diminishing binge eating as a chronic and recurrent behavior.

Two tDCS studies sought to determine the effect of direct current stimulation on food cravings in healthy individuals. In the study by Fregni, Orsati et al. (2008), 23 subjects were tested in a randomized, sham-controlled study, which targeted the DLPFC following the presentation of food items and of a movie depicting food items. Food cravings were assessed with ratings on the VAS before and after the presentation of food cues. Interestingly, they also measured the visual attention to food with an eye-tracking apparatus. They tested active tDCS of 2 mA for 20 minutes, with both electrode configurations (anodal stimulation of the left DLPFC, anodal stimulation of the right DLPFC) and sham tDCS, in a random order. Cravings were significantly induced by the presentation of food items. Active anodal tDCS of the right DLPFC significantly reduced food cravings compared to sham tDCS, and to anodal tDCS of the left DLPFC. After sham stimulation, cravings were increased by the presentation of food cues, whereas cravings did not increase after active stimulation (with both electrode configurations). Of note, the cathode electrode was placed on the opposite DLPFC in both configurations. Hence, these results suggest that both tDCS electrode configurations may have a reducing effect on the cravings induced by the presentation of food cues. Interestingly, the eye-tracking results demonstrated that subjects who were stimulated with active tDCS (anode/right DLPFC) focused less visually on food items after the stimulation, which indicates that an attentional shift induced by tDCS might contribute to decreased food cravings. Attentional processing seems to play an important role in reward, which involves PFC regions (Rossi, Pessoa, & Desimone, 2009). The other study investigated the effect of a 20-minute 2-mA tDCS session (anode over the right DLPFC) in 19 healthy adults experiencing food cravings (Goldman et al., 2011). Subjects were presented with visual food cues and rated their own sensations of craving on the VAS. Participants then received active or sham stimulation for 10 minutes and were asked to re-evaluate their craving intensity with the VAS, and again after completion of the whole 20-minute session. Participants were then presented with real palatable food items, which were available to eat. Consistent with the study from Fregni and colleagues, active tDCS decreased craving ratings compared to sham stimulation. Moreover, subjects were self-reportedly more able to resist food after tDCS, which suggests that active tDCS could increase a person's control over reward availability. Results from these two studies suggest that tDCS may be capable of decreasing the intensity of food cravings. However, the studies have certain limitations, as eating behaviors observed in laboratory settings are not necessarily representative of those encountered in the real world. Furthermore, the studies (tDCS and rTMS) investigated food cravings in healthy individuals experiencing food cravings (Fregni, Orsati et al., 2008; Goldman et al., 2011; Uher et al., 2005) and in individuals struggling with bulimia (Van den Eynde et al., 2010). Food cravings are observed in psychiatric conditions such as bulimia and binge-eating disorder, but are also reported in people dealing with obesity, visceral obesity, and/or metabolic syndrome (Després & Lemieux, 2006), without known psychiatric comorbidities. Hence, specific screening of patients is extremely important, and must take physiological measurements (such as body mass index and waist circumference) and psychiatric variables into account in order to provide valid results.

CONCLUSION

Addiction is a pathology of neuroadaptation. It is neurobiologically determined by the modulation of dopamine transmission, and modifications in mesocortico-limbic circuitry and, subsequently, in the excitability of prefrontal cortices. Various lines of research have identified the DLPFC as an important cerebral relay in normal and pathological behavioral output, which makes it a brain target of great interest for NIBS in drug addictions. tDCS and rTMS, applied over the DLPFC, are novel means to non-invasively modulate cortical excitability over a sustained period. Human studies provide concrete insight for the use of NIBS in reducing cravings and intake of addictive substances.

In this review, we report that NIBS can induce beneficial effects in various substance-related addictions. Although more studies and results are needed to characterize the mechanisms of action of NIBS in toning down addictive behaviors, actual results demonstrate its great potential in becoming an alternate therapeutic tool to present pharmacotherapies. One common mechanistic player is likely to be the dopamine pathways. Regardless of the substance abused, dopamine pathways are involved in the development of addiction. Neurobiological literature often refers to these pathways as the hedonic center of the brain, since their natural stimulation (physical accomplishment, tasting food, listening to music, etc.) will lead to the subjective experience of pleasure. Although the studied substances have different psychotropic effects and pharmacological properties, neurobiological data suggest that they all commonly activate the mesolimbic dopamine pathway and act on the NA in the basal forebrain, using dopamine directly as a neurotransmitter, or not (Nestler, 2005). While psychostimulants will act directly on dopamine transmission, several other drugs will modulate the activity of the opioid (alcohol, nicotine, and opiates) and cannabinoid systems within the same mesolimbic pathway (Nestler, 2005). Future studies are needed for further characterization of tDCS and rTMS on the dopamine pathways in patients with addiction.

Finally, as described previously, addiction comprises different stages, each with its own neurobiological substrates and behavioral outputs; intoxication, withdrawal and negative affect, preoccupation, and craving. Most studies on rTMS and tDCS are presently focused on craving, as this is mainly under the control of the PFC, which is a preferential brain target in NIBS protocols. However, since rTMS can theoretically exercise its influence on subcortical structures (Strafella et al., 2001, 2003), much has yet to be unveiled regarding its modulatory potential in addictive disorders at various, ideally earlier, stages of developing addiction.

Acknowledgments

This work was supported by the Canada Research Chair in Cognitive Neuroplasticity to SF; and a CRIUSMQ scholarship to AHB.

References

Amiaz, R., Levy, D., Vainiger, D., Grunhaus, L., & Zangen, A. (2009). Repeated high-frequency transcranial magnetic stimulation over the dorsolateral prefrontal cortex reduces cigarette craving and consumption. *Addiction, 104*(4), 653–660.

Avena, N., & Rada, P. (2008). Evidence for sugar addiction: Behavioral and neurochemical effects of intermittent, excessive sugar intake. *Neuroscience & Biobehavioral Reviews, 32,* 20–39.

Bechara, A. (2005). Decision making, impulse control and loss of willpower to resist drugs: A neurocognitive perspective. *Nature Neuroscience, 8*(11), 1458–1463.

Benowitz, N. L. (2009). Pharmacology of nicotine: Addiction, smoking-induced disease, and therapeutics. *Annual Review of Pharmacology and Toxicology, 49*(1), 57–71.

Benton, D. (2010). The plausibility of sugar addiction and its role in obesity and eating disorders. *Clinical Nutrition, 29,* 288–303.

Boggio, P., Liguori, P., Sultani, N., & Rezende, L. (2009). Cumulative priming effects of cortical stimulation on smoking cue-induced craving. *Neuroscience, 463,* 82–86.

Boggio, P., Sultani, N., Fecteau, S., & Merabet, L. (2008). Prefrontal cortex modulation using transcranial DC stimulation reduces alcohol craving: A double-blind, sham-controlled study. *Drug and Alcohol Dependence, 92,* 55–60.

Boutros, N. N., Lisanby, S. H., McClain-Furmanski, D., Oliwa, G., Gooding, D., & Kosten, T. R. (2005). Cortical excitability in cocaine-dependent patients: A replication and extension of TMS findings. *Journal of Psychiatry Research, 39*(3), 295–302.

Boutros, N. N., Lisanby, S. H., Tokuno, H., Torello, M. W., Campbell, D., & Berman, R. (2001). Elevated motor threshold in drug-free, cocaine-dependent patients assessed with transcranial magnetic stimulation. *Biological Psychiatry, 49*(4), 369–373.

Brody, A. L., Mandelkern, M. A., London, E. D., Childress, A. R., Lee, G. S., Bota, R. G., et al. (2002). Brain metabolic changes during cigarette craving. *Archives of General Psychiatry, 59,* 1162–1172.

Camprodon, J. A., Martínez-Raga, J., Alonso-Alonso, M., Shih, M. -C., & Pascual-Leone, A. (2007). One session of high frequency repetitive transcranial magnetic stimulation (rTMS) to the right prefrontal cortex transiently reduces cocaine craving. *Drug and Alcohol Dependence, 86*(1), 91–94.

Camus, M., Halelamien, N., Plassmann, H., Shimojo, S., O Doherty, J., Camerer, C., et al. (2009). Repetitive transcranial magnetic stimulation over the right dorsolateral prefrontal cortex decreases valuations during food choices. *European Journal of Neuroscience, 30*(10), 1980–1988.

Cho, S. S., & Strafella, A. P. (2009). rTMS of the left dorsolateral prefrontal cortex modulates dopamine release in the ipsilateral anterior cingulate cortex and orbitofrontal cortex. *PLoS One, 4*(8), e6725.

Conte, A., Attilia, M. L., Gilio, F., Iacovelli, E., Frasca, V., Bettolo, C. M., et al. (2008). Acute and chronic effects of ethanol on cortical excitability. *Clinical Neurophysiology: Official Journal of the International Federation of Clinical Neurophysiology, 119*(3), 667–674.

Cornish, J. L., & Kalivas, P. W. (2000). Glutamate transmission in the nucleus accumbens mediates relapse in cocaine addiction. *Journal of Neuroscience, 20,* 1–5.

Dackis, C. A., & O'Brien, C. (2001). Cocaine dependence: A disease of the brain's reward centers. *Journal of Substance Abuse Treatment, 21,* 111–117.

Davis, C., & Carter, J. C. (2009). Compulsive overeating as an addiction disorder. A review of theory and evidence. *Appetite, 53,* 1–8.

De Ridder, D., Vanneste, S., Kovacs, S., Sunaert, S., & Dom, G. (2011). Transient alcohol craving suppression by rTMS of dorsal anterior cingulate: An fMRI and LORETA EEG study. *Neuroscience Letters, 496*(1), 5–10.

Després, J. -P., & Lemieux, I. (2006). Abdominal obesity and metabolic syndrome. *Nature, 444* (7121), 881–887.

Eichhammer, P., Johann, M., Kharraz, A., Binder, H., Pittrow, D., Wodarz, N., et al. (2003). High-frequency repetitive transcranial magnetic stimulation decreases cigarette smoking. *Journal of Clinical Psychiatry, 64–8*, 951–953.

Fecteau, S., Fregni, F., Boggio, P. S., Camprodon, J. A., & Pascual-Leone, A. (2010). Neuromodulation of decision-making in the addictive brain. *Substance Use & Misuse, 45*(11), 1766–1786.

Fecteau, S., Knoch, D., Fregni, F., Sultani, N., Boggio, P., & Pascual-Leone, A. (2007). Diminishing risk-taking behavior by modulating activity in the prefrontal cortex: A direct current stimulation study. *Journal of Neuroscience, 27*(46), 12500–12505.

Feil, J., & Zangen, A. (2010). Brain stimulation in the study and treatment of addiction. *Neuroscience & Biobehavioral Reviews, 34*(4), 559–574.

Franken, I., Booij, J., & Vandenbrink, W. (2005). The role of dopamine in human addiction: From reward to motivated attention. *European Journal of Pharmacology, 526*(1–3), 199–206.

Fregni, F., Liguori, P., Fecteau, S., & Nitsche, M. (2008). Cortical stimulation of the prefrontal cortex with transcranial direct current stimulation reduces cue-provoked smoking craving: A randomized, sham-controlled study. *Journal of Clinical Psychiatry, 69*(1), 32–40.

Fregni, F., Orsati, F., Pedrosa, W., Fecteau, S., Tome, F. A. M., Nitsche, M. A., et al. (2008). Transcranial direct current stimulation of the prefrontal cortex modulates the desire for specific foods. *Appetite, 51*(1), 34–41.

Fregni, F., & Pascual-Leone, A. (2007). Technology Insight: Noninvasive brain stimulation in neurology—perspectives on the therapeutic potential of rTMS and tDCS. *Nature Clinical Practice. Neurology, 3*(7), 383–393.

Gearhardt, A. N., Yokum, S., Orr, P. T., Stice, E., Corbin, W. R., & Brownell, K. D. (2011). Neural correlates of food addiction. *Archives of General Psychiatry, 68*(8), 808–816.

George, M. S., Wassermann, E. M., Kimbrell, T. A., Little, J. T., Williams, W. E., Danielson, B. A., et al. (1997). Mood improvement following daily left prefrontal transcranial magnetic stimulation in patient with depression: A placebo-controlled crossover trial. *The American Journal of Psychiatry, 154*(12), 1752–1756.

Goldman, R. L., Borckardt, J. J., Frohman, H. A., O'Neil, P. M., Madan, A., Campbell, L. K., et al. (2011). Prefrontal cortex transcranial direct current stimulation (tDCS) temporarily reduces food cravings and increases the self-reported ability to resist food in adults with frequent food craving. *Appetite, 56*(3), 741–746.

Goldstein, R. Z., Moeller, S. J., & Volkow, N. D. (2011). Cognitive disruption in drug addiction: A focus on the prefrontal cortex. In B. Adinoff & E. A. Stein (Eds.), *Neuroimaging in addiction* (pp. 177–207). Chichester, UK: John Wiley & Sons, Ltd.

Goldstein, R. Z., & Volkow, N. D. (2002). Drug addiction and Its underlying neurobiological basis: Neuroimaging evidence for the involvement of the frontal cortex. *The American Journal of Psychiatry, 159*(10), 1642.

Goldstein, R. Z., & Volkow, N. D. (2011). Dysfunction of the prefrontal cortex in addiction: Neuroimaging findings and clinical implications. *Nature Reviews. Neuroscience, 12*(11), 652–669.

Herremans, S. C., Baeken, C., Vanderbruggen, N., Vanderhasselt, M. A., Zeeuws, D., Santermans, L., et al. (2012). No influence of one right-sided prefrontal HF-rTMS session on alcohol craving in recently detoxified alcohol-dependent patients: Results of a naturalistic study. *Drug and Alcohol Dependence, 120*(1–3), 209–213.

Herz, A. (1997). Endogenous opioid systems and alcohol addiction. *Psychopharmacology, 129* (2), 99–111.

Hillemacher, T., Heberlein, A., Muschler, M. A., Bleich, S., & Frieling, H. (2011). Opioid modulators for alcohol dependence. *Expert Opinion on Investigational Drugs, 20*(8), 1073–1086.

Höppner, J., Broese, T., Wendler, L., Berger, C., & Thome, J. (2011). Repetitive transcranial magnetic stimulation (rTMS) for treatment of alcohol dependence. *The World Journal of Biological Psychiatry, 12*, 57–62.

Hyman, S. E. (2007). Addiction: A disease of learning and memory. *Focus, 5*(2), 220.

Johann, M., Wiegand, R., Kharraz, A., Bobbe, G., Sommer, G., & Hajak, G. (2003). Transcranial magnetic stimulation for nicotine dependence. *Psychiatrische Praxis, 30*(Suppl. 2), S129–S131.

Kähkönen, S., Wilenius, J., Nikulin, V. V., Ollikainen, M., & Ilmoniemi, R. J. (2003). Alcohol reduces prefrontal cortical excitability in humans: A combined TMS and EEG study. *Neuropsychopharmacology, 28*(4), 747–754.

Kalivas, P. W. (2007a). Cocaine and amphetamine-like psychostimulants: Neurocircuitry and glutamate neuroplasticity. *Dialogues in Clinical Neuroscience, 9*(4), 389–397.

Kalivas, P. W. (2007b). Neurobiology of cocaine addiction: Implications for new pharmaco-therapy. *American Journal on Addictions, 16*(2), 71–78.

Kalivas, P. W., & O'Brien, C. (2007). Drug addiction as a pathology of staged neuroplasticity. *Neuropsychopharmacology, 33*(1), 166–180.

Kalivas, P. W., Volkow, N., & Seamans, J. (2005). Unmanageable motivation in addiction: A pathology in prefrontal-accumbens glutamate transmission. *Neuron, 45*(5), 647–650.

Kauer, J. A., & Malenka, R. C. (2007). Synaptic plasticity and addiction. *Nature Reviews. Neuroscience, 8*(11), 844–858.

Keck, M. E., Welt, T., Müller, M. B., Erhardt, A., Ohl, F., Toschi, N., et al. (2002). Repetitive transcranial magnetic stimulation increases the release of dopamine in the mesolimbic and mesostriatal system. *Neuropharmacology, 43*(1), 101–109.

Kenny, P. (2011a). Reward mechanisms in obesity: New insights and future directions. *Neuron, 69*, 664–679.

Kenny, P. J. (2011b). Common cellular and molecular mechanisms in obesity and drug addiction. *Nature Reviews. Neuroscience, 12*(11), 638–651.

Knoch, D., Gianotti, L. R. R., Pascual-Leone, A., Treyer, V., Regard, M., Hohmann, M., et al. (2006). Disruption of right prefrontal cortex by low-frequency repetitive transcranial magnetic stimulation induces risk-taking behavior. *Journal of Neuroscience, 26*(24), 6469–6472.

Ko, J. H., & Strafella, A. P. (2011). Dopaminergic neurotransmission in the human brain: New lessons from perturbation and imaging. *The Neuroscientist, 18–2*, 149–168.

Koob, G. (2011). Neurobiology of addiction. *Focus, 9*(1), 55–65.

Koob, G., & Kreek, M. J. (2007). Stress, dysregulation of drug reward pathways, and the transition to drug dependence. *The American Journal of Psychiatry, 164*(8), 1149–1159.

Koob, G., & Volkow, N. D. (2009). Neurocircuitry of addiction. *Neuropsychopharmacology Reviews, 35*, 217–238.

Krain, A., Wilson, A. M., Arbuckle, R., Castellanos, F. X., & Milham, M. P. (2006). Distinct mechanisms of risk and ambiguity: A meta-analysis of decision-making. *NeuroImage, 32*(1), 477–484.

Lang, N., Hasan, A., Sueske, E., Paulus, W., & Nitsche, M. A. (2007). Cortical hypoexcitability in chronic smokers? A transcranial magnetic stimulation study. *Neuropsychopharmacology, 33*(10), 2517–2523.

Lev-Ran, S., Balchand, K., Lefebvre, L., Araki, K. F., & Le Foll, B. (2012). Pharmacotherapy of alcohol use disorders and concurrent psychiatric disorders: A review. *Canadian Journal of Psychiatry. Revue Canadienne de Psychiatrie, 57*(6), 342–349.

Markou, A. (2008). Neurobiology of nicotine dependence. *Philosophical Transactions of the Royal Society, B: Biological Sciences, 363*(1507), 3159–3168.

Mishra, B. R., Nizamie, S. H., Das, B., & Praharaj, S. K. (2011). Efficacy of repetitive transcranial magnetic stimulation in alcohol dependence: A sham-controlled study. *Addiction, 105* (1), 49–55.

Muralidharan, K., Venkatasubramanian, G., Pal, P. K., & Benegal, V. (2008). Abnormalities in cortical and transcallosal inhibitory mechanisms in subjects at high risk for alcohol dependence: A TMS study. *Addiction Biology, 13*(3–4), 373–379.

Nahas, Z., Lomarev, M., Roberts, D. R., Shastri, A., Lorberbaum, J. P., Teneback, C., et al. (2001). *Biological Psychiatry, 50*(9), 712–720.

Nardone, R., Bergmann, J., Christova, M., Lochner, P., Tezzon, F., Golaszewski, S., et al. (2012). Non-invasive brain stimulation in the functional evaluation of alcohol effects and in the treatment of alcohol craving: A review. *Neuroscience Research*, 8 pages. In Press.

Nestler, E. J. (2005). Is there a common molecular pathway for addiction? *Nature Neuroscience, 8*(11), 1445–1449.

NIDA. (2012). *Cocaine: Abuse and addiction. Research report series.* NIH Publication Number 10-4166. http://www.drugabuse.gov/sites/default/files/rrcocaine.pdf.

Nitsche, M. A. (2003). Pharmacological modulation of cortical excitability shifts induced by transcranial direct current stimulation in humans. *The Journal of Physiology, 553*(1), 293–301.

Nitsche, M. A., Lampe, C., Antal, A., Liebetanz, D., Lang, N., Tergau, F., et al. (2006). Dopaminergic modulation of long-lasting direct current-induced cortical excitability changes in the human motor cortex. *European Journal of Neuroscience, 23*(6), 1651–1657.

Olsen, C. M. (2011). Natural rewards, neuroplasticity, and non-drug addictions. *Neuropharmacology, 61*(7), 1109–1122.

Pascual-Leone, A., Rubio, B., Pallardò, F., & Català (1996). Rapid-rate transcranial magnetic stimulation of left dorsolateral prefrontal cortex in drug-resistant depression. *The Lancet, 348*(9022), 233–237.

Philiastides, M. G., Auksztulewicz, R., Heekeren, H. R., & Blankenburg, F. (2011). Causal role of dorsolateral prefrontal cortex in human perceptual decision making. *Current Biology, 21* (11), 980–983.

Pitchers, K., Balfour, M., & Lehman, M. (2010). Neuroplasticity in the mesolimbic system induced by natural reward and subsequent reward abstinence. *Biological Psychiatry, 67*, 872–879.

Pogarell, O., Koch, W., Pöpperl, G., Tatsch, K., Jakob, F., Mulert, C., et al. (2007). Acute prefrontal rTMS increases striatal dopamine to a similar degree as d-amphetamine. *Psychiatry Research: Neuroimaging, 156*(3), 251–255.

Politi, E., Fauci, E., Santoro, A., & Smeraldi, E. (2008). Daily sessions of transcranial magnetic stimulation to the left prefrontal cortex gradually reduce cocaine craving. *American Journal on Addictions, 17*(4), 345–346.

Rose, J. E., McClernon, F. J., Froeliger, B., Behm, F. M., Preud'homme, X., & Krystal, A. D. (2011). Repetitive transcranial magnetic stimulation of the superior frontal gyrus modulates craving for cigarettes. *Biological Psychiatry, 70*(8), 794–799.

Rossi, A., Pessoa, L., & Desimone, R. (2009). The prefrontal cortex and the executive control of attention. *Experimental Brain Research, 192*, 489–497.

Russo, S. J., Dietz, D. M., Dumitriu, D., Morrison, J. H., Malenka, R. C., & Nestler, E. J. (2010). The addicted synapse: Mechanisms of synaptic and structural plasticity in nucleus accumbens. *Trends in Neurosciences, 33*(6), 267–276.

Russo, S., Mazei-Robison, M., Ables, J., & Nestler, E. J. (2009). Neurotrophic factors and structural plasticity in addiction. *Neuropharmacology, 56*, 73–82.

Schwartz, R. S., & Benowitz, N. L. (2010). Nicotine addiction. *The New England Journal of Medicine, 362*(24), 2295–2303.

Stagg, C. J., & Nitsche, M. A. (2011). Physiological basis of transcranial direct current stimulation. *The Neuroscientist, 17*(1), 37–53.

Stahl, S. M. (2005). Essential psychopharmacology, (2nd ed.). Cambridge University Press, 1–662.

Stice, E., Spoor, S., Ng, J., & Zald, D. H. (2009). Relation of obesity to consummatory and antic-ipatory food reward. *Physiology & Behavior, 97*(5), 551–560.

Stoeckel, L. E., Kim, J., Weller, R. E., Cox, J. E., Cook, E. W., & Horwitz, B. (2009). Effective connectivity of a reward network in obese women. *Brain Research Bulletin, 79*(6), 388–395.

Strafella, A. P., Paus, T., Barrett, J., & Dagher, A. (2001). Repetitive transcranial magnetic stim-ulation of the human prefrontal cortex induces dopamine release in the caudate nucleus. *The Journal of Neurosciences, 21*, 1–4.

Strafella, A. P., Paus, T., Fraraccio, M., & Dagher, A. (2003). Striatal dopamine release induced by repetitive transcranial magnetic stimulation of the human motor cortex. *Brain, 126*(12), 2609–2615.

Sulzer, D. (2011). How addictive drugs disrupt presynaptic dopamine neurotransmission. *Neuron, 69*(4), 628–649.

Sundaresan, K., Ziemann, U., Stanley, J., & Boutros, N. (2007). Cortical inhibition and excita-tion in abstinent cocaine-dependent patients: A transcranial magnetic stimulation study. *Neuroreport, 18*(3), 289–292.

Trigo, J. M., Martin-García, E., Berrendero, F., Robledo, P., & Maldonado, R. (2010). The endogenous opioid system: A common substrate in drug addiction. *Drug and Alcohol Dependence, 108*(3), 183–194.

Uher, R., Yoganathan, D., Mogg, A., & Eranti, S. (2005). Effect of left prefrontal repetitive tran-scranial magnetic stimulation on food craving. *Biological Psychiatry, 58*, 840–842.

Van den Eynde, F., Claudino, A. M., Mogg, A., Horrell, L., Stahl, D., Ribeiro, W., et al. (2010). Repetitive transcranial magnetic stimulation reduces cue-induced food craving in bulimic disorders. *Biological Psychiatry, 67*(8), 793–795.

Vengeliene, V., Bilbao, A., Molander, A., & Spanagel, R. (2009). Neuropharmacology of alco-hol addiction. *British Journal of Pharmacology, 154*(2), 299–315.

Volkow, N. D., Fowler, J. S., Wang, G. -J., Telang, F., Logan, J., Jayne, M., et al. (2010). Cog-nitive control of drug craving in brain reward regions in cocaine abusers. *NeuroImage, 49* (3), 2536–2543.

Volkow, N. D., Wang, G., & Baler, R. D. (2011). Reward, dopamine and the control of food intake: Implications for obesity. *Trends in Cognitive Sciences, 15*(1), 37–46.

Volkow, N. D., Wang, G. J., Fowler, J. S., Tomasi, D., & Baler, R. (2011). Food and drug reward: Overlapping circuits in human obesity and addiction. *Current Topics in Behavioral Neuro-sciences, 11*, 1–24.

Volkow, N. D., & Wise, R. A. (2005). How can drug addiction help us understand obesity? *Nature Neuroscience, 8*(5), 555–560.

Wagner, T., Valero-Cabre, A., & Pascual-Leone, A. (2007). Noninvasive human brain stimu-lation. *Annual Review of Biomedical Engineering, 9*(1), 527–565.

Ziauddeen, H., Farooqi, I. S., & Fletcher, P. C. (2012). Obesity and the brain: How convincing is the addiction model? *Nature Reviews. Neuroscience, 13*(4), 279–286.

Ziemann, U., Lönnecker, S., & Paulus, W. (1995). Inhibition of human motor cortex by etha-nol. A transcranial magnetic stimulation study. *Brain, 118*(6), 1437–1446.

PART IV

FUTURE PERSPECTIVES

Transcranial Electrical Stimulation to Enhance Cognitive Abilities in the Atypically Developing Brain

Beatrix Krause, Chung Yen Looi, and Roi Cohen Kadosh

Department of Experimental Psychology, University of Oxford, Oxford, UK

OUTLINE

INTRODUCTION

Cognitive loss or underdevelopment can cause a chain of severe consequences in an individual's life. Depending on the type and degree of the deficit, school performance may initially be low, but throughout development the external cognitive demands increase and therefore the child starts to lag more and more behind in the educational environment. Moreover, the chances for academic and occupational achievements become further and further reduced, and the rates of unemployment and depression increase (Parsons & Bynner, 2005; Stein, Blum, & Barbaresi, 2011). This downward spiral demonstrates how quality of life can be greatly compromised in individuals with poor cognitive abilities. Societal values, including physical, financial and social wellbeing, play a big role in an individual's quality of life. These factors affect an individual's competence and independence, freedom of choice and perceived situational control, work, leisure activities, education and productivity, and eventually, of course, emotional wellbeing – including satisfaction, self-esteem, status, and respect (Felce & Perry, 1995). In fact, academic achievement, such as childhood reading and mathematical abilities, are strongly linked with socioeconomic status, but also academic motivation, educational duration, and intelligence later at mid-age (i.e., around 40 years) (Ritchie & Bates, 2013).

The impact of academic achievement also stretches beyond the individual level. At the societal level, learning difficulties contribute to a high rate of unemployment. This results in a lack of tax payments and, furthermore, the need to treat the consequences, such as increased rates of obesity and depressive symptoms in affected individuals. In addition, the consequences of learning impairments cause further costs due to increased crime rates and drug abuse, and for special educational training, to remediate these deleterious effects (Gross, Jones, Raby, & Tolfree, 2006; Gross, Hudson, & Price, 2009; Matza, Paramore, & Prasad, 2005). For these reasons, it is pressing to find successful, and more efficient interventions in order to ameliorate learning disabilities and childhood developmental disorders.

Some of the most common types of child behavioral and cognitive developmental impairments are dyslexia, developmental dyscalculia (DD), attention deficit hyperactivity disorder (ADHD), and autism. Each of these is associated with profound cognitive impairments in at least one major domain of cognitive processing, or even combinations of these. The DSM-V states that learning disabilities involve a central nervous system (CNS)-based disorder that affects reading, writing, and/or mathematics, leading to severe underachievement on common psychometric tests that assess the cognitive domain in question. This is despite having an average IQ. However, it also states that such learning disabilities are more complex and require the consideration and evaluation of a range of environmental influences in order to assess the exact problem (American Psychiatric Association, 2013; Gilger & Kaplan, 2001; Rimrodt & Lipkin, 2011). Accordingly, the exact diagnosis and boundaries between the different types of learning disabilities are difficult, and the large variety of symptoms require different approaches for coping (Stein et al., 2011). There is significant overlap and a variety of comorbidities among different types of disorders, such that cognitive domains (for instance, working memory) are impaired in several different disorders but the general manifestations of the cognitive problems differ (Gilger & Kaplan, 2001; Willcutt et al., 2013). Learning difficulties in developmental disorders are generally associated with abnormalities in the trajectory of brain development, both at the functional and the structural level – examples of which we will discuss in more detail later.

If successful cognitive training is applied during developmental periods of high neural plasticity – i.e., sensitive periods – atypical brain functioning and development can be partially redirected, promoting structural reorganization (Knudsen, 2004). Plasticity is the capacity of the brain to change with experience, and can involve changes in the size or the number of neurons or synapses, the organization or conductivity of white matter connections, or enhanced vascularization (Zatorre, Fields, & Johansen-Berg, 2012). Conventional intervention methods involve individualized cognitive training, including, for example, one-on-one instructions, as well as computerized learning games (see, for instance, Cohen Kadosh, Dowker, Heine, Kaufmann, & Kucian, 2013). There is also a variety of cognitive enhancement methods that are suggested to modulate brain functioning, such as medication (in the case of ADHD, Ritalin™ is the most commonly prescribed drug), yoga and mindfulness meditation, computer training games, and physical exercise (Dresler et al., 2013).

Unfortunately, training cannot always be applied during periods of maximum learning capacity (see Fig. 16.1). It is also important to note that each individual has his or her own limit for cognitive capacity, which can be reached, but not necessarily exceeded, using cognitive training (Jolles & Crone, 2012). As a consequence, the deficit persists and limits the individual's academic success further. Given the importance of an individual's personal circumstances, existing levels of capacity for brain plasticity, and past history of intervention attempts, we need to find more successful interventions that can cater to a variety of deficits. We therefore need to target the neural substrate directly, in addition to the moderate improvement gained from conventional cognitive methods, to overcome the individual barriers of brain plasticity. Non-invasive brain stimulation has been suggested to have the capacity to reopen sensitive periods in developmental disorders (see, for example, Krause & Cohen Kadosh, 2013), by "releasing the brakes" of cortical inhibition (Hensch & Bilimoria, 2012).

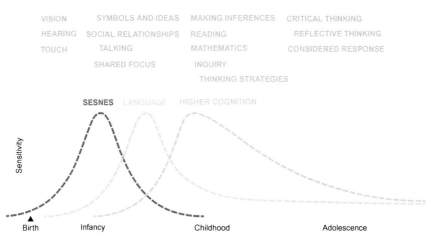

FIGURE 16.1   **The sensitive periods of the cortex for different cognitive functions peak at different time points in child development.** The curves symbolize the degree of sensitivity for learning; the flatter the curve, the less learning capacity the individual holds at a given stage of development. For example, senses develop early on during infancy, whereas language peaks later, and higher-level cognition matures throughout childhood. The differences in peaks must be taken into consideration for tES application. Parameters may need to be carefully adapted to a higher baseline capacity for plasticity, such that potential overstimulation can be avoided. *Figure reproduced from Bardin (2012), by permission from Macmillan Publishers Ltd.*

It has recently been suggested that we can use non-invasive brain stimulation techniques, such as transcranial electrical stimulation (tES), to improve developmental learning and/or behavioral deficits in children. Due to their cortical deficits, cognitive learning impairments that would benefit from such neuroenhancement techniques include, for example, dyslexia, DD, and ADHD (Cohen Kadosh, 2013; Krause & Cohen Kadosh, 2013; Vicario & Nitsche, 2013a). We suggest that a variety of developmental disorders, including autism, Down's syndrome, Williams syndrome, schizophrenia, and motor disorders involving cognitive deficits may also be improved by enhancing brain plasticity using tES in combination with successful behavioral training.

We will discuss these options in the light of implementing tES into pediatrics as a treatment and intervention method. In addition, we will provide an outlook on how tES could be used in a more practical environment: the school classroom. We will further outline important safety and ethical considerations, and present an overview of tES methodologies and its potential applications in this field of neurodevelopmental disorders. Finally, we will elaborate on the biological functioning of the techniques.

FORMS OF tES

As discussed in other chapters in this book (e.g., Chapter 2), tES is a relatively cheap, portable, and easy-to-administer non-invasive stimulation method that can be used to increase brain plasticity. Two or more electrodes are strapped onto the person's scalp surface by rubber bands, or are integrated into a whole-head cap, inducing a weak electrical current into the cortical surface under the electrodes (Im, Park, Shim, Chang, & Kim, 2012). The most frequently used current intensity in cognitive research settings is between 1 and 2 mA. The international or extended 10–20 system for EEG recording is used to localize the desired stimulation site on the individual head (Auvichayapat & Auvichayapat, 2011) (Figure 16.2). In the research setting, a sham condition can be applied, or even preprogrammed, which allows both subject- and experimenter-blinding. In the most commonly used sham condition, the stimulator delivers current for the initial 30 seconds but then ramps down and remains inactive while the participant is engaged in the training. Since skin sensations such as

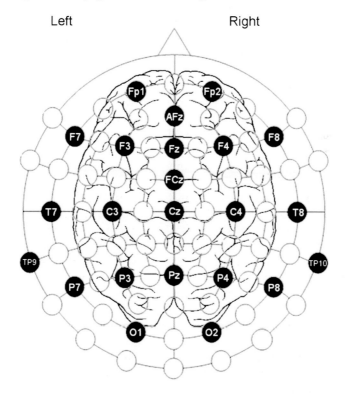

FIGURE 16.2   Electrode positions according to the international 10–20 system for EEG recording, based on the individual's head proportions.

tingling, itching, or a light stinging can occur during the initial period of the stimulation, the participant is unable to distinguish the real from the sham stimulation (Gandiga, Hummel, & Cohen, 2006).

Four major forms of tES can be distinguished: anodal and cathodal transcranial direct current stimulation (A-tDCS and C-tDCS, respectively), transcranial random noise stimulation (tRNS), and transcranial alternating current stimulation (tACS). In tDCS, the current flows from the anode to the cathode and thereby is likely to induce neuronal excitability under the anode (Nitsche & Paulus, 2001) and reductions in excitability under the cathode (Nitsche et al., 2003). In particular, A-tDCS usually leads to depolarization of neurons, whereas C-tDCS causes hyperpolarization, and therefore the inhibition of firing (Nitsche & Paulus, 2000). This means that activity can be enhanced in one area while reduced in another. An alternative approach is to stimulate (A-tDCS) one region and place the cathode over a neutral region on the scalp or the body, in order to affect only a single region. Such a neutral position can be the vertex or the forehead above the eyes, termed the supraorbital region (DaSilva, Volz, Bikson, & Fregni, 2011). Alternatively, some studies use the shoulder (deltoid muscle), the cheek (buccinator muscle), or the chin as a reference (Im et al., 2012). The choice of the placement of the reference electrode, however, affects the induced excitability under the stimulation electrode and may therefore have to be adjusted for the distance between the two electrodes (Moliadze, Antal, & Paulus, 2010).

tRNS induces current noise (e.g., high frequencies between 100 and 600 Hz) at a certain current intensity (e.g., 1.5 mA), and thereby enhances cortical excitability (Terney, Chaieb, Moliadze, Antal, & Paulus, 2008). The output from both electrodes is thus polarity unspecific, and the user can stimulate two regions at the same time – such as bilateral homologs in the frontal cortex. This method has been shown to have superior effects to A-tDCS and C-tDCS in certain cases, but not all (Fertonani, Pirulli, & Miniussi, 2011; Mulquiney, Hoy, Daskalakis, & Fitzgerald, 2011). tRNS has the advantage of causing less skin sensation, which allows more effective subject-blinding (Ambrus, Paulus, & Antal, 2010). The facilitatory processing effects of tRNS can be observed after just 10 minutes, and can have aftereffects of sustained excitability for at least 60 minutes post-stimulation after a single session (Terney et al., 2008). This electrical noise is hypothesized to increase excitability by a mechanism called "stochastic resonance," in which the noise increases the sensitivity to subthreshold stimuli on a background of ongoing neuronal activity, such that the firing threshold is reached more easily (Fertonani et al., 2011). The neuronal response to weak stimuli is therefore enhanced with the right amount of noise added. Excessive noise intensity however, can invert the enhancement effect and instead impair the neuron's capacity to detect signals amongst the noise (Moss, Ward, & Sannita, 2004).

The mechanism of tACS involves changes in the synchronicity of neurons by inducing sinusoidal wave-like currents in a fixed frequency range (for example, beta frequencies of 14–22 Hz), whereby different frequencies have different effects (Kanai, Chaieb, Antal, Walsh, & Paulus, 2008; Kanai, Paulus, & Walsh, 2010). The effect is based on alterations of the oscillatory pattern of the stimulated neurons (Thut, Miniussi, & Gross, 2012).

The advantage of tES over a similar non-invasive brain stimulation technique, called transcranial magnetic stimulation (TMS), is that it provides a better sham control. tES is not noticeably different from its sham condition (Gandiga et al., 2006), whereas TMS causes loud clicking noises for each administered pulse and, often, muscle twitches under the stimulation focus (Wagner, Valero-Cabre, & Pascual-Leone, 2007). Furthermore, the side effects that may easily identify real stimulation in tES studies are more flexibly manageable. For example, tACS can induce phosphenes, which in turn can be avoided with the right choice of stimulation parameters (for discussion, see Davis, Gold, Pascual-Leone, & Bracewell, 2013).

Previously, an advantage of TMS has been the increased stimulation focality, since electrode sizes for tES commonly start at a surface area of 4×4 cm. However, with the development of high-definition tDCS (HD-tDCS) it is now also possible to achieve more focal effects using tES (Datta, Elwassif, Battaglia, & Bikson, 2008). The disadvantage of this form is that expensive neuronavigation equipment may become necessary in order to localize the exact target stimulation site in each individual. In cases where there is a very focally restrained neurological deficit, this will be beneficial. Aside from the technical flexibility in tES usage, the choice of the stimulation region and the training applied during the sessions are crucial for the outcome of the intervention. We will therefore discuss some of the current applications and issues regarding such choices.

LEARNING AND tES

For successful cognitive processing, a multitude of cognitive subfunctions subserved by different brain areas are required to interact efficiently in order to produce meaningful output. The interaction between brain areas is therefore more important for the behavioral outcome than the efficient processing of a single brain region (Spencer-Smith & Anderson, 2009). Furthermore, the balance between cortical excitation and inhibition (E/I balance) is crucial for the capacity for plastic changes in synaptic connections, and therefore also determines the efficiency of information transfer in the brain (Turrigiano & Nelson, 2000). tES has the potential to modulate activity in whole networks rather than just a single region, and is thought to modulate different brain mechanisms, including E/I (Krause, Marquez-Ruiz, & Cohen Kadosh 2013; Polania, Paulus, Antal, & Nitsche, 2011). These features are highly useful, given the complexity of abnormalities observed in individuals with learning difficulties, and in order to enhance plasticity and long-term cortical reorganization. Even though in some cases the original source area in the deficient brain circuit might not be accessible to tES (e.g., subcortical regions, such as the thalamus), there is evidence that stimulation of later circuit areas in the processing chain can affect and improve the behavioral or cognitive outcome, even for extended periods of time (Benninger et al., 2010). Ideally, the stimulation will modify the whole network to adapt and function more efficiently.

Long-term potentiation (LTP) refers to the prolonged and enhanced activity between neurons that fire together in a Hebbian fashion. The formation of LTP is crucial for information storage (Turrigiano & Nelson, 2000), and is capable of inducing cortical reorganization (Hess & Donoghue, 1994). LTP only occurs when neurons receive sufficient activation, which is modulated by the excitatory neurotransmitter glutamate (Collingridge & Bliss, 1987). The inhibitory neurotransmitter gamma-aminobutyric acid (GABA) also plays an important role in LTP. GABAergic inhibition is viewed as a gatekeeper for LTP and plasticity processes, and its reduction can contribute to activity-dependent cortical reorganization (Hess & Donoghue, 1994). For example, a decrease in GABAergic inhibition is accompanied by a facilitation in practice-based learning, whereas an increase in GABA is associated with reduced learning effects (Floyer-Lea, Wylezinska, Kincses, & Matthews, 2006; Ziemann, Muellbacher, Hallett, & Cohen, 2001). The change in learning also varies with the degree of change in GABA (Stagg, Bachtiar, & Johansen-Berg, 2011). These neural learning-related functional processes are crucial to those with atypical cortical development. Regional levels of GABA and glutamate – i.e., cortical inhibition and excitation – can be artificially modulated using tES (Clark, Coffman, Trumbo, & Gasparovic, 2011; Stagg et al., 2009). tES can therefore be used to support the restoration of a network in order for it to become more efficient. This also demonstrates the importance of choosing the appropriate training task, as the brain is still required to make the effort to learn. Simultaneously, tES acts as a supporting facilitator and is crucial for the induction of change through the removing of inhibitory restraints (or decreasing facilitation) of the cortex. In the following sections, we will describe some of the methodological and parameter options that have been explored in tES research on cognitive training.

ENHANCING COGNITIVE ABILITIES WITH tES

A wide range of cognitive abilities, but also motor and perceptual functions, have been targeted using different tES methods in adults. Some of the most relevant cognitive abilities affected by childhood atypical development are working memory, filtering of irrelevant information, attentional processes, reading, speech production, numerical and arithmetic abilities, and also motor learning and visual perception or discrimination (for examples, see Table 16.1). In tES research, experimental tasks that target a highly specific aspect of a cognitive domain are typically used. The cognitive domains targeted are thereby known to be associated with metabolic activity in certain brain areas that are accessible to the stimulation. For example, numerical tasks can range from spatial numerical skills over subitizing or comparing quantities, to counting and computing, which all involve different brain areas to different degrees (Piazza, Mechelli, Butterworth, & Price, 2002). Furthermore, similar types of tasks may engage different brain areas depending on the strategy an individual uses to solve a given problem (Delazer et al., 2005; Rivera, Reiss, Eckert, & Menon, 2005). For example, while some people solve an arithmetic problem by performing the actual computation, another individual might retrieve certain substeps of the calculation from memory. It is therefore important for the optimization of intervention paradigms to combine tES with tasks that tap into the cognitive domain of interest. Importantly, the outcomes should have a meaningful impact on real-life numerical abilities.

A short-term cognitive improvement is of little value in clinical or school settings. What is needed instead is an intervention method that allows for long-term enhancement of cognitive abilities. In addition, it must be noted that the majority of research studies report response times and accuracy separately, and often it is response times in the order of milliseconds that improve, but not necessarily accuracy (see Pascual-Leone, Horvath, & Robertson, 2012). Therefore, depending on the desired outcomes, experimenters should be critical when integrating the latest scientific evidence into the design of more effective intervention programs. Moreover, in the case of a specific learning difficulty – for example, mathematical learning difficulty – it is important to understand that there is often a spectrum of severity, and individuals might differ in their impairments and/or have other co-morbidities, such as ADHD or dyslexia. Therefore, in order to enable successful training with meaningful outcomes for a given individual, these factors should be taken into consideration when designing an intervention. Ideally this will be achieved with the consultation of professionals (e.g., occupational therapists or teachers) who have experience with the previous treatment and impairments of the individual.

Furthermore, in order to achieve the optimal outcome for each individual, important tES methodological considerations involve the number of sessions and intersession intervals, the stimulation parameters (type, polarization, duration, intensity, electrode size, shape and position, frequency if applicable). This is because the resulting dosage and the electric

TABLE 16.1   Common Electrode Positions in Current Brain Stimulation Paradigms*

Electrode Position	Function	Brain Area Targeted	Stimulation	Reference(s)
LANGUAGE				
F3	Vocabulary and syntax	Left DLPFC	A-tDCS (reference contralateral supraorbital)	(Schneider & Hopp, 2011)
FC5	Speech, naming	Left inferior frontal gyrus (IFG)	A-tDCS (reference contralateral supraorbital)	(Holland et al., 2011)
CP5	Word retrieval	Superior temporal gyrus (STG; Wernicke's area)	A-tDCS (reference contralateral supraorbital)	(Fiori et al., 2011)
CP5	Associative language learning	Left posterior perisylvian area (Wernicke's)	A-tDCS (reference contralateral supraorbital)	(Floel, Rosser, Michka, Knecht, & Breitenstein, 2008)
CP5–CP6	Speech	Left superior temporal gyrus (STG; Wernicke's area)	Left-anodal, right-cathodal	(You, Kim, Chun, Jung, & Park, 2011)
T7/TP7–T8/ TP8 (extended 10–20 system)	Word reading efficiency	Left posterior temporal cortex	Left-anodal, right-cathodal	(Turkeltaub et al., 2012)
MEMORY				
P3–T5; P6–T4	Word recognition memory and visual attention	Bilateral temporoparietal junctions	A-tDCS	(Ferrucci et al., 2008)
T3–T4	Visual recognition memory	Bilateral temporal lobes	A-tDCS (external reference right deltoid muscle)	(Boggio et al., 2012)
WORKING MEMORY				
F3	3-back task	Left DLPFC	A-tDCS (reference contralateral supraorbital)	(Ohn et al., 2008; Teo, Hoy, Daskalakis, & Fitzgerald, 2011)

TABLE 16.1 Common Electrode Positions in Current Brain Stimulation Paradigms—cont'd

Electrode Position	Function	Brain Area Targeted	Stimulation	Reference(s)
F3	2-back task	Left DLPFC	A-tDCS (reference contralateral supraorbital)	(Mulquiney et al., 2011)
P3–P4	1- and 2-back span task	Posterior parietal cortex	Interaction between task and condition (RALC vs LARC)	(Sandrini, Fertonani, Cohen, & Miniussi, 2012)
P4	Impaired working memory recognition	Left parietal cortex	C-tDCS (reference contralateral cheek)	(Berryhill, Wencil, Branch Coslett, & Olson, 2010)
NUMERICAL ABILITIES				
F3–F4	Arithmetic learning, numerical automaticity	DLPFC	Left-anodal, right-cathodal	(Iuculano & Cohen Kadosh, 2013)
F3–F4	Arithmetic learning	DLPFC	TRNS to bilateral DLPFCs	(Snowball et al., 2013)
P3–P4	Basic numerical skills, numerical learning	Parietal cortex	Left-anodal, right-cathodal	(Iuculano & Cohen Kadosh, 2013)
P3–P4	Basic numerical skills, numerical learning	Parietal cortex	Right-anodal, left-cathodal	(Cohen Kadosh, Soskic, Iuculano, Kanai, & Walsh, 2010)
P3	Mental arithmetic	Left intraparietal sulcus (IPS)	A-tDCS (reference contralateral supraorbital)	(Hauser, Rotzer, Grabner, Merillat, & Jancke, 2013)
P3–P4	Approximate number sense (ANS)	Bilateral parietal lobes	Bilateral tRNS	(Cappelletti et al., 2013)
ATTENTION				
T4/Fz–F8/Cz	Stop-signal task	Right inferior frontal gyrus	A-tDCS (reference contralateral supraorbital)	(Ditye, Jacobson, Walsh, & Lavidor, 2012)

Continued

TABLE 16.1   Common Electrode Positions in Current Brain Stimulation Paradigms—cont'd

Electrode Position	Function	Brain Area Targeted	Stimulation	Reference(s)
P4	Flanker task	Left posterior parietal cortex	C-tDCS to PPC (reference contralateral supraorbital)	(Weiss & Lavidor, 2012)
EXECUTIVE PLANNING				
F3	Tower of London task	Left DLPFC	A-tDCS (reference contralateral supraorbital)	(Dockery, Hueckel-Weng, Birbaumer, & Plewnia, 2009)
INTELLIGENCE				
F3	Logical reasoning	Left middle frontal gyrus (MFG)	5-Hz tACS (reference vertex)	(Santarnecchi et al., 2013)
T3 (estimated location)	Logical problem solving	Right anterior temporal lobe	A-tDCS (cathode on left anterior temporal lobe)	(Chi & Snyder, 2012)

Examples of the choice of electrode positions for different types of cognitive tasks that are associated with certain cognitive regions. Note the variety of different cognitive tasks used for similar brain areas.

field induced in the cortex depend on these and related parameters (Guleyupoglu, Schestatsky, Edwards, Fregni, & Bikson, 2013; Peterchev et al., 2012). It is important to consider that tDCS-induced effects are also affected by individual differences, such as baseline performance, previous educational background, and even personality (see, for example, Berryhill & Jones, 2012; Pena-Gomez, Vidal-Pineiro, Clemente, Pascual-Leone, & Bartres-Faz, 2011; Tseng et al., 2012).

IMPROVING THE DEFICITS: EXAMPLES FOR LEARNING DEFICITS

Developmental cognitive difficulties are associated with atypical structural and functional patterns in the brains of the affected children, compared to typically developing children. This can be demonstrated, for instance in DD (Kucian et al., 2006; Price, Holloway, Rasanen, Vesterinen, & Ansari, 2007; Rykhlevskaia, Uddin, Kondos, & Menon, 2009), dyslexia (Stein & Walsh, 1997; Temple et al., 2003), and ADHD (Shaw et al., 2012). The neurodevelopmental deficits in some of these developmental disorders are very complex. We will therefore provide some simple results from different meta-analyses based on brain-imaging studies as examples of areas where target-specific tES intervention can be planned and applied.

Developmental Dyscalculia

Developmental dyscalculia refers to the severe difficulty in manipulating numerical information and performing arithmetic operations, which cannot otherwise be explained by cognitive dysfunctions, such as in intelligence, reading, or attention (Butterworth, Varma, & Laurillard, 2011). The usual prevalence of 6–7% (Butterworth et al., 2011) can rise to 26%, when taking into account the existence of several other weaker forms of arithmetic difficulties (Gross-Tsur, Manor, & Shalev, 1996). Individuals with DD usually have a poor prognosis for future employment and socio-economic status, unless a successful intervention technique can be applied to enhance their performance in the deficient modality (Gabrieli, 2009; Rimrodt & Lipkin, 2011; Stein et al., 2011). tES can be applied to impaired brain areas in order to enhance neural activation during cognitive (i.e., maths or reading) training. It is aimed to restore the abnormalities in structure and functioning to a normalized level, as it can lead to effective and long-lasting intervention effects, and can thereby possibly alter atypical development to typical development if intervention occurs early enough.

The core regions that are associated with DD consist of a wide fronto-parieto-occipital network, with structural abnormalities such as reduced gray matter in bilateral prefrontal and parietal areas, white matter reductions in right temporo-parietal networks, but also decreased functional activation in bilateral intraparietal sulci (IPS) in children during arithmetic tasks (Kucian et al., 2006; Mussolin et al., 2010; Price et al., 2007; Rykhlevskaia et al., 2009). The most consistent functional findings in DD children compared to typically developing children also involve reductions or increases in brain activity in multiple regions compared to typically developing children (Kaufmann, Wood, Rubinsten, & Henik, 2011; see also Table 16.2).

Using tES, the perspective is to enhance excitability in such underactivated areas, while suppressing excitability (i.e., inhibiting) in hyperactive areas. The choice of polarity over the stimulated region depends on the brain state of the receiver, and needs to complement the training methods applied. For example, if a child has very pronounced problems with approximate calculation, the area associated with reduced activity would be the left IPS and the left inferior frontal gyrus (IFG) (Kucian et al., 2006). One of these regions should be chosen as the stimulation site where either anodal tDCS or tRNS can be applied to enhance cortical excitability. Since

TABLE 16.2 Suggested Electrode Positions for Developmental Dyscalculia (DD) According to Neurodevelopmental Deficits*

Underactivation	Overactivation	Electrode Position
Left precuneus		C3–P3
Left IPS		P3
Right inferior parietal lobe		TP4
Left paracentral frontal lobe		C3
Left superior frontal gyrus		F3
Right middle frontal gyrus	Right superior frontal	F4
Left fusiform gyrus		T3
	Postcentral gyri	C3–P3, C4–P4
	Bilateral inferior parietal lobes (including right supramarginal gyrus)	TP3–4
	Paracentral frontal lobes	FCz, Cz

*Brain areas of atypical activation in developmental dyscalculia (DD), according to a meta-analysis of 19 functional MRI papers (Kaufmann et al., 2011). The right column shows approximate electrode positions according to the original 10–20 system for EEG recording (see Homan, Herman, & Purdy, 1987, for these areas to be stimulated by tES). Areas of underactivation are expected to benefit from excitatory stimulation (e.g., anodal tDCS or tRNS), whereas areas of overactivation require inhibitory cathodal tDCS. Electrode positions in the original 10–20 system are called T3, T4, T5, and T6, but have been relabeled as T7, T8, P7, and P8, respectively, in the extended 10–20 system. Measuring the proportions of the head surface provides approximations for the exact location of a cortical area, but since the electrodes are relatively large (typically 16–35 cm²), the localization in a millimeter range is abundant.

the atypical activity pattern in this case is mainly restricted to unilateral areas, anodal stimulation to these regions would be possible, with the reference electrode on the contralateral supraorbital area (above the right eye). However, it can be argued that reducing excitability in the same region of the contralateral hemisphere may be beneficial (see Chapter 12). It is therefore a matter of the specific hypothesis underlying the intervention. tRNS would be most applicable in cases where two brain regions, such as bilateral areas, are the stimulation targets (Snowball et al., 2013). The current level of the developmental status of the brain for a given task must be thoroughly assessed for each individual in order to define the appropriate stimulation site. This is crucial especially for children, whose regional recruitment of neural networks differs and changes throughout development (Cohen Kadosh, 2011; Johnson, 2011).

It is important to note here that cognitive loss similar to that observed in developmental disorders (such as DD) might occur through brain damage. For example, acalculia is comparable to DD but is acquired through neurological damage. Acalculia often comes with various comorbidities and deficits in other cognitive domains, as well as neurodegenerative diseases (Boller & Grafman, 1983). The same applies to the other way around: although an intervention design leads to beneficial effects of tES, using the same paradigm in DD may not lead to the same effects. The same applies to other cognitive deficits caused by either brain damage or neurodevelopmental disorders. Even though the symptoms can be similar in both cases, the neurological deficit may be different and will therefore interact differently with tES. This is because various factors, such as the type of damage and its occurrence as a function of age, are different. For example, the flow of the induced current of the stimulation applied to a damaged area is relatively unpredictable, as different tissue types have different properties (Datta, Baker, Bikson, & Fridriksson, 2011; see also Chapter 4).

Dyslexia

Dyslexia has a similar prevalence to dyscalculia and denotes severe difficulties in reading and text comprehension, despite an average IQ (Shaywitz, 2003). Individuals with dyslexia have deficits in fast temporal processing of speech and visual attention, which has been previously associated with an impairment in the magnocellular visual pathway (Stein & Walsh, 1997). Dyslexia has also been associated with reduced levels of activation in temporo-parietal areas, which are generally related to phonological processing and are therefore essential to speech and reading (Gabrieli, 2009; Temple et al., 2003). Reductions in brain activity were found in, for example, the middle temporal gyrus and the inferior and superior temporal gyri, as well as the middle occipital gyrus, compared to normal readers in a study using positron emission tomography (PET) (Paulesu et al., 2001). However, there were no over activations in dyslexic participants compared to control readers. An interesting finding was that, despite investigating groups with different native languages in their respective countries (English, French, and Italian), the pattern of brain activity was slightly different across the groups. The authors interpreted this as a result of different orthographies in the languages, leading to differences in terms of reading difficulty and performance. Furthermore, the observed areas of under-activation in the same subjects were also associated with reduced gray matter volumes, particularly in the inferior temporal cortex (Silani et al., 2005). In this area, the degree of reading impairment was significantly correlated with gray matter volume, such that inferior performance corresponded to higher gray matter density.

Most importantly, however, decreases in gray matter density were observed in the inferior frontal gyrus (IFG) and the middle temporal gyrus, the latter of which was directly adjacent to an area of increased gray matter density – the middle posterior temporal gyrus. These results have important implications for the use of tES. First of all, due to the potential for slight anatomical differences in reading disabilities across languages, the electrode placements have to be determined for each language group separately. The tES training and stimulation design should therefore also be individually adapted, such that the stimulation affects the specific impairment. Secondly, potentially hypoactive or underdeveloped brain areas may lie very close to hyperactive areas, such that larger electrodes may stimulate an area that would preferably be inhibited. Electrode size and positioning must therefore be carefully considered and based on the individual functional anatomy, in order to avoid accidental excitation or suppression of unintended areas. Lastly, the example of the cross-cultural reading study demonstrates that consistently reduced brain activity can largely co-occur with reduced gray matter volume in poor readers compared to normal readers. The subsequent decision to apply excitatory stimulation (e.g., A-tDCS or tRNS) is then made relatively simple and straightforward. The induction of excitability and enhancement of plasticity and LTP would be ideal in this case. However, we should be cautious not to generalize from this to other examples. Different analysis methods and task assessments may affect the interpretation of findings. This is similar in this case, where the stimulation design should be chosen based on the individual's exact reading problem and strong evidence on the associated brain functioning. Experimental data therefore always need to be carefully reviewed to establish the relationship between tasks, activation, and structural abnormalities in learning impairments, and to design a successful intervention strategy.

Some tES studies have successfully improved reading performance by stimulating left temporal areas (see, for example, Turkeltaub et al., 2012), but most studies so far have focused on language areas such as Broca's and Wernicke's areas, which are core regions in language production and reading abilities, among others (e.g., Cattaneo, Pisoni, & Papagno, 2011).

Attention Deficit Hyperactivity Disorder (ADHD)

The economic costs of the consequences of ADHD are particularly high, as they involve medical costs, including the treatment of psychiatric and medical comorbidities, as well as high levels of criminality and unemployment (Matza et al., 2005). tES is therefore an attractive potential intervention technique to alleviate some of the behavioral and cognitive problems associated with the disorder. In ADHD, the pattern of atypical brain development is complex and involves a variety of cortical and subcortical areas. Symptoms of impulsivity and attentional deficits are accompanied by delayed cortical maturation in right and, to a lesser degree, left prefrontal cortices (PFCs) (see, for example, Shaw et al., 2012). Underdevelopment of the right PFC is thought to cause ADHD-related deficits in response inhibition, whereas the DLPFC is responsible for the observed reductions in, for instance, divided attention, both of which are impaired in ADHD (e.g., Pasini, Paloscia, Alessandrelli, Porfirio, & Curatolo, 2007).

Krain and Castellanos (2006) discussed a range of available evidence, but also inconsistencies, for globally reduced brain volume, including gray (and white) matter reductions in the basal ganglia, the frontal cortex, and the cerebellum. Non-invasive stimulation of deep brain structures, such as the basal ganglia, is challenging at the moment, as there is no fixed protocol to reach such structures effectively. The effects of tES on the cerebellum are currently less clearly understood than on neocortical areas, but have already been shown to affect cognition, motor performance, and procedural learning (for a discussion, see Ferrucci & Priori, 2014) and may therefore improve ADHD deficits. In contrast, prefrontal areas are easily accessible with tES, and a wider range of experimental evidence regarding its effects on higher-level cognition is available that is relevant to ADHD intervention (see, for instance, Ditye et al., 2012; Hsu et al., 2011; Weiss & Lavidor, 2012). As demonstrated through magnetic resonance spectroscopy (MRS) measures of cortical glutamate and GABA, individuals with ADHD also show regional abnormalities in their levels of cortical excitation and inhibition, which have been related to their behavioral and cognitive symptoms (Arcos-Burgos et al., 2012; Carrey, MacMaster, Gaudet, & Schmidt, 2007; Edden, Crocetti, Zhu, Gilbert, & Mostofsky, 2012). It is therefore most practical to attempt to reduce the behavioral and cognitive disinhibition by modulating prefrontal and motor cortex excitability (Ditye et al., 2012; Jacobson, Ezra, Berger, & Lavidor, 2012). With the advancement of non-invasive brain stimulation techniques, we will hopefully be able to directly affect deeper brain structures in the future (see Chapter 19).

THE YOUNG AND PLASTIC BRAIN

Given the current uncertainty about the effects of tES on the developing brain, one might wonder why we should not wait until the child has reached an age at which stimulation is predictable and safe. Aside from the cumulative negative effect that learning disabilities have on the child's life, the other main reason for such intervention is the increased potential for plastic changes during child development. Animal research has shown that silent synapses in certain circuits of the developing rat brain can be made functional by the induction of LTP (Feldman, Nicoll, & Malenka, 1999). Furthermore, certain mechanisms of receptor functioning promote the interaction between LTP and LTD and thereby regulate experience-dependent changes in the circuits. However, these mechanisms decrease after the end of the sensitive period (Crair & Malenka, 1995). The effects of plasticity may therefore originate from the activation of silent synapses, the efficiency of which is subsequently regulated by LTP and LTD, causing plastic experience-dependent changes (Feldman et al., 1999). With development and maturation the cortical layer becomes thinner, such that cortical connections are relatively stable and less prone to flexible changes (Gogtay et al., 2004; Knudsen, 2004).

During a sensitive period, glutamatergic activity is crucial for the induction of cortical plasticity and reorganization (Schlaggar, Fox, & O'Leary, 1993). tES is therefore likely to support neural activity in networks that show deficient excitability. Such sensitive periods are also marked by an enhanced excitation/inhibition (E/I) balance, which can be modulated artificially even outside these periods. This can be achieved using a variety of different means, including neuromodulatory medication or certain kinds of training and enrichment, that can modify the E/I balance to allow higher levels of plasticity (Bavelier, Levi, Li, Dan, & Hensch, 2010). tES, as the current evidence demonstrates, has the potential to modulate this E/I balance during a later period, where there is normally a relatively high degree of stability in cortical synapses. This may be beneficial in adults, who have reached a relatively stable synaptic system, but also in children with atypical development, who have more stable or limited capacity for plasticity in critical brain regions (see Figs 16.1, 16.3). It is also important to note that such a trajectory in brain organization is linked to different domains of cognition that peak at different stages of child development in terms of the opening and closing times of their sensitive period (see Bardin 2012; McCain, Mustard, & McCuaig, 2011).

A DREAM COME TRUE: tES IN THE CLASSROOM?

At the moment, applying tES in the real classroom is an idea that requires further development. It might be more cumbersome to use it in groups where electrodes need to be fitted on each subject, and from the ethical point of view it might also cause discomfort or anxiety, especially in the case of children. New developments, such as wireless electrical stimulators (e.g. Starstim Neuroelectrics® stimulator (Barcelona, Spain) would make it possible to apply non-invasive electrical brain stimulation in the real-life classroom setting, where it is most relevant for real-life application. Compared to highly-controlled research settings, where participants mostly perform computer or paper-and-pencil tasks, wireless

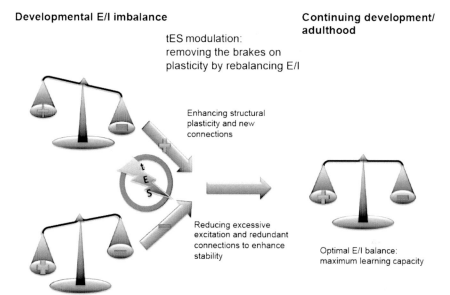

Developmental E/I imbalance

Continuing development/ adulthood

tES modulation: removing the brakes on plasticity by rebalancing E/I

Enhancing structural plasticity and new connections

t E S

Reducing excessive excitation and redundant connections to enhance stability

Optimal E/I balance: maximum learning capacity

FIGURE 16.3   tES is aimed to increase inhibition or reduce excitation during atypical brain development. Targeted tES thereby modulates the E/I balance and removes the brakes on learning and normal brain development, so that the rebalanced E/I system allows for maximal learning and consolidation throughout further development. The eventual brain dynamics can become more efficient due to tES intervention (see also Bavelier et al., 2010).

tES can be applied while children learn through educational instructions and explanations. A possibility is to even use the stimulation in a group of children, which may provide a more supportive environment under close attention of expert educators.

Using a wireless stimulator, the individual wears a head cap similar to a rugby cap (which can also be tailored to fit the child's personal taste) onto which the electrodes are mounted. The receiver can therefore move around freely in space and is not restrained by the wires. For example, this allows a child in the classroom to use the blackboard in front of the class. In addition, the cap ascertains that the electrodes are held in place and will not slip or lose connection to the scalp. It is more useful to apply the stimulation in an environment where the learning occurs directly, in order to enhance the ability to integrate new information. Depending on the desired outcome, simultaneous tES and training can be individually adapted by the administrator, and can be flexibly adjusted in terms of the content and the complexity of the task material. Depending on the desired outcome, the administrator can therefore determine whether to target global or more specialized cognitive functions. This type of intervention also minimizes the number of staff necessary for successful training, and the time needed to achieve the desired outcome. Depending on the type and intensity of the stimulation, the child might not even notice when the stimulation starts and therefore should not be affected by any discomfort (Looi and colleagues, personal communication). Overall, optimizing the use of tES by combining it with appropriate learning material offers the possibility for more effective learning, especially for those with learning difficulties.

POTENTIAL RISKS AND ETHICAL CONSIDERATIONS

The research using tES in child populations is currently extremely limited, and therefore definitive predictions about the tolerability of tES cannot be made until the field gains more experience (Kessler et al., 2013; Looi & Cohen Kadosh, personal communication). It is important to consider that, due to the smaller head size, the same dosage of tES is likely to have a more intensive effect on a child's brain than on an adult brain (Minhas, Bikson, Woods, Rosen, & Kessler, 2012). Some early studies, however, have indicated that young children from the age of 5 years onwards tolerate the stimulation well, even at higher intensities of 2 mA. Only minor side effects have been observed, such as tingling, itching, and mood changes (Andrade et al., 2013; Mattai et al., 2011; Schneider & Hopp, 2011). The current is typically ramped up and ramped down at the end of the stimulation period in order to increase tolerability or to avoid irritation, whereby the skin can gradually accommodate the change in current flow (Guleyupoglu et al., 2013).

In addition to concerns about tolerability, there is also a risk of cumulative effects of the stimulation – for example, daily administration of tDCS leads to higher cortical excitability than when the stimulation is applied every other day (Alonzo, Brassil, Taylor, Martin, & Loo, 2012). The duration of aftereffects is crucial for the purpose of rehabilitation and treatment, and the duration of the stimulation itself, as well as intersession intervals, affects the duration of such aftereffects (Monte-Silva, Kuo, Liebetanz, Paulus, & Nitsche, 2010). Individuals with a personal or family history of seizures should generally be excluded from tES studies or treatments. This is important because the enhancement in cortical excitability may increase the risk of seizures. It should be noted, however, that seizure thresholds could be experimentally down-modulated in epileptic children using C-tDCS (for a brief discussion, see Vicario & Nitsche, 2013b). In addition, patients with skull traumas or metal fragments stuck in their head area are at risk of side effects, due to the unpredictability of current flow. Similarly, neuro-active drugs might act on cortical excitability. In our opinion, for the current purpose of cognitive enhancement, individuals using any kind of medication should be excluded to avoid potential interactions with the stimulation, and in order to prevent cumulative effects of the stimulation (see Chapter 6). Moreover, it should be ascertained that if individuals have participated in any other brain stimulation research or treatment, the wash-out period is sufficiently long (Davis et al., 2013).

As Pascual-Leone and colleagues stated, "A system capable of such flexible reorganization harbors the risk of unwanted change" (Pascual-Leone, Amedi, Fregni, & Merabet, 2005). They warned of the consequences caused by practice or restraint, as well as by non-invasive brain stimulation to enhance neuroplasticity. Their warning is especially relevant during developmental periods of high levels of plasticity, as the effect and consequences of shaping a wrong pathway of synaptic connections can be difficult or impossible to reverse (Knudsen, 2004). Cognitive tES training effects in adults have been observed up to 6 months later (Cohen Kadosh et al., 2010; Snowball et al., 2013), which is highly advantageous for positive changes in behavior and cognition, but deleterious if the outcome is negative. As the long-term effects of tES are currently unclear in child populations, future studies should include follow-up assessments to monitor the longevity of tES-induced effects, and other potential side effects. It is important that researchers consider the potential consequences and adapt their research techniques to modulate brain plasticity efficiently and safely, with limited or no physical or psychological side effects.

When considering neural changes induced by tES, it is not only the intra-regional balance between excitation and inhibition that plays an important role in the behavioral outcome, but also interhemispheric and inter-regional connections, and interactions of excitation and inhibition (Pascual-Leone et al., 2005). For example, in a tDCS study in which subjects received stimulation either to their DLPFCs or their posterior parietal cortices, it was demonstrated that, for each region, certain aspects of numerical learning and competence were enhanced while others were compromised (Iuculano & Cohen Kadosh, 2013). This illustrates how unpredictable changes in plasticity can be. One region may become functionally stronger but consequently exhibit inhibitory effects on other regions, or might require more resources, compromising other brain regions, which is observable in behavioral deterioration (Brem, Fried, Horvath, Robertson, & Pascual-Leone, 2014; Pascual-Leone et al., 2012; see also Chapter 19). These consequences that could affect targeted and/or untargeted behavior must be avoided and careful monitoring carried out during periods of treatment, such that it can be terminated if necessary. In this respect, it is of great importance to prevent parents or adults from purchasing their own stimulators and trying out their own intervention ideas at home (for a more detailed discussion on the risks, see Cohen Kadosh, Levy, O'Shea, Shea, & Savulescu, 2012, and Chapter 3).

Similar to the issue of inter-regional effects of tES is the interpretation of the initial neural impairment. While some atypical patterns of brain functioning (in both function and structure) are indicative of the original cognitive impairments, mechanisms compensating for these symptoms may be present (see, for example, Fassbender & Schweitzer, 2006). These in turn are also associated with specific atypical patterns in the brain and can easily be mistaken for a to-be-stimulated brain area. Careful interpretation of the brain-deficit and brain-compensatory mechanisms for the specific cognitive deficit is therefore necessary to avoid the induction of maladaptive plasticity.

It is also important to note that brain areas mature at different speeds, and their peaks for plasticity occur at different time points during development (see Fig. 16.1). The cortex develops in a back-to-front fashion, in which simpler sensory areas mature first, followed by more complex processing and, eventually, higher cognitive abilities associated with prefrontal areas (Gogtay et al., 2004).

In terms of the safety and comfort of using tES, it is crucial to consider risks such as the induction of seizures, unwanted long-term cognitive changes, irritation or damage of the tissue, or feelings of discomfort during stimulation. The potential benefits in many cases might outweigh the low probability of these risks if safety guidelines are followed carefully (see also Chapter 18). Considering that the small cost of discomfort during stimulation (e.g., tingling or itching) might be returned with better future prospects, we suggest that tES should be tested as an intervention method in child populations with learning disabilities and behavioral disorders.

CONCLUSION

tES is a relatively new and promising tool that has the potential to reduce learning and behavioral deficits in adults, and to ameliorate developmental disorders. The adult experimental literature has grown large enough to provide promising results for a large variety of cognitive functions and behavioral improvements (see Chapters 12–15). With further refinements and more targeted application to child populations, tES is likely to redirect some of the developmental brain deficits during childhood and thereby benefit the child on a long-term basis. Similar to every novel method, tES-induced effects in such populations need to be established and carefully monitored in order to prevent accidental reductions in performance (Krause et al., 2013). For safety reasons, over-motivated parents should be educated on the infancy of this method and its potential negative consequences, to avoid misuse. We think that with adequate and careful safety considerations, tES is a promising method to modulate deficits in neural processing and therefore improve learning and behavioral deficits in both children and adults.

Acknowledgements

RCK is funded by the Wellcome Trust (WT 88378) and BK by the Economic and Social Research Council, the Deutscher Akademischer Austauschdienst (DAAD), and the Studienstiftung des Deutschen Volkes. We thank Michael Clayton for his comments.

References

Alonzo, A., Brassil, J., Taylor, J. L., Martin, D., & Loo, C. K. (2012). Daily transcranial direct current stimulation (tDCS) leads to greater increases in cortical excitability than second daily transcranial direct current stimulation. *Brain Stimulation, 5*(3), 208–213.

Ambrus, G. G., Paulus, W., & Antal, A. (2010). Cutaneous perception thresholds of electrical stimulation methods: Comparison of tDCS and tRNS. *Clinical Neurophysiology, 121*(11), 1908–1914.

American Psychiatric Association. (2013). *Diagnostic and statistical manual of mental disorders* (5th ed.). Arlington, VA: American Psychiatric Association.

Andrade, A. C., Magnavita, G. M., Allegro, J. V., Neto, C. E., Lucena, R. D., & Fregni, F. (2013). Feasibility of transcranial direct current stimulation use in children aged 5 to 12 years. *Journal of Child Neurology*, 8 September (epub ahead of print).

Arcos-Burgos, M., Londono, A. C., Pineda, D. A., Lopera, F., Palacio, J. D., Arbelaez, A., et al. (2012). Analysis of brain metabolism by proton magnetic resonance spectroscopy (1H-MRS) in attention deficit/hyperactivity disorder suggests a generalized differential ontogenic pattern from controls. *Attention Deficit and Hyperactivity Disorders, 4*(4), 205–212.

Auvichayapat, P., & Auvichayapat, N. (2011). Basic knowledge of transcranial direct current stimulation. *Journal of the Medical Association of Thailand, 94*(4), 518–527.

Bardin, J. (2012). Neurodevelopment: Unlocking the brain. *Nature, 487*(7405), 24–26.

Bavelier, D., Levi, D. M., Li, R. W., Dan, Y., & Hensch, T. K. (2010). Removing brakes on adult brain plasticity: From molecular to behavioral interventions. *The Journal of Neuroscience, 30* (45), 14964–14971.

Benninger, D. H., Lomarev, M., Lopez, G., Wassermann, E. M., Li, X., Considine, E., et al. (2010). Transcranial direct current stimulation for the treatment of Parkinson's disease. *Journal of Neurology, Neurosurgery, and Psychiatry, 81*(10), 1105–1111.

Berryhill, M. E., & Jones, K. T. (2012). tDCS selectively improves working memory in older adults with more education. *Neuroscience Letters, 521*(2), 148–151.

Berryhill, M. E., Wencil, E. B., Branch Coslett, H., & Olson, I. R. (2010). A selective working memory impairment after transcranial direct current stimulation to the right parietal lobe. *Neuroscience Letters, 479*(3), 312–316.

Boggio, P. S., Ferrucci, R., Mameli, F., Martins, D., Martins, O., Vergari, M., et al. (2012). Prolonged visual memory enhancement after direct current stimulation in Alzheimer's disease. *Brain Stimulation, 5*(3), 223–230.

Boller, F., & Grafman, J. (1983). Acalculia: Historical development and current significance. *Brain and Cognition, 2*(3), 205–223.

Brem, A. -K., Fried, P. J., Horvath, J. C., Robertson, E. M., & Pascual-Leone, A. (2014). Is neuroenhancement by noninvasive brain stimulation a net zero-sum proposition? *NeuroImage, 85*(Part 3), 1058–1068 (0).

Butterworth, B., Varma, S., & Laurillard, D. (2011). Dyscalculia: From brain to education. (Review). *Science, 332*(6033), 1049–1053

Cappelletti, M., Gessaroli, E., Hithersay, R., Mitolo, M., Didino, D., Kanai, R., et al. (2013). Transfer of cognitive training across magnitude dimensions achieved with concurrent brain stimulation of the parietal lobe. *The Journal of Neuroscience, 33*(37), 14899–14907.

Carrey, N. J., MacMaster, F. P., Gaudet, L., & Schmidt, M. H. (2007). Striatal creatine and glutamate/glutamine in attention-deficit/hyperactivity disorder. *Journal of Child and Adolescent Psychopharmacology, 17*(1), 11–17.

Cattaneo, Z., Pisoni, A., & Papagno, C. (2011). Transcranial direct current stimulation over Broca's region improves phonemic and semantic fluency in healthy individuals. *Neuroscience, 183,* 64–70.

Chi, R. P., & Snyder, A. W. (2012). Brain stimulation enables the solution of an inherently difficult problem. *Neuroscience Letters, 515*(2), 121–124.

Clark, V. P., Coffman, B. A., Trumbo, M. C., & Gasparovic, C. (2011). Transcranial direct current stimulation (tDCS) produces localized and specific alterations in neurochemistry: A (1)H magnetic resonance spectroscopy study. *Neuroscience Letters, 500*(1), 67–71.

Cohen Kadosh, K. (2011). What can emerging cortical face networks tell us about mature brain organisation? (Review). *Developmental Cognitive Neuroscience, 1*(3), 246–255.

Cohen Kadosh, R. (2013). Using transcranial electrical stimulation to enhance cognitive functions in the typical and atypical brain. *Translational Neuroscience, 4*(1), 20–33. http://dx.doi.org/10.2478/s13380-013-0104-7.

Cohen Kadosh, R., Dowker, A., Heine, A., Kaufmann, L., & Kucian, K. (2013). Interventions for improving numerical abilities: Present and future. *Trends in Neuroscience and Education, 2*(2), 85–93.

Cohen Kadosh, R., Levy, N., O'Shea, J., Shea, N., & Savulescu, J. (2012). The neuroethics of non-invasive brain stimulation. *Current Biology, 22*(4), R108–R111.

Cohen Kadosh, R., Soskic, S., Iuculano, T., Kanai, R., & Walsh, V. (2010). Modulating neuronal activity produces specific and long-lasting changes in numerical competence. *Current Biology, 20*(22), 2016–2020.

Collingridge, G. L., & Bliss, T. V. P. (1987). NMDA receptors – Their role in long-term potentiation. *Trends in Neurosciences, 10*(7), 288–293.

Crair, M. C., & Malenka, R. C. (1995). A critical period for long-term potentiation at thalamocortical synapses. *Nature, 375*(6529), 325–328.

DaSilva, A. F., Volz, M. S., Bikson, M., & Fregni, F. (2011). Electrode positioning and montage in transcranial direct current stimulation. *Journal of Visualized Experiments, 51,* e2744.

Datta, A., Baker, J. M., Bikson, M., & Fridriksson, J. (2011). Individualized model predicts brain current flow during transcranial direct-current stimulation treatment in responsive stroke patient. *Brain Stimulation, 4*(3), 169–174.

Datta, A., Elwassif, M., Battaglia, F., & Bikson, M. (2008). Transcranial current stimulation focality using disc and ring electrode configurations: FEM analysis. *Journal of Neural Engineering, 5*(2), 163–174.

Davis, N. J., Gold, E., Pascual-Leone, A., & Bracewell, R. M. (2013). Challenges of proper placebo control for non-invasive brain stimulation in clinical and experimental applications. *European Journal of Neuroscience, 38*(7), 2973–2977.

Delazer, M., Ischebeck, A., Domahs, F., Zamarian, L., Koppelstaetter, F., Siedentopf, C. M., et al. (2005). Learning by strategies and learning by drill–Evidence from an fMRI study. *NeuroImage, 25*(3), 838–849.

Ditye, T., Jacobson, L., Walsh, V., & Lavidor, M. (2012). Modulating behavioral inhibition by tDCS combined with cognitive training. *Experimental Brain Research, 219*(3), 363–368.

Dockery, C. A., Hueckel-Weng, R., Birbaumer, N., & Plewnia, C. (2009). Enhancement of planning ability by transcranial direct current stimulation. *The Journal of Neuroscience, 29*(22), 7271–7277.

Dresler, M., Sandberg, A., Ohla, K., Bublitz, C., Trenado, C., Mroczko-Wasowicz, A., et al. (2013). Non-pharmacological cognitive enhancement. *Neuropharmacology, 64,* 529–543.

Edden, R. A., Crocetti, D., Zhu, H., Gilbert, D. L., & Mostofsky, S. H. (2012). Reduced GABA concentration in attention-deficit/hyperactivity disorder. *Archives of General Psychiatry, 69* (7), 750–753.

Fassbender, C., & Schweitzer, J. B. (2006). Is there evidence for neural compensation in attention deficit hyperactivity disorder? A review of the functional neuroimaging literature. *Clinical Psychology Review, 26*(4), 445–465.

Felce, D., & Perry, J. (1995). Quality of life: Its definition and measurement. *Research in Developmental Disabilities, 16*(1), 51–74.

Feldman, D. E., Nicoll, R. A., & Malenka, R. C. (1999). Synaptic plasticity at thalamocortical synapses in developing rat somatosensory cortex: LTP, LTD, and silent synapses. *Journal of Neurobiology, 41*(1), 92–101.

Ferrucci, R., Mameli, F., Guidi, I., Mrakic-Sposta, S., Vergari, M., Marceglia, S., et al. (2008). Transcranial direct current stimulation improves recognition memory in Alzheimer disease. (Case Reports). *Neurology, 71*(7), 493–498

Ferrucci, R., & Priori, A. (2014). Transcranial cerebellar direct current stimulation (tcDCS): Motor control, cognition, learning and emotions. *NeuroImage, 5*(3), 918–923.

Fertonani, A., Pirulli, C., & Miniussi, C. (2011). Random noise stimulation improves neuroplasticity in perceptual learning. *The Journal of Neuroscience, 31*(43), 15416–15423.

Fiori, V., Coccia, M., Marinelli, C. V., Vecchi, V., Bonifazi, S., Ceravolo, M. G., et al. (2011). Transcranial direct current stimulation improves word retrieval in healthy and nonfluent aphasic subjects. *Journal of Cognitive Neuroscience, 23*(9), 2309–2323.

Floel, A., Rosser, N., Michka, O., Knecht, S., & Breitenstein, C. (2008). Noninvasive brain stimulation improves language learning. *Journal of Cognitive Neuroscience, 20*(8), 1415–1422.

Floyer-Lea, A., Wylezinska, M., Kincses, T., & Matthews, P. M. (2006). Rapid modulation of GABA concentration in human sensorimotor cortex during motor learning. *Journal of Neurophysiology, 95*(3), 1639–1644.

Gabrieli, J. D. (2009). Dyslexia: A new synergy between education and cognitive neuroscience. *Science, 325*(5938), 280–283.

Gandiga, P. C., Hummel, F. C., & Cohen, L. G. (2006). Transcranial DC stimulation (tDCS): A tool for double-blind sham-controlled clinical studies in brain stimulation. *Clinical Neurophysiology, 117*(4), 845–850.

Gilger, J. W., & Kaplan, B. J. (2001). Atypical brain development: A conceptual framework for understanding developmental learning disabilities. *Developmental Neuropsychology, 20*(2), 465–481.

Gogtay, N., Giedd, J. N., Lusk, L., Hayashi, K. M., Greenstein, D., Vaituzis, A. C., et al. (2004). Dynamic mapping of human cortical development during childhood through early adulthood. *Proceedings of the National Academy of Sciences of the United States of America, 101*(21), 8174–8179.

Gross, J., Hudson, J., & Price, D. (2009). *The long term costs of numeracy difficulties: Every child a chance trust.* London, UK: KMPG.

Gross, J., Jones, D., Raby, M., & Tolfree, T. (2006). *The long-term costs of literacy problems.* London, UK: Every Child a Chance (KMPG).

Gross-Tsur, V., Manor, O., & Shalev, R. S. (1996). Developmental dyscalculia: Prevalence and demographic features. *Developmental Medicine and Child Neurology, 38*(1), 25–33.

Guleyupoglu, B., Schestatsky, P., Edwards, D., Fregni, F., & Bikson, M. (2013). Classification of methods in transcranial Electrical Stimulation (tES) and evolving strategy from historical approaches to contemporary innovations. *Journal of Neuroscience Methods, 219*(2), 297–311.

Hauser, T. U., Rotzer, S., Grabner, R. H., Merillat, S., & Jancke, L. (2013). Enhancing performance in numerical magnitude processing and mental arithmetic using transcranial Direct Current Stimulation (tDCS). *Frontiers in Human Neuroscience, 7*, 244.

Hensch, T. K., & Bilimoria, P. M. (2012). Re-opening windows: Manipulating critical periods for brain development. *Cerebrum, 2012*, 11.

Hess, G., & Donoghue, J. P. (1994). Long-term potentiation of horizontal connections provides a mechanism to reorganize cortical motor maps. *Journal of Neurophysiology, 71*(6), 2543–2547.

Holland, R., Leff, A. P., Josephs, O., Galea, J. M., Desikan, M., Price, C. J., et al. (2011). Speech facilitation by left inferior frontal cortex stimulation. *Current Biology, 21*(16), 1403–1407.

Homan, R. W., Herman, J., & Purdy, P. (1987). Cerebral location of international 10–20 system electrode placement. *Electroencephalography and Clinical Neurophysiology, 66*(4), 376–382.

Hsu, T. Y., Tseng, L. Y., Yu, J. X., Kuo, W. J., Hung, D. L., Tzeng, O. J., et al. (2011). Modulating inhibitory control with direct current stimulation of the superior medial frontal cortex. *NeuroImage, 56*(4), 2249–2257.

Im, C. H., Park, J. H., Shim, M., Chang, W. H., & Kim, Y. H. (2012). Evaluation of local electric fields generated by transcranial direct current stimulation with an extracephalic reference electrode based on realistic 3D body modeling. *Physics in Medicine and Biology, 57*(8), 2137–2150.

Iuculano, T., & Cohen Kadosh, R. (2013). The mental cost of cognitive enhancement. *The Journal of Neuroscience, 33*(10), 4482–4486.

Jacobson, L., Ezra, A., Berger, U., & Lavidor, M. (2012). Modulating oscillatory brain activity correlates of behavioral inhibition using transcranial direct current stimulation. *Clinical Neurophysiology, 123*(5), 979–984.

Johnson, M. H. (2011). Interactive specialization: A domain-general framework for human functional brain development. *Developmental Cognitive Neuroscience, 1*(1), 7–21.

Jolles, D. D., & Crone, E. A. (2012). Training the developing brain: A neurocognitive perspective. *Frontiers in Human Neuroscience, 6*, 76.

Kanai, R., Chaieb, L., Antal, A., Walsh, V., & Paulus, W. (2008). Frequency-dependent electrical stimulation of the visual cortex. *Current Biology, 18*(23), 1839–1843.

Kanai, R., Paulus, W., & Walsh, V. (2010). Transcranial alternating current stimulation (tACS) modulates cortical excitability as assessed by TMS-induced phosphene thresholds. *Clinical Neurophysiology, 121*(9), 1551–1554.

Kaufmann, L., Wood, G., Rubinsten, O., & Henik, A. (2011). Meta-analyses of developmental fMRI studies investigating typical and atypical trajectories of number processing and calculation. *Developmental Neuropsychology, 36*(6), 763–787.

Kessler, S. K., Minhas, P., Woods, A. J., Rosen, A., Gorman, C., & Bikson, M. (2013). Dosage considerations for transcranial direct current stimulation in children: A computational modeling study. *PloS One, 8*(9), e76112.

Knudsen, E. I. (2004). Sensitive periods in the development of the brain and behavior. *Journal of Cognitive Neuroscience, 16*(8), 1412–1425.

Krain, A. L., & Castellanos, F. X. (2006). Brain development and ADHD. *Clinical Psychology Review, 26*(4), 433–444.

Krause, B., & Cohen Kadosh, R. (2013). Can transcranial electrical stimulation improve learning difficulties in atypical brain development? A future possibility for cognitive training. *Developmental Cognitive Neuroscience, 6*, 174–196.

Krause, B., Marquez-Ruiz, J., & Cohen Kadosh, R. (2013). The effect of transcranial direct current stimulation: A role for cortical excitation/inhibition balance? *Frontiers in Human Neuroscience, 7*, 602.

Kucian, K., Loenneker, T., Dietrich, T., Dosch, M., Martin, E., & von Aster, M. (2006). Impaired neural networks for approximate calculation in dyscalculic children: A functional MRI study. *Behavioral and Brain Functions, 2*, 31.

Mattai, A., Miller, R., Weisinger, B., Greenstein, D., Bakalar, J., Tossell, J., et al. (2011). Tolerability of transcranial direct current stimulation in childhood-onset schizophrenia. *Brain Stimulation, 4*(4), 275–280.

Matza, L. S., Paramore, C., & Prasad, M. (2005). A review of the economic burden of ADHD. *Cost Effectiveness and Resource Allocation, 3*, 5.

McCain, M. N., Mustard, J. F., & McCuaig, K. (2011). *Early years study 3: Making decisions, taking action.* Toronto, Canada: Margaret & Wallace McCain Family Foundation.

Minhas, P., Bikson, M., Woods, A. J., Rosen, A. R., & Kessler, S. K. (2012). Transcranial direct current stimulation in pediatric brain: A computational modeling study. *Conference proceedings: Annual International Conference of the IEEE Engineering in Medicine and Biology Society. IEEE Engineering in Medicine and Biology Society. Conference, 2012,* 859–862.

Moliadze, V., Antal, A., & Paulus, W. (2010). Electrode-distance dependent after-effects of transcranial direct and random noise stimulation with extracephalic reference electrodes. *Clinical Neurophysiology, 121*(12), 2165–2171.

Monte-Silva, K., Kuo, M. F., Liebetanz, D., Paulus, W., & Nitsche, M. A. (2010). Shaping the optimal repetition interval for cathodal transcranial direct current stimulation (tDCS). *Journal of Neurophysiology, 103*(4), 1735–1740.

Moss, F., Ward, L. M., & Sannita, W. G. (2004). Stochastic resonance and sensory information processing: A tutorial and review of application. *Clinical Neurophysiology, 115*(2), 267–281.

Mulquiney, P. G., Hoy, K. E., Daskalakis, Z. J., & Fitzgerald, P. B. (2011). Improving working memory: Exploring the effect of transcranial random noise stimulation and transcranial direct current stimulation on the dorsolateral prefrontal cortex. *Clinical Neurophysiology, 122*(12), 2384–2389.

Mussolin, C., De Volder, A., Grandin, C., Schlogel, X., Nassogne, M. C., & Noel, M. P. (2010). Neural correlates of symbolic number comparison in developmental dyscalculia. *Journal of Cognitive Neuroscience, 22*(5), 860–874.

Nitsche, M. A., Nitsche, M. S., Klein, C. C., Tergau, F., Rothwell, J. C., & Paulus, W. (2003). Level of action of cathodal DC polarisation induced inhibition of the human motor cortex. *Clinical Neurophysiology, 114*(4), 600–604.

Nitsche, M. A., & Paulus, W. (2000). Excitability changes induced in the human motor cortex by weak transcranial direct current stimulation. *The Journal of Physiology, 527*(Pt 3), 633–639.

Nitsche, M. A., & Paulus, W. (2001). Sustained excitability elevations induced by transcranial DC motor cortex stimulation in humans. *Neurology, 57*(10), 1899–1901.

Ohn, S. H., Park, C. I., Yoo, W. K., Ko, M. H., Choi, K. P., Kim, G. M., et al. (2008). Time-dependent effect of transcranial direct current stimulation on the enhancement of working memory. *Neuroreport, 19*(1), 43–47.

Parsons, S., & Bynner, J. (2005). *Does numeracy matter more?* London, UK: NRDC.

Pascual-Leone, A., Amedi, A., Fregni, F., & Merabet, L. B. (2005). The plastic human brain cortex. *Annual Review of Neuroscience, 28,* 377–401.

Pascual-Leone, A., Horvath, J. C., & Robertson, E. M. (2012). Enhancement of normal cognitive abilities through noninvasive brain stimulation. In R. Chen & G. C. Rothwell (Eds.), *Cortical connectivity* (pp. 207–249). New York, NY: Springer.

Pasini, A., Paloscia, C., Alessandrelli, R., Porfirio, M. C., & Curatolo, P. (2007). Attention and executive functions profile in drug naive ADHD subtypes. *Brain & Development, 29*(7), 400–408.

Paulesu, E., Demonet, J. F., Fazio, F., McCrory, E., Chanoine, V., Brunswick, N., et al. (2001). Dyslexia: Cultural diversity and biological unity. *Science, 291*(5511), 2165–2167.

Pena-Gomez, C., Vidal-Pineiro, D., Clemente, I. C., Pascual-Leone, A., & Bartres-Faz, D. (2011). Down-regulation of negative emotional processing by transcranial direct current stimulation: Effects of personality characteristics. *PloS One, 6*(7), e22812.

Peterchev, A. V., Wagner, T. A., Miranda, P. C., Nitsche, M. A., Paulus, W., Lisanby, S. H., et al. (2012). Fundamentals of transcranial electric and magnetic stimulation dose: Definition, selection, and reporting practices. *Brain Stimulation, 5*(4), 435–453.

Piazza, M., Mechelli, A., Butterworth, B., & Price, C. J. (2002). Are subitizing and counting implemented as separate or functionally overlapping processes? *NeuroImage, 15*(2), 435–446.

Polania, R., Paulus, W., Antal, A., & Nitsche, M. A. (2011). Introducing graph theory to track for neuroplastic alterations in the resting human brain: a transcranial direct current stimulation study. *NeuroImage, 54*(3), 2287–2296.

Price, G. R., Holloway, I., Rasanen, P., Vesterinen, M., & Ansari, D. (2007). Impaired parietal magnitude processing in developmental dyscalculia. *Current Biology, 17*(24), R1042–R1043.

Rimrodt, S. L., & Lipkin, P. H. (2011). Learning disabilities and school failure. (Review). *Pediatrics in Review/American Academy of Pediatrics, 32*(8), 315–324

Ritchie, S. J., & Bates, T. C. (2013). Enduring links from childhood mathematics and reading achievement to adult socioeconomic status. *Psychological Science, 24*(7), 1301–1308.

Rivera, S. M., Reiss, A. L., Eckert, M. A., & Menon, V. (2005). Developmental changes in mental arithmetic: Evidence for increased functional specialization in the left inferior parietal cortex. *Cerebral Cortex, 15*(11), 1779–1790.

Rykhlevskaia, E., Uddin, L. Q., Kondos, L., & Menon, V. (2009). Neuroanatomical correlates of developmental dyscalculia: Combined evidence from morphometry and tractography. *Frontiers in Human Neuroscience, 3*, 51.

Sandrini, M., Fertonani, A., Cohen, L. G., & Miniussi, C. (2012). Double dissociation of working memory load effects induced by bilateral parietal modulation. *Neuropsychologia, 50*(3), 396–402.

Santarnecchi, E., Polizzotto, N. R., Godone, M., Giovannelli, F., Feurra, M., Matzen, L., et al. (2013). Frequency-dependent enhancement of fluid intelligence induced by transcranial oscillatory potentials. *Current Biology, 23*(15), 1449–1453.

Schlaggar, B. L., Fox, K., & O'Leary, D. D. (1993). Postsynaptic control of plasticity in developing somatosensory cortex. *Nature, 364*(6438), 623–626.

Schneider, H. D., & Hopp, J. P. (2011). The use of the bilingual aphasia test for assessment and transcranial direct current stimulation to modulate language acquisition in minimally verbal children with autism. *Clinical Linguistics & Phonetics, 25*(6–7), 640–654.

Shaw, P., Malek, M., Watson, B., Sharp, W., Evans, A., & Greenstein, D. (2012). Development of cortical surface area and gyrification in attention deficit/hyperactivity disorder. *Biological Psychiatry, 72*(3), 191–197.

Shaywitz, S. (2003). *Overcoming dyslexia.* New York, NY: Vintage Books.

Silani, G., Frith, U., Demonet, J. F., Fazio, F., Perani, D., Price, C., et al. (2005). Brain abnormalities underlying altered activation in dyslexia: A voxel based morphometry study. *Brain, 128*(Pt 10), 2453–2461.

Snowball, A., Tachtsidis, I., Popescu, T., Thompson, J., Delazer, M., Zamarian, L., et al. (2013). Long-term enhancement of brain function and cognition using cognitive training and brain stimulation. *Current Biology, 23*(11), 987–992.

Spencer-Smith, M., & Anderson, V. (2009). Healthy and abnormal development of the prefrontal cortex. *Developmental Neurorehabilitation, 12*(5), 279–297.

Stagg, C. J., Bachtiar, V., & Johansen-Berg, H. (2011). The role of GABA in human motor learning. *Current Biology, 21*(6), 480–484.

Stagg, C. J., Best, J. G., Stephenson, M. C., O'Shea, J., Wylezinska, M., Kincses, Z. T., et al. (2009). Polarity-sensitive modulation of cortical neurotransmitters by transcranial stimulation. *The Journal of Neuroscience, 29*(16), 5202–5206.

Stein, D. S., Blum, N. J., & Barbaresi, W. J. (2011). Developmental and behavioral disorders through the life span. (Review). *Pediatrics, 128*(2), 364–373

Stein, J., & Walsh, V. (1997). To see but not to read; The magnocellular theory of dyslexia. *Trends in Neurosciences, 20*(4), 147–152.

Temple, E., Deutsch, G. K., Poldrack, R. A., Miller, S. L., Tallal, P., Merzenich, M. M., et al. (2003). Neural deficits in children with dyslexia ameliorated by behavioral remediation: Evidence from functional MRI. *Proceedings of the National Academy of Sciences of the United States of America, 100*(5), 2860–2865.

Teo, F., Hoy, K. E., Daskalakis, Z. J., & Fitzgerald, P. B. (2011). Investigating the role of current strength in tDCS modulation of working memory performance in healthy controls. *Frontiers in Psychiatry, 2*, 45.

Terney, D., Chaieb, L., Moliadze, V., Antal, A., & Paulus, W. (2008). Increasing human brain excitability by transcranial high-frequency random noise stimulation. *The Journal of Neuroscience, 28*(52), 14147–14155.

Thut, G., Miniussi, C., & Gross, J. (2012). The functional importance of rhythmic activity in the brain. *Current Biology, 22*(16), R658–R663.

Tseng, P., Hsu, T. Y., Chang, C. F., Tzeng, O. J., Hung, D. L., Muggleton, N. G., et al. (2012). Unleashing potential: Transcranial direct current stimulation over the right posterior parietal cortex improves change detection in low-performing individuals. *The Journal of Neuroscience, 32*(31), 10554–10561.

Turkeltaub, P. E., Benson, J., Hamilton, R. H., Datta, A., Bikson, M., & Coslett, H. B. (2012). Left lateralizing transcranial direct current stimulation improves reading efficiency. *Brain Stimulation, 5*(3), 201–207.

Turrigiano, G. G., & Nelson, S. B. (2000). Hebb and homeostasis in neuronal plasticity. *Current Opinion in Neurobiology, 10*(3), 358–364.

Vicario, C. M., & Nitsche, M. A. (2013a). Transcranial direct current stimulation: A remediation tool for the treatment of childhood congenital dyslexia? *Frontiers in Human Neuroscience, 7*, 139.

Vicario, C. M., & Nitsche, M. A. (2013b). Non-invasive brain stimulation for the treatment of brain diseases in childhood and adolescence: State of the art, current limits and future challenges. (Review). *Frontiers in Systems Neuroscience, 7*, 94

Wagner, T., Valero-Cabre, A., & Pascual-Leone, A. (2007). Noninvasive human brain stimulation. *Annual Review of Biomedical Engineering, 9*, 527–565.

Weiss, M., & Lavidor, M. (2012). When less is more: Evidence for a facilitative cathodal tDCS effect in attentional abilities. *Journal of Cognitive Neuroscience, 24*(9), 1826–1833.

Willcutt, E. G., Petrill, S. A., Wu, S., Boada, R., Defries, J. C., Olson, R. K., et al. (2013). Comorbidity between reading disability and math disability: Concurrent psychopathology, functional impairment, and neuropsychological functioning. *Journal of Learning Disabilities, 46*(6), 500–516.

You, D. S., Kim, D. Y., Chun, M. H., Jung, S. E., & Park, S. J. (2011). Cathodal transcranial direct current stimulation of the right Wernicke's area improves comprehension in subacute stroke patients. *Brain and Language, 119*(1), 1–5.

Zatorre, R. J., Fields, R. D., & Johansen-Berg, H. (2012). Plasticity in gray and white: Neuroimaging changes in brain structure during learning. *Nature Neuroscience, 15*(4), 528–536.

Ziemann, U., Muellbacher, W., Hallett, M., & Cohen, L. G. (2001). Modulation of practice-dependent plasticity in human motor cortex. *Brain: A Journal of Neurology, 124*(Pt 6), 1171–1181.

A Brief Guide to the Scientific Entrepreneur

Souhile Assaf[1,2] and Joseph Kerr[2]

[1]Medtrode Inc., London, Ontario, Canada
[2]XLR Imaging Unit 116, Stiller Centre, London, Ontario, Canada

OUTLINE

INTRODUCTION

The use of electricity from various sources to treat pain and attempt to modulate brain function has been around for thousands of years. Modern neuromodulation dates to the early 1960s, with the first deep brain stimulation, followed in 1967 by spinal cord stimulation. Although spinal cord stimulation for the treatment of neuropathic pain is now well established, deep brain stimulation (DBS) has been growing as a treatment for movement disorders. More recently, DBS has been approved by regulators, or is in clinical trial stages, for treating depression, obsessive-compulsive disorders, and epilepsy. Peripheral nerve stimulation and in particular vagal nerve stimulation are also being used or evaluated to treat the latter disorders. While hundreds of thousands of patients already benefit from these neuromodulation treatments, they still represent a very small percentage of the total market size.

Although the above modes of neurostimulation are slowly replacing destructive surgical treatments such as cutting or ablating neuronal tissue, they are in themselves invasive. Moreover, while these newer methods do offer the advantage of being somewhat reversible compared to ablation, they also entail a cumbersome surgical implantation procedure of a high maintenance device. Another problem is that they compete with existing drug treatments, and their approvals are usually limited to drug-resistant or intractable cases.

In contrast to the above invasive procedures, less invasive or non-invasive neurostimulation devices are available or being developed. Electroconvulsive therapy (ECT) has been used since the 1930s, and was approved by the Food and Drug Administration (FDA) for depression treatment in 1979. Cortical stimulation using surface electrodes or magnetic coils (transcranial magnetic stimulation, TMS) to treat pain was introduced in the 1990s (Tsubokawa, Katayama, Yamamoto, Hirayama, & Koyama, 1993).

TMS cortical stimulation has taken a leap forward with the FDA approval of its use to treat depression. TMS best fits the non-invasive neuromodulation, since it can be performed without anesthesia and on an outpatient basis. It is not only a relatively safe treatment but also well tolerated by patients. Transcranial direct current stimulation (tDCS) has also proven to be relatively safe and well tolerated by human subjects. Although there are not any devices approved by the FDA for clinical treatment, experiments with human volunteers support promising clinical applications.

As more non-invasive neurostimulation devices and treatments are developed and the hardware becomes smaller and more user-friendly, the authors predict that their market will surpass that for implantable deep brain stimulation.

MARKET SIZE AND DYNAMICS

Neuromodulation is one of the fastest growing medical device market sectors. Current sales of neuromodulation devices are worth approximately $3 billion dollars, with forecasts predicting an annual growth of 15% through until 2015. After that point the market will grow steadily, driven by increased adoption rates, an aging population, and the introduction of new and innovative therapies. New non-invasive neurostimulation devices, including transcranial magnetic or electrical stimulators, as therapies or assistive devices, will also be introduced. An example is the multichannel wireless device developed at Neuroelectrics.

The business landscape is currently dominated by three global players: Medtronic, St Jude's, and Boston Scientific. Noteworthy is the fact that these market leaders are companies with a long history in cardiovascular implants; the neuromodulation market is following the pattern of the interventional cardiology market in the 1970s, addressing an initially low adoption rate, high development costs, and stringent regulatory barriers. These companies are well positioned for the challenges and have the additional advantage of already owning significant patent portfolios in the areas of neurostimulation leads and implantable stimulators developed for cardiac pacing.

A second layer of companies comprises new entries that were able to develop a novel therapeutic approach protected by unique patents. An example is Cyberonics, which has a patent portfolio in the area of vagal stimulation for treating depression and epilepsy. The third and most interesting layer, and what lies below the "tip of the iceberg", is an ever-increasing number of small innovative companies and spin-offs from universities and research institutions that are developing novel neuromodulation treatments for stroke, brain injury, and cognitive disorders such as memory and dyscalculia.

Several companies are currently supplying devices for transcranial stimulation, including Neuroelectrics, Neuroconn, Soterix, and others. The devices are currently valuable research tools, and are not sold to the general public. On the other hand, some companies, such as foc.us, have recently started marketing tDCS devices that are not FDA approved. The marketing literature of these companies steers away from significant therapeutic benefit claims, although users are buying the devices to increase focus and thereby performance in video gaming. Complications and related legal cases will result from the use of scientific papers to suggest benefits without relating the research technique, parameters, and findings to the current used and placements in the devices being sold.

The remainder of this chapter addresses this "third layer" of innovation, and provides a guide to neuromodulation scientists on the pathway to commercializing their findings and intellectual property.

COMMERCIALIZATION PATHWAYS

There is a wealth of publications on the various commercial pathways available, from discovery through to market entry. A good online summary is provided by Youtie, Hicks, Shapira, and Horsely (2011). Another useful resource, dedicated to financing inventors and monetizing their inventions, is authored by Nathan Myhrvold, CEO of Intellectual Ventures (Myhrvold, 2010).

Figure 17.1 summarizes the most common pathways from a research finding to commercialization. The path the scientist ultimately takes is dependent on the intellectual property (IP) ownership policy at the scientists' institution. In a country such as Canada, policies range from total ownership by the institution, as is the case for National Research Councils (NRCs) and most of the universities, to complete ownership by the scientist as is the case at the University of Waterloo. Ownership of IP can have a great impact on financial gain by the scientist, and it is said that the greatest concentration of technology millionaires is among those who own their intellectual property.

DISCLOSURE AND EVALUATION

Disclosure rules differ, and scientists must take into consideration their institute's policy on the need for and mechanisms of disclosure of inventions. After disclosure, technology transfer offices at most institutes get involved in deciding upon commercialization pathways. The first step in the disclosure process is to ensure that the scientist and the institute understand the invention. An attempt is made to understand what is

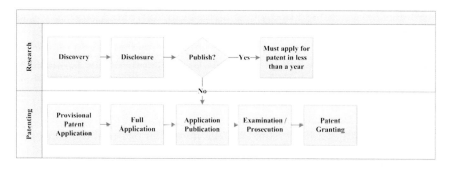

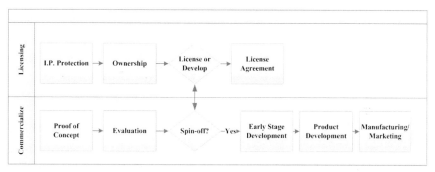

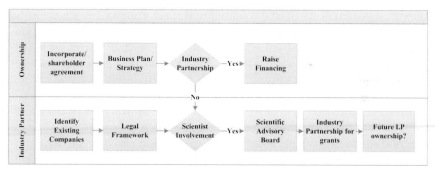

FIGURE 17.1   A schematic of pathways from scientific discovery to commercialization of a device.

novel about it, and its possible utility. The second step is to determine what else needs to be done at this early stage of development to demonstrate the value of the invention. The third step is to evaluate the commercial applications, and what products or treatments will be enabled by the invention. This is a significant step, because it will determine how excited your technology transfer office is about the invention and whether it wants to dedicate resources to patent and commercialize it. A scientist must keep in mind that hundreds of disclosures are made and most institutes have a limited budget, so many of them will not proceed to the patent and commercialization stage. There will be a number of potentially valuable inventions that are ignored, as only patents that have a real prospect of being licensed will be pursued. This depends on the proficiency and the resources of the specific technology transfer office. Typically, they will be guided by the answers they formulate to these questions:

1. Is the invention novel, as confirmed by a patent search?
2. How difficult is it to demonstrate the invention or proof the concept?
3. Will industry value the invention and be willing to license it and invest resources to develop it into a product?

Scientists will also have to evaluate the value of dedicating their time to pursuing commercialization by asking these questions:

1. Am I interested in championing the technology and doing additional work to prove the concept or build a prototype?
2. Am I willing to dedicate some time, at the cost of my other research activities, to work with the licensee to develop it further?
3. What's in it for me, including research funds from the licensee and royalties that I can consider as future income?

If the conclusion to the above set of questions is that there is a potential market for the invention and the scientist or the institute wishes to proceed further, a patent is filed. The scientist will meet with and work with the patent attorney to explain why the invention is novel, and the non-obviousness of it. The patent attorney will then conduct a prior art search and see if any prior art exists, which a patent examiner can use to discount the claims. The patent attorney will also ensure that the inventor has not publically disclosed or published the invention, thereby disqualifying it from being patented. Typically, the inventor is encouraged to file a provisional patent prior to publication, which effectively sets a priority date for a period of 1 year during which a full application can be filed. The provisional patent is not published by the patent office, whereas a full application will eventually be published prior to examination of the patent.

LICENSING

Subsequent to evaluating and protecting the invention, licensing is the primary vehicle by which companies acquire rights to intellectual property owned by universities and research institutions. A license can be exclusive or non-exclusive to all or some of the technology. A license can also specify the field of use and the period of the agreement.

From a business point of view, the institution and the scientist must ensure that the license agreement has a "Due Diligence" section which details the effort that the licensee will make to develop the technology. The agreement should also specify the involvement of the university and/or the inventors in the development process, and how they will gain from commercialization of the invention. It is essential for scientists to ensure that their invention will not be licensed by a large company that can afford to pay the license fee and bank the invention in case it needs it at a later date. Scientists would be well advised to seek smaller companies that have an appetite for early stage development and whose success depends on developing the technology further.

SPIN-OFFS

Spin-offs are new companies founded to commercialize intellectual property created at an academic and research institution. This is not the most common commercialization pathway at universities, and in the United States less than 5% of all inventions are used to set up new companies (according to statistics from the Association of University Technology Managers). Starting a company takes an enormous amount of time and energy. However, there is a great deal of personal satisfaction and financial gain to inventors if their invention is commercialized by a company they helped start. Since universities are usually partners with the scientists in these spin-offs, they offer more commercialization expertise than industrial partners. Cleveland Clinic is one of the best incubators for neuromodulation spin-offs, since it is willing to commit capital and human resources to take their innovations to market. The payoff to Cleveland Clinic is huge, as exemplified by the recent sale of the neuromodulation company Intelect Medical to Boston Scientific for $78 million. Medical technology companies such as Boston Scientific are increasingly taking early equity stakes in companies, like the stake they already have in intellectual property. Sometimes larger medical device firms make an early investment in a start-up in return for a right to eventually acquire the company at a certain price. Alternatively, they may have an agreement or option to acquire exclusive licenses or marketing rights. Such exclusive deals allow them to shut out competitors. Another advantage for the industry partner is that an equity stake also allows it the opportunity to influence the start-up's technology.

Some spin-offs are started by founders who spend many years providing prototypes or assemblies at little or no cost to university researchers. Financial support during this stage comes from granting agencies. Both authors of this chapter are affiliated with a company called XLR Imaging, which was spun out by Robarts Research Institute at the University of Western Ontario. For 5 years the company supplied research-grade MRI coils to researchers all over the world. Since each coil was custom made, there was no economy of scale or "cookie cutter" manufacturing involved. The company needed government grants to sustain it. While this early-stage seeding of the market with research devices may not have generated massive revenue, it helped the company to fine-tune product development and explore new clinical applications. The same company is now focused on a clinical-grade pediatric coil benefitting from product standardization. In Europe, programs funded by the European Commission or other national programs can play a similar role.

FUNDING SPIN-OFFS

Financing is the biggest challenge to successful launch of a university spin-off. The inability to raise finance for a new venture, or starting a spin-off that is not adequately financed, is a serious impediment to commercialization. This results in a large proportion of inventions left on the researcher's bench and unlikely ever to get to market. As detailed by Sørheim, Widding, Oust, and Madsen (2011) in their work "Funding of university spin-off companies: a conceptual approach to financing challenges," investors are also reluctant to invest in early-stage companies because of the level of uncertainty compared with other investments.

At the earliest spin-off stage it is not uncommon for founders, their family and friends to provide start -up capital. This allows the spin-off to start IP protection and begin pitching the opportunity to potential investors. In the USA, many states have funds that will invest at the early stage to promote innovation. In Canada, provincial and federal funding is available but the trend is to match private funding rather than seed the spin-off.

Public funding falls into three categories: grants, loans, and tax initiatives. Traditionally, most funding takes the form of grants, where the money given does not have to be repaid. However, to force researchers to have a vested interest in the use of capital, there are emerging schemes where governments take a role in providing loans, instead of grants, to medical device start-up companies. Complementing these two forms of funding, in most countries there are tax breaks for the research and development activities of companies. While the funding available through government programs is always in flux, depending on the governing party, budgets, and political priorities, there is always funding available for the commercialization of technology.

Many scientists and researchers will likely already be familiar with government funding programs for science and research, which will help them navigate the wide variety of programs available to help commercialize their products.

These funding options should help entrepreneurs develop their technology and product to a stage where an investor is willing to provide capital to the business. Accordingly, to help decide what type of funding suits the business best, entrepreneurs should determine what the money will be used for.

Funding is used for additional design, testing, and development costs, and often a business will need to hire an employee to help with these goals. Money can also be used to purchase necessary equipment, materials, and prototypes. Moreover, as mentioned below, a business will often need paid help for its regulatory (often FDA) clearance. Funds can also be used to help with intellectual property protection. Determining where the money is spent will help a business decide which government programs to apply to.

Because many government programs require either an academic or an industry partner, it is helpful for a researcher or small business to identify other companies that can provide complementary or necessary skills, such as testing, regulatory advice, or design and development.

Government Programs

Research and development funding is available from the European Union and national governments. We will use the programs available in Canada, which the authors are familiar with, as an example of national programs.

The following is a breakdown of the types of funding available in Canada. The programs available in Canada should be indicative of other funding schemes available across the world.

- Federal Funding (grants)
  - Fund research (principally from IRAP and NSERC)
  - Fund prototypes (IRAP and NSERC)
  - Fund hiring of employees (MITAC)
  - Fund regulatory applications (Local Innovation Centres)
- Artical I. Tax Incentives (Both Federal and Provincial)
  - Credits for research and development

Angel Investors

The second level of investment is likely to come from "angel" investors. These are affluent individuals who provide capital for start-ups in exchange for ownership equity. The trend is for these angel investors to organize themselves into "angel groups" and pool their investments, which typically focus on local companies. Angels fill the gap in spin-off financing between seed funding by founders and venture capital.

Angel investors are usually retired entrepreneurs or executives. They are also investing in mentoring the founders, and will invest their experience and networks in addition to funds. Founders will meet these investors face to face at investor conferences and symposia, and pitch directly to them.

A NESTA study in 2009 estimated that there were up to 6000 angel investors in the UK with an average investment size of £42,000. The same study indicated that 35 percent of investments produced returns of between one and five times the initial investment.

Venture Capital

The next level of financing is usually venture capital, which occurs after the seed-funding round as a growth-funding round. This is sometimes referred to as "Series A Round." Venture capital is really private equity, although not all private equity is venture capital. It is a subset of financing targeted for new companies with a limited operating history that are too small to raise capital from banks or traditional investors. These companies would not have reached the point where they are able to complete a debt offering or initial public offering (IPO). In exchange for the high risk that venture capitalists assume, they usually have control over company decisions. Their interest is in generating a huge return through an IPO or trade sale of the company. If they cannot realize this within the 5- to 7-year timeframe they usually target, they may abandon the project – leaving the university and the founders with nowhere to go, since they no longer control their IP.

REGULATORY PATHWAYS

A key phase in commercializing neuromodulation technology is obtaining clearance to market (or sell) the device from a regulatory body in the country where the product will be sold. In addition to this clearance, manufacturers must also register their devices with the appropriate regulatory body (getting a "medical device license"). Regulatory approval can be a very complex process that varies from country to country.

With any medical device, and in particular those based on neuromodulation, the developer must undertake careful planning and execution throughout all of the product development phases so that a regulatory clearance can happen easily and quickly (Mehta [2008] and Whitmore [2004] provide valuable guides to the design, development, and commercialization of medical devices, and assist applicants in meeting all the quality management requirements for a regulatory clearance and/or ISO 13845 certification). This section will give an overview of the regulatory pathways for getting clearance to market and how to register a neuromodulation device, so that the regulatory submission can be planned for early in the development of the business.

FDA 510k and CE Marking

For most companies, the largest markets for their products are the US and the EU, which require an FDA Pre-Market Notification (510k) or Pre-Market Approval (PMA) submission, or CE mark, respectively, for clearance to market a medical device. The CE marking system covers a wide variety of products, and requires compliance with a Quality Management System (QMS); however, an FDA clearance will also help a submission in any other country, since many of the requirements are similar (such as a QMS). The process for an FDA submission is discussed here.

FDA 510k/PMA Process for Neuromodulation Devices

The first step in regulatory approval is to determine into which FDA class a product falls. The FDA classifies devices according to risk and efficacy. Invasive devices are class III devices, while non-invasive devices are class II. This is an important classification, since class II devices may be eligible for approval without the need for clinical trials. Most class II devices are eligible to be approved based on proving that they are essentially similar to a device previously approved by the FDA.

Most neuromodulation devices are currently restricted to FDA class III, since they are considered "those that support or sustain human life, are of substantial importance in preventing impairment of human health, or which present a potential, unreasonable risk of illness or injury." It is important to classify a device correctly, since a class III device requires far more data to support a submission. With time, as they are proven safe through use, neuromodulation devices might change classification – similar to the case of high-field MR equipment, which has mostly been re-classified as class II.

Once classified, the process to obtain an FDA clearance to market (a 510k or PMA) for a neuromodulation device will follow these steps:

1. Pre-Market – Classify your device (II or more likely III)
   a. Class II – 510k Pre-Market Notification Submission (510k)
      i. Identify non-PMA predicate devices (for a class II device)
   b. Class III – Pre-Market Approval Submission (PMA)
      i. Perform clinical studies required for PMA (and some 510k submissions)
      ii. Obtain an Investigational Device Exemption (IDE, if required to do studies)
2. Post-Market
   a. Quality Management System Audits
      i. ISO 13485:2003
   b. Post-Market Surveillance.

510k Pre-Market Notification (Class I or II)

The key purpose of a 510k submission is to show that a class I or II device is "substantially equivalent" to another device that is proven safe, and does not require a PMA. An important element in showing "equivalence" is the use of a predicate device, thereby showing a product similarly safe. Performance and design data should be also submitted to show that the device being submitted and the predicate devices operate in largely the same way.

Pre-Market Approval (Class III and Those Devices Where "Substantial Equivalence" is Not Found)

A PMA requires data to show that a medical device is "safe and effective" before it can be cleared to market. Clinical studies are often required to show the safety and effectiveness of a class III product. In order to perform the clinical trials required for a PMA, a company can obtain an "investigational device exemption" (IDE) so that it can test the product legally. Based on the data obtained in these studies, the applicant should use good scientific practice and writing to prove that the device is safe.

Post-Marketing Requirements

Regardless of the classification, once a device is cleared to market, the FDA requires the manufacturer to have both a QMS and Medical Device Reporting (MDR) (FDA Documents 21CFR820.30 and 21CFR803.1). The implementation of ISO 13485:2003 should allow a company to satisfy these requirements. Such a system will also take into account the required documentation for manufacturing and also post-marketing surveillance of a product to document any safety issues.

Registering Your Device/Getting a Medical Device "License"

Once a device is cleared to market, a company must also register with the appropriate authority before it can sell its device. The authority varies between countries.

United States

Registration with the FDA is required after a 510k or PMA submission, and a list of manufactured devices must be submitted with this registration.

European Union

Neuromodulation products fall under the European Medical Device Directive, and therefore, like the FDA, still require a company to "classify" your device with your CE marking and also to register it with a "competent authority" in the country where the device is sold, such as the MHRA in the UK. In the EU, most neuromodulation products will likely be considered "Class III" and fall under the category of "Active Implantable Medical Device" (AIMD) (defined in directives 93/42/EEC 90/383/EEC respectively)

Canada

Health Canada will administer a "medical device license" when a product is cleared to be sold. Once this happens, the company must also get an "establishment license" and register with Health Canada. Health Canada requires ISO 13485:2003 for clearance to market.

Japan

In order to market a device in Japan, a company needs to provide a submission document for its product to the Pharmaceuticals and Medical Devices Agency (PMDA), and to register to be an "accredited foreign manufacturer." The PMDA also requires ISO 13485:2003 for these clearances and registrations.

Preparing for a Regulatory Clearance

Most companies will undertake a regulatory submission without necessarily having planned for a submission. The simplest way to prepare is to ensure that the company is following Good Manufacturing Practices (GMP, and likely ISO 13485:2003), which will speed up the documentation required for an FDA or CE submission. An ISO consultant can help a company through this task, as it is a very involved process.

Regulatory Clearance in Emerging Markets

China and India are two particularly strong emerging markets for medical devices, and the regulatory environment is evolving along with these two countries' development. In China the current regulatory body is called the State Food and Drug Administration (SFDA), while in India there are registration requirements for devices that fall under the Drugs and Cosmetic Rules. The best idea here is to hire a local consultant to help guide the business through the regulatory maze for these countries.

CONCLUSIONS

The market for neurostimulation devices that modulate brain function and neuronal disorders is one of the fastest growing medical device markets. Neurostimulation devices and treatments can be grouped into invasive devices, which involve implanting a stimulator or electrode, and non-invasive devices, which stimulate the nervous system without the need for surgical implantation. The potential market for non-invasive neurostimulation is much larger, but is dependent on developing and commercializing effective treatments approvable by regulatory bodies such as the FDA. This chapter provides a brief guide for scientists wishing to transfer their findings from the laboratory to the marketplace. The chapter covers the protection of intellectual property, commercialization strategies, and financing available from various agencies.

References

Mehta, S. S. (2008). *Commercializing successful biomedical technologies*. Cambridge, UK: Cambridge University Press.

Myhrvold, N. (2010). The big idea: Funding eureka! *Harvard Business Review*, March 2010.

Sørheim, R., Widding, L. O., Oust, M., & Madsen, O. (2011). Funding of university spinoff companies: A conceptual approach to financing challenges. *Journal of Small Business and Enterprise Development*, *18*(1), 58–73.

Tsubokawa, T., Katayama, Y., Yamamoto, T., Hirayama, T., & Koyama, S. (1993). Chronic motor cortex stimulation in patients with thalamic pain. *Journal of Neurosurgery*, *78*, 393–401.

Whitmore, E. (2004). *Development of FDA-regulated medical products – Prescription drugs, biologics and medical devices*. Milwaukee, United States: American Society for Quality, Quality Press.

Youtie, J., Hicks, D., Shapira, P., & Horsely, T. (2011). Pathways from discovery to commercialization: Using web sources to track small and medium-sized enterprise strategies in emerging nanotechnologies. *The Selected Works of Diana Hicks*. http://works.bepress.com/diana_hicks/26.

18

The Neuroethics of Transcranial Electrical Stimulation

Neil Levy[1,2] and Julian Savulescu[2]

[1]Florey Institute of Neuroscience and Mental Health, Melbourne,
Victoria, Australia
[2]Oxford Centre for Neuroethics, University of Oxford, Oxford, UK

INTRODUCTION

According to the materialist view almost all thinkers accept today, the brain gives rise to the mind. Activity in the brain is the sole cause of personality, thought, belief, desire, and behavior. Subtle differences in brain activity may cause profound differences in mental states. The activity of the brain arises from and is influenced by a wide range of causes – genetic, social, environmental, and, by way of top-down processes, through the exercise of "voluntary" agency. While the causes of brain activity (and so personality, thought, perception, desire, etc.) are diverse, there is a final common pathway: neuronal electrical activity. Increasingly, brain activity is coming to be deliberately altered through the use of pharmacology, surgery, and the application of technology. Different interventions into the brain have different effects on the person, and thus raise different issues. They may have different risks, promise different benefits, or be more or less permanent. They may be used, or used mainly, as a treatment for dysfunctions (which may be more or less severe) or to enhance the capacities of persons who are already functioning at or above normal levels. For these reasons, it is helpful to focus discussion on a narrow range of interventions, used for particular purposes. However, the "holy grail" of brain (and so mind) modification is the co-ordinated, strategic non-invasive control of single-neuron electrical activity.

In this chapter, we focus on one important technology that is an early step towards targeted control of neuronal activity: transcranial electrical stimulation (tES). tES refers to a family of non-invasive means of stimulating the brain using direct current, alternating current, or random noise. While tES does not target single-neuron activity, it is anatomically focused and modifies neuronal firing non-invasively. We will focus on enhancement because it is far more controversial than treatment – no one begrudges a suffering person the alleviation of their suffering. tES, we shall argue, is, from an ethical perspective, an almost ideal enhancer. It neatly avoids nearly all of the main worries that have been raised concerning other (potential) enhancers. We do not aim to show that these worries are, in general, misplaced: we aim to show that they do not rule out all enhancements because there is *at least* one cognitive enhancer which is immune to them all. However, we will raise one major objection which is almost unique to electrical stimulation as an enhancement.

THE TREATMENT/ENHANCEMENT DISTINCTION

Before moving on to discuss enhancement proper, it is important to say something about the treatment/enhancement distinction, thought to be so central to the evaluation of new technologies. When tES is used for the treatment of disease, there is an established ethical process (research ethics review) by which it can be tested, as well as a willingness to employ it as treatment of disease or disorder. Deployment in clinical practice would be governed by the standard principles of medical ethics – that treatment is given in the best interests of the patient, that appropriate valid consent be given, that it represents a just allocation of community resources when it is publicly funded, and so on.

When tES is employed to enhance the capacities of persons, it is far more controversial. The distinction between treatment and enhancement has played a central role in ethical debate around the acceptability of genetic selection and enhancement. For Michael Sandel, for instance, whereas both treatments and enhancements intervene in nature, the latter (alone) "represent a boundless bid for mastery and domination" over nature, thereby expressing a limitless hubris (Sandel, 2007, pp. 46–47). This concern is echoed by thinkers as diverse as the neo-Marxist Jürgen Habermas (2003) and the conservative bioethicist Leon Kass (2002). Yet this distinction between disease and health, treatment and enhancement, is morally irrelevant, we now argue. We will begin with an illustrative case.

Teresa Lewis died on the 24th of September 2010, after being given a lethal injection at the Greensville Correctional Centre in Virginia. The 41-year-old was convicted of plotting to kill her husband, Julian Lewis, and her stepson, Charles Lewis. She persuaded two men to carry out the murders in return for sex and money. The two men received life sentences. The execution went ahead in spite of protests from lawyers, celebrities, and others who argued that she should have been given clemency because of her low IQ. Under US law, anyone with an IQ of 70 avoids the death penalty. Lewis was judged to have an IQ of 72 (Jensen et al., 2012).

In Virginia, there is a law that prohibits the execution of intellectually disabled people. Intellectual disability is a medical diagnosis. General intelligence, or g, naturally varies in a normal distribution within a given, defined population. For western populations, it famously follows a bell curve with a mean of 100 and a standard deviation of 15 points. Intellectual disability for medical, legal, and social purposes is arbitrarily defined as an IQ two standard deviations below the mean (below 70). Around 2% of people have an intellectual disability.

If Lewis' IQ had been 3 points lower, 69, she would still be alive today. Those 3 points make no discernible difference to functional capacity. For all intents and purposes, the abilities and competencies of a person with an IQ of 69 would be the same as those of a person of 70.

Of course, the law must draw lines, and there will inevitably be cases which fall on either side of the line, with drastic consequences. The law has been based on a scientific, medical definition of what constitutes disability. But the definition of disease and disability is completely ill-suited to this application. It is a statistical concept, where a line has been drawn arbitrarily at two standard deviations from the mean. It could have been drawn at 3 standard deviations, in which case more people would have been liable for execution in Virginia, or at 1 standard deviation, in which case Lewis would be alive. Such lines are chosen based on the benefits and harms of drawing them, and other ethical principles. Most importantly, one's "natural" position on a statistical curve is not *in itself* of moral significance. Everyone ages, and everyone dies. The fact that these occurrences are "normal" does not make them any less bad. Deafness, impotence for men, loss of memory, and loss of reproductive capacity in women are all statistically normal with advanced age, but that does not make them less bad.

Our definition of disease evolved to serve various functions, including who should have excuses due to illness, receive support, and be objects of medical research and treatment. Its use to determine treatment should not be independent from its effects on wellbeing.

There are various different conceptions of disease and disability. The one that cost Lewis her life is an objectivist conception statistically based on normal species functioning, according to which a condition is a disease if it deviates sufficiently from what is statistically normal in a species (Boorse, 1977, 1997). Yet there are good reasons to revise our concept of disability away from this statistical conception to one which serves the goals we require of it. In the case of medical care, such a concept of disability would be one that is related to our wellbeing (Kahane & Savulescu, 2009).

In legal terms, disability should be defined in terms of legal competence – competence to make free and informed judgments about one's actions. The confused idea that there is a deep, clear distinction between disease and normality (that can be scientifically or medically defined) infects debate about human enhancement. If we increase the IQ of someone with an IQ of 69 it is a treatment, and so many people believe is permissible. If we increase the IQ of someone with an IQ of 72 it is an enhancement, and thus fundamentally ethically different. But this is nonsense. The effects are virtually identical, and it is very hard to see *any* moral difference (let alone a hubristic desire for dominion over nature).

When a new intervention like tES arrives that can affect brain function directly, the important question is not whether it is treating a disease, but what its effects on wellbeing are. Failure to address this point head on can cause benevolent (or avaricious) doctors and other professionals to pathologize normal variation to enable enhancements to be employed as treatments.

This may help to explain the apparently growing epidemic of mental illness. Depression is the fourth leading cause of disability and disease worldwide. The World Health Organization projects that it will be leading cause in developed countries by 2020. Over 20 million people in the US suffer from Social Anxiety Disorder – they get anxious in social situations.

There is about a 15% chance of suffering each of these during your lifetime. Worse, this epidemic is spreading to our children. Around 12% of New Zealand children are medicated for attention deficit hyperactivity disorder (ADHD) (3–9% in the UK). The meteoric rise in mental illness is due, at least in part, to three factors: increased willingness to diagnose mental illness, relaxation of diagnostic criteria, and the invention of new mental diseases for people to suffer from.

The *Diagnostic and Statistical Manual of Mental Disorders* (DSM) produced by the American Psychiatric Association lays down the criteria for mental disease. A new fifth edition is imminent. The initial draft for comment included shyness, substance use (making it the same as dependence), and eccentric behavior as disorders. Even grieving for a relative could be a disorder: persistent complex bereavement disorder. Changes in the definition of alcoholism mean that 40% of American college students are alcoholics.

The American Psychiatric Association considered (but dropped) plans for attenuated psychosis syndrome and Internet addiction as psychiatric disorders. It has expanded the definition of ADHD without the usual ADHD symptoms by adding "ADHD not elsewhere classified."

Premenstrual tension is now an official mental health disorder: DSM-V calls it "premenstrual dysphoric disorder." There is also "disruptive mood dysregulation disorder in children". As it stands prior to revision, the DSM already includes "hypoactive sexual desire disorder" (HSDD) to describe low libido.

We are redefining unwanted or less than optimal states, which are nevertheless normal, as diseases. And this has led to the overtreatment of some people and the medicalization of social problems. Professor Allen Frances, who chaired the previous edition DSM, even admitted that childhood epidemics of autism, bipolar disorder, and attention deficit disorder had led to widespread mislabeling and medicating.

Part of the reason for the explosion of diagnoses of mental disease is because it is often difficult to get effective drugs and other medical treatments unless you are ill or suffering from a disease – partly because insurance companies and governments typically refuse to fund enhancements. Society steadfastly refuses to medicate or enhance normal people, even when their situation can be significantly improved. So, to give them the drug you must call them diseased or disordered.

The fact is that a substantial proportion of mental health promotion consists in the quite legitimate enhancement of normality. Disease, like cancer, Parkinson's disease, or diabetes, is associated with visible pathology. Even "hard" psychiatric diseases, like schizophrenia or manic depression, have not so far been associated with any clear pathology, though they probably will at a cellular level one day. One might be skeptical that any clear pathology will ever be found for many of the modern psychiatric disorders, like "social anxiety" and "premenstrual dysphoric disorder." These may be variants of normal.

But it is important to recognize that just because something is normal it is not a reason to retain it. One target of enhancement is poor impulse control. Over 40 years of psychological research has shown that 3-year-old children who are unable to delay gratification, unable to exercise self-control in the face of temptation, and have poor impulse control, face significant obstacles for the rest of their life, whatever they want to do (Moffitt et al., 2011). They are more likely to end up in prison and at the bottom of the socio-economic scale. They will have fewer friends and less motivation to succeed, and the latter feature is more closely correlated with academic success than IQ (Baumeister & Tierney, 2011). If you can improve impulse control, you will make that child's life better – much better. Poor impulse control is not a disease. It's the lower end of a spectrum.

What is exciting about tES and other forms of non-invasive brain stimulation is that they hold the hope of changing brain activity directly and precisely, rather than through the intermediaries of drugs with broad physiological effects, or through surgery.

Some of this explosion of diagnosis of mental disorder is a product of a legitimate concern about the wellbeing of people, coupled with the fact that we now have the tools to improve it. This is enhancement through the back door; enhancement under the thin disguise of treatment. tES will be an increasingly attractive way to modify brain activity.

In asking whether the use of tES is justifiable, we should not ask: is it treating a disease? Rather, we should ask: is it improving wellbeing?

As well as being conceptually confused, pathologizing normality has various costs. It can:

- increase stigma, alter self-perception and esteem
- lower the sense of responsibility
- provide an excuse and encourage a sense of powerlessness
- be an inappropriate use of public resources
- invite compensation

We should ask not whether tES is a treatment for a disease (or invent a new disease for which it could be a treatment), but rather whether its application will improve wellbeing.

COGNITIVE ENHANCEMENT: THE NEUROETHICAL DEBATE

In the previous section, we argued that the treatment–enhancement distinction is morally irrelevant. However, we will now grant, for argument's sake, that there is a morally relevant distinction between treatment and enhancement. We do so because so doing makes the case for tES stronger: we aim to show that the use of tES can be morally unproblematic even in the most controversial cases – even if it is an enhancement, it avoids the problems that beset some other interventions. Thus we shall focus on tES utilized as an enhancement in those who are already functioning at, or even above, existing levels. Our aim is to show that even given the cogency of the treatment–enhancement distinction, the objections to the use of tES are not compelling; this clears the way for our favored view according to which tES is permissible if it improves the wellbeing of users.

Why are cognitive enhancements controversial? Many reasons have been offered in the literature. In this section, we shall outline the most common objections to their use. We shall focus the discussion initially on the most common cognitive enhancers, psychopharmaceuticals.

The potential cognitive enhancers that have received the most attention in the literature are pharmaceuticals designed for the treatment of medical conditions, utilized off-label in people who do not suffer from those conditions. The issue was first raised, in a sustained manner, with reference to selective serotonin reupake inhibitors, like Prozac. SSRIs were approved for the treatment of depression, which can be an extremely severe, even life-threatening, condition. In his book *Listening to Prozac*, Peter Kramer (1993) claimed that many patients wanted to continue on Prozac even when it is was no longer medically indicated, or in the absence of diagnosable depression. They took it to stabilize mood, or to feel more confident. They wanted to feel "better than well." They wanted the success in relationships or careers they felt they owed to the drug.

A number of bioethicists reacted to the off-label use of SSRIs with concern. They raised a number of worries about the use of medications to alter brain function, when such uses were not medically indicated. Some of these worries centered on obviously and uncontroversially important issues, such as the potential long-term risks of the use of psychopharmaceuticals. Others depended for their force on controversial philosophical views about the nature of humanity. The following annotated list is by no means comprehensive, but covers most of the more common ethical concerns.

Safety

Just as treatments are acceptable only if their (weighted) benefits outweigh their (weighted) costs, so the ethical assessment of the use of enhancements requires a positive weighted benefit/cost ratio. Many people think that benefits have a diminishing marginal utility: the higher the level at which a person is performing, the less an increment in performance is worth to them (it is worth remarking, however, that this claim may not be true in all contexts: a scientist striving for a Nobel Prize may regard a small chance of a slight increase in, say, fluid intelligence as worth a large risk of ill health, whereas most ordinary people may think that the risks would need to be very much smaller for the small benefit to be worthwhile). If it is true that benefits have a diminishing utility, the weighted benefit/cost ratio would need to be very high for the use of enhancements to be ethically unproblematic.

All pharmaceuticals carry some risks. SSRIs, for instance, are associated with a range of side effects, mainly mild to moderate (e.g., weight gain, insomnia, sexual dysfunction). There have been reports of severe side effects in some cases, such as suicidal ideation. The most commonly used cognitive enhancers today also present potential safety risks. For instance, methylphenidate, a drug used for the treatment of attention deficit hyperactivity disorder but reportedly widely used for enhancement purposes by students, has been associated with rare but serious adverse events, including cardiac arrest.

Authenticity

Whereas it is uncontentious that safety is a pressing concern when assessing the ethical permissibility or advisability of the use of cognitive enhancers, concerns over authenticity are far more controversial. However, though the concern is difficult to articulate clearly, its force is widely felt.

The worry is that the enhancement is in some sense an alien intrusion into the person. Carl Elliot, who has done more than anyone else to articulate the concern, claims that though enhancements may bring us benefits, these benefits come at the cost of taking ourselves further away from who we genuinely are. Elliot outlined the worry initially with regard to Prozac:

> It would be worrying if Prozac altered my personality, even if it gave me a better personality, simply because it isn't *my* personality. This kind of personality change seems to defy an ethics of authenticity. *(Elliott, 1998, p. 182)*

The underlying concern is that each of us has an authentic self, an essence or a set of characteristics, developing which represents authenticity for us. An enhancer obscures that authentic self, substituting something foreign in its place. The resulting person might be better, but would not be truly *me*.

Elliot has also expressed a related worry in terms of the proper relationship between the person and his or her world. The authentic person understands her place in that world; understands how her life is going and how well she is doing at her basic projects. The risk of enhancements is that they may substitute a false picture for the clear-eyed grasp of reality. Suppose, for instance, that someone takes Prozac because the failure of his marriage, or the drabness of his daily life makes him sad. If Prozac boosts his mood, it may make him better off in one dimension of his life, but this boost comes at the cost of wisdom. The inauthentic individual, trapped in a loveless marriage or mired in dumb conformity, *should* experience a malaise: a malaise is the only adequate response to an existence that is without point. All going well, this malaise ought to be a spur to correcting the problems with the life; the enhancer might cover up the problems and thereby preclude meaningful change.

Indeed, Elliot argues, even if meaningful change is impossible, the person might still be better off suffering than medicated. It is better to know that your life is meaningless than not to know; to that extent, Prozac comes at a cost to the person. Of course, this might be a cost worth paying in particular cases.

Cheating

A number of ethicists have raised the worry that the use of cognitive enhancement constitutes a kind of cheating. The best analogy might be with the use of performance enhancers in sport. The use of these enhancers is strictly regulated. Given these regulations, and on the assumption that most sportspeople abide by them, the person who takes a performance enhancer and is undetected has an unearned and unfair advantage over other competitors. It is unfair because the performance boost provided by the enhancer is unavailable to competitors who abide by the rules. It is cheating just because the boost in performance is produced by a violation of the rules.

It is controversial whether the use of performance enhancers is really unethical. It might be argued, for instance, that the notion of fairness is difficult to apply with regard to elite competition, because the differences between athletes will be as arbitrary and unearned in the absence of performance enhancers as in their presence. Small differences in muscle composition might explain why one athlete consistently outperforms another, but the genetic and environmental factors that explain these differences will not have been earned by the athlete. Nevertheless, many people do regard performance enhancement as impermissible in sport; these people may regard cognitive enhancement as equally problematic, at least in some contexts.

There are many circumstances in which rewards are distributed to people in ways that are sensitive to their performance on measures of cognition. The most obvious is, of course, school and university examinations, and the distribution of rewards (grants, prestige, employment opportunities) to researchers. Many kinds of professional employment, from law to medicine to software design and finance, seek and reward performance in the cognitive domain. All of these spheres are explicitly or implicitly spheres of competition, governed by rules both formal and informal. They are all spheres in which individuals may therefore be able to cheat – garner an unearned and unfair advantage by violating the rules. We have already seen how researchers utilize modafinil in a manner that might be regarded by some as cheating (Maher, 2008). There is also evidence (albeit mostly anecdotal) that students utilize cognitive enhancers to boost performance in university examinations; Ritalin and Adderall, prescribed for the treatment of ADHD, are both reported to be in common use for this purpose (Forlini & Racine, 2009).

In part, the concern about cheating is related to the concern about authenticity: the achievement on an enhancer will not be the person's "own." In this way, enhancement causes alienation from the true person and his labor or achievements. The product is partly due to the enhancer, and pharmaceutical companies become responsible for the result or outcome.

Social Justice

Related to, but distinct from, these worries are concerns about social justice. These concerns are, we believe, the most serious. They are the most serious both in that we take them to be the strongest objections to the use of enhancements (assuming that safety issues can be set aside), and because if they succeed their implications are among the most far-reaching. Whereas worries about authenticity, for instance, might render the use of enhancements unwise or costly, these worries do not seem sufficient to support a ban on their use. The harms they threaten, if they are indeed genuine, are harms to the person using the enhancer. If the person is a competent adult, these are harms to which they seem to have the right to consent. Social justice concerns are different. If the harms they portend are genuine, they are harms to third parties – indeed, to vulnerable third parties. For that reason, these concerns might actually justify a prohibition on the use of cognitive enhancers.

The social justice concerns arise from the costs and limited availability of enhancements. Though cognitive enhancers need not be expensive, a small expense is sufficient to place them out of the reach of many millions of people. This raises the prospect that cognitive enhancement will be available only, or at least mainly, to those who are already very much better off than average. Moreover, intelligence positively correlates with affluence. Higher socio-economic status is already associated with higher intelligence (Hunt, 1995), and even when we restrict our attention to the normal range of weights, thereby excluding children born into extreme poverty, birth-weight, which reflects the nutritional and health status of the mother, is correlated with IQ (Matte, Bresnahan, Begg, & Susser, 2001). The benefits from cognitive enhancement might therefore flow almost exclusively to those who need them least, while those who are most disadvantaged do not benefit at all.

The world we live in today is more unequal than at any previous time in human history, and this inequality is increasing (Persson & Savulescu, 2012a). But if cognitive enhancements become widely available, we can expect the gap to grow ever greater, both between countries, and between the wealthy and less wealthy citizens within countries. Many people think inequality is bad all by itself, or, at the very least, that inequality must be justified (for instance, by the economic efficiencies it sometimes brings). The fact that cognitive enhancements seem likely to exacerbate inequality might therefore be a sufficient reason to regulate or even prohibit these technologies. Moreover, there are potential costs associated with inequality which can strengthen concerns centered on it. A growing gap between the elite and the rest might diminish feelings of social solidarity, on both sides. Some commentators blamed the London riots of 2011 in part on the sense that many less-affluent people felt that they had no stake in the society around them. For their part, elites may no longer feel they are in the same boat as the poor, so different are they from one another, and this might translate into a reduced willingness to contribute to the general welfare. They might demand a lowering of tax rates, failing which they might move their assets offshore. They might refuse to contribute to campaigns which aim to alleviate famine and the effects of natural disasters around the world. They may regard the poor as natural slaves (in Aristotle's phrase), who are born to serve their needs. Nothing less than the future of democracy might be at stake in the debate over cognitive enhancement.

Positional Goods

The final worry we will mention concerns positional goods. For many enhancements, while it is true that they bring particular benefits to individuals who adopt them early, widespread adoption leads to these benefit evaporating. This is due to the fact that benefits may depend on an individual's *relative* performance, not her *absolute* performance. Suppose, for instance, a high-intelligence individual enhances her IQ by two points. In a competitive environment in which most of her peers are similarly intelligent – say, Harvard Law School – this relatively small boost might make a big difference to her examination scores (which are partially comparative) and to her chance of success in landing a lucrative position at a prestigious law firm. However, her comparative advantage obviously disappears if the cognitive enhancer she uses is also employed by her classmates. In that case, everyone expends resources (their time plus whatever money is required to acquire the enhancer; the resources involved in producing the enhancer) in a fruitless quest for advantage. Like Alice's Red Queen, the widespread use of enhancements leaves us running just to stay in the same place.

Though we believe that some of the concerns outlined above rest on philosophical mistakes (see Savulescu [2006] and Levy [2007] for discussion), they deserve to be taken seriously. Some of them might indeed prove formidable problems that ought to be taken into account in regulating particular cognitive enhancers or in formulating social policies. However, we shall suggest that tES may be the perfect cognitive enhancer, in as much as though many enhancers can avoid one or more of these worries, tES may be alone in neatly sidestepping all these concerns. We shall address the worries one by one and then introduce two new ones which we take to be the most serious concerns about the development of tES.

THE PERFECT ENHANCER?

Safety

The tES apparatus is comparatively simple to assemble, and the parts are widely and cheaply available. These facts make it quite feasible for home use by amateurs. Indeed, self-experimentation with tES is a thriving cottage industry, with plans for the apparatus available online (there are kits for those seeking a shortcut) and groups of interested lay people swapping stories and experiences. These facts make tES unique: there is no other comparable new technology that is within easy reach of lay people. They also entail unique safety concerns. They raise the possibility that individuals or unscrupulous business people may attempt to apply tES without an adequate understanding of the function of the brain regions involved or the best parameters for stimulation (for further discussion, see Chapter 3).

However, though these facts raise genuine safety concerns, the actual risks seem to be low (Arul-Anandam, Loo, & Sachdev, 2009). Unlike transcranial magnetic stimulation (TMS), there are no reports of seizures in individuals who have participated in tES. Some mild side effects of untrained use have been reported, including dizziness and vision disturbances, but these appear to resolve rapidly. There is a genuine possibility of serious brain damage, but animal studies indicate that damage occurs only with current densities orders of magnitude higher than those supplied by off-the-shelf kits (Bikson, Datta, & Elwassif, 2009). Given the current state of our knowledge, even in the uncontrolled environment of the hobbyist the risk of long-lasting harm seems to be relatively small.

Of course, we cannot yet rule out the possibility of perhaps subtle side effects, since the scientific study of tES is in its infancy, but it seems as though risk/benefit ratios favor the use of tES by competent adults. Much greater caution ought to be exercised with regard to its use by children and adolescents (for further discussion, see Cohen Kadosh, Levy, O'Shea, Shea, & Savulescu, 2012). Little is yet known about the potential effects of tES on the developing brain (Krause & Cohen Kadosh, 2013). There are as yet no guidelines for its use in children. Again, there is a genuine risk that unscrupulous business people might exploit vulnerable individuals by, for example, offering parents tES without the proper training to use it (though the risk seems more acute with regard to its application as a treatment than an enhancement: parents may be desperate to find a cure for a cognitive deficit in their children, and their desperation may lead them to act without critically scrutinizing the claims of third parties).

The potential safety concerns involved with the use of tES in the developing brain, and related issues (for instance, concerning the potential for enhancement of one function of the developing brain to come at the cost of decreased performance with regard to other functions; see Iuculano & Cohen Kadosh, 2013 for an example of this scenario in adults), make its use as an enhancer in this population premature. As noted above, assessing the advisability of the use of an enhancer depends on its weighted benefit/cost ratio, but making that calculation requires knowledge we do not currently possess, with regard to the potential costs and to their probability. Differences between the mature and the developing brain entail that we cannot gain this knowledge by studying the former alone. Animal models are of limited utility, too, since many of the functions of interest (mathematical cognition, linguistic processing, and so on) are uniquely human. For this reason, we believe that it is necessary to gather the data on the risks and benefits of stimulating the developing brain *directly*, by testing tES on children and adolescents. The potential benefits of, for example, greater mathematical abilities justify careful research. It is worth noting, moreover, that this research is also justified from a treatment perspective, since tES seems to have great promise as a treatment for identifiable dysfunctions, such as dyscalculia. The potential to treat impairments justifies the use of techniques the acute and chronic risks of which are as yet not fully known, by making the weighted benefit/cost ratio higher. If the use of tES as a treatment proves safe in the developing brain, research on its application as a cognitive enhancer can proceed with greater confidence. However, it should be noted that the typically and atypically developed brain might be qualitatively different from one another, so further research in the former population will be required even after safety is established in the latter.

Authenticity

Worries about authenticity are difficult to assess, because the concept of authenticity is so amorphous. Indeed, it is likely that there is no unified concept of authenticity: rather, there are (at least) two concepts of authenticity, which are quite different in the demands they make on the self (Levy, 2011). One concept of authenticity emphasizes self-creation – i.e., the deliberate attempt to shape one's self, from one's goals and aspirations to one's personality (DeGrazia, 2000). There is not even a *prima facie* worry that enhancement might threaten authenticity of this sort, since enhancements can be used in the quest deliberately to shape the self. Enhancement can be a threat only to authenticity conceived in a rival manner, according to which authenticity consists in being true to, rather than reshaping, one's somehow pre-given self.

It is certainly quite plausible that notions of selfhood incorporate some kind of narrative condition, according to which an authentic self is a self of which we can make some kind of narrative sense. If this is correct, too rapid and too dramatic changes in personality traits or other dispositions might be disruptive of our sense of self. If tES were a magic bullet, it might threaten authenticity in this kind of way.

However, no cognitive enhancer is a magic bullet. There is no suggestion or possibility that applying tES to oneself might suddenly transform one's personality or one's cognitive dispositions. Rather, tES appears to make ordinary processes of learning and practice somewhat more effective. Applying tES to the prefrontal cortex facilitates the acquisition of mathematical know-how (Snowball et al., 2013), for instance. From the phenomenological perspective, the increase in capacity will not be experienced as disruptive; rather, it will be experienced in the way learning is always experienced – as the gradual acquisition of knowledge and capacity. It requires input by the subject to change brain state and knowledge – cognitive enhancement makes it easier to learn, but it does not provide knowledge or skill. In this regard, tES is like every other cognitive enhancer. Further, there seems no proprietary phenomenology associated with tES (hence the fact that researchers can use placebo-controlled paradigms in comparing tES to sham stimulation). This fact may distinguish tES from some other enhancers, and may make the former feel less disruptive of self and identity to users.

It is possible that the newly acquired capacities will be somewhat disruptive of personal narratives. Consider the English major who has thought of himself as bad at maths, but now finds himself keeping pace with the rest of the class with no more difficulty – perhaps even slightly less difficulty – than the rest of his classmates. Though he will need to rewrite his narrative, it does not seem as though the revision can be dramatic enough to count as disruptive of the self. The very fact that it is mediated, necessarily, through learning and effort ensures that it can be relatively easily incorporated into the ongoing story of his life. It is worth pointing out that there are multitudes of (largely anecdotal) reports of similar effects being achieved by more traditional means: the person who is bad at languages or can't draw, and who thinks of herself as having deficits in these areas, but who blossoms given the right kind of teaching or guidance. We have no more reason to think that tES is disruptive of the authentic self than these teaching methods.

As we saw above, worries about authenticity are often combined with worries about how enhancements might cut the person off from a genuine understanding of his or her place in the world. "Happy pills" might undercut the ability to appreciate the problems one confronts, and thereby to respond to them. So far as we can see, this kind of worry arises only for affective enhancers. If a cognitive enhancement works, there need be nothing of which the enhanced person is ignorant.

Cheating

Many of the considerations just cited to allay concerns that tES threatens authenticity will do double duty to show that tES need not constitute cheating. The use of any effective means to an end can constitute cheating, of course: if there is some context in which people compete to achieve that end, and that context is rule-governed, then use of the means is cheating just because the rules prohibit it. But of course that the use of (say) tES would violate the rules were the rules to prohibit its use is simply tautological. The charge of cheating is interesting only if there is something inherent in the means that makes it use unfair. In that case, this unfairness may be a reason to have rules prohibiting its use. We shall therefore focus on this question: is there some good reason (other than concerns about social justice, authenticity, and safety) to think that the use of tES should be prohibited in competitive contexts (such as examinations at school or university)?

Prima facie, it might seem that the use of tES would be unfair in the latter sense of cheating, which we mentioned before, even were it not against the rules. To see this, consider two agents, one of whom uses tES while studying for her math examination and one of whom does not. The following facts might be true: each agent exerted just as much effort and was just as talented as the other. Furthermore, it might be true that prior to the date at which the first agent began to use tES, each was as skilled in the domain as the other. But, assuming that tES is an effective cognitive enhancer, it might be true that the first agent did better than the second in the exam, only because she used tES. In that case, it seems, the second agent has a complaint: the competition was unfair because the other competitor was enhanced. The result is down to the tES, not the agent herself.

However, even in such a "pure" case, it is not clear that the advantage gained by tES is different in kind from other cognitive enhancements: exercise, "micronaps," nutrition, or caffeine. If these effective interventions are safe and accessible, the fact that some people choose not to employ them is their responsibility. Questions of fairness return to issues of safety and access.

When we broaden the context from the two rivals, this charge is even more difficult to sustain. It is difficult to sustain because even if the stipulated facts are true of the two rivals, there is little likelihood that they are true of all other competitors. Rather, they are likely to differ – in talents, in capacity for hard work, in the educational opportunities they have been offered, in social backgrounds, and so on – in many ways over which they lack control, but which cause them to be better or worse mathematicians. There seems no more reason to worry about tES than these other factors. Indeed, it is very plausible that there is less reason to worry about tES than other factors. Unjust social arrangements probably have a bigger causal role to play in differences in mathematical achievement than tES is likely to, whether through differential access to education, or through stereotype threat (Spencer, Steele, & Quinn, 1999).

However, it might be objected that the fact that there are already many sources of unfairness in the world is no reason to add further sources. We believe that this is no reason to prohibit tES. If it is not objectionable on other grounds, rather, it is a reason to ensure that it is as widely available as possible (on the supposition, to which we shall soon turn, that it can be made widely available). If tES is made available for everyone, those people who fail to take advantage of it seem to have no stronger grounds for complaints of unfairness than do people who fail to take advantage of the library. Of course, it is quite likely that different people will get different degrees of enhancement from identical courses of tES, even coupled with identical training regimes, but that is true of the use of vitamins, exercise, libraries, and computing in enhancing cognition too.

It is even possible that cognitive enhancements may play a role in reducing unfairness. We will discuss this issue under the closely related heading of social justice, to which we now turn.

Social Justice

We see questions of unequal access and growing inequality as the most significant ethical obstacles to cognitive enhancers. Since enhancement technologies are often expensive, they are available only to those who are already better off. They may therefore play a role in increasing already significant inequality.

Clearly, worries of this sort are most pressing when there are significant barriers to access for those who lack resources. These barriers may be cost, or they may be a combination of legal and cost barriers (when patent restrictions prevent governments of less-developed countries from making generic pharmaceuticals available at a low cost to their populations, for instance). Pharmaceuticals used as enhancers may be costly even if the per dose cost is low, if repeated or even constant doses are required for continuing effects (as seems to be true of methylphenidate and modafinil, for instance).

Though the tES apparatus is financially out of reach of the many millions of people who live in poverty around the world, the cost of building the apparatus is actually relatively low. It may easily be assembled by a technician for less than US$800, using plans that are already available for use. Once assembled, it may be reused an indefinite number of times on an indefinite number of people. So while the cost of the unit is prohibitive for many people, the cost of use may be extremely small. Further, the effects of tES appear to be long-lasting: repeated use of the apparatus, once a training course has been completed, may not be necessary. For these reasons, there seem few barriers to the use of tES even in impoverished countries. If tES is effective, any state might choose to provide it for its population.

Further, cognitive enhancement in general and tES in particular may have important social and economic *benefits*. Higher intelligence appears to be protective against social and economic misfortunes (Gottfredson 1997, 2004) and to promote health (Batty, Deary, & MacIntyre, 2007; Whalley & Deary, 2001) and educational achievement.

Individual cognitive capacity (estimated by IQ scores) is positively correlated with income (Rowe, Vesterdal, & Rodgers, 1998). In a very controversial book (although the controversy is irrelevant to the use to which we put it here), Herrnstein and Murray (1994) argue that a 3-point increase in IQ would have the following effects:

Poverty rate	**−25%**
Males in jail	−25%
High school dropouts	−28%
Parentless children	−20%
Welfare recipiency	−18%
Out-of-wedlock births	−15%

One study estimated the increase in income from 1 additional IQ point to be 1.763% (Schwartz, 1994), while a later study put it at 2.1% for men and 3.6% for women (Salkeverl, 1995). The annual gain per IQ point (for the US) would be on the order of US$55 − 65 billion, 0.4–0.5% of GDP. Fitting "national IQ" to GDP shows an exponential relationship with moderate correlation, suggesting that a 5-point IQ increase is worth a 40% GDP increase (1 point = 8.2% GDP) (Dickerson, 2006). Fitting economic product to IQ estimated from educational testing in different US states also shows a similar relationship (Kanazawa, 2006). Improved IQ even at the top end may have beneficial social effects. Patent production does not appear to be a competitive endeavor, but rather a sign of real creativity and wealth production. One study found a doubling of the number of patents in the top quartile compared to the bottom quartile (corresponding to about 7.5 and 3.8 times the base rate of the population). This suggests that not only do the top performers do well professionally; they also add more per capita to the economy (Park, Lubinski, & Benbow, 2008).

Further, cognitive enhancement may be used to reduce inequality (Savulescu, 2006). This is due to the fact that, at least with regard to existing psychopharmaceuticals, the benefits seem to be subject to a diminishing return: the better one's baseline cognitive capacities prior to their use, the smaller the benefit derived. For instance, while Ritalin (methylphenidate) has been shown to enhance spatial working memory and sustained attention in healthy adults, the better the individual performed on working memory tasks prior to ingestion, the smaller the benefit to him or her (Mehta et al., 2000). There is evidence for a similar declining marginal utility of modafinil (Randall, Shneerson, & File, 2005). This diminishing marginal benefit may be a function of their mode of action: they may improve the efficiency of the underlying neural processes. Recent results indicate that tES is subject to the same decline in return (Looi, Duta, Huber, Nuerk, & Cohen Kadosh, 2013; Tseng et al., 2012).

Positional Goods

We conclude this review by returning to the question of whether enhancements, if widely adopted, would leave us no better off than before, and therefore be a waste of scarce resources. Insofar as an enhancement is expected to bring comparative benefits, the worry has bite. However, not all goods are positional; we do not value all goods (only) because of the advantage they give us over others. IQ is a case in a point. People do value IQ because it can be expected to give them a comparative advantage, but they also take an intrinsic satisfaction in the exercise of their intelligence. Wisdom and understanding are at least partially their own reward.

Indeed, widespread enhancement may have a multiplier effect on the search for truth. Because the scientific enterprise is, very importantly, a shared enterprise, in which progress is made by the mutual cooperation and criticism of independent researchers, we can expect its progress to increase substantially if enhancement is shared. Insofar as individual researchers gain satisfaction from being involved in the successful pursuit of truth, widespread enhancement will lead to more, and not less, satisfaction for individuals.

Of course, the economic and social benefits, which flow to individuals and to society as a whole, increase massively when enhancement is on a broader scale. So while it is true that some individuals will be motivated by the search for comparative advantage, and that these individuals may be disappointed, this fact does not entail that enhancement is not a valuable good. Perhaps those who seek a competitive edge alone will be able to take an intrinsic satisfaction from their newfound cognitive powers, even if they do not achieve the end they sought.

Moral Enhancement

We have so far discussed the use of tES to enhance wellbeing, but in principle it could be used to enhance moral behavior. Already, cognitive behavioral therapy, neurofeedback, and methylphenidate are being used to improve impulse control in violent offenders (Raine, 2013), and anti-libidinal agents to reduce libido in paedophiles. Whether interventions such as tES should be used for such moral enhancement has been the subject of vigorous debate (Harris, 2011; Harris & Chan, 2010; Persson & Savulescu, 2012a).

TWO IMPORTANT OBJECTIONS

The Distant Future: The Slippery Slope, Freedom, and the Self

tES is non-invasive and affects the basic currency of the brain and mind: electrical activity. It is, at this time, crude, stimulating relatively large areas of the brain, and the impact on human behavior in real-life situations is still to be seen. It is also likely to be relatively benign – lowering the threshold of neuronal firing and so making learning easier. But, from a wider perspective, it is a step towards the "holy grail" of neuroscience: strategic control of single-neuronal activity. It is not inconceivable that neuronal electrical activity could, in the future, be more and more precisely controlled. Once neuronal activity was under external control, the brain would be under external control, and so the mind and person would be under external control. Freedom would be annihilated. Indeed, with perfect single-neuronal control, there would be real issues of authenticity, cheating, and alienation between the pre-existing person and subsequent brain activity and human behavior.

Such precise control would raise utterly different concerns to those that are leveled at tES as it is currently used. The worry that attempted enhancements, including moral enhancements, might undermine freedom is an old worry (Burgess, 1962; Harris, 2011). While tES at present does not represent a major threat to freedom, it is one of a family of technologies that could one day be used for perfect mind control.

This is a deep and important worry. Some might argue that so bad is this slope, either in steepness or in final outcome, that such research should never go ahead. One way to respond to such worries is to ensure that such technologies are always under the voluntary control of the person whose mind is being affected (Savulescu & Persson, 2012). In this way, individuals might be able to use this technology to enhance achievement of their goals, by staving off addictions or improving impulse control, or even enhance their own values, starting with what they believe to be good and right. Indeed, if freedom to remove desires for grossly immoral ends were possible, and control limited to that end, then the price might be worth paying in terms of promotion of welfare (Persson & Savuelscu, 2012b).

There is of course, enormous capacity for abuse, both by the person involved and by other malevolent actors.

Individuals could descend into an Experience Machine-like existence. First described by Nozick (1974), the Experience Machine allows individuals to dial up any life they like. The machine then stimulates the brain to give the experience of that life, be it President, despot, star footballer, or novelist. All the while the subject is sitting in a chair. The film *The Matrix* was based on this idea.

Of course, such precise mind control could be used for perfect moral or immoral control. The specter of whole human races with small electrical caps or helmets precisely controlling their every thought, belief, desire, and behavior is one endpoint of this project – a subject well-suited to future science fiction movies.

While such scenarios are at present science fiction, they speak to the profound potential power of this family of technologies and stress the importance of early, vigorous, wide-ranging, deep, and professional dialogue about the development and growing potential of technologies that directly modify the brain, and so the mind.

CONCLUSION

None of the usual ethical arguments against the use of tES is compelling, we have claimed. For this reason, its use ought to be permissible if it genuinely improves the wellbeing of users. In replying to the objections, we have made a preliminary case for the claim that it has a positive effect on wellbeing (for instance, by pointing out that cognitive capacities are intrinsically valuable, as well as by citing evidence that better capacities produce individual and social goods). We do not claim that the positive case for their use is overwhelming or definitive. However, respect for autonomy and the liberty of individuals entails that it does not need to be: the burden is on those who would prohibit competent individuals from using tES if they wish. This burden cannot be shouldered by opponents of tES.

Opponents of cognitive enhancement typically seem to think that either all cognitive enhancements are permissible or unproblematic, or none are. We believe this is mistaken: while some cognitive enhancements, in some contexts, genuinely raise issues of serious concern, others do not. Assessment of the ethical permissibility or advisability of their use must therefore proceed piecemeal, assessing particular technologies, in specific circumstances. Though we have not attempted to show this here, we believe that several cognitive enhancements pass reasonable tests for permissibility and advisability, for particular uses. For these enhancements, though there are potential costs and risks associated with their use, the potential benefits outweigh the risks.

For tES, existing evidence indicates that the potential costs and risks – while by no means non-existent – are few, and the potential benefits greater than with regard to other cognitive enhancements. For tES, we suggest, the case in favor of permissibility is overwhelming. Should competent individuals choose to utilize the technology for enhancement, their choice can be a rational and autonomous one, and interference with it would be unjustified on any grounds. In the case of children, we should await long-term safety data. But the door remains open to its future use as a cognitive enhancer augmenting conventional education.

We have also positioned tES on a continuum of interventions that aim to control brain behavior precisely. Such a project does raise important ethical issues. We briefly considered two important objections related to the slippery slope and the possibility of undermining human freedom. While we do not see that such objections pertain to tES as it exists now, they are important reminders of the need for continuous real-time, scientifically collaborative ethical reflection and monitoring. What today seems ideal may in the future be seen as the first step towards the abyss. tES, almost more than any other technology, seeks to influence the very nature of our humanity: our brain and its activity.

References

Arul-Anandam, A., Loo, C., & Sachdev, P. (2009). Transcranial direct current stimulation – What is the evidence for its efficacy and safety? *Medicine Reports, 1*, 58, 27.

Batty, G. D., Deary, I. J., & MacIntyre, S. (2007). Childhood IQ in relation to risk factors for premature mortality in middle-aged persons: The Aberdeen children of the 1950s study. *Journal of Epidemiology and Community Health, 61*, 241–247.

Baumeister, R. F., & Tierney, J. (2011). *Willpower: Rediscovering the greatest human strength.* London: Penguin Books.

Bikson, M., Datta, A., & Elwassif, M. (2009). Establishing safety limits for transcranial direct current stimulation. *Clinical Neurophysiology, 120*(2009), 1033–1034.

Boorse, C. (1977). Health as a theoretical concept. *Philosophy of Science, 44*, 542–573.

Boorse, C. (1997). A rebuttal on health. In J. M. Humber & R. F. Almeder (Eds.), *What is disease?* (pp. 3–143). Totowa, NJ: Humana Press.

Burgess, A. (1962). *A clockwork orange.* London, UK: William Heinemann Ltd.

DeGrazia, D. (2000). Prozac, enhancement, and self-creation. *Hastings Center Report, 30,* 34–40.

Dickerson, R. E. (2006). Exponential correlation of IQ and the wealth of nations. *Intelligence, 34,* 291–295.

Elliott, C. (1998). The tyranny of happiness: Ethics and cosmetic psychopharmacology. In E. Parens (Ed.), *Enhancing human traits. Ethical and social implications.* Washington, DC: Georgetown University Press.

Forlini, C., & Racine, E. (2009). Autonomy and coercion in academic "Cognitive Enhancement" using methylphenidate: Perspectives of key stakeholders. *Neuroethics, 2,* 163–177.

Gottfredson, L. S. (1997). Why *g* matters: The complexity of everyday life. *Intelligence, 24,* 79–132.

Gottfredson, L. S. (2004). Life, death, and intelligence. *Journal of Cognitive Education and Psychology, 4,* 23–46.

Habermas, J. (2003). *The future of human nature.* Cambridge: Polity Press.

Harris, J. (2011). Moral enhancement and freedom. *Bioethics, 25,* 102–111.

Harris, J., & Chan, S. (2010). Moral behavior is not what it seems. *Proceedings of the National Academy of Science, 107,* E183.

Herrnstein, R. J., & Murray, C. (1994). *The bell curve: Intelligence and class structure in American life.* New York: Free Press.

Hunt, E. (1995). The role of intelligence in modern society. *American Scientist, 83,* 356–368.

Iuculano, T., & Cohen Kadosh, R. (2013). The mental cost of cognitive enhancement. *The Journal of Neuroscience, 33,* 4482–4486.

Jensen, V., Barrientos, L., & Niemand, A. Women and criminal offending: Individual level perspectives. In V. Jensen (Ed.), (2012). *Women criminals* (pp. 53–80). Santa Barbara, CA: ABC-CLIO.

Kadosh, R. C., Levy, N., O'Shea, J., Shea, N., & Savulescu, J. (2012). The neuroethics of non-invasive brain stimulation. *Current Biology, 22,* R108–R111.

Kahane, G., & Savulescu, J. (2009). The welfarist account of disability. In K. Brownlee & A. Cureton (Eds.), *Disability and disadvantage* (pp. 14–53). Oxford, UK: Oxford University Press.

Kanazawa, S. (2006). IQ and the wealth of states. *Intelligence, 34,* 593–600.

Kass, L. (2002). *Life, liberty and the defense of dignity: The challenge for bioethics.* San Francisco, CA: Encounter Books.

Kramer, P. D. (1993). *Listening to prozac.* London: Fourth Estate.

Krause, B., & Cohen Kadosh, R. (2013). Can transcranial electrical stimulation improve learning difficulties in atypical brain development? A future possibility for cognitive training. *Developmental Cognitive Neuroscience, 6,* 176–194.

Levy, N. (2007). *Neuroethics: Challenges for the 21st century.* Cambridge, UK: Cambridge University Press.

Levy, N. (2011). Enhancing authenticity. *Journal of Applied Philosophy, 28,* 308–318.

Looi, C. Y., Duta, M., Huber, S., Nuerk, H. -C., & Cohen Kadosh, R. (2013). Stimulating the brain while playing a computer-based maths game to enhance domain-specific and domain-general cognitive abilities. In *Proceedings of the 5th international conference on non-invasive brain stimulation, Leipzig, Germany.*

Maher, B. (2008). Look who's doping. *Nature, 452,* 674–675.

Matte, T. D., Bresnahan, M., Begg, M. D., & Susser, E. (2001). Influence of variation in birth weight within normal range and within sibships on IQ at age 7 years: Cohort study. *British Medical Journal, 323,* 310–314.

Mehta, M. A., Owen, A. M., Sahakian, B. J., Mavaddat, N., Pickard, J. D., & Robbins, T. W. (2000). Methylphenidate enhances working memory by modulating discrete frontal and parietal lobe region in the human brain. *Journal of Neuroscience, 20,* RC65.

Moffitt, T. E., Arseneault, L., Belsky, D., Dickson, N., Hancox, R., Harrington, H. L., et al. (2011). A gradient of childhood self-control predicts health, wealth, and public safety. *Proceedings of the National Academy of Sciences of the United States of America, 108,* 2693–2698.

Nozick, R. (1974). *Anarchy, state and utopia.* New York, NY: Basic Books.

Park, G., Lubinski, P., & Benbow, C. P. (2008). Ability differences among people who have commensurate degrees matter for scientific creativity. *Psychological Science, 19,* 957–961.

Persson, I., & Savulescu, J. (2012a). *Unfit for the future: The need for moral enhancement.* Oxford, UK: Oxford University Press.

Persson, I., & Savulescu, J. (2012b). Moral enhancement, freedom and the god machine. *The Monist, 95*(3), 399–421.

Raine, A. (2013). *The anatomy of violence: The biological roots of crime.* London, UK: Penguin.

Randall, D. C., Shneerson, J. M., & File, S. E. (2005). Cognitive effects of modafinil in student volunteers may depend on IQ. *Pharmacology, Biochemistry, and Behavior, 82,* 133–139.

Rowe, D. C., Vesterdal, W. J., & Rodgers, J. L. (1998). Herrnstein's syllogism: Genetic and shared environmental influences on IQ, education, and income. *Intelligence, 26,* 405–423.

Salkever, D. S. (1995). Updated estimates of earnings benefits from reduced exposure of children to environmental lead. *Environmental Research, 70,* 1–6.

Sandel, M. (2007). *The case against perfection.* Harvard, MA: Harvard University Press.

Savulescu, J. (2006). Justice, fairness and enhancement. *Annals of the New York Academy of Sciences, 1093,* 321–338.

Savulescu, J., & Persson, I. (2012). Moral enhancement, freedom and the god machine. *The Monist, 95,* 399–421.

Schwartz, J. (1994). Societal benefits of reducing lead exposure. *Environmental Research, 66,* 105–124.

Snowball, A., Tachtsidis, I., Popescu, T., Thompson, J., Delazer, M., Zamarian, L., et al. (2013). Long-term enhancement of brain function and cognition using cognitive training and brain stimulation. *Current Biology, 23*(11), 987–992.

Spencer, S. J., Steele, C. M., & Quinn, D. M. (1999). Stereotype threat and women's math performance. *Journal of Experimental Social Psychology, 35,* 4–28.

Tseng, P., Hsu, T.-Y., Chang, C.-F., Tzeng, O. J. L., Hung, D. L., Muggleton, N. G., et al. (2012). Unleashing potential: Transcranial direct current stimulation over the right posterior parietal cortex improves change detection in low-performing individuals. *The Journal of Neuroscience, 32,* 10554–10561.

Whalley, L. J., & Deary, I. J. (2001). Longitudinal cohort study of childhood IQ and survival up to age 76. *British Medical Journal, 322*(7290), 819–822.

19

The Future Usage and Challenges of Brain Stimulation

Roi Cohen Kadosh

Department of Experimental Psychology, University of Oxford, Oxford, UK

OUTLINE

INTRODUCTION

The current book starts with an overview of the past, by providing a brief history of how transcranial electrical stimulation has been used to enhance cognition and improve health. The rest of the book discusses current knowledge in the field, and provides an excellent overview of different lines of research, such as those in animals, healthy humans, and patients. The aim of this last chapter is to discuss further directions for research in the field of transcranial electrical stimulation (tES).

Over the different chapters it becomes clear that research using tES has demonstrated improvements in different cognitive and non-cognitive functions, ranging from perception and motor movement to attention, working memory, language, and mathematical abilities. These results show that such improvements are not limited to typical populations but can also affect young adults and the elderly, and neurological and psychiatric patients. These results are indeed promising, but suffer from some limitations that have been discussed in various of these chapters, as well as elsewhere (Pascual-Leone, Horvath, & Robertson, 2012; Rothwell, 2012). Some of these limitations include low sample size, artificial tasks with reduced ecological validity, lack of consistency in the montage that led to the enhancement effects, and need for replication. I will not extend the discussion on these points, as they are rather trivial and are not limited to the current field. Instead I will discuss what I perceive as the directions in which the field of tES should, and hopefully will, go. It was difficult deciding which sections to include in this respect, and I have chosen to limit our discussion to 10 sections. I will conclude the chapter with a brief discussion of the challenges that the field is facing.

NEURODEVELOPMENT

tES is used currently to examine the improvement of cognitive performance, for a brief or long period of time, in young adults and elderly. However, its application in younger populations is sparse. Stimulating the child or adolescent brain is a double-edged sword. On the one hand the child brain is more plastic than the adult brain (Anderson, Spencer-Smith, & Wood, 2011; Gogtay et al., 2004), and therefore stimulation at this stage could lead to remarkable and stronger effects, especially when plastic changes would be desirable due to atypical development. On the other hand, this same reason – that the child brain has a greater degree of plasticity – is a cause for concern; namely, that stimulation may substantially change the balance between different brain regions and brain networks, and might lead to a subsequent impairment of the trained and/or non-trained abilities. It is a dilemma whether one should aim to use tES in the pediatric population, and I have discussed this elsewhere (Krause & Cohen Kadosh, 2013). I think that such a decision should be made by weighing the potential risk versus the potential gain (Maslen, Douglas, Cohen Kadosh, Levy, & Savulescu, 2014). For this reason, I recommend that studies on typically developing children should not be run at this stage. However, studies are desperately needed for those with detrimental atypical development, as the consequences of such development negatively impact such children's current life and future. It is an open question at this stage what type of stimulation, montage, and dose would be optimal in their case, as such knowledge is currently limited even when one aims to stimulate the adult brain. However, further tES experiments in this population, along with parallel research using neuroimaging techniques, computational modeling, and preclinical studies, could provide better understanding of the optimal sites for stimulation as a function of development and cognitive abilities, and stimulation efficacy and risk.

ECOLOGICAL VALIDITY AND TRANSFER

Nowadays, most tES studies (as well as studies in other fields) are run in a controlled laboratory setting and on tasks that have little to do with everyday life activities. This is, of course, clearly warranted at the first stage of exploratory research in order to assess the efficacy of tES on human behavior, and to give greater understanding of the biological and cognitive mechanisms that are affected as a function of tES. However, there is a need to expand this line of research toward more ecological settings and tasks that might be more closely related to everyday life. In this case, the combination of tES with other fields, such as education or neurology, is very promising, and would allow assessment of the effect of tES in a more real-life situation. For example, improvement in learning language or improving SAT/intelligence quotient (IQ) scores would provide a demonstration of the real applicability of tES. Of course, one of the caveats is that such improvement cannot allow us to pinpoint the cognitive function(s) and biological mechanisms that have been affected. My answer for this is that we should not forget what is the ultimate goal: to improve human behavior and life. Of course, a better cognitive and neural understanding can further aid us to reach this goal. However, achieving our goal does not necessarily depend on better mechanistic knowledge. Once this goal is achieved, we can redirect our research focus to identify the reasons (e.g., the relevant cognitive/biological mechanisms). One might argue that we should not use tES without a clear understanding of the mechanistic operation, whether cognitive or biological. However, this is not the case when looking at other fields. For example, MRI scanners are used quite successfully for research and clinical applications based on theories that we still do not have a clear understanding of (such as quantum mechanics). Similarly, scurvy was at one time common among sailors, pirates, and others aboard ships at sea. James Lind, a Scottish surgeon in the Royal Navy, proved that scurvy can be treated with fresh fruits in experiments he described in his 1753 book, *A Treatise of the Scurvy* (Krebs, 2013). It would have been ridiculous to wait until the exact mechanism was revealed (lack of vitamin C), two centuries later, to treat this illness. The final example is even more relevant: the current situation with deep brain stimulation (DBS) is the same, in that mechanisms of action are largely unknown but DBS is used worldwide for treating neurological and psychiatric disorders (Kringelbach, Jenkinson, Owen, & Aziz, 2007). Likewise, I do not see any objection if cognitive abilities can be improved in the first instance by using tES. Rather, I believe that achieving this goal could facilitate research in different fields and allow us to shed light on the potential mechanisms.

Another closely related issue in cognitive enhancement and training is the issue of transfer (Taatgen, 2013). Currently, there is mixed evidence from tES-paired training studies that either found or did not find transfer of tES-training benefits to another task. One of the issues regarding this lack of consistency is the difficulty of selecting appropriate training and transfer tasks, and of identifying which cognitive functions and brain regions are tapped by the training material. In other words, the limitation might not be the limited ability of tES to induce transfer, but rather a suboptimal experimental design. Therefore, this potential limitation that has been put forward in the past is not limited to tES but is a generic problem in the field of rehabilitation and cognitive enhancement (Taatgen, 2013). Indeed, some studies have shown that tES can even further increase the chance of transfer in paradigms that have struggled to show transfer without stimulation (Cappelletti et al., 2013; Looi, Duta, Huber, Nuerk, & Cohen Kadosh, 2013). How such improvement occurs at the neural level is still unknown. Further studies are needed to examine the multifaceted issue of transfer effects, and their possible enhancement using tES. Such knowledge will have important applications for improving human behavior in typical and atypical populations.

THE IMPACT OF tES

Another current caveat for the observed results so far is the issue of impact. Is a tES-induced improvement in performance in the order of tens of milliseconds or few percentage points significant for our everyday life (Pascual-Leone et al., 2012; Walsh, 2013)? We can, of course, suggest events in which a few milliseconds can make a difference, such as car accidents, professional sports, playing a musical instrument, or on the battlefield. Nevertheless, our everyday activities are less affected by such small increments in our behavior. It is important to note that not *all* the findings are at the level of milliseconds – for example, improvements have been shown of 1.25 s in arithmetic problem-solving (Snowball et al., 2013), 3 s in solving logic reasoning tasks (Santarnecchi, Feurra, Galli, Rossi, & Rossi, 2013), and up to 50% average reduction in resting tremor amplitude in patients with Parkinson's disease (Brittain, Probert-Smith, Aziz, & Brown, 2013), enhanced working memory capacity (Looi et al., 2013), or qualitative change in behavior (Cohen Kadosh, Soskic, Iuculano, Kanai, & Walsh, 2010). However, such effects are currently the exception rather than the rule. The low level of improvement might be attributed to several factors. This might include suboptimal task difficulty, lack of adjunct cognitive training, and infrequent repetitions of brain stimulation. As discussed, most studies nowadays are still at the proof-of-concept stage, and this might hamper the possibility of examining real-life situations in which the significance of the effects could be examined.

So far, tES studies have focused on cognitive tasks that produce quantitative effects, begging the question of what other fields of research might benefit from involvement of tES techniques. Notably, tES studies have mainly neglected fields of research that produce more qualitative effects. One such field that has shown promise is social neuroscience, including moral behavior (Ruff, Ugazio, & Fehr, 2013; M. Lavidor and J. Savulescu, personal communication).

INDIVIDUAL DIFFERENCES

Whether or not the effects prove to be robust in daily life, so far various studies have provided evidence for neuroenhancement due to tES at the behavioral and neural levels. However, one unresolved question, which has important implications for the translation of tES, replication, and neuroethics, is the issue of individual differences. Namely, it is unclear how tES affects brain and behavior as a function of individual differences at these levels. Some research has provided initial answers to this pending question (see, for example, Antal et al., 2010; Tseng et al., 2012). While further research in this direction is definitely needed, one of the issues is that research so far has examined the effect of tES after categorizing the group of subjects rather than investigating parametric changes in phenotype (Tseng et al., 2012) or genotype (Antal et al., 2010). The few studies that have examined the efficacy of tES as a function of individual differences have compared dichotomous variables, such as high vs low attention abilities (Tseng et al., 2012). This "extreme groups approach" is warranted at earlier stages of research to examine possible differences, but subsequently impairs reliability and replication (Preacher, Rucker,

MacCallum, & Nicewander, 2005). Instead, future research is needed to see how *variation* in human performance is linked to improvement in cognitive abilities. One view is that those with lower abilities will have more room to improve. However, this is not necessarily the case. For example, in the case of education it has been shown that those with greater cognitive ability will also benefit more from schooling, which is one of the most acceptable methods for cognitive enhancement. If two children with different cognitive abilities in a given topic are entering the same class, it is more likely that the child with the higher ability will maintain his or her superior performance and the gap between the children will further increase (Duncan et al., 2007). If tES leads to improvement in those who are already well off cognitively it will lead to neuroethical problems, as it will increase natural inequality rather than reducing it. Methods of enhancement, such as tES, that could reduce the cognitive inequality due to gaps in biological (e.g., reduced gray matter, or suboptimal brain functions, suboptimal neuronal oscillations) or environmental (e.g., socioeconomic) backgrounds would allow more equal opportunities for effective learning. Such a balance in improvement of cognitive abilities would be an important step toward a fairer and more equal society.

I have focused so far on individual differences at the behavioral level. However, individual differences at the neural level can be used as a target to reduce inequality. This can occur at different levels, from structural and functional differences to genetic and neurochemical differences, such as cortical excitation/inhibition ratio level (e.g., Krause, Márquez-Ruiz, & Cohen Kadosh, 2013; Meinzer, Lindenberg, Antonenko, Flaisch, & Flöel, 2013). This will require a better understanding of the connection between behavior and brain as a function of individual differences, and of how we could modify a neural system in order to push it toward an optimal level. In this respect it must be noted that, on the one hand, stimulation of one or more brain regions might be more advantageous to those with low cognitive abilities, and this might be due to differences in the recruitment of these brain regions by this population (e.g., Grabner et al., 2007; Rivera, Reiss, Eckert, & Menon, 2005). On the other hand, it might well be that targeting a different brain region will be more beneficial to those with high cognitive abilities. Such differences in the efficacy of tES might be due to qualitative and quantitative differences in individuals' brain–behavioral relationships, and differences in the usage of strategies to solve a given problem as a function of *a priori* ability (Dowker, Flood, Griffiths, Harriss, & Hook, 1996; Lemaire, 2010; Pesenti, 2005; Pesenti et al., 2001). Therefore, careful experimentation, combined with a better understanding of the brain–behavior relationship and cognitive processes, would allow greater advancement in the efficacy of tES and its effect as a function of individual differences.

COGNITIVE AND NEURAL COST

We aim to improve human behavior and brain functions; however, we usually neglect the fact that such improvement might be associated with cognitive and/or neural cost. The brain receives a fixed supply of oxygen and nutrients, and shifting the balance by increasing or decreasing the levels of excitation and inhibition in a given area of the brain might come at the cost of other brain regions and affect the behavior of other domains (Brem, Fried, Horvath, Robertson, & Pascual-Leone, 2014; Krause et al., 2013; Pascual-Leone et al., 2012). This view, which is similar to concerns regarding the use of cognitive enhancing drugs (Greely et al., 2008; Hyman, 2011), has not been examined so far in a thorough fashion, although some evidence has been documented at the behavioral level (Iuculano & Cohen Kadosh, 2013). I would like to note that, while I am focusing here on tES, to the best of my knowledge the same also applies to transcranial magnetic stimulation and DBS. That is, it is currently unknown whether there is any mental cost that is associated with cognitive or physical improvement.

As mentioned earlier, one option is to consider the potential gain versus the potential risk. That is, if someone is impaired in a given cognitive function (e.g., speech production), they might be willing to sacrifice other abilities to some degree in order to regain their impaired function (see Chapter 18). Similarly, some might want to increase their average or above-average cognitive capacities in order to enhance their function at work or improve the results of their study (e.g., improve their exam results by a few points in order to gain acceptance to a prestigious programme at the University of Cambridge). In such cases the usage of tES is subjective, and to some degree could be justified (depending of course how keen one is to study at the University of Cambridge). However, it is not clear who should make the decision regarding whether such usage is warranted, especially in the case of patients or people with reduced cognitive abilities who cannot provide their own consent (Maslen et al., 2014).

In contrast to this view of cognitive and neural cost, another scenario might be that the changes in one brain region will lead to proportional changes in other brain regions, thus meaning that changes will be distributed and therefore relatively negligible. In such a scenario, the brain would have no difficulties in adapting to such changes while maintaining similar levels of behavior in other domains.

It is difficult, however, to attempt to examine the extent of potential cognitive/neural costs of tES. The range of cognitive abilities that can be examined in a given experiment is limited logistically, and this is without taking into account abilities outside the cognitive domain, such as emotional and social skills. One possibility is to guide such research by examining how stimulation changes the stimulated brain region and various brain

This could help researchers to narrow down significantly the potential behavioral indices, and to employ behavioral tasks affected brain regions. Combining tES with methods such as resting-state functional magnetic resonance imaging (Keeser et al., 2011; Meinzer et al., 2012, 2013; Polanía, Paulus, & Nitsche, 2012), electroencephalography (Neuling, Rach, & Herrmann, 2013; Zaehle, Rach, & Herrmann, 2010; Zaehle, Sandmann, Thorne, Jancke, & Herrmann, 2011), magnetoencephalography (Soekadar et al., 2013; Venkatakrishnan, Contreras-Vidal, Sandrini, & Cohen, 2011), or near infrared spectroscopy (Snowball et al., 2013) can be excellent candidates for such an approach.

MILITARY USE

It is natural that, when discussing human enhancement, defense forces would be interested in examining the applicability of such tools for improving performance in future battlefields and headquarters (Academy of Medical Sciences, British Academy, Royal Academy of Engineering, and Royal Society, 2012). tES in this respect is no exception, and the number of defense forces investing research money in this field is increasing. These projects could range from enhancing the abilities of snipers and drone operators, to improving sustained attention, social skills, and problem-solving and reasoning.

Collaboration between scientists and the military can cause a level of discomfort to some scientists, who should eventually decide where to draw their own line and decide which projects, if any, it is morally right to engage with from the scientist's perspective. I, of course, will not attempt to serve as a moral compass in this case; this should be a personal decision, being one where there is no clear distinction between right and wrong. However, if consulted, my opinion is that projects that are likely to yield benefits for the wider public should not be dismissed outright. Some projects, such as improving problem-solving and reasoning abilities (in which I am involved) or improving social skills, can be easily translated to everyday life activities and in some cases can save lives (e.g., improving sustained attention of airport traffic controllers or lorry drivers).

SPORT

As a potential enhancement in healthy subjects, tES raises issues familiar to ethicists from discussions of pharmacological interventions (Cohen Kadosh, Levy, O'Shea, Shea, & Savulescu, 2012). Without delving into a long discussion on the neuroethical implications of using tES for cognitive and physical enhancement (Cohen Kadosh et al., 2012; Hamilton,

Messing, & Chatterjee, 2011), tES could plausibly be used to improve performance in sports and thus raises ethical questions akin to those surrounding doping in sport (Schermer, 2008). tES has a unique feature that makes this issue more pressing: unlike most pharmaceutical enhancements, currently it is not possible to detect that tES has been used to enhance an individual's cognitive or non-cognitive abilities (Davis, 2013). At present, in professional sport, blood and urine samples are routinely used to establish whether performance enhancers have been used.

A previous study has shown that tES can increase muscle endurance and decrease muscle fatigue in normal subjects (Cogiamanian, Marceglia, Ardolino, Barbieri, & Priori, 2007). Professional athletes who use tES to decrease muscle fatigue might have an important advantage, especially when there is increased load on their muscles, as in some of the most prestigious sporting events, (e.g., Tour de France, Football World Cup, Olympic Games). Similarly, tES has been shown to improve motion perception (Antal et al., 2004) – an important ability in a wide variety of sports, such as football, basketball, and baseball. For example, a goalkeeper who receives stimulation to area MT+ (also known as visual area V5), an extrastriate cortical area known to mediate motion processing (Born & Bradley, 2005; Pascual-Leone & Walsh, 2001), could exhibit improved performance and make fewer mistakes. Such a method of enhancement might, of course, be enthusiastically endorsed by some sports fans!

Another aspect of tES in sport is its application to improve mental preparation before the game. Currently, mental preparation is moderated mostly by sport psychologists. However, some have suggested that tES might be used to generate that feeling of effortless concentration that characterizes outstanding performance (Adee, 2012). Moreover, in the same way that behavioral intervention alone (compared to behavioral intervention with tES) seems to have limited capacity in improving human performance (Cappelletti et al., 2013; Cohen Kadosh, 2013; Krause & Cohen Kadosh, 2013; Reis, Prichard, & Fritsch, 2014), a similar argument can be made for mental preparation techniques that aim to improve athletic performance.

Although we cannot yet be confident that the findings cited above have ecological validity, they provide a potential field of use that scientists and policymakers should be aware of, and that I anticipate will receive considerable attention in the future (for a similar discussion, see Banissy & Muggleton, 2013; Cohen Kadosh, 2013).

COMBINATION WITH OTHER METHODS

At the moment, most tES studies are run in their purest possible form: that is, stimulating a given brain region to see its effect on behavior or a simple physiological measure (motor-evoked potential). However, combining tES with other methods and fields can enrich the basic understanding of the biological and cognitive mechanisms implicated, and may lead to more efficient protocols for stimulation and subsequent enhancement. Neuroimaging is one such method, as it can offer us insights into changes that are induced by tES from the neurochemical to the functional level (for reviews, see Dayan, Censor, Buch, Sandrini, & Cohen, 2013; Hunter, Coffman, Trumbo, & Clark, 2013; Venkatakrishnan & Sandrini, 2012). However, other methods that are less utilized include genetic expression as a function of tES, the combination of tES with DBS electrode recordings, and the effect of *a priori* anatomical, neural, and neurochemical correlates on the efficacy of tES.

Another combination that has been used, although to date to a very small degree, is that of tES with pharmacological manipulations (see Chapter 6). While most tES studies involve healthy adults and focus on motor tasks, there is room for further combinations to assess how interaction between drugs and tES can modulate and further enhance neuroplasticity and efficacy of training. This issue is related to state-dependency of the neural system, because CNS-acting drugs may change the responsiveness of the brain to electrical intervention, similar to the effect of psychological tasks (Feurra et al., 2013).

OPTIMIZATION

Chapter 4 provides an excellent review of the different ways in which tES can be optimized, by taking into account individual differences in brain anatomy. Others have also suggested that individual differences in brain functions, such as cortical excitability, should be taken into account in tES studies, as they may affect the efficacy of stimulation (Krause et al., 2013). Identifying sources of interindividual variability will allow adjustment of stimulation protocols, potentially leading to prolongation and strengthening of the effects of tES (M. Nitsche, personal communication). Similarly, it will also be vital to develop new stimulation montages to better focus the stimulation and perhaps steer the current to the desired sites as a function of individual subjects' brain anatomy (Tecchio et al., 2013) (M. Bikson and D. Terhune, personal communication). Notably, such approaches are time consuming and currently expensive. Future development of cheap and easy-to-use methods to improve optimization would increase the likelihood of using them outside the laboratory.

The combination of tES with brain–computer interfaces is another direction to further optimize stimulation. For example, coupling behavioral measurements with EEG recording can help to assess neuronal oscillations, and specifically to determine which frequency might serve as the optimal neural marker of performance. This, in turn, can be used to design protocols for transcranial alternating current stimulation (tACS) to entrain those optimal EEG performance markers and thus improve online behavior in the most efficient way.

Another approach to optimization is to target a network of brain regions, rather than a single brain region as is commonly the case with tES. Stimulating a network that is engaged in the cognitive function one would like to improve could allow us the ability to increase the strength between the network's regions and the overall network (G. Ruffini, personal communication).

The effect of tES is assumed to stem largely from cortical brain regions close to the electrodes (see Chapter 4). However, it may be possible to use tES to affect subcortical brain regions. This would greatly increase the applicability of tES to additional cognitive domains, as well as neurological and psychiatric conditions (D. Terhune, personal communication). However, targeting subcortical regions is a challenge that, to date, has barely begun to be tackled. Stimulating cortical brain regions that are remotely connected to those subcortical structures seems to be one potential way to bypass such a challenge (Takano et al., 2011).

HOME USE

This last section is probably the "hot potato," subject to considerable debate in the field and, to some degree, even in this book (see Chapters 3 and 18): should tES eventually be used at home? Some concerns have been demonstrated, with regard to safety and knowledge of stimulation, which could lead to an increased risk when tES is used by amateurs (Bikson, Bestmann, & Edwards, 2013; Fitz & Reiner, 2013; Santarnecchi et al., 2013; see also Chapter 3). Others have expressed their view that the risk is over-exaggerated, along with the implications of the results from tES (Walsh, 2013), but at the same time have neglected several points that challenge their view (Chapter 3). In addition, the latter perspective did not take into account future directions that could lead to results with more ecological validity and that will increase the likelihood of amateur use of tES. In addition, safety studies are still lacking, especially longitudinal studies that examine the changes that have occurred as a result of repeated usage of tES (A. Antal, personal communication).

It is a fact that home use of tES does exist. This is due not only to companies that are making easy money from public enthusiasm, but also to an increasing "do-it-yourself" (DIY) culture of those who build their own machines and try to improve their mental ability (see, for example, this video at YouTube: http://www.youtube.com/watch?v=6V64IXFg9yc).

Independent of the varying views of future home use of tES, scientists might agree that at the moment we are still not ready for this stage; indeed, others have articulated this elsewhere (Bikson et al., 2013; Fitz & Reiner, 2013; Santarnecchi et al., 2013; see also Chapter 3. In face of the growing usage of tES by the public, I would like to suggest that if we cannot beat them we should join them. The idea, of course, is not to market devices for profit, but to engage with home users to ameliorate the current lack of knowledge and potential risk while at the same time providing training and examining the changes that occur to their brains as a function of tES. This could include a longitudinal assessment to examine changes in cognitive and brain functions. Of course, it is hard to find a good control for those subjects, but the effect of frequency of usage, and daily dose, would be able to shed some light on the risk of tES for home use, as well as its potential ecological validity. Such a combination could reduce the risk of home use tES (due to the training that will be provided by scientists), and allow a unique insight into the risk and gain from such use.

CONCLUSIONS

The different sections in this chapter provide a glimpse of the challenges that the field of tES is likely to encounter, and future directions. While I limited us to 10 strands that currently pose a challenge and should be examined in future research, I acknowledge that other lines of research are equally needed, as indicated in the various book chapters. These future directions for upcoming research are exciting, will increase our basic knowledge, and will have important impacts on society. The future appears full of intellectual and experimental stimulation.

Acknowledgments

I would like to thank Michal Lavidor, Julian Savulescu, Michael Nitsche, Marom Bikson, Devin Terhune, Giulio Ruffini, and Andrea Antal for their suggestions.

I am most grateful to Simone Rossi for reviewing this chapter and the many excellent additions to it. I would like to thank the different contributors to this book for their very kind suggestions, and interaction on future directions. Some of these have been included, but others were not due to lack of space. I am grateful for this openness and willingness to share their views. I would like to thank Jackie Thompson for proofreading, and the Wellcome Trust (WT88378) for its support.

References

Academy of Medical Sciences, British Academy, Royal Academy of Engineering, and Royal Society (2012). *Human enhancement and the future of work: Report from a joint workshop.* Available online at, http://www.acmedsci.ac.uk/p47prid102.html.

Adee, S. (2012). Zap your brain into the zone: Fast track to pure focus. *New Scientist*, 33, February 6.

Anderson, V., Spencer-Smith, M., & Wood, A. (2011). Do children really recover better? Neurobehavioural plasticity after early brain insult. *Brain*, *134*, 2197–2221.

Antal, A., Chaieb, L., Moliadze, V., Monte-Silva, K., Poreisz, C., Thirugnanasambandam, N., et al. (2010). Brain-derived neurotrophic factor (BDNF) gene polymorphisms shape cortical plasticity in humans. *Brain Stimulation*, *3*, 230–237.

Antal, A., Nitsche, M. A., Kruse, W., Hoffmann, K. -P., & Paulus, W. (2004). Direct current stimulation over V5 enhances visuomotor coordination by improving motion perception in humans. *Journal of Cognitive Neuroscience*, *16*, 521–527. http://refhub.elsevier.com/B978-0-12-404704-4.00019-3/rf0030.

Banissy, M. J., & Muggleton, N. G. (2013). Transcranial direct current stimulation in sports training: Potential approaches. *Frontiers in Human Neuroscience*, *7*.

Bikson, M., Bestmann, S., & Edwards, D. (2013). Neuroscience: Transcranial devices are not playthings. *Nature*, *501*, 167.

Born, R. T., & Bradley, D. C. (2005). Structure and function of visual area MT. *Annual Review of Neuroscience*, *28*, 157–189.

Brem, A. -K., Fried, P. J., Horvath, J. C., Robertson, E. M., & Pascual-Leone, A. (2014). Is neuroenhancement by noninvasive brain stimulation a net zero-sum proposition? *NeuroImage*, *85*(Part 3), 1058–1068.

Brittain, J. -S., Probert-Smith, P., Aziz, T. Z., & Brown, P. (2013). Tremor suppression by rhythmic transcranial current stimulation. *Current Biology*, *23*, 436–440.

Cappelletti, M., Gessaroli, E., Hithersay, R., Mitolo, M., Didino, D., Kanai, R., et al. (2013). Transfer of cognitive training across magnitude dimensions achieved with concurrent brain stimulation of the parietal lobe. *The Journal of Neuroscience*, *33*, 14899–14907.

Cogiamanian, F., Marceglia, S., Ardolino, G., Barbieri, S., & Priori, A. (2007). Improved isometric force endurance after transcranial direct current stimulation over the human motor cortical areas. *European Journal of Neuroscience*, *26*, 242–249.

Cohen Kadosh, R. (2013). Using transcranial electrical stimulation to enhance cognitive functions in the typical and atypical brain. *Translational Neuroscience*, *4*, 20–33.

Cohen Kadosh, R., Levy, N., O'Shea, J., Shea, N., & Savulescu, J. (2012). The neuroethics of non-invasive brain stimulation. *Current Biology*, *22*, R108–R111.

Cohen Kadosh, R., Soskic, S., Iuculano, T., Kanai, R., & Walsh, V. (2010). Modulating neuronal activity produces specific and long lasting changes in numerical competence. *Current Biology*, *20*, 2016–2020.

Davis, N. J. (2013). Neurodoping: Brain stimulation as a performance-enhancing measure. *Sports Medicine*, *43*, 649–653.

Dayan, E., Censor, N., Buch, E. R., Sandrini, M., & Cohen, L. G. (2013). Noninvasive brain stimulation: From physiology to network dynamics and back. *Nature Neuroscience*, *16*, 838–844.

Dowker, A., Flood, A., Griffiths, H., Harriss, L., & Hook, L. (1996). Estimation strategies of four groups. *Mathematical Cognition*, *2*, 113–135.

Duncan, G. J., Dowsett, C. J., Claessens, A., Magnuson, K., Huston, A. C., Klebanov, P., et al. (2007). School readiness and later achievement. *Developmental Psychology*, *43*, 1428–1446.

Feurra, M., Pasqualetti, P., Bianco, G., Santarnecchi, E., Rossi, A., & Rossi, S. (2013). State-dependent effects of transcranial oscillatory currents on the motor system: What you think matters. *The Journal of Neuroscience*, *33*, 17483–17489.

Fitz, N. S., & Reiner, P. B. (2013). The challenge of crafting policy for do-it-yourself brain stimulation. *Journal of Medical Ethics*. http://dx.doi.org/10.1136/medethics-2013-101458, Jun 3.

Gogtay, N., Giedd, J. N., Lusk, L., Hayashi, K. M., Greenstein, D., Vaituzis, C. A., et al. (2004). Dynamic mapping of human cortical development during childhood through early adulthood. *Proceedings of the National Academy of Sciences of the United States of America, 101,* 8174–8179.

Grabner, R. H., Ansari, D., Reishofer, G., Stern, E., Ebner, F., & Neuper, C. (2007). Individual differences in mathematical competence predict parietal brain activation during mental calculation. *NeuroImage, 38,* 346–356.

Greely, H., Sahakian, B., Harris, J., Kessler, R. C., Gazzaniga, M., Campbell, P., et al. (2008). Towards responsible use of cognitive-enhancing drugs by the healthy. *Nature, 456,* 702–705.

Hamilton, R., Messing, S., & Chatterjee, A. (2011). Rethinking the thinking cap. *Neurology, 76,* 187–193.

Hunter, M. A., Coffman, B., Trumbo, M., & Clark, V. (2013). Tracking the neuroplastic changes associated with transcranial direct current stimulation: A push for multimodal imaging. *Frontiers in Human Neuroscience, 7,* 495.

Hyman, S. E. (2011). Cognitive enhancement: Promises and perils. *Neuron, 69,* 595–598.

Iuculano, T., & Cohen Kadosh, R. (2013). The mental cost of cognitive enhancement. *The Journal of Neuroscience, 33,* 4482–4486.

Keeser, D., Meindl, T., Bor, J., Palm, U., Pogarell, O., Mulert, C., et al. (2011). Prefrontal transcranial direct current stimulation changes connectivity of resting-state networks during fMRI. *The Journal of Neuroscience, 31,* 15284–15293.

Krause, B., & Cohen Kadosh, R. (2013). Can transcranial electrical stimulation improve learning difficulties in atypical brain development? A future possibility for cognitive training. *Developmental Cognitive Neuroscience, 6,* 176–194.

Krause, B., Márquez-Ruiz, J., & Cohen Kadosh, R. (2013). The effect of transcranial direct current stimulation: A role for cortical excitation/inhibition balance? *Frontiers in Human Neuroscience, 7,* 602.

Krebs, J. (2013). *Food: A very short introduction.* Hampshire: Oxford University Press.

Kringelbach, M. L., Jenkinson, N., Owen, S. L. F., & Aziz, T. Z. (2007). Translational principles of deep brain stimulation. *Nature Reviews Neuroscience, 8,* 623–635.

Lemaire, P. (2010). Cognitive strategy variations during aging. *Current Directions in Psychological Science, 19,* 363–369.

Looi, C. Y., Duta, M., Huber, S., Nuerk, H. -C., & Cohen Kadosh, R. (2013). Stimulating the brain while playing a computer-based maths game to enhance domain-specific and domain-general cognitive abilities. In: *5th International conference on non-invasive brain stimulation, Leipzig, Germany.*

Maslen, H., Douglas, T., Cohen Kadosh, R., Levy, N., & Savulescu, J. (2014). The regulation of cognitive enhancement devices: Extending the medical model. *Journal of Law and Bioethics,* (in press).

Meinzer, M., Antonenko, D., Lindenberg, R., Hetzer, S., Ulm, L., Avirame, K., et al. (2012). Electrical brain stimulation improves cognitive performance by modulating functional connectivity and task-specific activation. *The Journal of Neuroscience, 32,* 1859–1866.

Meinzer, M., Lindenberg, R., Antonenko, D., Flaisch, T., & Flöel, A. (2013). Anodal transcranial direct current stimulation temporarily reverses age-associated cognitive decline and functional brain activity changes. *The Journal of Neuroscience, 33,* 12470–12478.

Neuling, T., Rach, S., & Herrmann, C. S. (2013). Orchestrating neuronal networks: Sustained after-effects of transcranial alternating current stimulation depend upon brain states. *Frontiers in Human Neuroscience, 7,* 161.

Pascual-Leone, A., Horvath, J. C., & Robertson, E. M. (2012). Enhancement of normal cognitive abilities through noninvasive brain stimulation. In R. Chen & J. C. Rothwell (Eds.), *Cortical connectivity* (pp. 207–249). Berlin: Springer-Verlag.

Pascual-Leone, A., & Walsh, V. (2001). Fast backprojections from the motion to the primary visual area necessary for visual awareness. *Science, 292,* 510–512.

Pesenti, M. (2005). Calculation abilities in expert calculators. In J. I. D. Campbell (Ed.), *Handbook of mathematical cognition* (pp. 413–430). New York: Psychology Press.

Pesenti, M., Zago, L., Crivello, F., Mellet, E., Samson, D., Duroux, B., et al. (2001). Mental calculation in a prodigy is sustained by right prefrontal and medial temporal areas. *Nature Neuroscience, 4,* 103–107.

Polanía, R., Paulus, W., & Nitsche, M. A. (2012). Reorganizing the intrinsic functional architecture of the human primary motor cortex during rest with non-invasive cortical stimulation. *PLoS One, 7,* e30971.

Preacher, K. J., Rucker, D. D., MacCallum, R. C., & Nicewander, W. A. (2005). Use of the extreme groups approach: A critical reexamination and new recommendations. *Psychological Methods, 10,* 178–192.

Reis, J., Prichard, G., & Fritsch, B. (2014). Improving functions in the typical brain: Motor system. In R. Cohen Kadosh (Ed.), *The stimulated brain.* Amsterdam: Elsevier (in press).

Rivera, S. M., Reiss, A. L., Eckert, M. A., & Menon, V. (2005). Developmental changes in mental arithmetic: Evidence for increased functional specialization in the left inferior parietal cortex. *Cerebral Cortex, 25,* 1779–1790.

Rothwell, J. C. (2012). Clinical applications of noninvasive electrical stimulation: Problems and potential. *Clinical EEG and Neuroscience, 43,* 209–214.

Ruff, C. C., Ugazio, G., & Fehr, E. (2013). Changing social norm compliance with noninvasive brain stimulation. *Science, 342,* 482–484.

Santarnecchi, E., Feurra, M., Galli, G., Rossi, A., & Rossi, S. (2013). Overclock your brain for gaming? Ethical, social and health care risks. *Brain Stimulation, 6,* 713–714.

Schermer, M. (2008). On the argument that enhancement is "cheating" *Journal of Medical Ethics, 34,* 85–88.

Snowball, A., Tachtsidis, I., Popescu, T., Thompson, J., Delazer, M., Zamarian, L., et al. (2013). Long-term enhancement of brain function and cognition using cognitive training and brain stimulation. *Current Biology, 23,* 987–992.

Soekadar, S. R., Witkowski, M., Cossio, E. G., Birbaumer, N., Robinson, S. E., & Cohen, L. G. (2013). *In vivo* assessment of human brain oscillations during application of transcranial electric currents. *Nature Communications, 4,* 2032.

Taatgen, G. A. (2013). The nature and transfer of cognitive skills. *Psychological Review, 120,* 439–471.

Takano, Y., Yokawa, T., Masuda, A., Niimi, J., Tanaka, S., & Hironaka, N. (2011). A rat model for measuring the effectiveness of transcranial direct current stimulation using fMRI. *Neuroscience Letters, 491,* 40–43.

Tecchio, F., Cancelli, A., Cottone, C., Tomasevic, L., Devigus, B., Zito, G., et al. (2013). Regional personalized electrodes to select transcranial current stimulation target. *Frontiers in Human Neuroscience, 7,* 131.

Tseng, P., Hsu, T. -Y., Chang, C. -F., Tzeng, O. J. L., Hung, D. L., Muggleton, N. G., et al. (2012). Unleashing potential: Transcranial direct current stimulation over the right posterior parietal cortex improves change detection in low-performing individuals. *The Journal of Neuroscience, 32,* 10554–10561.

Venkatakrishnan, A., Contreras-Vidal, J. L., Sandrini, M., & Cohen, L. G. (2011). Independent component analysis of resting brain activity reveals transient modulation of local cortical processing by transcranial direct current stimulation. *Conference proceedings: ... Annual International Conference of the IEEE Engineering in Medicine and Biology Society. IEEE Engineering in Medicine and Biology Society. Conference, 8102–8105.*

Venkatakrishnan, A., & Sandrini, M. (2012). Combining transcranial direct current stimulation and neuroimaging: Novel insights in understanding neuroplasticity. *Journal of Neurophysiology, 107,* 1–4.

Walsh, V. Q. (2013). Ethics and social risks in brain stimulation. *Brain Stimulation*, 6, 715–717.

Zaehle, T., Rach, S., & Herrmann, C. S. (2010). Transcranial alternating current stimulation enhances individual alpha activity in human EEG. *PLoS One, 5*, e13766.

Zaehle, T., Sandmann, P., Thorne, J., Jancke, L., & Herrmann, C. (2011). Transcranial direct current stimulation of the prefrontal cortex modulates working memory performance: Combined behavioural and electrophysiological evidence. *BMC Neuroscience, 12*, 2.

Index

Note: Page numbers followed by *f* indicate figures and *t* indicate tables.

CPI Antony Rowe
Eastbourne, UK
November 20, 2014